Jonathan L. Benumof, M.D.

Professor of Anesthesia
University of California, San Diego
La Jolla, California

Anesthesia for

Thoracic Surgery

1987

W. B. SAUNDERS COMPANY
Harcourt Brace Jovanovich, Inc.

Philadelphia London Toronto
Montreal Sydney Tokyo

W. B. SAUNDERS COMPANY
Harcourt Brace Jovanovich, Inc.

210 West Washington Square
Philadelphia, PA   19105

Library of Congress Cataloging-in-Publication Data

Benumof, Jonathan, 1942–

Anesthesia for thoracic surgery.

1. Chest—Surgery.   2. Anesthesia.   I. Title.
   [DNL: 1. Anesthesia.   2. Thoracic Surgery.   WF 980
   B478a]

RD536.B46 1988   617'.96754   87–9790

ISBN 0–7216–1374–8

Editor: Carol Trumbold
Developmental Editor: Kathleen McCullough
Designer: Terri Siegel
Production Manager: Bob Butler
Manuscript Editor: Roger Wall
Illustration Coordinator: Lisa Lambert
Indexer: Nancy Weaver and Nelle Garricht

Anesthesia for Thoracic Surgery   ISBN   0–7216–1374–8

Last digit is the print number: 9   8   7   6   5   4   3   2   1

To
Sherrie, Benjamin, and Sarah
my loving family

PREFACE

Noncardiac thoracic surgery has become an important surgical subspecialty. Compared with pre–1940 levels of thoracic surgery, when only three pneumonectomies and 30 esophagogastrectomies had been reported worldwide, today's combined national noncardiac thoracic surgery caseload has been estimated to be approximately 120,000 to 130,000 cases per year.[1,2] In addition, the caseload, especially for pulmonary resections, can be expected to increase steadily in the next decade.[1,2]

The increase in the noncardiac thoracic surgery caseload has been accompanied by many advances in anesthesia practice that can greatly improve the care of patients undergoing thoracic surgery. Some of the more important recent advances have been in the understanding of the physiology of one-lung ventilation (the determinants of hypoxic pulmonary vasoconstriction; see chapters 3, 4, and 8), preoperative evaluation (staging of tumors, physiologic function testing; see chapter 5), monitoring (oximetry, capnography; see chapter 7), choice of anesthesia (new narcotics, isoflurane; see chapter 8), fiberoptic bronchoscopy (to position double-lumen tubes; see chapter 9), nondependent lung CPAP (see chapter 11), high-frequency ventilation (see chapter 12), providing anesthesia for laser resection of airway tumors (see chapter 13), and utilization of epidural narcotics (see chapter 20). The reports of these advances are presently scattered throughout the applied respiratory physiology, critical care, anesthesiologic, surgical, and medical literature in such diverse forms as letters to the editor, original studies, and clinical reports. This book gathers all of these recent advances into one convenient educational resource.

This book is intended to be a complete textbook for the subspecialty of anesthesia for thoracic surgery. I have assumed that such anesthesia is administered by individuals who have advanced beyond basic considerations and have the ability to safely administer anesthesia for straightforward, uncomplicated cases. For example, the section on double-lumen tubes assumes the reader has the ability to perform laryngoscopy, and the recommendation to insert a pulmonary artery catheter, or arterial line, or to administer epidural narcotics assumes the reader has knowledge of how to insert the appropriate catheters.

The book covers the entire perioperative period. The first section, basic considerations, provides information that should help resolve any perspective or comprehension difficulties that arise in later chapters. Sections two through five go through the perioperative period in the temporal sequence that they occur in practice: preoperative considerations, intraoperative considerations (for all routine cases and for special cases), and postoperative considerations. In all areas of the book, respiratory considerations are given much more attention than any other considerations, since thoracic surgery is predominantly required for respiratory problems and predominantly impairs respiratory function. In most areas, the book is oriented toward anesthesia for lung resections, since they are by far the most common thoracic surgery procedure.[1,2]

I greatly enjoyed writing this book. The reason that it was so enjoyable was that I was able to concentrate on communicating information and my editorial assistant, Ms. Allyn Charney, did everything else. She typed every word of every chapter, and each chapter underwent many revisions. In these early stages, she did not let bad sentences stand, or misspelled words and incomplete references filter through. In the latter stages, she completely took care of the many details of getting the manuscript publication-ready: letters of permission, reproduction of materials, packaging the manuscript, and dealing with illustrators and publishing people. Allyn allowed me to concentrate on communication, and that made the writing a labor of love.

Acknowledgement of several other people is necessary. I owe much to Dr. Mark Scheller for reviewing the entire book in the latter stages of preparation. I thank Drs. Roderick Calverly, James Gibbons, William Mazzei, Theodore Sanford, James Harrell, Clarence Ward, and Jordan Katz for kindly reviewing individual chapters in earlier stages. Finally, I would like to thank Dr. Lawrence Saidman for two things. First, for kindly agreeing to write a thoughtful Foreword. Second, as chairman of my department for the past 12 years, he helped to create an environment that allowed me to grow scientifically and clinically, so that someday I could be in a position to write a complete book on anesthesia for thoracic surgery.

REFERENCES

1. Melton LJ III, McGoon DC, O'Fallon WM: Population-based requirements for thoracic surgery. J Thorac Cardiovasc Surg 82:729–737, 1981.
2. Rutkow IM: Thoracic and cardiovascular operations in the United States, 1979 to 1984. J Thorac Cardiovasc Surg 92:181–185, 1986.

FOREWORD

LAWRENCE J. SAIDMAN, MD

A STEP FORWARD

One has only to look at the content of anesthesia journals 20 years ago to recognize that remarkable changes have occurred in the management of patients undergoing thoracic surgery. Just 20 years ago, the use of invasive monitoring was infrequent, double-lumen tubes were a curiosity, monitoring of arterial blood gases was unavailable in most circumstances, clinically useful oximetry was not yet developed, ventilators were unreliable, and most intensive care units were special nursing units rather than true multidisciplinary critical care units. The effects of most anesthetics on pulmonary circulation were not yet known, and maneuvers such as PEEP and CPAP, now considered commonplace, were as yet unconceived. The intervening 20 years have seen development of all these advances. The specialty of thoracic anesthesia has emerged, to at least as great an extent as any clinical subspecialty, as a scientifically based discipline wherein the physiologic consequences of airway and lung manipulation and pharmacologic side effects of drugs are used as the basis for what is done to each patient. In other words, hardly a clinical maneuver or a therapeutic decision is made today that is not founded on some basic research or clinical development that has occurred over the past 15 to 20 years. The specialty and its practitioners in every sense epitomize modern anesthesia and contemporary anesthesiologists.

Dr. Benumof is, among all experts in the area, perhaps the best equipped, as a consequence of training, research experience, and clinical expertise, to author such a textbook. His career in anesthesia encompasses nearly 20 years—the same time period during which rapid progress has occurred in the specialty of thoracic anesthesia. His research interests have, in one way or another, centered about the physiology, pharmacology, and clinical science having to do with patients undergoing thoracic anesthesia. Examples of his research interests include studies of the determinants of distribution of pulmonary blood flow during one-lung ventilation—including anesthetics, vasoactive drugs and mechanical maneuvers, ways to manage patients undergoing one-lung ventilation, pulmonary artery pressure monitoring, and characterization of tracheobronchial anatomy, which convincingly provides evidence that fiberoptic bronchoscopy, rather than a luxury to be used occasionally, is of crucial importance for ensuring proper placement of double-lumen endotracheal tubes. Not only are his research interests pertinent but also are his clinical training and his clinical interest. He has, in his career at University of California San Diego, directed the respiratory care unit and been the principal individual in the department identified as a "thoracic surgery anesthesiologist."

This textbook covers the entire subject of thoracic anesthesia, from its history to a description of the implements used in the specialty, to management of the patient pre-, intra-, and postoperatively, including such special situations as the management of pulmonary complications, mechanical ventilation, and postoperative pain. Although it draws extensively on an understanding of physiology and pharmacology, it is principally a textbook for clinicians. As such, the emphasis is to provide a step-by-step approach to the management of clinical problems.

Although other texts on thoracic anesthesia have been produced over the years, and at the time of their production were contemporaneous, most of them had the single major disadvantage of being multiple-authored rather than single-authored, as is this text. Inherent disadvantages in multiple authorship of any textbook are a lack of consistent approach toward problems, a lack of uniformity of editorial style, a lack of knowledge of the totality of the subject by any one author, and unnecessary and, at times, frequent redundancy in the presentation of much of the material. In addition, because individuals vary in their opinions about certain subjects, conflicting thoughts regarding management may emerge, which, more often than not, will be confusing rather than illuminating to the readers.

Finally, I take special and to some extent proprietary pride in seeing this project come to fruition. Many of the studies underlying the material in the book were performed at the University of California San Diego while I was department chairman and, though entirely a result of Jon's creativity and energies, I have been privileged to be privy to many of the ideas while they were only a thought—before they were finally expressed in the laboratory. The tedium of many a long-distance jog was broken by his excited discourse of research in progress. What little influence I have had on his development as a complete academician is one of the special treats offered me as chairman. Jon has fully matured, and this book—a confirmation of his growth and accomplishments—truly represents "A Step Forward"in the management of patients undergoing thoracic surgery.

CONTENTS

1

BASIC CONSIDERATIONS

History of Anesthesia for Thoracic Surgery

1

I. INTRODUCTION

Modern anesthesia practice for thoracic surgery has a deep physiologic and pharmacologic basis, is often technically demanding and complex, and requires extensive monitoring. The know-how to administer a modern anesthetic agent for thoracic surgery was acquired mainly during the twentieth century in irregular periods of advancement. A good deal of this irregularity was caused by the two world wars, especially World War II, which created large populations of patients with chest injuries. The urgent need to care for these patients adequately greatly stimulated the growth of both surgery and anesthesia, and, in particular, it stimulated the development of the thoracic anesthesia subspecialty (see section III).

The role and importance of each advancement can be best understood if there is an appreciation of what constitutes modern anesthesia practice for thoracic surgery. Consequently, this chapter will first briefly describe where we are today (by summarizing a typical modern anesthetic for a typical thoracic surgical procedure), and then the main body of the chapter will trace how we got there (by describing the historical evolution toward that modern anesthetic practice).

II. WHERE ARE WE TODAY? BRIEF SUMMARY OF MODERN ANESTHETIC PRACTICE FOR THORACIC SURGERY

Today, a patient with a disease that can be treated by thoracic surgery (i.e., surgery on all structures within the thorax but excluding cardiac surgery or surgery requiring cardiopulmonary bypass) will usually have an accurate preoperative anatomic diagnosis (see chapter 5), and all major organ systems will have been prepared for anesthesia and surgery (see chapter 6). Consequently, it is now unusual to have an alteration in diagnosis or in treatment plan following the induction of anesthesia or the incision for elective thoracic surgery. Figure 1–1 summarizes the very common and/or very important components of modern intraoperative anesthesia practice for thoracic surgery.[1, 2]

Most patients are primarily anesthetized with a halogenated drug (see chapter 8). The induction of anesthesia may be accomplished rapidly and with hemodynamic stability by the administration of short-acting intravenous anesthetic drugs (barbiturates, narcotics, sedatives) and anesthetic adjuvants (muscle relaxants, lidocaine, vasoactive drugs). Following relaxation with a nondepolarizing drug and the monitoring of relaxation with a neuromuscular blockade

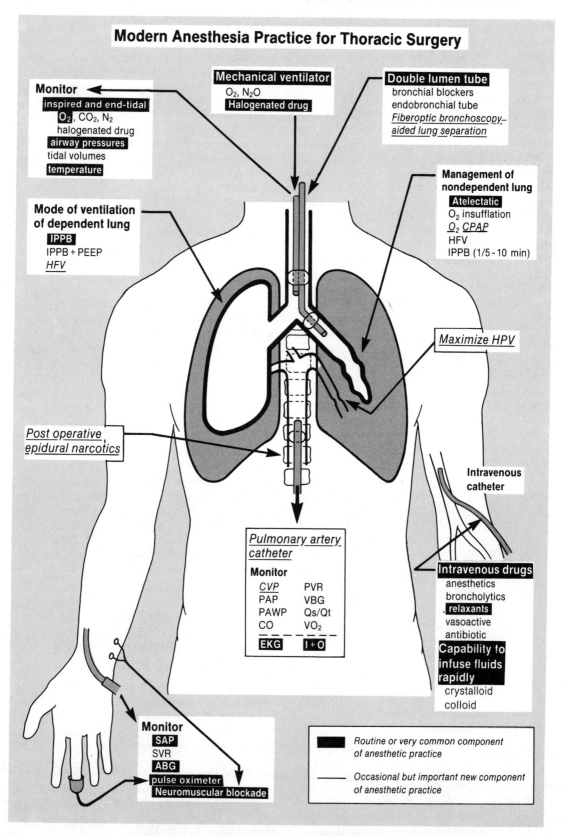

Figure 1–1. Modern anesthesia practice for thoracic surgery.

monitor, a double-lumen endotracheal tube is inserted (see chapter 9). Whenever necessary throughout the procedure, the position of the double-lumen tube may be very precisely and accurately positioned with the aid of a pediatric fiberoptic bronchoscope. The double-lumen tube will be connected to a reliable volume-limited mechanical ventilator. Attached to the double-lumen tube-connector apparatus are monitors that are used to measure end-tidal and inspired oxygen, carbon dioxide, nitrogen, and halogenated drug concentrations. The airway pressure and tidal volume to both lungs and to each lung separately will be measured, allowing the calculation of whole and independent lung compliance (see chapter 7).

The double-lumen tube allows for differential and independent management of the operative and nonoperative lungs (see chapters 11 and 12). The operative lung will most often simply be made atelectatic (one-lung ventilation); however, if oxygenation is a problem during atelectasis of the operative lung, the operative lung may be insufflated with oxygen, statically distended with small amounts of constant positive airway pressure (CPAP), made to oscillate slightly with high-frequency ventilation (HFV), or very occasionally expanded with an intermittent positive-pressure breath (IPPB). Each one of these operative lung management modalities greatly facilitates the performance of thoracic surgery in the opened hemithorax, since the nonmoving operative lung allows the surgeon to have a quiet operative field. In addition, the operative lung may be optimally managed by avoiding known causes of inhibition of operative lung hypoxic pulmonary vasoconstriction (HPV) (which diverts blood flow away from the operative lung). Finally, if hypoxemia is a severe and persistent problem, the operative lung may be conventionally ventilated with intermittent positive-pressure breathing (return to two-lung ventilation). The nonoperative lung may be managed with conventional intermittent positive-pressure breathing alone or in conjunction with positive end-expiratory pressure (PEEP). Alternatively, the nonoperative lung can be occasionally managed with high-frequency ventilation, as in surgery of the major conducting airways or the presence of a major bronchopleural fistula.

The patient's overall and specific organ well-being will be followed by a variety of monitors (see chapter 7). Routinely, the patient will have the electrocardiogram (EKG) continuously displayed, with input (from intravenous fluids) and output (from nasogastric and urinary catheters

as well as blood loss from the operative field) (I & O) frequently tallied. The vast majority of patients will have an indwelling arterial catheter, which will continuously display the phasic systemic arterial pulse pressure (SAP) and from which frequent intermittent arterial blood gas (ABG) samples may be drawn. Additionally, a pulse oximeter is routinely placed on a finger or toe and continuously displays heart rate and systemic arterial oxygen saturation. A central venous catheter (index of right heart filling pressure) will often be inserted to monitor intravascular volume status (central venous pressure, or CVP). However, if the overall cardiovascular status is questionable or at high risk (i.e., the patient is at risk for myocardial ischemia and/or failure), a pulmonary artery catheter may be inserted, which will allow measurement of pulmonary arterial pressure (PAP), pulmonary artery wedge pressure (PAWP) (index of left heart filling pressure), frequent determination of cardiac output (CO), pulmonary vascular resistance (PVR), systemic vascular resistance (SVR), and venous blood gases (VBG), which will allow for calculation of right to left transpulmonary shunt ($\dot{Q}_s/\dot{Q}_t$) and oxygen consumption ($\dot{V}O_2$). If the patient does not breathe adequately postoperatively, a sophisticated reliable mechanical ventilator will provide respiratory support (see chapter 19). Finally, an epidural catheter is often placed preoperatively or immediately postoperatively to provide postoperative analgesia with epidural opioids (see chapter 20). The routine or very common components of this modern anesthesia practice are enclosed in a box in Figure 1–1, with the occasional, but still very important, new components of anesthesia practice underlined.

III. HOW DID WE GET THERE? HISTORICAL EVOLUTION OF MODERN ANESTHETIC PRACTICE FOR THORACIC SURGERY

It would be impossible to list all of the many wonderful medical discoveries and accomplishments that have contributed to the evolution of modern anesthesia practice for thoracic surgery. Consequently, this chapter will concentrate on events that were especially important and relevant to the development of anesthesia for thoracic surgery as a subspecialty and will not describe, or will simply just mention, events that were important to the overall development of anesthesia as a broad discipline.[3-7]

Figure 1–2 summarizes the evolution of mod-

Evolution of Modern Anesthesia Practice for Thoracic Surgery

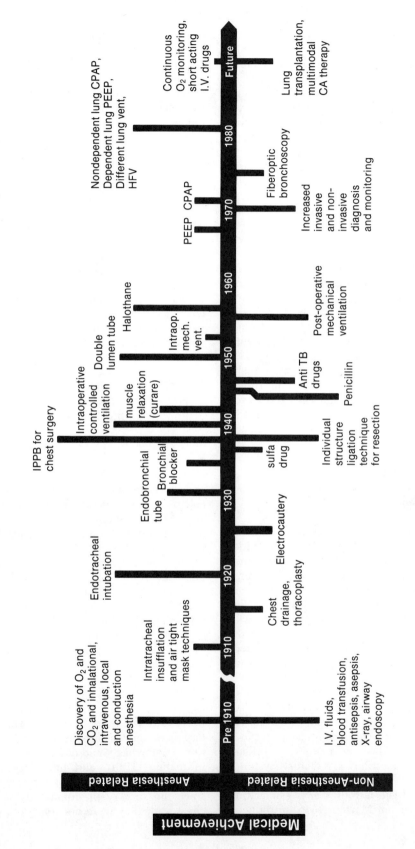

Height of Bars = Relative importance of achievement

Figure 1–2. *Evolution of modern anesthesia practice for thoracic surgery.*

ern anesthesia practice for thoracic surgery. On the x-axis of the figure is the passage of time in decades. The y-axis lists medical achievements according to whether they were primarily anesthesia related (positive y-axis) or nonanesthesia related (negative y-axis). The height of the medical accomplishment above or below the x-axis indicates its relative importance in the evolution of modern thoracic anesthesia practice. This history/time chart emphasizes change in conceptual approach by listing achievements only when they were first clinically established, although in almost all instances the real "first" and background for the achievement was provided by earlier workers, often using animals, or in single isolated cases or institutions (see the following text).

As can be seen from Figure 1–2, the sequential ability to intubate the trachea, to administer controlled intermittent positive-pressure breathing under relatively light anesthesia (curare and halothane), and to separate the lungs in order to manage the two lungs differentially dominates the anesthesia-related evolution. The development of antibiotics and of ligation techniques for individual structures for lung resection dominates the nonanesthesia-related evolution. Most of these major advances were made during World War II.

A. Pre–1910: Basic Medical Accomplishments Advancing All Types of Surgery

Prior to 1910 many basic and important discoveries were made that permitted the initial overall development of surgery as a discipline. Primarily anesthesia-related medical accomplishments included discovery of oxygen, carbon dioxide, and inhalational, intravenous, local, and conduction anesthesia. Primarily nonanesthesia-related medical accomplishments included the administration of intravenous fluids, including blood transfusion, the use of antisepsis, asepsis, the discovery of x-rays, and airway endoscopy. The names of a few of the persons responsible for these medical accomplishments, which are important to all aspects of modern medicine, are Andreas Vesalius (1555, described thoracic anatomy), William Harvey (1628, described circulatory system), Joseph Priestley (1772, discovered O_2 and N_2O), Horace Wells (1844, introduced N_2O inhalation anesthesia), William Morton (1846, introduced ether inhalation anesthesia), Louis Pasteur (1860–1880, described bacterial origin of infection), Joseph Lister (1867, introduced antisepsis), Robert Koch (1878–1882, introduced bacterial culture), Ernst von Bergmann (1886, introduced asepsis), Alfred Kirstein (1895, first used direct vision laryngoscope), Wilhelm Conrad von Roentgen (1895, discovered x-rays), Karl Landsteiner (1900, described ABO blood groups), and Chevalier Jackson (1907, greatly extended endoscopy).

Although these advancements permitted the development of surgery as a discipline, thoracic surgery was still in a remedial stage and was confined to extrathoracic chest wall procedures. Open-chested intrathoracic surgery could not be performed because of the still unsolved "pneumothorax problem" (mediastinal shift and paradoxical respiration; see chapter 4). The extrathoracic chest wall procedures that were performed at this time (see section B) were with ventilatory techniques that did not include endotracheal intubation (see section C).

B. 1900–1920: Extrathoracic Chest Wall Procedures Were Performed To Treat Infective Lung Disease

From 1900 to 1920 empyema and tuberculosis were the main indications for thoracic surgery. The former was treated by rib resection and drainage, and the latter primarily by lung collapse. This was usually achieved by creating an artificial pneumothorax, but a number of patients required division of adhesions so that the lung could retract, and some were selected for the more aggressive treatment of phrenic nerve avulsion. Thoracoplasty was introduced in 1912 by Morriston Davies but was considered hazardous at first and, thus, was performed infrequently. However, as both experience and expertise were acquired after World War I, the procedure greatly gained in popularity. In addition, infrequent thoracotomies were also performed for lung resection and the removal of tumors using a very quickly applied total lesion snare or tourniquet technique. The subsequent necrosis of the lesion required removal several days later and was usually associated with infection, hemorrhage, and/or air leak. Endotracheal intubation, IPPB, and lung separation techniques were not yet in use for anesthesia, and since the surgery predominantly involved the chest wall, they were not really required.

C. 1900–1920: Ventilatory Techniques for Chest Wall Procedures Did Not Include Endotracheal Intubation

Around 1910 these types of chest wall operations were managed with two different ventilatory techniques. The first involved intratracheal insufflation anesthesia. This was first described by two American physiologists, James Meltzer and John Auer. They demonstrated in animals that if gas is blown under pressure into the trachea through a narrow catheter, and allowed to escape around it, satisfactory gas exchange could be achieved. Charles Elsberg expanded on Meltzer and Auer's insufflation method for surgery in patients by using Chevalier Jackson's laryngoscope (1907) to deliver the respiratory gases (air-ether). This technique usually rendered the patient apneic and became a very popular choice for chest surgery in the United States in 1914 and for head and neck surgery in Britain following its introduction there by the ear, nose, and throat surgeon Robert Kelley. Indeed, Elsberg was able to further promote the technique by being asked to write the chapter on anesthesia for thoracic surgery in the 1914 edition of Gwathmay's textbook *Anesthesia*. It should be noted that insufflation of gases during bronchoscopy, now largely superseded by the injector technique of Sanders (1967), is a modern derivative of this technique. Although laryngoscopy was a prerequisite for intratracheal insufflation, the value of endotracheal intubation, which would have allowed for the use of intermittent positive-pressure ventilation to solve the open chest "pneumothorax problem," simply did not occur to these individuals.

The second ventilatory method for intrathoracic operations was primarily used during World War I (1914 to 1918) and consisted of administration of nitrous oxide and oxygen via spontaneous respirations through an airtight mask with a positive end-expiratory pressure of 5 to 7 mm Hg and intravenous morphine added for additional analgesia. Endotracheal intubation, although possible (see next section), was not used for chest operations, even on casualties, because it required expertise not readily available, and since deeper anesthesia was required, cardiovascular collapse was feared. The airtight mask ventilatory method continued to be used a great deal for chest surgery for another decade after the war. Individuals responsible for the development of the nitrous

oxide/oxygen/morphine anesthesia technique and apparatus included Charles Peter, J. A. Heidbrink, James T. Gwathmay, Elmer I. McKesson, and George W. Crile.

D. 1920s: Beginning of Significant Use of Endotracheal Intubation

The history of endotracheal intubation is closely related to the history of laryngoscopy. In the area of laryngoscopy and endotracheal intubation (and, perhaps, positive-pressure ventilation) there were several "firsts," but they were forgotten or discarded as a result of contemporary criticism. Consequently, the date of introduction of these new techniques or apparatuses was often controversial.

Prior to the 1920s, attempts at laryngoscopy and/or endotracheal intubation were sporadic and short lived (with the exception of Chevalier Jackson's laryngoscope for throat and neck surgery). Charles Kite first used an endotracheal tube in resuscitation of drowned victims in 1788. Manuel Garcia, a singing teacher, used indirect laryngoscopy in 1855. Around 1880 George Fell, Joseph O'Dwyer, and William Macewen practiced blind oral intubation, and in 1893 Fell attached a bellows system to the intubating cannulae to achieve resuscitative lung expansion by positive pressure. Rudolph Matas, a surgeon, applied some of the Fell-O'Dwyer blind techniques and apparatus to the treatment of traumatic pneumothorax, and a few other surgeons at this time (1895 to 1900) adopted the Fell-O'Dwyer blind intubation-bellows apparatus for use in surgery (see introduction of intermittent positive-pressure breathing into thoracic anesthesia in section F). A direct vision laryngoscope for endotracheal intubation developed by Kirstein in 1895 was not used by anyone in surgery.

During and after World War I (1916 to 1928) Ivan W. Magill and Stanley Rowbotham were prompted by the need to provide safe operating conditions for maxillofacial surgery on injured servicemen to develop the technique of endotracheal intubation; this work pioneered contemporary endotracheal anesthesia. At first, wide-bore rubber tubes were passed by blind nasal and oral intubation, a technique that did not require either laryngoscopy or deep anesthesia. Nevertheless, this technique was little used for chest wall procedures with nitrous oxide/oxygen/morphine anesthesia during this period. In fact, despite his own remarkable skill at both blind nasal and orotracheal intubation, Magill expressed the following view as late as 1928 in a communication to the Anaesthetic Section of the Royal Society of Medicine: "Operations on the thorax, such as thoracoplasty and pulmonary decortication, give better results when nitrous oxide or ethylene and oxygen are administered by means of a face-piece. The condition of the patient after operation is ample compensation for the difficulty sometimes entailed in maintaining airtight apposition of the mask. Moreover, an efficient apparatus provides for positive ventilation of the lungs without the necessity for intubation."[6]

However, within 2 to 4 years of this statement, Gale and Waters in the United States and Magill in the United Kingdom, all of whom understood the value of endotracheal intubation and were aware of Chevalier Jackson's work with direct laryngoscopy, began the natural marriage of direct laryngoscopy with endotracheal intubation, and direct orotracheal intubation soon became increasingly used in the following years. This was a very important step because it was prerequisite to the use of intermittent positive-pressure ventilation, which would prove, a decade later, to be the solution to the "pneumothorax problem."

The ability to perform laryngoscopy and endotracheal intubation more routinely logically led to the capability of separating the two lungs with various endobronchial tubes and bronchial blockers during the 1930s (see Tables 1–1 and 1–2). Although these devices proved to be extremely valuable following 1940 (see section F), their use at this particular time was still restricted to a few experts in a few centers. Other than the ability to separate the two lungs, the development of anesthesia for thoracic surgery between 1930 and 1940 was relatively insignificant. Following this relatively static period and World War II, thoracic surgery and anesthesia for thoracic surgery greatly changed; operations on the chest wall dramatically decreased, and major operations within the thorax dramatically increased.

E. 1940–1950: Decline in Chest Wall Procedures To Treat Infective Lung Disease

As with all infectious diseases, the development of antibiotics completely changed the clinical course of infective chest diseases. The treatment of lung abscess, bronchiectasis, and empyema was revolutionized in the post–World War II period by the use of sulfonamides (introduced by May and Baker in 1938 for the control of hemolytic streptococcal infections) and the availability of penicillin for civilian use (the antibiotic effects of penicillin were first described by Alexander Fleming in 1929). The discovery of streptomycin in 1943, para-aminosalicylic acid in 1946, and isoniazid in 1952 had equally profound effects on the treatment of tuberculosis. Because of the discovery of these antibiotics, pulmonary tuberculosis and bronchiectasis were treated surgically far less often, whereas resection for malignant disease became more and more common (see the following section), a trend that has certainly continued to the present time.[6]

Table 1–1. Development of Single-Lumen Endobronchial Tubes[3]

Date	Name	Distinctive Characteristics	Bronchial Intubation Technique*
1932	Gale and Waters	Carinal cuff that only when inflated to give airtight seal excludes other main bronchus. Unstable.	Blind
1936	Magill	Right and left tube with large endobronchial cuff. Right tube has terminal wire spiral.	Intubating bronchoscope
1955	Macintosh and Leatherdale	Left endobronchial tube, angulated at carina. Tracheal as well as endobronchial cuff. Incorporated tracheal suction stem. Good stability.	Blind
1957	Gordon and Green	Right endobronchial tube with tracheal and bronchial cuffs. Carinal hook. Bronchial cuff has slot in lateral wall.	Blind or intubating bronchoscope
1958	Pallister	Left endobronchial tube with one tracheal and two bronchial cuffs.	Intubating bronchoscope
1958	Machray	Left endobronchial tube similar to the left-sided Magill tube but has a shorter bronchial cuff.	Intubating bronchoscope

*Prior to availability of fiberoptic bronchoscopy

Table 1–2. Development of Endobronchial Blockers[3]

Date	Name	Distinctive Characteristics	Bronchial Intubation Technique*
		Simple Bronchial Blocker	
1938	Craford	Gauze pack inserted into affected bronchus.	Intubating bronchoscope under topical analgesia
1936	Magill	Rubber suction catheter with a small inflatable bronchial cuff.	Bronchoscope
1943	Vernon	Similar to Magill catheter but larger and with cuff covered with gauze or woven nylon.	Bronchoscope
		Combined Endotracheal Tube Plus Bronchial Blocker	
1953	Sturtzbecher	Essentially an endotracheal tube with an incorporated suction catheter plus blocker cuff.	Blind—blocker directed into diseased bronchus with wire stylet
1954	Vellacott	Right-sided endobronchial tube with bronchial cuff that blocks upper lobe orifice, plus tracheal cuff; an orifice in left lateral wall between cuffs.	Intubating bronchoscope
1955	Macintosh and Leatherdale	Cuffed endotracheal tube with an angulated cuffed suction catheter blocker incorporated for left bronchus blockade.	Blind
1958	Green	Right-sided tube similar to Vellacott tube but with carinal hook.	Blind or intubating bronchoscope
1981	Ginsberg	Modern clear plastic endotracheal tube with second smaller "kangaroo" lumen for balloon-tipped bronchial blocker.	Blind

*Prior to availability of fiberoptic bronchoscopy.

F. 1938–1950: Emergence of Intrathoracic Lung Resection for Malignancy

Several events around 1938 resulted in an explosion of growth of intrathoracic surgery. These were both nonanesthesia- and anesthesia-related. The major nonanesthesia-related advance was the development of techniques for dissecting and ligating individual structures at the hilum of the lung. Prior to 1930, lung resection was only occasionally performed using a quickly applied total lesion snare or a tourniquet technique. The technique required two surgical stages: one to snare the lesion, and then another several days later to remove the necrotic tissue. Consequently, the technique was fraught with dangers of infection, hemorrhage, and air leak, and it always resulted in significant morbidity and mortality. The first successful pneumonectomy using the snare technique was carried out by Rudolf Nisson in Germany in 1931 for bronchiectasis. Cameron Haight and John Alexander in 1932 performed the first successful pneumonectomy in the western hemisphere using the same technique in a patient with bronchiectasis. In 1933 Evarts Graham performed a left snare pneumonectomy on a physician with squamous cell carcinoma, and the individual survived 30 years.[8] No patient

had survived a total pneumonectomy for a malignant tumor of the lung prior to Dr. Graham's operation.

Although everyone recognized that Dr. Graham's success was a milestone, the development of the individual structure (bronchus, pulmonary artery, pulmonary vein) ligation technique in the 1930s was much more important because it greatly reduced the incidence and risk of postoperative bronchial leaks and tension pneumothorax, pulmonary hemorrhage (from either artery or vein), and infection from residual necrotic tissue. The individual structure ligation technique for lobectomy was extensively used by Edward Churchill starting in 1938. W. F. Rienhoff performed the first pneumonectomy using the individual ligation technique in the late 1930s. The work of these early surgeons laid the groundwork for the performance of lung resection as it is done today.[8] These early attempts at intrathoracic procedures during the 1930s were aided by the introduction of an endobronchial tube for one-lung anesthesia by J. W. Gale and R. M. Waters in 1932, and by the introduction of an endobronchial tube, bronchoscope, and bronchial blocker by Magill in 1936 (see Tables 1–1 and 1–2 for the subsequent development of endobronchial tubes and bronchial blockers).

The anesthesia-related advances that contributed to the explosive growth in thoracic surgery around 1938 consisted of the development of intermittent positive-pressure breathing (IPPB) for chest surgery, which, combined with the introduction of muscle relaxation with curare in 1942, led to the ability to easily control ventilation in the intraoperative period. Prior to this time, the primary difficulty in performing intrathoracic procedures was known as "the pneumothorax problem" (see chapter 4). As soon as the chest of a spontaneously breathing patient was opened, the lung in question not only collapsed but also moved up and down violently with each struggling breath (mediastinal flap and paradoxical respirations). Within a few minutes, the patient became cyanotic and hypotensive, and, unless the chest was closed quickly, the patient would die. These were extremely poor conditions under which to make a diagnosis and to undertake treatment. The single most important factor enabling thoracic surgery to advance rapidly was the solution to this pneumothorax problem by artificial rhythmic inflation of the lungs (through controlled ventilation with IPPB) after the patient had been rendered apneic (by muscle relaxation).

The successful introduction of IPPB for the management of intrathoracic operations first required the development of laryngoscopy, endotracheal intubation, and adequate bellows or pump machinery. Many early attempts to solve the "pneumothorax problem" failed because they lacked one of these essential components. In trying to avoid atelectasis, Ernst Sauerbruch in Germany during 1893 to 1904 did his early thoracotomies in an airtight chamber with the pressure reduced 7 mm Hg below atmospheric pressure, while the patient's head and the anesthetist were outside in atmospheric air (negative-pressure breathing). This was followed in 1904 by a positive-pressure breathing chamber of another German, Ludolph Brauer. Brauer's method was essentially the same as the constant positive airway pressure (CPAP) method introduced by Gregory et al in 1971[9] but used more complicated machinery. The positive-pressure breathing method of Brauer slowly replaced the negative-pressure breathing cabinet of Sauerbruch. Sauerbruch, who was without a doubt the most dominant influence in (European) thoracic surgery at this time, was extremely resistant to the change from negative-pressure to positive-pressure breathing in spite of the obvious clinical failure of his method of spontaneous negative-pressure breathing to permit prolonged surgery. In fact, Sauerbruch's spontaneous negative-pressure breathing method remained in widespread use until World War II and indeed appeared as the recommended method in an English textbook in 1937, of which he was coauthor. However, at the end of Sauerbruch's career he advocated Brauer's positive-pressure breathing technique. Neither Sauerbruch's nor Brauer's breathing chamber techniques involved endotracheal intubation.

There was also considerable interest in the United States in developing positive-pressure breathing, and the development of positive-pressure breathing was closely related to the development of endotracheal intubation (see section D). In the 1880s, George Fell popularized the use of bellows for resuscitation (compression leading to positive pressure), and O'Dwyer designed a hooked metal intubating cannula. In 1895 Theodore Tuffier, a French surgeon, used a cuffed O'Dwyer tube and rhythmic positive pressure with PEEP for thoracic surgery. In 1898, Rudolph Matas clearly recognized that the Fell-O'Dwyer apparatus could revolutionize thoracic surgery and used their apparatus in thoracic surgery. Indeed, in 1899 Matas wrote, "The procedure that promises the most benefit in preventing pulmonary collapse in operations on the chest is the artificial inflation of the lung and the rhythmical maintenance of artificial respiration by a tube in the glottis directly connected with a bellows. Like other discoveries, it is not only elementary in its simplicity, but the fundamental ideas involved in this important suggestion have been lying idle before the eye of the profession for years. It is curious that surgeons should have failed to apply for so long a time the suggestions of the physiological laboratory, where the bellows and tracheal tubes have been in constant use from the days of Magendie to the present in practicing artificial respiration in animals."[7] In 1899 Matas's colleague P.W. Parham stated, "so imbued am I with its (the apparatus) great value that I believe no surgeon now would be justified in attempting a thoracic resection without having the Fell-O'Dwyer apparatus at hand. I believe it will revolutionize the field of surgery, making possible operations in the chest that would otherwise clearly be too hazardous."[7] It is strange that pioneer thoracic surgeons like Tuffier, Matas, and Parham neglected to try Kirstein's laryngoscope for endotracheal intubation and preferred instead to depend entirely upon blind oral digital methods that appeared uncertain and unhygienic even to their colleagues. In 1905 Janeway and Green from New

York described a cuffed endotracheal tube and a pump for experimental chest surgery. In 1910, Dorrance from Philadelphia described cuffed endotracheal tubes and a pump for chest surgery. However, none of these early American "firsts" in intubation-bellows or pump systems attracted considerable attention.

The history of IPPB as we know and use it today began in 1916 when Giertz, a former assistant to Sauerbruch, conducted experiments in animals showing that rhythmic inflation of the lungs was more effective than either negative pressure or continuous positive-pressure ventilation. In 1934, Guedel, using ether anesthesia, was the first to routinely manually control respiration intraoperatively in intubated patients. In 1934, Frenckner, a Swedish ear, nose, and throat surgeon, described the first experimental model "Spiropulsater" ventilator for chest operations. The Frenckner positive-pressure "Spiropulsater" respirator was first used by Clarence Crafoord in surgery in Stockholm in 1938, and this really was the dawn of the modern era of mechanical intermittent positive-pressure breathing. The controlled IPPB ventilation concept was further promoted by Waters and simplified by Guedel in this country in the late 1930s and by Nosworthy in England in 1941. All three advocated controlled breathing by intermittent pressure on the reservoir bag of a closed cyclopropane anesthesia circuit. Although ether and cyclopropane, which were the most widely used inhalation anesthetics at that time, were safe and potent (and therefore permitted controlled respiration to a certain extent), they were also highly explosive and therefore precluded the use of electrocautery. Controlled positive-pressure breathing really became routinely possible during entire intrathoracic procedures with the introduction of muscle relaxation with curare in 1942 by H. R. Griffith. Curare had the great advantages of inducing apnea, diminishing reflexes, and, most importantly, allowing the unrestricted use of electrocautery.

Thus, the late 1930s and early 1940s witnessed the advent of manual and mechanical controlled ventilation in paralyzed patients. Despite the fact that Crafoord's results were enthusiastically accepted in Scandinavia, and despite the efforts of Guedel, Waters, and Nosworthy and the introduction of muscle relaxation, a significant portion of the British and American anesthesia community continued to use the older methods of continuous positive pressure by mask and intratracheal insufflation during the 1940s.

The slow acceptance by American and British anesthetists of intraoperative controlled IPPB caused mechanical ventilators to first be used extensively and routinely outside the operating room. The catastrophic Copenhagen polio epidemic of 1952 led to a crash production program of Engstrom volume ventilators. In 1955, Björk and Engstrom in Sweden first described the use of their ventilator for postoperative respiratory care of poor-risk thoracic surgery patients. The Jefferson ventilator was developed on John Gibbons's thoracic surgery service in Philadelphia and was introduced in 1957 as the first American ventilator for controlled ventilation. The clear-cut efficacy of mechanical ventilators outside of the operating room soon convinced anesthetists to use these machines to control IPPB ventilation reliably in the operating room, and operating room mechanical ventilators became commonplace in the 1960s and 1970s.

G. 1950s and 1960s: Development of Double-Lumen Endotracheal Tubes

The development of double-lumen tubes was a response to the fast-growing capabilities in thoracic surgery, which now required faster, surer, and simpler methods of separating the two lungs and of causing the lung under operation to be atelectatic. The Björk and Carlens bronchospirometric double-lumen tube was first used during anesthesia in 1950. In the next two decades several different types of double-lumen tubes with varying capabilities were introduced (see Table 1–3). Until the advent of fiberoptic bronchoscopy, the method of placement of these tubes within the tracheobronchial tree was essentially blind. Fiberoptic bronchoscopy now allows for these tubes to be placed and for the position of tubes to be checked under direct vision repeatedly with extreme precision and very low risk (see section K).

H. 1956: Introduction of Halogenated Inhalation Anesthetic Drugs

The introduction of halothane in England in 1956 by M. Johnstone was the result of a search for an inhalational anesthetic that would meet many needs that remain unfulfilled by previ-

Table 1–3. Development of Double-Lumen Endobronchial Tubes[3]

Date	Name	Distinctive Characteristics	Bronchial Intubation Technique*
1950	Carlens	Double-lumen catheter with two inbuilt curves. Tracheal and a bronchial cuff for left main bronchus, carinal hook and cross-sectional shape—oval in horizontal plane.	Blind
1959	Bryce-Smith	Modification of the Carlens catheter with no carinal hook. Cross-sectional shape—oval in horizontal plane.	Blind
1960	Bryce-Smith and Salt	Right-sided version of the Bryce-Smith tube, possessing slit in endobronchial cuff, no carinal hooks.	Blind
1960	White	Right-sided version of the Carlens catheter, possessing slit in endobronchial cuff and a carinal hook.	Blind
1962	Robertshaw	Right and left double-lumen tubes. Modification of the Carlens catheter with a larger lumen and hence low resistance to gas flows; slotted right endobronchial cuff; no carinal hooks. Cross-sectional shape—D-shaped in the horizontal plane.	Blind
1979	National Catheter Corporation	Right and left Robertshaw–type disposable double-lumen tube made of clear tissue implantable plastic with low-pressure high-volume cuffs.	Blind

*Prior to availability of fiberoptic bronchoscopy.

ously used drugs. It was nonflammable (which ether and cyclopropane were not) and therefore allowed the use of electrocautery; it allowed high concentrations of oxygen to be used (which nitrous oxide obviated); it was thought to be inert; it had limited solubility in water and fat (as opposed to ether and chloroform); it did not react with alkali used for CO_2 absorption (as did trichloroethylene); it was tolerated reasonably well by the heart; and it produced a smooth induction and awakening. By 1959, the use of halothane was widespread in both the United States and the rest of the world. This signaled the beginning of the era of nonflammable, inhalational anesthetics. Although halothane was initially thought to have no toxicity, it now appears that hepatic toxicity is a real, but very rare, entity. Fortunately, other halogenated drugs have been developed, such as isoflurane, which have all the desirable properties of halothane and appear not to cause any tissue toxicity.

I. 1970s: Increased Invasive and Noninvasive Monitoring

The 1970s witnessed a phenomenal explosive increase in monitoring patients intra- and postoperatively. Almost all of the monitors shown in Figure 1–1 were introduced during this period. The use of these monitors has allowed for the diagnosis of major patient problems that heretofore were impossible to make with certainty (such as the diagnosis of cardiac failure by pulmonary artery pressure monitoring). The monitors (oxygenation and ventilation monitors, neuromuscular blockade monitors) also refine the specificity of, and can quantitate, many diagnoses that previously were possible to make but without great precision or accuracy.

J. 1970s: Introduction of PEEP and CPAP into Clinical Practice

PEEP was introduced into clinical practice almost 20 years ago[10] and has proved to be a rapid and relatively high-benefit, low-risk method for increasing the oxygenation capability of severely diseased lungs. CPAP was introduced a few years later to treat spontaneously breathing infants with idiopathic respiratory distress syndrome.[9] Since then the use of CPAP and PEEP to treat patients with respiratory disease can almost be characterized as routine, because these are the primary therapeutic mechanisms by which the inspired oxygen concentration can be reduced below toxic levels.

K. 1975: Introduction of Fiberoptic Bronchoscopy

Direct examination of the tracheobronchial tree with flexible fiberoptic bronchoscopy has greatly facilitated the diagnosis, staging, and management of pulmonary neoplasms as well as many other lung diseases.[11] With particular reference to thoracic anesthesia, the fiberoptic bronchoscope now allows for placement of double-lumen and endobronchial tubes and bronchial blockers with great precision and accuracy and at low risk to the patient. Prior to the advent of the fiberoptic bronchoscope, these instruments were placed blindly (see Table 1–3). Consequently, their exact position was often precarious, and they sometimes malfunctioned, preventing collapse of the nondependent lung and ventilation of the dependent lung. Today, the fiberoptic bronchoscope, although expensive, is considered to be a high-priority piece of equipment for an individual practicing anesthesia for thoracic surgery.

L. 1980s: Use of Nondependent Lung CPAP, Dependent Lung PEEP, Differential Lung Ventilation, High-Frequency Ventilation

The ability to place double-lumen tubes easily and accurately and at low risk (in part due to the development of the fiberoptic bronchoscope) has led to the ability to manage the two different lungs specifically according to their individual pathology. Thus, the nondependent lung may be statically distended by low levels of CPAP (using oxygen), which greatly enhances oxygenation during one-lung ventilation. The dependent lung may be ventilated in the conventional manner, but with the addition of PEEP, thereby correcting a low ventilation-to-perfusion situation that may exist owing to dependent lung compression by the mediastinum, abdominal contents, and positioning effects. Use of these two ventilation modalities together is termed differential lung ventilation.[12] Similarly, in the intensive care unit, patients with predominantly unilateral adult respiratory distress syndrome have been treated with differential lung ventilation.[13] High-frequency ventilation may be the treatment of choice for some patients with major bronchopleural fistulas and for some patients having surgery on major conducting airways. High-frequency ventilation is efficacious for major bronchopleural fistulas because it involves low airway pressures, which minimize air leaks from the fistulas. High-frequency ventilation is efficacious for surgery on major conducting airways because it requires that only a small catheter pass through the surgeon's operative field; consequently, the anastomosis of a major conducting airway is made much easier.

IV. THE FUTURE

The focus of present research will determine to a large extent the type of advances that will be made in the near future. Prevention of lung carcinoma is probably the most important consideration, and efforts to discourage smoking will certainly continue to increase. Since early detection of lung carcinoma by radiologic and cytologic methods has limited potential (high cost, low yield), the future of screening for lung carcinoma may lie in developing sensitive cellular markers. Indeed, development of specific antisera to tumor antigens, and radiolabeling of these antibodies may serve not only for early detection but also for early therapy.[14] It appears likely that we will witness an increase in availability and use of continuous monitors of oxygenation, ventilation, and acid-base balance. In addition, it is likely that very short-acting narcotics, sedatives, and relaxants will be available in the near future. Since the most important cause of failure of resectional surgery to cure patients of thoracic carcinoma is mediastinal and extrathoracic metastatic disease, much effort will go into making the diagnosis of metastatic disease, and we will likely witness improvement in such noninvasive procedures as computed tomography and magnetic resonance imaging. Interest will continue to be high in multimodal therapy (chemotherapy, irradiation, laser and surgical excision) of carcinoma of both the lung and the esophagus. Finally, lung transplantation should begin to achieve a reasonable degree of success in the next two to three decades.

V. SUMMARY

Anesthesia for thoracic surgery has gone through a remarkable evolution over the last 50 years. We have moved from performing simple chest wall surgery without a secure airway in poorly monitored patients who were deeply anesthetized with inherently dangerous techniques to performing extremely complicated intrathoracic procedures, with firm control over each lung independently, in very well-monitored patients who are moderately anesthetized with inherently safe techniques. Consequently, the present mortality rate of a pneumonectomy and of a lobectomy is only 6 and 3 per cent, respectively.[15] Conversely, with non–small cell lung carcinoma and no hilar or mediastinal node involvement, a 90 per cent 5-year survival rate may now be expected following definitive resection.[16] These figures compare extremely favorably with a mortality of 52 per cent for a lobectomy for bronchiectasis in 1922.[8] Considering the fact that the first modern pneumonectomy was performed only 50 years ago, thoracic anesthesia represents a subspeciality that has had a rapid and dramatic development.

REFERENCES

1. Benumof JL: Monitoring respiratory function during anesthesia. In Saidman LJ, Smith NT (eds): Monitoring During Anesthesia. 2nd ed. Boston, Butterworth Publishers, 1983, pp 35–78.
2. Alfery DD, Benumof JL: Anesthesia for thoracic surgery. In Miller R (ed): Anesthesia. New York, Churchill Livingstone, 1981, pp 925–980.
3. Lee JA, Atkinson RS: The history of anesthesia. In Lee JA, Atkinson RS (eds): A Synopsis of Anesthesia. 7th ed. Baltimore, Williams & Wilkins Co., 1973, pp 1–24.
4. Lee JA, Atkinson RS: Anesthesia for thoracic surgery. In Lee JA, Atkinson RS (eds): A Synopsis of Anesthesia. 7th ed. Baltimore, Williams & Wilkins Co., 1973, pp 599–633.
5. Kaplan JA: Development of thoracic anesthesia. In Kaplan JA (ed): Thoracic Anesthesia, New York, Churchill Livingstone, 1982, pp 3–8.
6. Gothard JWW, Branthwaithe MA: History. In Gothard JWW, Branthwaite MA (eds): Anesthesia for Thoracic Surgery. Oxford, Blackwell Scientific Publications, 1982, pp 1–8.
7. Rendell-Baker L: History of anesthesia for thoracic surgery. In Mushin WW (ed): Thoracic Anesthesia. Oxford, Blackwell Scientific Publications, 1963, pp 598–661.
8. Brewer LA III: The first pneumonectomy. J Thorac Cardiovasc Surg 88:810–826, 1984.
9. Gregory GA, Kitterman JA, Phibbs RH, et al: Treatment of the idiopathic respiratory distress syndrome with continuous positive airway pressure. N Engl J Med 284:1333, 1971.
10. Ashbaugh DG, Bigelow DB, Petty TL, et al: Acute respiratory distress in adults. Lancet 2:319, 1967.
11. Sackner MA: Bronchofiberoscopy. Am Rev Respir Dis 111:62–88, 1975.
12. Benumof JL: One-lung ventilation: Which lung should be PEEPed? Anesthesiology 56:161–163, 1982.
13. Kvetan V, Carlon GC, Howlan WS: Acute pulmonary failure in assymetric lung disease: Approach to management. Crit Care Med 10:114, 1982.
14. Benfield JR, Yellin A: New horizons for lung cancer. Surg Rounds April:26–52, 1985.
15. Ginsberg JR, Hill DL, Eagan TR, et al.: Modern thirty-day operative mortality for surgical resections in lung cancer. J Thorac Cardiovasc Surg 86:654–658, 1983.
16. Denis CA, Pairolero CP, Vergstralh JE, et al: Roentgenographically occult lung cancer. J Thorac Cardiovasc Surg 86:373–380, 1983.

Thoracic Anatomy

2

I. INTRODUCTION

Understanding thoracic anatomy is important to the thoracic anesthetist for several reasons. First, knowledge of thoracic anatomy is important in diagnosing and understanding the physiologic and therapeutic implications of thoracic lesions. Second, the anesthesiologist should understand how surgery will proceed (patient position, incisions, intrathoracic procedures) because surgical requirements often dictate anesthetic requirements. Third, an appreciation of anatomy should allow the anesthesiologist to anticipate and to prepare for intraoperative complications. Fourth, understanding thoracic anatomy is an integral part of the safe and successful use of regional anesthesia and pain relief. This chapter first discusses the anatomy of the thoracic wall, then the anatomy of the airway and lung parenchyma, and finally the anatomy of the mediastinum. Special pediatric anatomy is considered in chapter 17.

II. THE THORACIC WALL[1–4]

A. Bones and Cartilage

The thoracic bones and cartilages are covered with muscles. The anterior muscles are the pectoralis major and minor and serratus anterior (Fig. 2–1), and the lateral and posterior muscles are the latissimus dorsi, rhomboid major and minor, serratus posterior, and trapezius (Fig. 2–2).

The thoracic bones and cartilages consist of the sternum, 10 pairs of ribs and costal cartilages (together termed costae), two pairs of ribs without cartilage, and 12 thoracic vertebrae and their intervertebral disks (Figs. 2–3 and 2–4). Together these bones and cartilages surround a cavity that is reniform in cross section; the cavity has a narrow thoracic inlet at the neck and a much larger thoracic outlet facing the abdominal cavity. The inlet is surrounded by the manubrium of the sternum, the first ribs, and the first thoracic vertebrae. The inlet is roofed by bilateral thickened endothoracic fascia, called Sibson's fascia, and subadjacent parietal pleurae that project upward into the base of the neck. The outlet is formed by the xiphoid process, fused costal cartilages of ribs 7 to 10, the anterior portions of the eleventh rib, the shaft of the twelfth rib, and the body of the twelfth thoracic vertebrae. The anterior margin of the outlet is at the level of the tenth thoracic, the lateral limits at the second lumbar, and the posterior margin at the twelfth thoracic vertebrae. The outlet is therefore higher at its anterior margin than at its posterior limit and reaches its lowest level in the lateral aspect near the midaxillary line. It is sealed off from the abdominal cavity by the diaphragm.

The size and shape of the thorax is largely determined by the ribs and the costal cartilages. The relations of ribs and their costal cartilages to the sternum and to each other vary at different levels. The upper seven pairs of ribs articulate directly with the sternum by way of costal cartilages and are therefore called "true" or

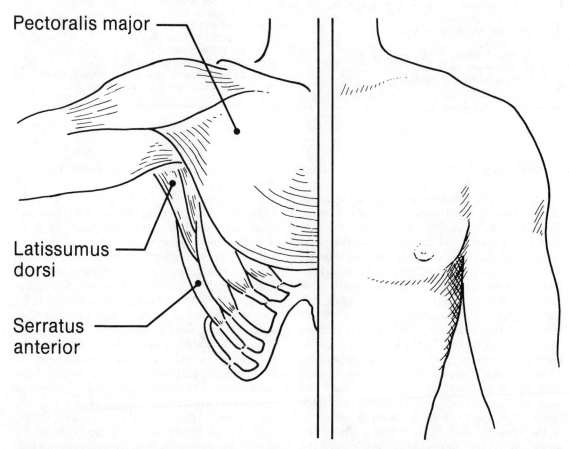

Pectoralis major

Latissumus
dorsi

Serratus
anterior

Figure 2–1. The important anterior thoracic wall muscles are the pectoralis major and minor (which is underneath the pectoralis major and is not shown) and the serratus anterior. The important lateral thoracic wall muscle is the latissimus dorsi. Corresponding surface features are shown on the right. The fifth intercostal space is just below the inferior border of the pectoralis major.

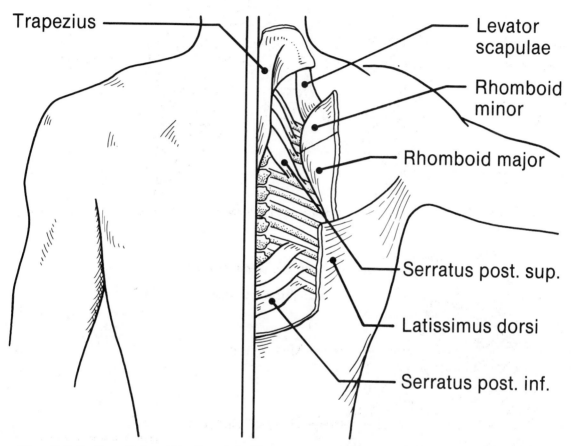

Trapezius

Levator
scapulae

Rhomboid
minor

Rhomboid major

Serratus post. sup.

Latissimus dorsi

Serratus post. inf.

Figure 2–2. The important posterior thoracic wall muscles are the latissimus dorsi, rhomboid major and minor, serratus posterior superior (post. sup.) and inferior (post. inf.), and trapezius. The corresponding surface markings are shown on the left.

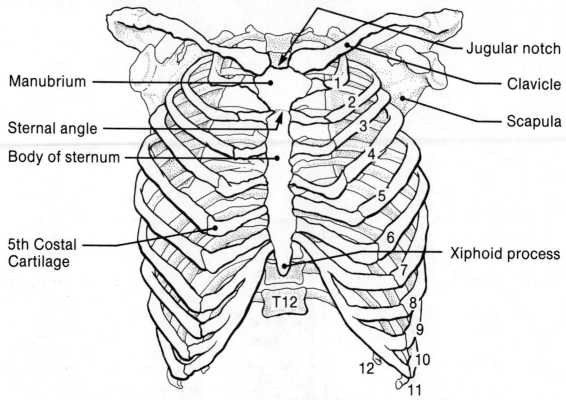

Figure 2–3. Anterior view of the bones and cartilages of the thorax. The ribs are numbered according to their vertebral origin.

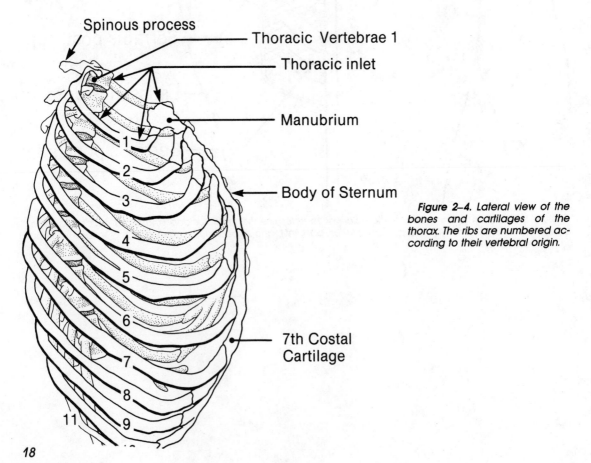

Figure 2–4. Lateral view of the bones and cartilages of the thorax. The ribs are numbered according to their vertebral origin.

vertebrosternal ribs. In contrast, the lower five pairs are called "false" ribs, since they do not articulate with the sternum at all. Of the false ribs, three pairs, the eighth, ninth, and tenth, are called the vertebrocostal ribs, since their associated cartilages articulate with immediately supradjacent cartilages. The remaining pairs, 11 and 12, terminate in cartilaginous tips, which are embedded in the muscles of the abdominal wall. Since the only articulation of these latter two ribs is with the vertebrae, they are called vertebral ribs. The flexibility of the rib-vertebral and rib-sternal joints permit the "bucket-handle" or "pump-handle" movements of breathing.

B. The Diaphragm

The diaphragm is a dome-shaped musculofibrous septum that separates the thoracic from the abdominal cavity: Its convex upper surface forms the floor of the thoracic cavity, and its concave undersurface forms the roof of the abdominal cavity. Its peripheral part consists of muscular fibers that originate from the circumference of the thoracic outlet and converge to be inserted into a large central tendon. The central tendon is C-shaped and concave toward the vertebrae (Fig. 2–5). The central tendon is perforated a little to the right of the midline and at the level of the lower border of the

eighth thoracic vertebra by the inferior vena cava. The esophageal opening lies in the muscular part of the diaphragm near the midline at the level of the tenth thoracic vertebra. The aorta passes posteriorly through the diaphragm as it lies on the front of the body of the twelfth thoracic vertebra. The abdominal surface of the diaphragm is closely applied to the liver, the fundus of the stomach, the spleen, and the right and left kidneys and suprarenal glands. The upper surface lies in relation to the right and left lungs and pleura and to the heart and pericardium.

C. The Intercostal Spaces

The intercostal spaces between the ribs are the main surgical pathway to the thorax. The muscles of the intercostal spaces themselves are arranged in three layers corresponding to the three layers of the lateral abdominal wall (Figs. 2–6 and 2–7). From a surgical approach, the first layer of tissue to be encountered within the intercostal space is the external intercostal muscle, which passes downward and forward from the lower border of one rib to the upper border of the rib below and extends from the tubercle of the rib posteriorly to the neighborhood of the costochondral junction in front. The next layer of muscle is called the internal intercostal muscle and extends from the sternum to

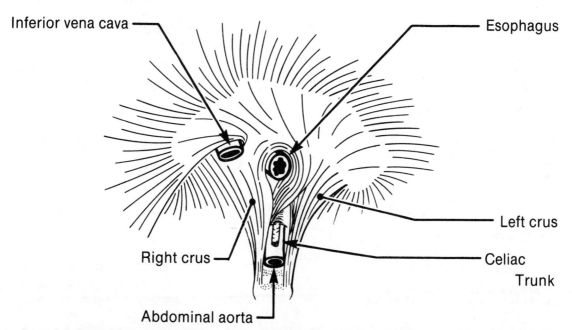

Figure 2–5. *The diaphragm is viewed from below. The muscular part of the diaphragm consists of the peripheral part, a left and right crus. The muscular part of the diaphragm inserts onto a C-shaped (concave posteriorly) central tendon. The diaphragm is pierced by the inferior vena cava, the esophagus, and aorta.*

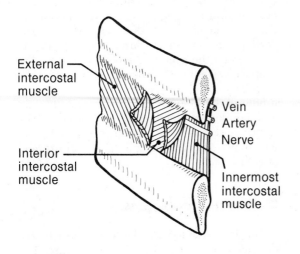

External intercostal muscle

Interior intercostal muscle

Vein
Artery
Nerve

Innermost intercostal muscle

Figure 2–6. *The muscle layers of the intercostal space, from external to internal aspect, are the external intercostal, the interior intercostal, and the innermost intercostal muscles. Between the interior and innermost intercostal muscle at the caudad aspect of each rib is the intercostal vein, artery, and nerve; the vein is most cephalad, and the nerve is most caudad.*

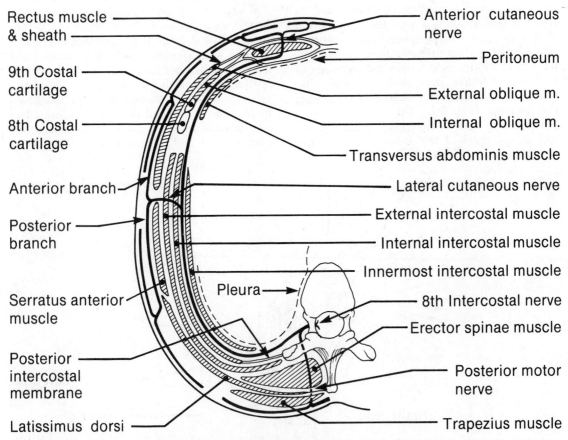

Rectus muscle & sheath

9th Costal cartilage

8th Costal cartilage

Anterior branch

Posterior branch

Serratus anterior muscle

Posterior intercostal membrane

Latissimus dorsi

Pleura→

Anterior cutaneous nerve

Peritoneum

External oblique m.

Internal oblique m.

Transversus abdominis muscle

Lateral cutaneous nerve

External intercostal muscle

Internal intercostal muscle

Innermost intercostal muscle

8th Intercostal nerve

Erector spinae muscle

Posterior motor nerve

Trapezius muscle

Figure 2–7. *Distribution of the eighth intercostal nerve to show its relationships in both its thoracic and abdominal courses to the muscle layers of the body wall. See text for full discussion of the anatomy of the intercostal space.*

the angle of the rib posteriorly and then is replaced by the posterior intercostal membrane. The muscle fibers run obliquely downward and backward. The innermost layer of muscle is called the innermost intercostal and is often incomplete with slips of muscle linked by membranous tissue. The endothoracic fascia, which is equivalent to the transversalis fascia of the abdominal wall, is no more than a fine layer of areolar connective tissue between the intercostal muscles and the parietal pleura.

In each intercostal space lies a neurovascular bundle comprising, from above downward, the intercostal vein, the intercostal artery, and the intercostal nerve, protected externally by the costal groove of the upper rib (Fig. 2–6). Posteriorly, this bundle lies between the pleura and the posterior intercostal membrane, but at the angle of the rib it passes between the internal and innermost intercostal muscles (Figs. 2–6 and 2–7). Each intercostal nerve first branches off into a posterior motor-cutaneous nerve, then into a lateral cutaneous nerve, which arises in the midaxillary line and itself gives off an anterior and posterior branch, and then finally into an anterior cutaneous nerve (Fig. 2–7).

Since the major intercostal vessels and nerves lie in close relation to the lower border of each rib, incisions near this level are to be avoided. A preferable site is along the upper margin of each rib. Although accessory nerves and vessels may be sectioned at this level, there is negligible loss of sensation. It is equally important, however, to understand that the overlap of adjacent nerves is so great that paralysis and complete anesthesia are seldom produced within one intercostal space incision unless its nerve and the nerves in the intercostal space above and below are all severed.

D. The Relation of the Thoracic Wall to the Pleura and Lungs

For surgical purposes, the lungs and pleura may be considered to be coextensive with their respective costal, mediastinal, and diaphragmatic surfaces separated only by a film of serous fluid. Thus, the pleural borders can be considered to be the lung borders and are formed by the continuity of the surfaces of costal, mediastinal, and diaphragmatic pleurae.

The anterior, inferior, and posterior borders of the pleurae may be related to the overlying structures of the thoracic cage (Figs. 2–8 and 2–9). The anterior pleural borders of the pulmonary cupulae are separated by visceral structures at the base of the neck. As they descend medially behind the sternum, they come to oppose one another at the sternal angle. The right anterior border continues downward, close to the midline. At the lower limits of the body of the sternum it diverges laterally along the sixth or seventh costal cartilage to become the inferior pleural border. The left anterior pleural border may follow a similar course, but more commonly it diverges laterally at the fourth costal cartilage, lies at the lateral sternal margin at the fifth, and still further laterally at the sixth cartilage, and then diverges laterally with increasing severity at the seventh costal cartilage. The lateral displacement of the left anteropleural border between the fourth and sixth costal cartilage forms the cardiac notch.

The inferior borders of both pleural sacs diverge laterally along the seventh costal cartilage and then cross ribs 8, 9, and 10. Their lowest level is reached about the middle of the eleventh rib in the midaxillary line. From this point they follow an almost horizontal course, cutting across the twelfth rib to meet the posterior border at the twelfth thoracic vertebra. The posterior pleural borders ascend alongside or in front of the bodies of the thoracic vertebrae until they diverge superiorly near the pulmonary cupula.

Knowledge of the surface relations of lobes and fissures of the lungs is important in percussion, auscultation, roentgen evaluation of the pulmonary field, and the decision where to make the thoracic incision (Figs. 2–8 and 2–9). The horizontal fissure of the right lung (which separates the right upper from the right middle lobe) lies under the fourth rib anteriorly and continues horizontally laterally so that it cuts underneath the downsloping fifth rib at the anterior axillary line. The oblique fissure of the right lung (which separates the right middle from the right lower lobe) lies under the sixth rib. The oblique fissure of the left lung (which separates the left upper lobe and lingula from the left lower lobe) also lies under the sixth rib.

III. THE AIRWAY AND LUNG[1, 2, 4, 5]

A. Trachea

In adults, the trachea extends from its attachment to the lower end of the cricoid cartilage, at the level of the sixth cervical vertebra, to its

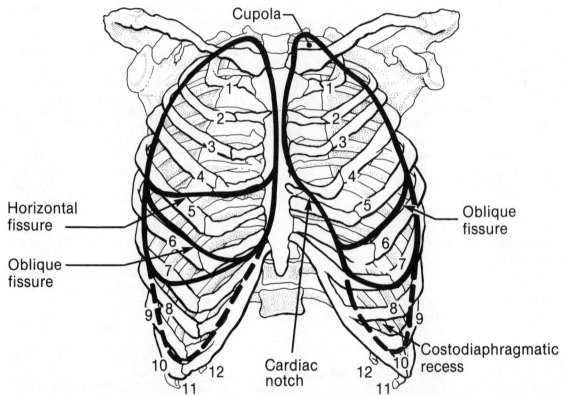

Figure 2–8. Anterior view of the thorax showing the relationship of the pleura and lungs to the thoracic wall. The oblique fissure runs nearly parallel to the sixth rib. The space between the inferior border of the lung at end exhalation and the inferior pleural surface (dashed line) is called the costodiaphragmatic recess. The top of the lung is called the cupola. The ribs are numbered according to their vertebral origin.

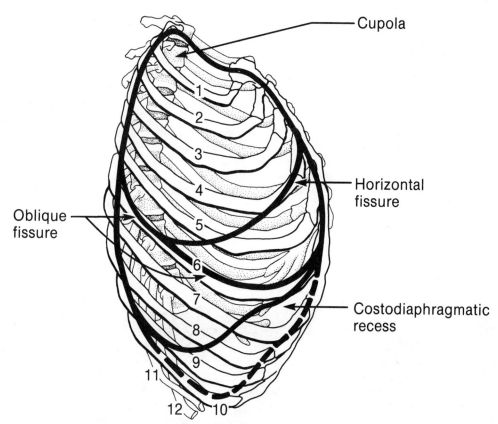

Figure 2–9. Lateral view of the thorax showing the relationship of the pleura and lungs to the thoracic wall. The oblique fissure runs nearly parallel to the sixth rib. The space between the inferior border of the lung at end exhalation and the inferior pleural surface (dashed line) is the costodiaphragmatic recess. The top of the lung is termed the cupola. The ribs are numbered according to their vertebral origin.

termination at the bronchial bifurcation at the level of the fifth thoracic vertebra. The adult trachea is approximately 6 inches long, of which 2 inches lie above the suprasternal notch; this portion is somewhat greater (nearly 3 inches) when the neck is fully extended. The diameter of the trachea correlates with the size of the subject, and a good working rule is that it has the same diameter as the patient's index finger. The patency of the trachea is due to a series of 16 to 20 C-shaped cartilages joined vertically by fibroelastic tissue and closed posteriorly by the unstriped trachealis muscle. The cartilage at the tracheal bifurcation is the keel-shaped carina, which is seen as a very obvious sagittal ridge when the trachea is inspected broncho-scopically. A finding of the sharp edge of the carina becoming flat usually denotes enlarge-ment of the hilar lymph nodes or gross distor-tion of the pulmonary anatomy by fibrosis, tumor, or some other pathology.

The trachea lies exactly in the midline in the cervical part of its course (but within the thorax it is deviated slightly to the right by the arch of the aorta). Tracheal relations to other organs in the neck are shown in Figure 2–10. Ante-riorly, the trachea is bounded by muscles, pre-tracheal fascia, and thyroid gland; laterally, by the pretracheal fascia and the carotid sheaths; and posteriorly, by the esophagus and vertebral bodies. The esophagus is in the midline be-tween the trachea and vertebral bodies. Tra-cheal and esophageal relations in the superior mediastinum are discussed in section IV and are shown in Figure 2–11.

B. Main Bronchi

The adult trachea bifurcates at the level of the fifth thoracic vertebra into right and left mainstem bronchi. The right main bronchus is shorter, wider, and more vertically placed than the left mainstem bronchus. The right main-stem bronchus is shorter than the left because it gives off its upper lobe bronchus after a course of only 2.0 cm, whereas the left mainstem bronchus gives off its upper lobe bronchus after a course of 5.0 cm. The right mainstem bron-chus is wider than the left because it supplies

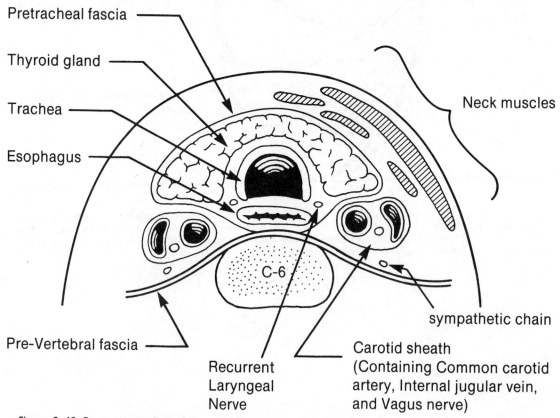

Figure 2–10. Transverse section of the neck through C-6 showing the fascial planes and the contents of the pretracheal fascia. The trachea begins at this level.

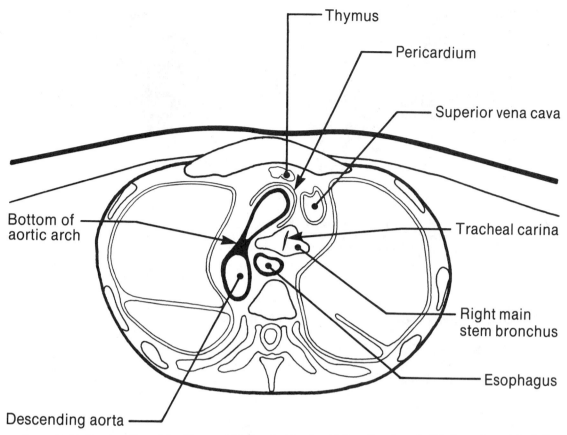

Figure 2–11. *Cross section of the thorax at the level of tracheal bifurcation (usually fifth thoracic vertebra). The pulmonary artery (not shown) lies just caudad to this level.*

a larger lung, and it is more vertically placed (at 25° to the vertical compared with 45° on the left) because the left bronchus has to extend laterally behind the aortic arch to reach its lung hilum. Obviously, inhaled foreign bodies or a bronchial aspirating catheter are far more likely to go to the wider and more vertically placed right bronchus than the narrower and more obliquely placed left mainstem bronchus.

C. Hilar Anatomy

From an anatomic surgical standpoint, knowledge of hilar anatomy is extremely important (Figs. 2–12 and 2–13). On the right side, the azygos vein marks the uppermost aspect of the hilar structures. From top to bottom on the right are the right mainstem bronchus, the main pulmonary artery, and then the right superior pulmonary vein. On the left side, the aortic arch marks the superior aspect of the hilum, and from top to bottom there is first the left

pulmonary artery, the left main bronchus, and then the left superior pulmonary vein. In both hilar regions, the most anterior structure is the superior pulmonary vein, behind which is the main pulmonary artery, and the most posterior structure is the mainstem bronchus.

D. Lung Lobes and Fissures (Figs. 2–8 and 2–9)

The right lung is composed of three lobes—the upper, middle, and lower—and is the larger of the two lungs. The left lung is composed of two lobes, the upper and lower. Two fissures are present on the right. The oblique fissure (major fissure) separates the lower lobe from the upper and middle lobes, and the horizontal fissure separates the upper from the middle lobe. On the left is the single major fissure dividing the upper and lower lobes.

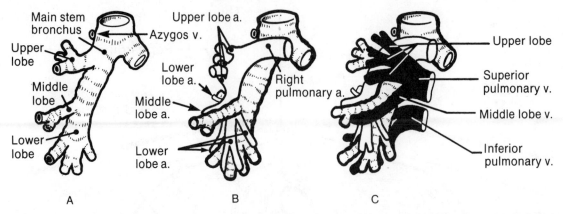

Figure 2–12. Anatomy of the right hilum. A, Bronchi. B, Bronchi and pulmonary arteries. C, Bronchi, pulmonary arteries, and veins. From top to bottom are azygos vein, bronchus, pulmonary artery, and superior pulmonary vein. From anterior to posterior are the superior pulmonary vein, pulmonary artery, and bronchus. a. = artery, v. = vein.

E. Bronchopulmonary Segments

Each lobe of the right and left lungs is subdivided into several individual anatomic units, the bronchopulmonary segments. The general pattern is that of 18 segments—10 in the right lung and 8 in the left lung. Each bronchopulmonary segment has its own bronchus, artery, and vein and consists of all of the lung that is distal to the third bifurcation. The bronchopulmonary segment names and numbers as seen from the conducting airway view are shown in Figure 2–14, and as seen from an external lung view, they are shown in Figures 2–15 and 2–16.

F. The Air Spaces

The tracheobronchial tree has 23 generations of branches. The successive subdivisions of the bronchial tree are bronchi, bronchioles, respiratory bronchioles, alveolar ducts, atria, alveolar sacs, and alveoli (Fig. 2–17). From the second to the eleventh generation the airways are called bronchi, and from the twelfth to approximately the seventeenth generation the airways are called bronchioles. The reason that there is a change in name of the airways at the eleventh generation is that there is an important anatomic change that occurs at this level; cartilage disappears from the walls of these 1-mm

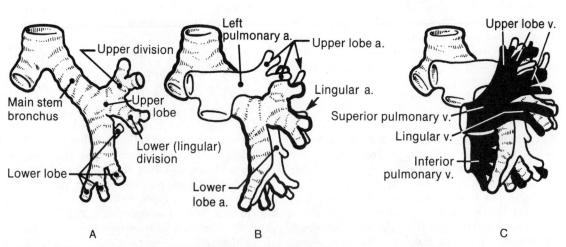

Figure 2–13. Anatomy of the left hilum. A, Bronchi. B, Bronchi and pulmonary arteries. C, Bronchi, pulmonary arteries, and veins. From top to bottom are aortic arch, pulmonary artery, bronchus, and superior pulmonary vein. From anterior to posterior are superior pulmonary vein, pulmonary artery, and bronchus (a. = artery; v. = vein).

Bronchopulmonary Segments

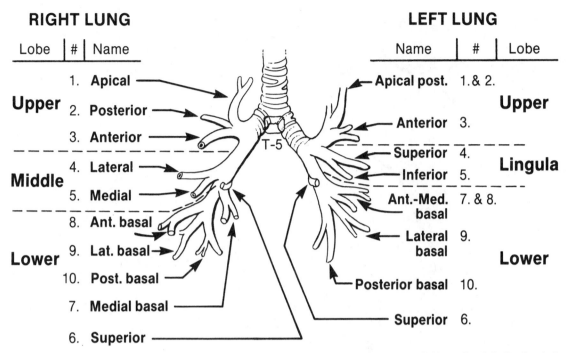

Lobe	#	Name
	1.	**Apical**
Upper	2.	**Posterior**
	3.	**Anterior**
Middle	4.	**Lateral**
	5.	**Medial**
	8.	**Ant. basal**
Lower	9.	**Lat. basal**
	10.	**Post. basal**
	7.	**Medial basal**
	6.	**Superior**

RIGHT LUNG

LEFT LUNG

Name	#	Lobe
Apical post.	1. & 2.	**Upper**
Anterior	3.	
Superior	4.	**Lingula**
Inferior	5.	
Ant.-Med. basal	7. & 8.	**Lower**
Lateral basal	9.	
Posterior basal	10.	
Superior	6.	

Figure 2–14. *The bronchopulmonary segments. There are ten on the right and eight on the left. On the left, segments 1 and 2 are combined into one apical posterior segment and segments 7 and 8 are combined into one anterior medial segment (ANT = anterior; LAT = lateral; MED = medial; POST = posterior).*

Right Lung Bronchopulmonary Segments

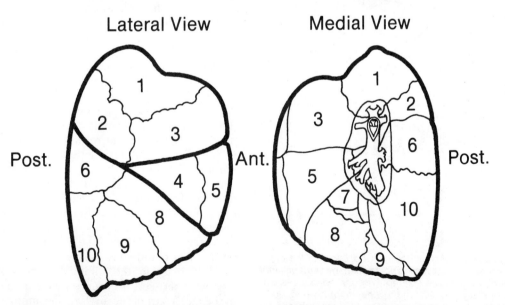

Figure 2–15. *The bronchopulmonary segments of the right lung as seen from a lateral and medial view. The key of the numbering is given in Figure 2–14 (ANT = anterior; POST = posterior).*

Left Lung Bronchopulmonary Segments

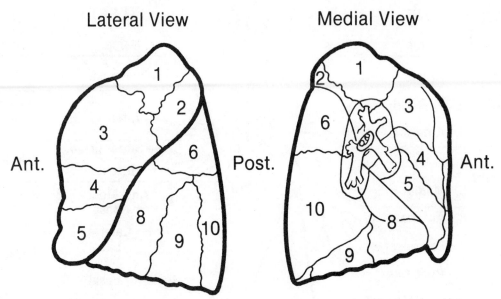

Figure 2–16. The bronchopulmonary segments of the left lung as seen from a lateral view and a medial view. The key of the numbering is given in Figure 2–14 (ANT = anterior; POST = posterior).

diameter air passages, and structural rigidity ceases to be the principal factor in maintaining patency. Fortunately, at this level the air passages leave their fibrous sheath and become embedded directly in the lung parenchyma.

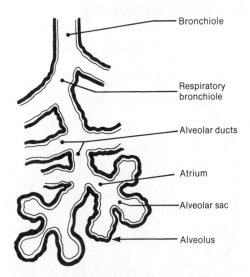

Figure 2–17. The successive subdivisions of the bronchial tree are bronchi (2nd to 11th generation—not shown), bronchioles (12th to 17th generation), respiratory bronchioles (17th to 18th generation), alveolar ducts (19th to 20th generation), atrium (21st generation), alveolar sacs (22nd generation), and alveoli (23rd generation).

Elastic recoil of the alveolar septa is then able to hold the air passages open like the guy ropes of a bell tent. Similarly, the patency of the alveolar duct is also maintained by the retraction of the surrounding alveolar septa. The caliber of airways and alveolar ducts beyond the eleventh generation is, therefore, mainly influenced by lung volume. The destruction of alveolar septa in individuals with emphysema renders the bronchioles and alveolar ducts more liable to closure. Each bronchiole with its subdivisions is termed a primary lung lobule.

The respiratory bronchioles occur at the seventeenth generation. All generations above the respiratory bronchioles are considered to be in the conductive zone, and all generations below the respiratory bronchioles are considered to be in the transition and respiratory zones.

At each dichotomous division the diameter of the airway decreases but at a rate that is less than the increase in the number of airways, so that the summed cross-sectional area at any given level increases and the airway resistance decreases down the airway tree. Reduction in diameter at each division below the bronchiole level is less than before, so that there is a very rapid increase in the summed cross-sectional area with respect to distance down the airway in the distal part of the airway. The approximate distribution of total lung volume for the adult human lung is shown in Table 2–1.[6]

Table 2–1. Approximate Distribution of Total Lung Volume in Milliliters (ml) for an Adult Human Lung at Three-Fourths Total Lung Capacity*

Zones	Air Channels	Compartments Tissue		Blood	
Conducting	Bronchi 170	Walls Septa Fibers	Arteries 150		Veins 250
Transition	Respiratory bronchioles Alveolar ducts 1500	Lymph 200	Arterioles 60		Venules 120
Respiratory	Alveoli 3150	Barrier 150		Capillaries 140	

*Total lung volume = 5700 ml.

The alveolar surfaces are lined with a layer of water and a surface tension–reducing material called surfactant (see chapter 3 for the physiology' of surfactant). The type II alveolar pneumocytes are responsible for the secretion of surfactant. The alveolar water/surfactant lining layer is continuous with the tracheobronchial tree surface lining layer.

In the distal bronchial tree, the Clara cells are throught to secrete a surface tension–reducing material that lines the bronchioles and is consistent in appearance with surfactant. Smokers have been demonstrated to have a decrease in the number of Clara cells and an increase in the number of mucous-producing goblet cells (normally located in the proximal bronchial tree).[7] The hypothesis has been advanced[7] that the disappearance of Clara cells and their replacement by goblet cells may result in the bronchioles becoming lined by a film of mucus. Replacement of the surfactant layer by a film of mucus would render the bronchioles unstable, and they would close unduly easily and open with greater difficulty, leading to functional obstruction.

There are several unusual bronchiolar and/or alveolar ventilation pathways, and these are collectively termed collateral ventilation. There are four known pathways of collateral ventilation. First, interalveolar communications (pores of Kohn) exist in most species and may range from 8 to 50 per alveolus and may increase with age and with the development of obstructive lung disease. Second, there are distal bronchiole to alveolar communications (channels of Lambert). Third, there are connections between respiratory bronchioles to terminal bronchioles from adjacent lung segments (channels of Martin) in healthy dogs and in humans with lung disease. Fourth, the functional characteristics of interlobar collateral ventilation through interlobar connections have recently been described in dogs,[8] and these interlobar connec-

tions have been observed in humans.[9] The role of these collateral ventilation pathways may be to prevent or to minimize atelectasis and alveolar hypoxia.

G. Pulmonary Arteries and Veins[10]

The pulmonary artery and mainstem bronchus of each lung are next to one another as they enter the parenchyma of the lung. As these structures enter the lung, they carry with them an invagination of the visceral pleura as a connective tissue sheath. The pulmonary artery branches in similar fashion to, and follows very closely, the bronchial tree. Distal to the bronchiolar level (eleventh generation), the penetration of pleural tissue stops and both the arteries and bronchi are attached directly to the lung substance.

The pulmonary artery finally gives rise to precapillary branches of variable length, which then break up into capillary nets that course over the rounded surface of the alveoli. As in the bronchial tree, arterial branches decrease in diameter at each dichotomy down to the precapillary branches, while the summed cross-sectional area increases. Although the two trees are similar, the arteries branch somewhat more profusely than the bronchi do, especially peripherally, where they give off branches to supply alveoli on respiratory bronchioles as well as immediately adjacent alveoli of neighboring alveolar sacs.

The pulmonary veins arise from capillaries at alveolar duct junctions, as well as on respiratory bronchioles, on the pleura and in connective tissue septae. Those veins that start within the acinus course centrifugally to the periphery of the lobule. There they join veins running between the lobules at right angles. The interlobular veins are therefore situated away from the conducting airways and arteries. Unlike arteries, veins do not have a perivascular space, so that veins within the lung are connected directly to the lung substance and are held open by elastic forces. The veins only came together with the arteries and airways as these three structures approach the hilum. Casts of arteries and veins show that the venous system has a larger volume than the arterial system (ratio 2:1) and at any given level has a larger cross-sectional area. The larger cross-sectional area of the veins results in a very low resistance system, which can still function with the low driving pressure available.

H. The Pulmonary Capillaries

1. Alveolar Sheet Arrangement

The pulmonary capillaries usually arise at right angles from the pulmonary arterioles. The pulmonary capillaries have been classically described as long branching tunnels lying adjacent to the alveoli (Fig. 2–18A).[11] However, in reality, the capillaries spread out over the alveolar surface in a complex, interconnecting pattern, which is confined to or contained within the

two dimensions of the alveolar surface plane (Fig. 2–18B).[11] Because of these anatomic characteristics, the geometry of the pulmonary capillaries has been likened to the appearance of an underground parking garage as viewed from within the garage (Fig. 2–19).[11] The top and bottom of the garage are flat endothelial surfaces, which are held together and supported by columns, or "posts," of connective tissue (Figs. 2–18B and 2–19). An alveolus is on the other side of each of the endothelial surfaces. The connective tissue columns between the endothelial plates have been called posts because of their structural support function as well as "struts" because they require one alveolus on one side of the capillary to expand if the alveolus on the other side of the capillary collapses. The connective tissue posts occupy the circular clear spaces between the interlacing capillary network seen in Figure 2–18B.

The endothelial surfaces form the boundaries of the mainly two-dimensional capillary, and blood flow through this two-dimensional world has been called sheet flow.[12] In this model, red blood cells must wind their way around and amongst the posts, much as a car would negotiate the garage in bumper-to-bumper traffic

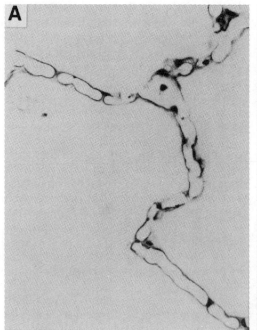
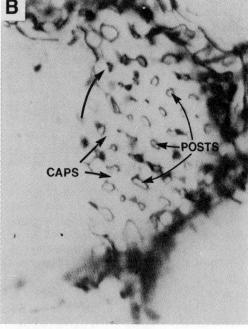

Figure 2–18. A, A classical histologic view of a pulmonary capillary surrounded on each side by an alveolus; the capillary appears as a long, branching tunnel. B, A histologic view of a pulmonary capillary bed cut tangential to the rounded surface of an alveolus; the pulmonary capillaries (CAPS) spread out in a complex, interconnecting pattern. Individual capillaries divide and meet around connective tissue posts, which join the two possible endothelial plates together. See text for futher explanation. (Reproduced with permission from Fung YC: The microcirculation as seen by a red cell. Microvasc Res 10:246–264, 1975.)

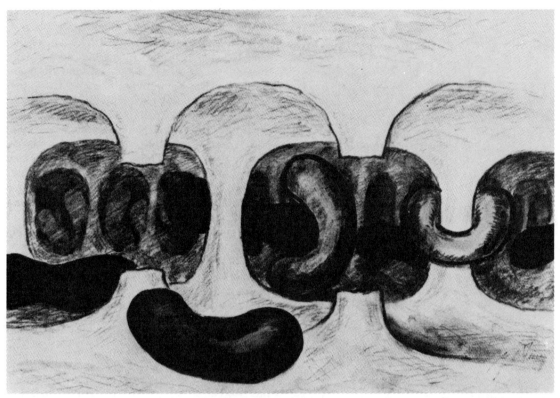

Figure 2–19. *Imaginary view of the inside of a pulmonary capillary as it might appear to a red blood cell. The view is similar to that seen when one stands inside a modern underground parking garage. Endothelial plates form the top and bottom of the garage, and the plates are held together and supported by connective tissue columns or "posts." On the other side of each of the endothelial surfaces would be an alveolus, which is not shown. (Reproduced with permission from Fung YC: The microcirculation as seen by a red cell. Microvasc Res 10:246–264, 1975.)*

(Fig. 2–19). The sheet flow theory of the pulmonary microcirculation is consistent with experimental data and, in brief, disassociates resistance from flow, as these two terms are normally related by Poiseuille's formula for fluid dynamics in a cylinder.[12] The precise flow pattern from post to post has been modeled as a function of the perfusion pressure.[13]

The sheet flow theory suggests that the capillaries may occupy up to half the surface of an alveolar wall and thereby expose an enormous capillary surface area to the alveolar gas for gas exchange. Previous estimates in humans have suggested that alveolar blood vessels (primarily capillaries) have a luminal surface area on the order of 80 m². [14] However, these early calculations of surface area assumed a more or less regular rounded shape of capillaries having smooth luminal surfaces. It is now evident that the capillary surfaces are not smooth but are covered with irregular complex projections.[15] The projections are approximately 300 nm in diameter and may reach 3000 nm in length.

Some projections came to blunt ends, while others bud, branch, or reflect back on the main body of the cell. The size and density of the endothelial projection meshwork is such that an eddy flow of cell-free plasma occurs along the endothelial lining cell.[16] This feature has extremely important implications for the exchange of metabolites between endothelium and blood (see the section Pulmonary Metabolism and Synthesis in chapter 3).[16] The endothelial cells also contain a large population in plasmalemmal (pinocytotic) vesicles (Fig. 2–20), many of which communicate freely with the vascular lumen (see the figures in Pietra[17] and Szidon[18]). These endothelial vesicles and cavities function both as mass carriers of fluid and solutes across the endothelium and as generators of transendothelial channels by fusion and fission with each other and with both endothelial domains (vascular and tissular). Therefore, owing to the presence of endothelial vesicles and the endothelial projections into the lumen of the capillary, it would appear that the true surface area

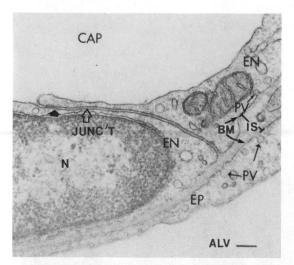

Figure 2–20. Electron photomicrograph of an alveolar capillary membrane. (EN = endothelium; EP = epithelium; CAP = capillary; ALV = alveolus; PV = plasmalemma vesicles [pointed to by thin dark arrows]; IS = interstitial space [indicated by bars]; BM = basement membrane [indicated by middle-sized dark arrows]; Junc't = loose endothelial junction [indicated by large open and dark arrows]). (Modified with permission from Pietra GG: The basis of pulmonary edema with emphasis on ultrastructure. In Thurlbeck WM [ed.]: The Lung: Structure, Function and Disease. Baltimore, The Williams & Wilkins Co., 1978, pp. 215–234). See text for explanation and function of the plasmalemma vesicles. See Figure 2–21 for a schematic of the arrangement of endothelial cells, loose junctions, basement membranes, interstitial space, and epithelial cells shown in this figure.

of capillary endothelial cells (at least for metabolism) is much larger than previously estimated.

2. Ultrastructure of Pulmonary Capillary–Interstitial Space–Alveolar Area

A cross-section through any capillary channel shown in Figure 2–24 would reveal a vascular channel lined by endothelium that usually contains one, or at most, two or three red blood cells.[17] A schematic of the ultrastructural appearance of an alveolar septum is shown in Figure 2–21.[19] Capillary blood is separated from alveolar gas by a series of anatomic layers: capillary endothelium, endothelial basement membrane, interstitial space, epithelial basement membrane, and alveolar epithelium (of the type I pneumocyte).

On one side of the alveolar septum (the thick, upper [see Fig. 2–21], fluid- and gas-exchange side), the epithelial and endothelial basement membranes are separated by a space of variable

thickness containing connective tissue fibrils, elastic fibers, fibroblasts, and macrophages. This connective tissue is the "backbone" of the lung parenchyma and forms a continuum with the connective tissue sheaths around the conducting airways and blood vessels. Thus, the pericapillary perialveolar interstitial space is continuous with the interstitial tissue space that surrounds terminal bronchioles and vessels, and both spaces constitute the connective tissue space of the lung. There are no lymphatics in the interstitial space of the alveolar septum. Instead, lymphatic capillaries first appear in the interstitial space surrounding terminal bronchioles, small arteries, and veins.

The opposite side of the alveolar septum (the thin, down [see Fig. 2–21], gas-exchanging only side) contains only fused epithelial and endothelial basement membranes. The interstitial space is thus greatly restricted on this side owing to fusion of the basement membranes. Interstitial fluid cannot separate the endothelial and epithelial cells from one another, and as a result the space and distance barrier to fluid movement from the capillary to alveolar compartment is reduced and is composed only of the two cell linings with their associated basement membranes.[20, 21]

Between the individual endothelial and epithelial cells are holes or junctions that provide a potential pathway for fluid to move from the intravascular space to the interstitial space and finally from the interstitial space to the alveolar space. The junctions between endothelial cells are relatively large and are therefore termed "loose"; the junctions between epithelial cells are relatively small and are therefore termed "tight." Pulmonary capillary permeability (K) is a direct function of and essentially equivalent to the size of the holes in the endothelial and epithelial linings (see chapter 3).

I. Lymphatic System[22]

A superficial lymphatic plexus drains the visceral pleura, and a deep plexus, lying alongside the pulmonary vessels, drains the bronchi but does not reach beyond the alveolar ducts into the more distal spaces. Consequently, these microscopic vessels have been called "juxtaalveolar lymphatic capillaries." Both of these lymphatic plexuses drain into progressively more proximal lymph node stations (Fig. 2–22). The stations, in sequence, consist of pulmonary lymph nodes, the bronchopulmonary lymph

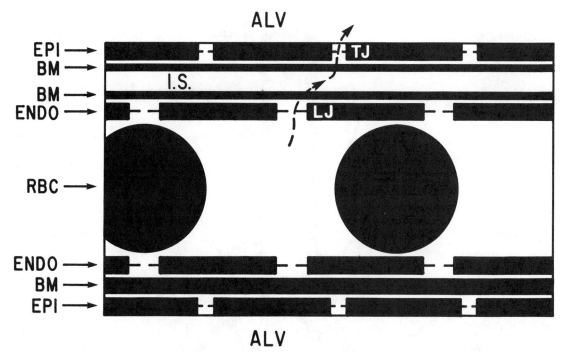

ALV

ALV

Figure 2–21. Schematic summary of the ultrastructure appearance of the pulmonary capillary. (RBC = red blood cell; ENDO = endothelium; BM = basement membrane; IS = interstitial space; EPI = epithelium; LJ = loose junction; TJ = tight junction; ALV = alveolus). The upper side of the capillary has the endothelial and epithelial basement membranes separated by an interstitial space, whereas the lower side of the capillary contains only fused endothelial and epithelial basement membranes. The dashed arrows indicate a potential pathway for fluid to move from the intravascular space to the interstitial space (through loose junctions in the endothelium) and from the interstitial space to the alveolar space (through tight junctions in the epithelium). (Modified with permission from Fishman AP: Pulmonary edema: The water-exchanging function of the lung. Circulation 46:390–408, 1972, and by permission of the American Heart Association, Inc.)

nodes placed at the points of bifurcation of the larger bronchi, tracheobronchial lymph nodes, right and left paratracheal (mediastinal) lymph nodes, and scalene and deep cervical lymph nodes. In an attempt to better define prognosis with lung cancer, the lymph node stations have been numbered 1 through 13, with 1 being the highest mediastinal and 13 being the most peripheral or segmental node station.[23] The stations of the lymph chain on either side drain into right and left lymphatic vessels. Most often the right and left lymphatic vessels open directly and independently into the junction between the internal jugular and subclavian veins on either side. However, the right vessel may drain into the main right lymphatic duct, and the left vessel may empty into the thoracic duct.

Malignant disease in the right lung spreads mainly up the lymph node chain on the same side.[22] The superior tracheobronchial nodes, being the regional lymph node station, are readily involved. From there the lymphatic pathway leads up to the paratracheal and finally to the right scalene or inferior deep cervical nodes. In contrast, when malignant disease involves the left lung, contralateral lymphatic spread occurs frequently in addition to proximal ipsilateral spread.[22] In addition, malignant lesions of the left lower lobe can also spread subdiaphragmatically through para-aortic nodes to the abdomen. The malignant dissemination of left lower lobe tumors by both contralateral and subdiaphragmatic spread are a reason, at least in part, why left lower lobe bronchial carcinoma has the worst prognosis of all the lobar carcinomas.[22]

J. Bronchial Arteries and Veins[24]

The bronchial arterial system arises from the systemic circulation and accounts for approximately 1 per cent of the cardiac output. The origins of the bronchial arteries are variable and include the aorta, intercostal arteries, and, oc-

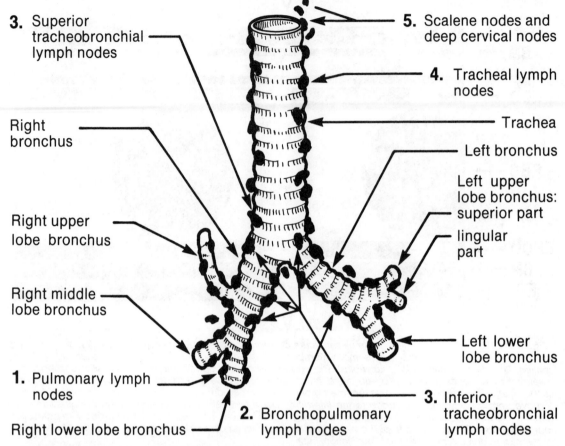

3. Superior tracheobronchial lymph nodes

5. Scalene nodes and deep cervical nodes

4. Tracheal lymph nodes

Right bronchus

Trachea

Left bronchus

Left upper lobe bronchus: superior part

lingular part

Right upper lobe bronchus

Right middle lobe bronchus

Left lower lobe bronchus

1. Pulmonary lymph nodes

2. Bronchopulmonary lymph nodes

3. Inferior tracheobronchial lymph nodes

Right lower lobe bronchus

Figure 2–22. The trachea and bronchi and associated lymph nodes. Lymph flows from 1 (pulmonary lymph nodes) to 2 (bronchopulmonary lymph nodes) to 3 (inferior and superior tracheobronchial lymph nodes) to 4 (tracheal lymph nodes) to 5 (scalene nodes and deep cervical nodes).

casionally, the subclavian or innominate arteries. On the right, the major source is from the first or, at times, the second right aortic intercostal artery. Distally on the right as well as on the left the other bronchial arteries take their origin directly from the aorta, the level of origin varying between the third and the eighth thoracic vertebra. The bronchial arteries to either side enter the hilus of the lung and form a communicating arc around the main bronchus. From here, the main arterial divisions radiate along the longitudinal axis of the major bronchi in close apposition to the bronchial wall. The vessels follow the course of the bronchus and divide, as do the bronchi. Discrete bronchial arterial branches can be identified as far as third to fifth order bronchi. Networks of intercommunicating vessels are often present on the bronchial walls. Throughout their course the bronchial arteries give off the vasa vasorum of the pulmonary arteries.

The bronchial veins form two distinct systems. The superficial bronchial veins, which constitute a relatively small system, drain the main and lobar bronchi and empty into the azygos vein on the right side and into the hemiazygos and mediastinal veins on the left side. The deep venous effluent of segmental and distal bronchi, which constitutes a relatively large system, empties into the pulmonary veins. It has been estimated that two thirds of the bronchial blood supply empties into the pulmonary veins (the deep system), and one third empties into the bronchial vein–azygos system (the superficial system). Since the deep bronchial circulation by-passes the lungs and empties into the left heart without being oxygenated, it is a normally present source of right-to-left shunting (approximately 0.7 per cent of the cardiac output).

The bronchial circulation undergoes brisk local development with new vessel formation in certain pulmonary and bronchial disease conditions. These conditions include prolonged infections, cavitation, neoplastic vessel growth, and atelectasis of the lung. The proliferation of the bronchial circulation under the previously mentioned pathologic conditions is often responsible for repeated, sometimes serious, episodes of hemoptysis. In addition, right-to-left shunting will be increased anytime there is increased bronchial blood flow.

Several connections between the pulmonary and bronchial systems have been demonstrated in men and in guinea pigs. Pulmonary artery–to–bronchial artery, capillary-to-capillary, and vein-to-vein as well as bronchial artery–to–pulmonary vein connections exist. Thus, almost any part of the lung may potentially be supplied by blood from either artery and be drained by either set of veins. The bronchial artery–to–pulmonary vein connections are very important, particularly in such lesions as pulmonary stenosis and pulmonary embolism. Under these two circumstances, bronchial collateral supply of tissues distal to blocked arteries helps to maintain a normal ventilation-perfusion ratio.

IV. THE MEDIASTINUM[1, 2, 4]

A. Divisions of the Mediastinum

The mediastinum is a wide organ-filled septum between the two pleural sacs. It is divided, somewhat arbitrarily for the purposes of description, into an upper and lower part by a plane that extends from the sternal angle (the angle of Louis) across the upper level of the pericardium to the lower border of the fourth thoracic vertebra (Fig. 2–23). The upper part is named the superior mediastinum, and the lower part is subdivided into three parts—the anterior mediastinum in front of the pericardium, the middle mediastinum containing the heart and pericardium, and the posterior mediastinum behind the pericardium (Fig. 2–23).

The superior mediastinum is bounded above by the thoracic inlet, below by the plane of the superior limit of the pericardium, anteriorly by the manubrium, posteriorly by the upper four thoracic vertebrae, and laterally by the mediastinal pleura of the two lungs. It contains the aortic arch, the innominate artery, the thoracic portions of the left common carotid and left

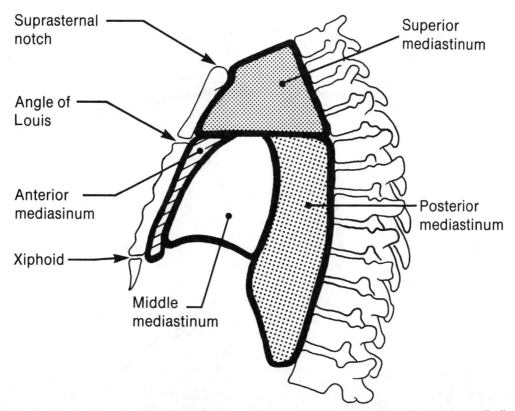

Figure 2–23. The mediastinum is divided up into a superior and inferior mediastinum. The inferior mediastinum is divided up into anterior, middle, and posterior mediastinum. See text for further explanation.

subclavian arteries, the innominate veins, the upper halves of the superior vena cava and trachea and esophagus, the thoracic duct, the remains of the thymus, the recurrent laryngeal and phrenic nerves, and some lymph nodes. The anterior mediastinum is bounded anteriorly by the body of the sternum and posteriorly by the parietal pericardium, and it extends downward as far as the diaphragm. The anterior mediastinum does not contain any vital structures. The middle mediastinum is the broadest part of the interpleural mediastinal septum and contains the heart, which is enclosed in the pericardium, the ascending aorta, the lower half of the superior vena cava with the azygos vein opening into it, the pulmonary artery dividing into its two branches, the right and left pulmonary veins, and the phrenic nerves. The posterior mediastinum is an irregularly shaped mass running parallel with the vertebral column, and because of the slope of the diaphragm, it extends caudally beyond the pericardium. It is bounded anteriorly by the

pericardium and more caudally by the diaphragm, posteriorly by the vertebral column from the lower border of the fourth to the twelfth thoracic vertebrae, and on either side by the mediastinal pleura. It contains the thoracic part of the distending aorta, the azygos and hemiazygos veins, the bifurcation of the trachea and the two bronchi, the esophagus, the thoracic duct, and many large lymph nodes.

B. Mediastinal Relations of the Trachea, Esophagus, Aorta, and Pulmonary Trunk (for Cervical Tracheal and Esophageal Relations See Section III)

From the thoracic inlet to the tracheal bifurcation, the thoracic esophagus remains in intimate relationship with the posterior wall of the trachea and the prevertebral fascia (Figs. 2–10, 2–11, and 2–24). Just above the tracheal bifurcation the esophagus is to the right of the aorta. This anatomic positioning can cause a notch

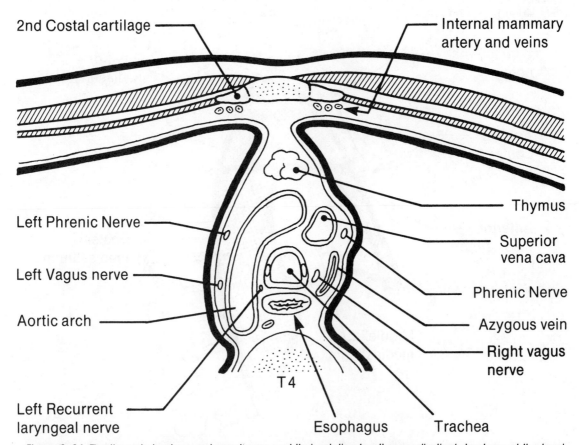

Figure 2–24. *The thoracic trachea and esophagus and their relation to other mediastinal structures at the level of the fourth thoracic vertebra. See Figure 2–11 for a cross section at a slightly lower level and Figure 2–10 for a cross section at a somewhat higher level.*

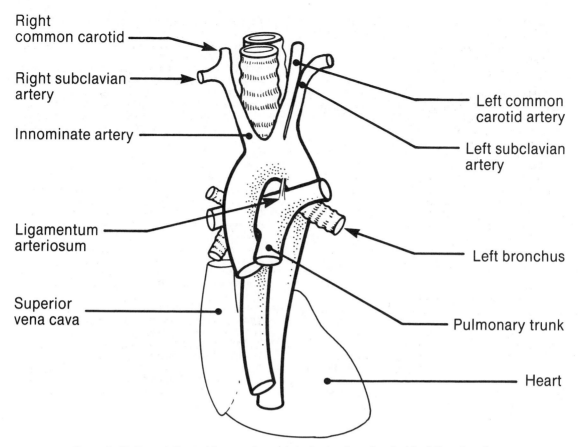

Right common carotid

Right subclavian artery

Innominate artery

Ligamentum arteriosum

Superior vena cava

Left common carotid artery

Left subclavian artery

Left bronchus

Pulmonary trunk

Heart

Figure 2–25. The relations of the great vessels to the trachea. See text for full explanation.

indentation in the esophageal left lateral wall on the barium swallow radiograph. Immediately below this notch the esophagus crosses both the bifurcation of the trachea and the left mainstem bronchus. From there down it passes over the posterior surface of the subcarinal lymph nodes, and then descends over the pericardium of the left atrium. From below the aortic arch, the esophagus lies to the right of and then in front of the descending thoracic aorta, the transition occurring at the level of the eighth thoracic vertebra. Posteriorly, the thoracic esophagus follows the curvature of the spine and remains in close contact with the vertebral bodies. From the eighth thoracic vertebra downward the esophagus moves anteriorly away from the spine and passes through the esophageal hiatus of the diaphragm in front of the aorta.

Figure 2–25 shows the relationship of the aorta, the pulmonary arteries, the tracheal bifurcation, and the esophagus to each other. The pulmonary trunk, which arises from the right ventricle, lies at first slightly in front of the ascending aorta and then to its left side before dividing into the left and right pulmonary arteries. The left pulmonary artery is connected to the concavity of the arch of the aorta by the ligamentum arteriosum, which represents the obliterated ductus arteriosus of the fetus. The ascending aorta becomes the arch of the aorta at the level of the manubrial-sternal joint, so that the arch lies entirely within the superior mediastinum. The arch passes backward and to the left and gives off in turn the innominate artery (which divides behind the sternal-clavicular joint into the right subclavian and right common carotid arteries) and the left common carotid and left subclavian arteries. The innominate and left common carotid arteries are located at first in front of the trachea and then past to its right and left sides, respectively.

REFERENCES

1. Ellis H, McLarty M: Anatomy for Anaesthetists. 2nd ed. Philadelphia, F. A. Davis Co, 1968.
2. Gray H, Goss CM: Gray's Anatomy. 27th ed. Philadelphia, Lea and Febiger, 1959.

3. Blevins CE: Anatomy of the thorax and pleura. In Shields TW (ed): General Thoracic Surgery. Philadelphia, Lea and Febiger, 1983, pp 43–60.
4. Moffat DB: Anatomical aspects of thoracic anesthesia. In Mushin WW (ed): Thoracic Anesthesia. Oxford, Blackwell Scientific Publications, 1963, pp 143–175.
5. Shields TW: Surgical anatomy of the lungs. In Shields TW (ed): General Thoracic Surgery. 2nd ed. Philadelphia, Lea and Febiger, 1983, pp 61–71.
6. Weibel ER: Anatomical distribution of air channels, blood vessels, and tissue in the lung. In Arcangeli P (ed): Normal Values for Respiratory Function in Man. Milano, Italy, Panminerva Medica, 1970, p 242.
7. Ebert RV, Terracio MJ: The bronchiolar epithelium in cigarette smokers. Observations with the scanning electron microscope. Am Rev Resp Dis 111:4, 1975.
8. Scanlon TS, Benumof JL: Demonstration of interlobar collateral ventilation. J Appl Physiol 46:658, 1979.
9. Kent EM, Blades B: The surgical anatomy of the pulmonary lobes. J Thorac Surg 12:18, 1971.
10. Horsfield K: Functional morphology of the pulmonary circulation. In Cumming G, Bonsignore G (eds): Pulmonary Circulation in Health and Disease. New York, Plenum Press, 1980, pp 1–18.
11. Fung YC: The microcirculation as seen by a red cell. Microvasc Res 10:246–264, 1975.
12. Fung YC, Sobin SS: Theory of sheet flow in lung alveoli. J Appl Physiol 26:472–488, 1969.
13. West JB, Schneider AM, Mitchell M: Recruitment in networks of pulmonary capillaries. J Appl Physiol 39:976–984, 1975.
14. Fishman AP: Dynamics of the pulmonary circulation. In Hamilton WF (ed): Handbook of Physiology, Section 2: Circulation. Baltimore, Williams & Wilkins Co, 1963, pp 1667–1743.
15. Heath D, Smith P: The pulmonary endothelial cell. Thorax 34:200–208, 1979.
16. Smith U, Ryan JW: Electron microscopy of endothelial components of the lungs: Correlations of structure and function. Fed Proc 32:1957–1966, 1973.
17. Pietra GG: The basis of pulmonary edema with emphasis on ultrastructure. In The Lung: IAP Monograph No. 19. Baltimore, Williams & Wilkins Co, 1978, chapter 12, pp 215–234.
18. Szidon JP, Pietra GG, Fishman AP: The alveolar-capillary membrane and pulmonary edema. N Engl J Med 286:1200–1204, 1972.
19. Fishman AP: Pulmonary edema: The water exchanging function of the lung. Circulation 46:390–408, 1972.
20. Low FN: Lung interstitium, development, morphology, fluid content. In Staub NC (ed): Lung Water and Solute Exchange. New York, Dekker, 1978, pp 17–48.
21. Weibel ER: Morphological basis of alveolar-capillary gas exchange. Physiol Rev 53:419, 1973.
22. Nohl-Oser HC: An investigation of the anatomy of the lymphatic drainage of the lungs. Ann R Coll Surg Engl 51:157, 1972.
23. Tisi GM, Friedman PJ, Peters RN, et al: Official American Thoracic Society statement adopted by the American Thoracic Society board of directors, November 1981. Clinical staging of primary lung cancer. Am Rev Resp Dis 127:659–664, 1983.
24. Blasi A: Bronchial circulation: Anatomical viewpoint. In Cumming G, Bonsignore G (ed): Pulmonary Circulation in Health and Disease. New York, Plenum Press, 1980, pp 19–26.

General Respiratory Physiology and Respiratory Function During Anesthesia

3

I. RESPIRATORY PHYSIOLOGY
A. Introduction
B. Normal (Gravity-Determined) Distribution of Perfusion, Ventilation, and the Ventilation-Perfusion Ratio
   1. Distribution of Pulmonary Perfusion
   2. Distribution of Ventilation
   3. Distribution of the Ventilation-Perfusion Ratio
C. Other (Nongravitational) Important Determinants of Pulmonary Vascular Resistance and Blood Flow Distribution
   1. Cardiac Output
   2. Alveolar Hypoxia
   3. Lung Volume
   4. Alternate (Nonalveolar) Pathways of Blood Flow Through the Lung
D. Other (Nongravitational) Important Determinants of Pulmonary Compliance, Resistance, and Lung Volume
   1. Pulmonary Compliance
   2. Airway Resistance
   3. Different Regional Lung Time Constants
   4. Work of Breathing
   5. Lung Volumes, the Functional Residual Capacity, and the Closing Capacity
      a. LUNG VOLUMES AND THE FUNCTIONAL RESIDUAL CAPACITY
      b. AIRWAY CLOSURE AND CLOSING CAPACITY
      c. THE RELATIONSHIP BETWEEN THE FUNCTIONAL RESIDUAL CAPACITY AND THE CLOSING CAPACITY
E. Oxygen and Carbon Dioxide Transport
   1. Alveolar and Dead Space Ventilation and Alveolar Gas Tensions
   2. Oxygen Transport
      a. THE OXYGENHEMOGLOBIN DISSOCIATION CURVE
      b. THE EFFECT OF $\dot{Q}_s/\dot{Q}_t$ ON THE P_aO_2
      c. THE EFFECT OF $\dot{Q}_t$ AND $\dot{V}O_2$ ON C_aO_2
      d. THE FICK PRINCIPLE
   3. Carbon Dioxide Transport
   4. The Bohr and Haldane Effects
F. Pulmonary Vascular Reflexes
G. Pulmonary Metabolism and Synthesis
H. Other Special Lung Functions
   1. Reservoir for the Left Ventricle
   2. Protective Function
   3. Nutrition

II. RESPIRATORY FUNCTION DURING ANESTHESIA
A. Introduction
B. Effect of Anesthetic Depth of Respiratory Pattern
C. Effect of Anesthetic Depth of Spontaneous Minute Ventilation

D. Effect of Pre-existing Respiratory Dysfunction on the Respiratory Effects of Anesthesia
E. Effect of Special Intraoperative Conditions on the Respiratory Effects of Anesthesia
F. Mechanisms of Hypoxemia During Anesthesia
   1. Malfunction of Equipment
      a. MECHANICAL FAILURE OF ANESTHESIA APPARATUS TO DELIVER OXYGEN TO THE PATIENT
      b. MECHANICAL FAILURE OF ENDOTRACHEAL TUBE: MAINSTEM BRONCHUS INTUBATION
   2. Hypoventilation
   3. Hyperventilation
   4. Decrease in FRC
      a. SUPINE POSITION
      b. INDUCTION OF GENERAL ANESTHESIA—CHANGE IN THORACIC CAGE MUSCLE TONE
      c. PARALYSIS
      d. LIGHT OR INADEQUATE ANESTHESIA AND ACTIVE EXPIRATION
      e. INCREASED AIRWAY RESISTANCE
      f. THE SUPINE POSITION, IMMOBILITY AND EXCESSIVE INTRAVENOUS FLUID ADMINISTRATION
      g. HIGH INSPIRED OXYGEN CONCENTRATION AND ABSORPTION ATELECTASIS
      h. SURGICAL POSITION
      i. VENTILATION HISTORY
      j. DECREASED REMOVAL OF SECRETIONS (DECREASED MUCOCILIARY FLOW)
   5. Decreased Cardiac Output and Increased Oxygen Consumption
   6. Inhibition of Hypoxic Pulmonary Vasoconstriction (HPV)
   7. Paralysis
   8. The Involvement of Mechanisms of Hypoxemia in specific diseases
G. Mechanisms of Hypercapnia and Hypocapnia During Anesthesia
   1. Hypercapnia
      a. HYPOVENTILATION
      b. INCREASED DEAD SPACE VENTILATION
      c. INCREASED CARBON DIOXIDE PRODUCTION
      d. INADVERTENT SWITCHING OFF OF A CARBON DIOXIDE ABSORBER
   2. Hypocapnia
H. Physiologic Effects of Abnormalities in the Respiratory Gases
   1. Hypoxia
   2. Hyperoxia (Oxygen Toxicity)
   3. Hypercapnia
   4. Hypocapnia

I. RESPIRATORY PHYSIOLOGY

A. Introduction

Understanding normal respiratory physiology is prerequisite to understanding mechanisms of impaired gas exchange during any type of anesthesia and surgery. Toward this end, the normal (gravity-determined) distribution of perfusion and ventilation, the major nongravitational determinants of resistance to perfusion and ventilation, the transport of the respiratory gases, and the pulmonary reflexes and special functions will be presented first in this chapter. These processes and concepts will then be utilized in the discussion of the general mechanisms of impaired gas exchange during anesthesia and surgery.

B. Normal (Gravity-Determined) Distribution of Perfusion, Venfilation, and the Ventilation-Perfusion Ratio

1. Distribution of Pulmonary Perfusion

Contraction of the right ventricle imparts kinetic energy to the blood in the main pulmonary artery. Most of the kinetic energy in the main pulmonary artery is dissipated in climbing a vertical hydrostatic gradient, and the absolute pressure in the pulmonary artery (P_{pa}) decreases 1 cm H_2O per centimeter of vertical distance up the lung (Fig. 3–1). At some great enough height above the heart, P_{pa} becomes zero (atmospheric), and still higher in the lung the P_{pa} becomes negative.[1] In this region alveolar pressure (P_A) then exceeds P_{pa} and pulmonary venous pressure (P_{pv}) (which is very negative at this vertical height). Since the pressure outside the vessels is greater than the pressure inside the vessels, the vessels in this region of the lung are collapsed and there is no blood flow (zone 1, $P_A > P_{pa} > P_{pv}$). Since there is no blood flow, no gas exchange is possible, and the region functions as alveolar dead space or "wasted" ventilation. Little or no zone 1 exists in the lung under normal conditions, but the amount of zone 1 lung may be greatly increased if P_{pa} is reduced, as in oligemic shock, or if P_A is increased, as in positive-pressure ventilation.

Further down the lung absolute P_{pa} becomes positive and blood flow will begin when P_{pa} exceeds P_A (zone 2, $P_{pa} > P_A > P_{pv}$). At this vertical level in the lung, P_A exceeds P_{pv}, and blood flow is determined by the mean P_{pa}-P_A difference rather than the more conventional

$P_{pa} - P_{pv}$ difference (see the following).[2] The zone 2 blood flow–alveolar pressure relationship has the same physical characteristics as a river waterfall flowing over a dam (Fig. 3–2). The height of the upstream river (before reaching the dam) is equivalent to P_{pa}, and the height of the dam is equivalent to P_A. The rate of water flow over the dam is only proportional to the difference between the height of the upstream river and the dam (P_{pa}-P_A), and it does not matter how far below the dam the downstream river bed (P_{pv}) is. This phenomenon has various names, including the "waterfall," "Starling resistor," "Weir" (dam made by beavers), and "sluice" effect. Since mean P_{pa} increases down this region of the lung but mean P_A is relatively constant, the mean driving pressure (P_{pa}-P_A) increases linearly, and therefore mean blood flow increases linearly.

However, it should be noted that respiration and pulmonary blood flow are cyclic phenomena. Therefore, absolute instantaneous P_{pa}, P_{pv}, and P_A are changing all the time, and the relationships between P_{pa}, P_{pv}, and P_A are dynamically determined by the phase lags between the cardiac and respiratory cycles. In other words, the upstream and downstream blood flows actually approach and leave, respectively, the respiratory dam as a wave, with the crest being equal to systolic pressure and the trough being equal to diastolic pressure; the respiratory dam is actually going up and down in a manner depending on whether positive or negative pressure ventilation is being used (Fig. 3–2B). Consequently, a given point in zone 2 may actually be in either a zone 1 or 3 condition at a given moment depending on whether the patient is in respiratory systole or diastole or cardiac systole or diastole.

A simple numerical example will further illustrate this point (the example assumes the alveolar pressure is constant). In a man of ordinary height, the distance between the top (apex) and the bottom (base) of the lung is about 30 cm. If the main pulmonary trunk is midway between the apex and the base in the erect position, there is a column of blood 15 cm high between the pulmonary trunk and arterioles in the apex and a similar column of blood between it and arterioles in the base. A column of blood 15 cm high is equivalent to a column of mercury 11 mm high. If the absolute pressure in the main pulmonary artery is 22/9 mm Hg, there is an adequate pressure to produce apical flow during systole, when apical pressure would be $22 - 11 = 11$ mm Hg (zone 2 or 3) but not

The Four Zones of the Lung

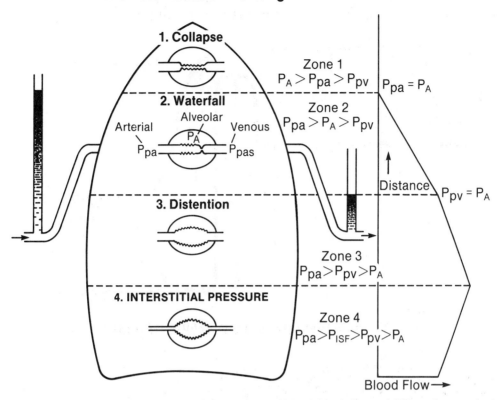

Figure 3–1. *This schematic diagram shows the distribution of blood flow in the upright lung. In zone 1, alveolar pressure (P_A) exceeds pulmonary artery pressure (P_{pa}), and no flow occurs because the intra-alveolar vessels are collapsed by the compressing alveolar pressure. In zone 2, arterial pressure exceeds alveolar pressure, but alveolar pressure exceeds pulmonary venous pressure (P_{pv}). Flow in zone 2 is determined by the arterial–alveolar pressure difference (P_{pa}-P_A) and has been likened to an upstream river waterfall over a dam (see Fig. 3–2). Since P_{pa} increases down zone 2 and P_A remains constant, the perfusion pressure increases, and flow steadily increases down the zone. In zone 3, pulmonary venous pressure exceeds alveolar pressure, and flow is determined by the arterial–venous pressure difference (P_{pa}-P_{pv}), which is constant down this portion of the lung. However, the transmural pressure across the wall of the vessel increases down this zone so that the caliber of the vessels increases (resistance decreases), and therefore flow increases. Finally, in zone 4, pulmonary interstitial pressure becomes positive and exceeds both pulmonary venous pressure and alveolar pressure (see Fig. 3–4). Consequently, flow in zone 4 is determined by the arterial–interstitial pressure difference (P_{pa}-P_{ISF}). (Redrawn by permission from West JB: Ventilation/Blood Flow and Gas Exchange. 4th Edition. Oxford, Blackwell Scientific Publications, 1985.)*

during diastole, when it would be $9 - 11 = -2$ mm Hg (zone 1). The blood pressure at the base would be $22 + 11/9 + 11$, or 33/20 mm Hg (see zone 3 as follows). Of course, simultaneous and perhaps irregular changes in alveolar pressure would considerably complicate this type of analysis.

Still lower down in the lung there is a vertical level where P_{pv} becomes positive and also exceeds P_A. In this region blood flow is governed by the pulmonary arteriovenous pressure difference (P_{pa}-P_{pv}) (zone 3, $P_{pa} > P_{pv} > P_A$), for in this zone both of these vascular pressures exceed the P_A, and the capillary systems are thus permanently open, and blood flow is continuous. In descending zone 3, gravity causes both

absolute P_{pa} and P_{pv} to increase at the same rate so that the perfusion pressure (P_{pa}-P_{pv}) is unchanged. However, the pressure outside the vessels, namely pleural pressure (P_{pl}), increases less than P_{pa} and P_{pv} so that the transmural distending pressures (P_{pa}-P_{pl} and P_{pv}-P_{pl}) increase down zone 3, the vessel radii increase, vascular resistance decreases, and blood flow therefore further increases.

Finally, whenever pulmonary vascular pressures are extremely high, as they would be in a severely volume-overloaded patient, a severely restricted and constricted pulmonary vascular bed and an extremely dependent lung (far below the vertical level of the left atrium), and in patients with pulmonary embolism and

Zone 2 Waterfall Phenomenom
Static Mean Pressure Condition

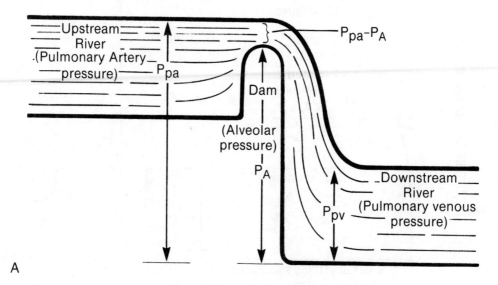

A

Dynamic Instantaneous Pressure Condition

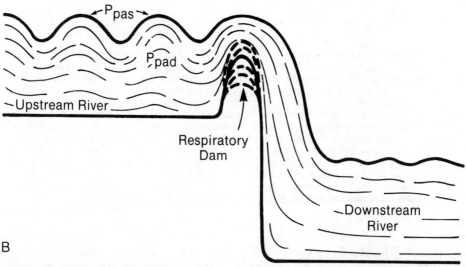

B

Figure 3–2. The relationships among pulmonary artery, alveolar, and venous pressures have the same charac-teristics as an upstream river flowing over a dam (as a waterfall) to a downstream river. *A,* Schematic diagram representing the conditions when just static mean pressures are considered. The pressure head for the upstream river to flow over the dam is the difference between pulmonary artery pressure (P_{pa}) and alveolar pressure (P_A). The rate of flow of the upstream river over the dam is independent of the pressure in the downstream river, namely, the pulmonary venous pressure (P_{pv}). *B,* Schematic diagram representing conditions when dynamic instantaneous pressures are considered. The upstream river actually approaches the respiratory dam as a wave, since there is a pulmonary artery systolic (P_{pas}) and pulmonary artery diastolic (P_{pad}) pressure. The downstream river actually leaves the respiratory dam as a wave, since there is a left atrial systolic and diastolic pressure. In addition, the respiratory dam is actually going up and down according to the respiratory cycle. The phase lag between P_{pas} and P_{pad}, the venous fluctuations, and the height of the respiratory dam are dependent on the timing between the respiratory and cardiac cycles and on whether respiration is by positive or negative pressure mechanisms. Depending on these phase lags, a given point in zone 2, as defined by mean static conditions, may actually transiently be in zone 1 or 3.

mitral stenosis, fluid may transudate out of the pulmonary vessels into the pulmonary interstitial compartment. Transudated pulmonary interstitial fluid may significantly alter the distribution of pulmonary blood flow. In order to understand how pulmonary interstitial fluid can determine the distribution of pulmonary perfusion, it is helpful to review the mechanism of how pulmonary interstitial fluid is formed, stored, and cleared.

The concepts of a continuous connective tissue sheath–alveolar septum interstitial space and of a negative interstitial space pressure gradient are prerequisite to understanding interstitial fluid kinetics (Fig. 3–3). After entering the lung parenchyma, both the bronchi and arteries run within a connective tissue sheath that is formed by an invagination of the pleura at the hilum and that ends at the level of the bronchioles (Fig. 3–3A). Thus, there is a potential perivascular and peribronchial space, respectively, between the arteries and the bronchi and the connective tissue sheath. The negative pressure in the pulmonary tissues surrounding the perivascular connective tissue sheath exert a radial outward traction force on the sheath. The radial traction creates a negative pressure within the sheath, and the negative pressure is transmitted to the bronchi and arteries, which tends to hold them open and increase their diameters (Fig. 3–3).[2] The alveolar septum interstitial space is the space between the capillaries and alveoli (or more precisely, the space between the endothelial and epithelial basement membranes) and is continuous with the interstitial tissue space that surrounds the larger arteries and bronchi (Fig. 3–3A) (also see chapter 2). Studies indicate that the alveolar interstitial pressure is also uniquely negative but not as much as the negative interstitial space pressure around the larger arteries and bronchi.[3]

The forces governing net transcapillary-interstitial space fluid movement are as follows: The net transcapillary flow of fluid (F) out of pulmonary capillaries is equal to the difference between pulmonary capillary hydrostatic pressure (P_{inside}) and the interstitial fluid hydrostatic pressure ($P_{outside}$) and to the difference between the capillary colloid oncotic pressure (π_{inside}) and the interstitial colloid oncotic pressure ($\pi_{outside}$). These four forces will produce a steady state fluid flow (F) during a constant capillary permeability (K). The equation that expresses these forces is written as follows:

$$F = K[(P_{inside} - P_{outside}) - (\pi_{inside} - \pi_{outside})] \quad (1)$$

K is a capillary filtration coefficient expressed in ml/min/mm Hg/100 g. The filtration coefficient is the product of the effective capillary surface area in a given mass of tissue and the permeability per unit surface area of the capillary wall to filter the fluid. Under normal circumstances, and at a vertical height in the lung that is at the junction of zones 2 and 3, the intravascular colloid osmotic pressure (about 26 mm Hg) acts to keep water in the capillary lumen, and working against this force, the pulmonary capillary hydrostatic pressure (about 10 mm Hg) acts to force water across the loose endothelial junctions into the interstitial space. If these were the only operative forces, the interstitial space, and consequently the alveolar surfaces, would be constantly dry, and there would be no lymph flow. In fact, alveolar surfaces are moist, and lymphatic flow from the interstitial compartment is constant (approximately 500 ml/day). This can be explained in part by the $\pi_{outside}$ (8 mm Hg) and in part by the negative $P_{outside}$ (approximately 8 mm Hg). Negative (subatmospheric) interstitial space pressure would promote, by suction, a slow loss of fluid across the endothelial holes.[4] Indeed, extremely negative pleural (and perivascular hydrostatic) pressure, such as might occur in a vigorously spontaneously breathing patient with an obstructed airway, can cause pulmonary interstitial edema.[5] Relative to the vertical level of the junction of zones 2 and 3, as lung height decreases (lung dependency), absolute P_{inside} increases, and fluid has a propensity to transudate; as lung height increases (lung nondependency), absolute P_{inside} decreases, and fluid has a propensity to be reabsorbed. However, fluid transudation induced by an increase in P_{inside} is limited by a concomitant dilution of proteins in the interstitial space and therefore a decrease in $\pi_{outside}$.[6] Any change in the size of the endothelial junctions, even if the above four forces remain constant, will change the magnitude and perhaps even the direction of fluid movement; increased size of endothelial junctions (increased permeability) promotes transudation, and decreased size of endothelial junctions (decreased permeability) promotes reabsorption.

There are no lymphatics in the interstitial space of the alveolar septum. Instead, lymphatic capillaries first appear in the interstitial space sheath surrounding terminal bronchioles and small arteries. Interstitial fluid is normally removed from the alveolar interstitial space into the lymphatics by a "sump" (pressure gradient) mechanism, which is caused by the presence of the more negative pressure surrounding the

Continuous Connective Tissue Sheath-
Alveolar Septum Interstitial Space

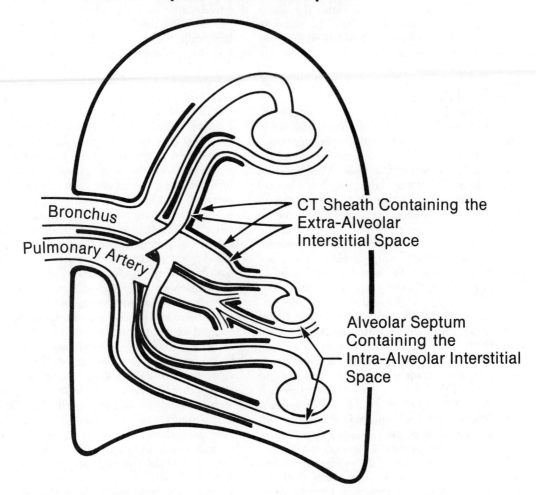

A

Interstitial Fluid Moves From Alveolar Septum
To Connective Tissue Space Via Three Mechanisms

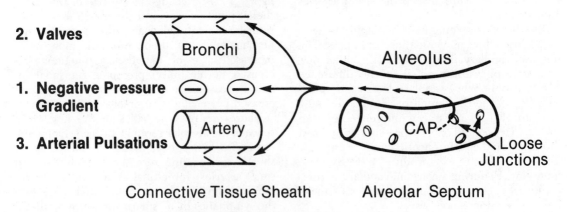

B

Continuous Interstitial Space

Figure 3–3 See legend on opposite page

larger arteries and bronchi.[7, 8] The sump mechanism is aided by the presence of valves in the lymph vessels. In addition, since the lymphatics run in the same sheath as the pulmonary arteries, they are exposed to the massaging action of the arterial pulsations. The differential negative pressure, the lymphatic valves, and the arterial pulsations all help to propel the lymph proximally toward the hilum and central venous circulation depot (Fig. 3–3*B*).

When flow of interstitial fluid through the endothelial holes is excessive and cannot be cleared adequately by lymphatics, it will accumulate in the interstitial connective tissue compartment around the large vessels and airways, forming peribronchial and periarteriolar edema fluid cuffs. The transudated pulmonary interstitial fluid fills the pulmonary interstitial space and may eliminate the normally present negative and radially expanding interstitial tension on the extra-alveolar pulmonary vessels (Fig. 3–4*B*). The expansion of the pulmonary interstitial space by fluid causes pulmonary interstitial pressure (P_{ISF}) to become positive and exceed P_{pv} (zone 4, $P_{pa} > P_{ISF} > P_{pv} > P_A$).[9, 10] In addition, the vascular resistance of extra-alveolar vessels may be increased at a very low volume (i.e., the residual volume), where the tethering action of the pulmonary tissue on the vessels is also lost, causing P_{ISF} to increase positively (see lung volume discussion below).[11, 12] Consequently, zone 4 blood flow is governed by the arterio-interstitial pressure difference (P_{pa}-P_{ISF}), which is less than the P_{pa}-P_{pv} difference, and therefore zone 4 blood flow is less than zone 3 blood flow. In summary, zone 4 is a region of the lung that has transudated a large amount of fluid into the pulmonary interstitial compartment or is possibly at a very low lung volume. Both these circumstances produce a positive interstitial pressure, causing extra-alveolar vessel compression, increased extra-alveolar vascular resistance, and decreased regional blood flow.

Following filling of the pulmonary interstitial compartment with edema fluid, fluid from the

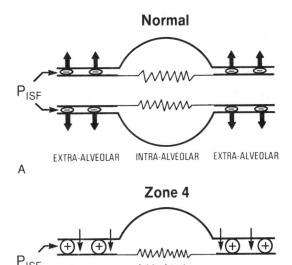

Figure 3–4. *This figure shows the effect of pulmonary interstitial fluid pressure (P_{ISF}) on extra-alveolar vessels. In normal lungs (A) a negative P_{ISF} around the extra-alveolar vessels tethers or keeps them open. When either pulmonary interstitial fluid accumulates or lung volume is extremely low, P_{ISF} may become positive, exceed both pulmonary venous and alveolar pressure, and create a zone 4 (B) of the lung (where flow is proportional to the pulmonary artery pressure–pulmonary interstitial pressure difference). (Modified with permission from Benumof JL: The pulmonary circulation. In Kaplan JA (ed.): Thoracic Anesthesia. New York, Churchill Livingstone, 1983, chapter 7.)*

interstitial space, under an increased driving force (P_{ISF}), will cross the relatively impermeable epithelial wall holes, and the alveolar space will fill. Intra-alveolar edema fluid will additionally cause alveolar collapse and atelectasis, thereby promoting further fluid accumulation.

It should now be evident that as P_{pa} and P_{pv} increase, three important changes take place in the pulmonary circulation, namely, recruitment or opening of previously unperfused vessels, distention or widening of previously perfused vessels, and transudation of fluid from very

Figure 3–3. A, *Schematic diagram of the concept of a continuous connective tissue sheath–alveolar septum interstitial space. The entry of the mainstem bronchi and pulmonary artery into the lung parenchyma invaginates the pleura at the hilum, forming a surrounding connective tissue sheath (heavy black line). The connective tissue sheath ends at the level of the bronchioles. The space between the pulmonary arteries and bronchi and the connective tissue sheath constitutes the extra-alveolar interstitial space. The connective tissue sheath–extra-alveolar interstitial space is continuous with the alveolar septum interstitial space. The alveolar septum interstitial space is contained within the endothelial and epithelial basement membranes of the capillaries and alveoli, respectively. B, Schematic diagram showing how interstitial fluid moves from the alveolar septum interstitial space to the connective tissue interstitial space. The mechanisms are via a negative pressure gradient ("sump"), presence of one-way valves in the lymphatics, and the massaging action of arterial pulsations.*

distended vessels.[13, 14] Thus, as mean P_{pa} increases, zone 1 arteries may beome zone 2 arteries, and as mean P_{pv} increases, zone 2 veins may become zone 3 veins. The increase in both mean P_{pa} and P_{pv} distends zone 3 vessels according to their compliance and decreases the resistance to flow through them. Zone 3 vessels may become so distended that they leak fluid and become converted to zone 4 vessels. In general, recruitment is the principal change as P_{pa} and P_{pv} increase from low to moderate levels; distention is the principal change as P_{pa} and P_{pv} increase from moderate to high levels of vascular pressure; and finally, transudation is the principal change as P_{pa} and P_{pv} increase from high to very high levels.

2. Distribution of Ventilation

Gravity also causes vertical P_{pl} differences that cause, in turn, regional alveolar volume, compliance, and ventilation differences. The vertical gradient of P_{pl} can be best understood by thinking of the lung as a plastic bag filled with semifluid contents; in other words, it is a viscoelastic structure. Without the presence of a supporting chest wall, the effect of gravity on the contents of the bag would cause the bag to bulge outward at the bottom and inward at the top (it would assume a globular shape). With the lung inside the supporting chest wall, the lung cannot assume a globular shape. However, gravity still exerts a force on the lung to assume a globular shape; the force creates a relatively more negative pressure at the top of the pleural space (where the lung pulls away from the chest wall) and a relatively more positive pressure at the bottom of the lung (where the lung is compressed against the chest wall) (Fig. 3–5). The magnitude of this pressure gradient is determined by the density of the lung. Since the lung is about one quarter of the density of water, the gradient of P_{pl} (in cm H_2O) will be about one quarter of the height of the upright lung (30 cm). Thus, P_{pl} increases positively by $30/4 = 7.5$ cm H_2O from the top to the bottom of the lung.[15]

Since P_A is the same throughout the lung, the P_{pl} gradient causes regional differences in transpulmonary distending pressures (P_A-P_{pl}). Since P_{pl} is most positive (least negative) in the dependent basilar lung regions, alveoli in these regions are more compressed and therefore are considerably smaller than superior, relatively noncompressed apical alveoli (there is an approximately fourfold alveolar volume differ-

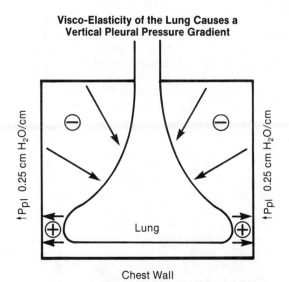

Visco-Elasticity of the Lung Causes a Vertical Pleural Pressure Gradient

Figure 3–5. This schematic diagram of the lung within the chest wall shows the tendency of the lung to assume a globular shape due to the lung's visco-elastic nature. The tendency of the top of the lung to collapse inward creates a relatively negative pressure at the apex of the lung, and the tendency of the bottom of the lung to spread outward creates a relatively positive pressure at the base of the lung. Thus, pleural pressure increases by 0.25 cm of H_2O per centimeter of lung dependency. (Modified with permission from Benumof JL: Respiratory physiology and respiratory function during anesthesia. In Miller RD (ed.): Anesthesia. 2nd ed. Churchill Livingstone, New York, 1983, chapter 32.)

ence).[16] If the regional differences in alveolar volume are translated over to a pressure-volume curve for normal lung (Fig. 3–6), the dependent small alveoli are on the midportion and the nondependent large alveoli are on the upper portion of the S-shaped pressure-volume curve. Since the different regional slopes of the composite curve are equal to the different regional lung compliances, dependent alveoli are relatively compliant (steep slope), and nondependent alveoli are relatively noncompliant (flat slope). Thus, the majority of the tidal volume is preferentially distributed to dependent alveoli, since they expand more per unit pressure change than nondependent alveoli.

3. Distribution of the Ventilation-Perfusion Ratio

Figure 3–7 shows that both blood flow and ventilation (both on the left-hand vertical axis) increase linearly with distance down the normal upright lung (horizontal axis, reverse polarity).[17] Since blood flow increases from a very low value and increases more rapidly than ventila-

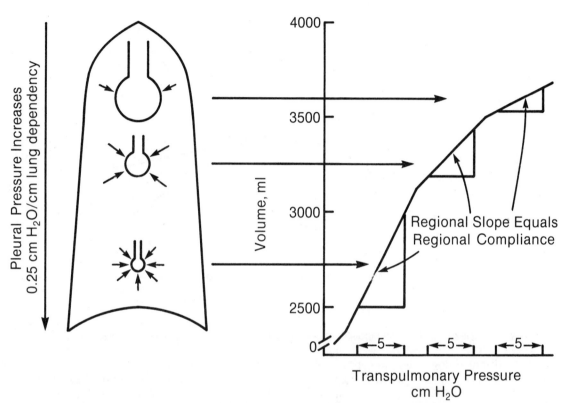

Figure 3–6. Pleural pressure increases 0.25 cm H_2O every centimeter down the lung. The increase in pleural pressure causes a fourfold decrease in alveolar volume. The caliber of the air passages also decreases as lung volume decreases. When regional alveolar volume is translated over to a regional transpulmonary pressure–alveolar volume curve, small alveoli are on a steep (large slope) portion of the curve, and large alveoli are on a flat (small slope) portion of the curve. Since the regional slope equals regional compliance, the dependent small alveoli normally receive the largest share of the tidal volume. Over the normal tidal volume range (lung volume increases by 500 ml from 2500 [normal FRC] to 3000 ml), the pressure–volume relationship is linear. Lung volume values in this diagram relate to the upright position. (Modified with permission from Benumof JL: Respiratory physiology and respiratory function during anesthesia. In Miller RD (ed.): Anesthesia. 2nd ed. Churchill Livingstone, New York, 1983, chapter 32.)

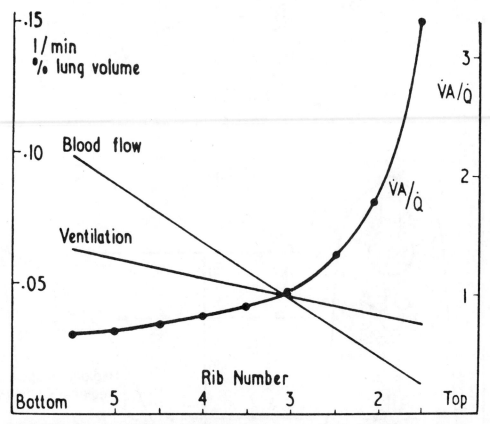

Figure 3–7. Distribution of ventilation and blood flow (left-hand vertical axis) and the ventilation-perfusion ratio (right-hand vertical axis) in normal upright lung. Both blood flow and ventilation are expressed in L/min per cent alveolar volume and have been drawn as smoothed out linear functions of vertical height. The closed circles mark the ventilation-perfusion ratios of horizontal lung slices (three of which are shown in Fig. 3–8). A cardiac output of 6 L/min and a total minute ventilation of 5.1 L/min were assumed. (Reproduced with permission from West JB: Ventilation/Blood Flow and Gas Exchange. 4th ed. Oxford, Blackwell Scientific Publications, 1985.)

tion with distance down the lung, the ventilation-perfusion ($\dot{V}_A/\dot{Q}$) ratio (right-hand vertical axis) decreases rapidly at first, then more slowly.

The $\dot{V}_A/\dot{Q}$ ratio best expresses the amount of ventilation relative to perfusion in any given lung region. Thus, alveoli at the base of the lung are somewhat overperfused in relation to their ventilation $\dot{V}_A/\dot{Q} > 1$). Figure 3–8 shows the calculated ventilation ($\dot{V}_A$) and blood flow ($\dot{Q}$) in L/min, $\dot{V}_A/\dot{Q}$ ratio, and the alveolar (P_{O_2} and P_{CO_2} in mm Hg for horizontal slices from the top (7 per cent of lung volume), middle (11 per cent of lung volume), and bottom (13 per cent of lung volume) of the lung.[18] It can be seen that the P_AO_2 increases by over 40 mm Hg from 89 mm Hg at the base to 132 mm Hg at the apex, while the P_{CO_2} decreases by 14 mm Hg from 42 mm Hg at the bottom to 28 mm Hg at the top. Thus, in keeping with the regional $\dot{V}_A/\dot{Q}$, the bottom of the lung is relatively hypoxic and hypercarbic compared with the top of the lung.

Recently, Wagner and colleagues[19] have described a method of determining the continuous distribution of $\dot{V}_A/\dot{Q}$ ratios within the lung based on the pattern of elimination of a series of intravenously infused inert gases. Gases of differing solubility are dissolved in physiologic saline solution and infused into a peripheral vein until a steady state is achieved (20 minutes). Toward the end of the infusion period, samples of arterial and mixed expired gas are collected, and total ventilation and cardiac output are measured. For each gas the ratio of arterial to mixed venous concentration (retention) and the ratio of expired to mixed venous concentration (excretion) are calculated, and retention-solubility and excretion-solubility curves are drawn. The retention/excretion–solubility curves can be regarded as a "fingerprint" of the particular distribution of ventilation-perfusion ratios that give rise to it.

Figure 3–9A shows the type of distribution found in young normal subjects breathing air in the semirecumbent position.[20] The distributions

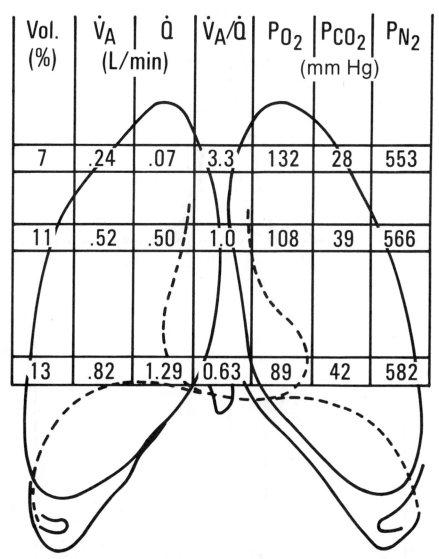

Vol. (%)	$\dot{V}_A$ (L/min)	$\dot{Q}$ (L/min)	$\dot{V}_A/\dot{Q}$	P_{O_2} (mm Hg)	P_{CO_2} (mm Hg)	P_{N_2} (mm Hg)
7	.24	.07	3.3	132	28	553
11	.52	.50	1.0	108	39	566
13	.82	1.29	0.63	89	42	582

Figure 3–8. *The ventilation-perfusion ratio ($\dot{V}_A/\dot{Q}$) and the regional composition of alveolar gas. Values for the regional flow ($\dot{Q}$), ventilation ($\dot{V}_A$), P_{O_2} and P_{CO_2} are derived from Figure 3–7. P_{N_2} has been obtained by what remains from the total gas pressure (which, including water vapor, equals 760 mm Hg). The volumes (vol [%]) of the three lung slices are also shown. Compared with the top of the lung, the bottom of the lung has a low ventilation-perfusion ratio and is relatively hypoxic and hypercarbic. (Reproduced with permission from West JB: Regional differences in gas exchange in the lung of erect man. J Appl Physiol 17:893, 1962.)*

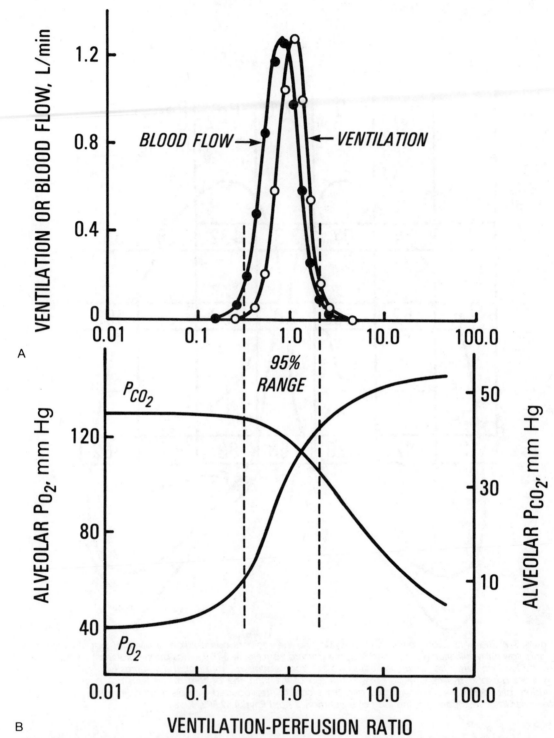

Figure 3–9. A, The average distribution of ventilation-perfusion ratios in young, semirecumbent normal subjects. The 95 per cent range covers ventilation-perfusion ratios from 0.3 to 2.1 (between dashed lines). The corresponding variations of P_{O_2} and P_{CO_2} in the alveolar gas can be seen in B. (Reproduced with permission from West JB: Blood flow to the lung and gas exchange. Anesthesiology 41:124, 1974.)

of both ventilation and blood flow are relatively narrow. The upper and lower 95 per cent limits shown (vertical interrupted lines) correspond to $\dot{V}_A/\dot{Q}$ ratios of 0.3 and 2.1, respectively. Notice these young normal subjects had no blood flow perfusing areas with very low $\dot{V}_A/\dot{Q}$ ratios nor did they have any blood flow to unventilated or shunted areas ($\dot{V}_A/\dot{Q} = 0$) or unperfused areas ($\dot{V}_A/\dot{Q} = \infty$). Figure 3–9 also shows alveolar P_{O_2} and P_{CO_2} in respiratory units having different $\dot{V}_A/\dot{Q}$ ratios. It can be seen that within the 95 per cent range of $\dot{V}_A/\dot{Q}$ ratios (0.3 to 2.1), the P_{O_2} ranges from 60 to 123 mm Hg while the corresponding P_{CO_2} range is 44 to 33 mm Hg.

C. Other (Nongravitational) Important Determinants of Pulmonary Vascular Resistance and Blood Flow Distribution

1. Cardiac Output

The passive effect of changes in cardiac output on the pulmonary circulation are as fol-
lows.[21] As cardiac output increases, pulmonary vascular pressures increase (Fig. 3–10). Since the pulmonary vasculature is distensible, an increase in pulmonary artery pressure increases the radius of the pulmonary vessels, causing pulmonary vascular resistance to decrease. Exactly the opposite effect applies to the passive effect of a decrease in cardiac output on the pulmonary circulation. As cardiac output decreases, pulmonary vascular pressures decrease. The decrease in pulmonary vascular pressure reduces the radius of the pulmonary vessels, causing pulmonary vascular resistance to increase.

Understanding the relationship among pulmonary vascular resistance, pulmonary artery pressure, and cardiac output during passive events is a prerequisite to recognition of active vasomotion in the pulmonary circulation (Fig. 3–11). Active vasoconstriction occurs any time cardiac output decreases and pulmonary artery pressure either remains constant or increases. Increased pulmonary artery pressure and pulmonary vascular resistance have been found to be "a universal feature of acute respiratory

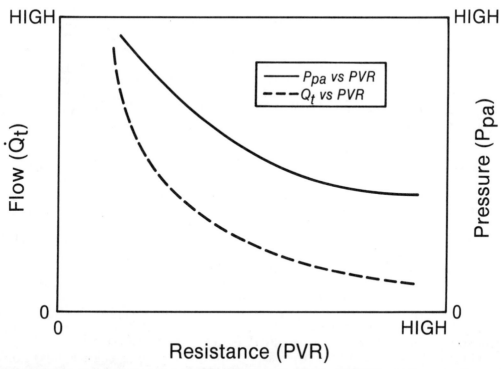

Figure 3–10. Passive changes in pulmonary vascular resistance (PVR) as a function of pulmonary artery pressure (P_{pa}) and pulmonary blood flow ($\dot{Q}_t$) (PVR = $P_{pa}/\dot{Q}_t$). As flow increases, pulmonary artery pressure also increases, but to a lesser extent, so that resistance decreases. As flow decreases, pulmonary artery pressure also decreases, but to a lesser extent, so that resistance increases. (Reproduced with permission from Fishman AP: Dynamics of the pulmonary circulation. In Hamilton WF (ed.): Handbook of Physiology. Section 2: Circulation. Vol. 2. Bethesda, American Physiological Society, 1963, pp. 1667–1743.)

The Pulmonary Circulation and Vasomotion

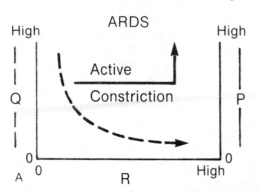

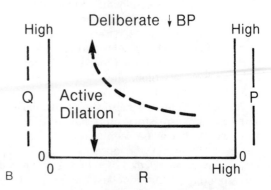

Figure 3–11. *The pulmonary circulation and vasomotion. Relationships among flow (Q), pressure (P), and resistance (R) and the pulmonary circulation in the adult respiratory distress syndrome (ARDS) (A) and during deliberate hypotension (↓ BP) (B). Active vasoconstriction is present in the pulmonary circulation whenever cardiac output decreases and pressure remains constant or increases; these findings are common in ARDS. Active vasodilation is present in the pulmonary circulation whenever cardiac output increases and pressure remains constant or decreases; these findings are often present with deliberate hypotension. (Modified with permission from Benumof JL: The pulmonary circulation. In Kaplan JA (ed.): Thoracic Anesthesia. New York, Churchill Livingstone, 1983, chapter 7.)*

failure."[22] Active pulmonary vasoconstriction can increase P_{pa} and P_{pv}, thereby contributing to the formation of pulmonary edema, and in that way have a role in the genesis of the adult respiratory distress syndrome.[23] Active vasodilation occurs any time cardiac output increases and the pulmonary artery pressure either remains constant or decreases. When deliberate hypotension is achieved with sodium nitroprusside, cardiac output often remains constant or increases, but pulmonary artery pressure decreases, and therefore, so does pulmonary vascular resistance.

2. Alveolar Hypoxia

Alveolar or environmental hypoxia of in vivo and in vitro whole lung, unilateral lung, lobe, or lobule of lung causes localized pulmonary vasoconstriction. This phenomenon is called hypoxic pulmonary vasoconstriction (HPV) and is present in all mammalian species.

Since the HPV response occurs primarily on the pulmonary arterioles of about 200-μm diameter, these vessels are advantageously situated anatomically in very close relation to the small bronchioles and alveoli, which permits rapid and direct detection of alveolar hypoxia. Indeed, it has been shown that blood may actually become oxygenated in small pulmonary arteries owing to the ability of oxygen to diffuse directly across the small distance between the contiguous air spaces and vessels.[24] This direct

access that gas in the airways has to small arteries makes possible a very rapid and localized vascular response to changes in gas composition.

There are two major theories as to how alveolar hypoxia may cause pulmonary vasoconstriction.[25–29] First, alveolar hypoxia may cause the release of vasoconstrictor substance(s) into the pulmonary interstitial compartment where the substance(s) may then cause vasoconstriction. In the past 10 years many vasoactive substances have been proposed as the mediators of HPV (e.g., prostaglandins, catecholamines, serotonin, histamine, angiotensin, and bradykinin), but none has been proved to be involved primarily in the process. Second and/or alternatively, hypoxia also appears to stimulate directly metabolic activity of pulmonary vascular smooth muscle and to accelerate production of ATP, whereas in systemic vascular beds the action of hypoxia on metabolism is depressant. Low oxygen tension also maintains the membrane of pulmonary vascular smooth muscle cells in a state of partial depolarization and influences the role of calcium in excitation-contraction coupling.[19] Thus, alveolar hypoxia may directly cause ion fluxes that cause or contribute to the vasoconstriction. In summary, HPV may be due to either a direct action of alveolar hypoxia on pulmonary vasculature or an alveolar hypoxia-induced release of a vasoactive substance(s). These two mechanisms for the production of HPV are not necessarily mutually exclusive.

There are three ways in which HPV operates in humans. First, life at high altitude or whole-lung respiration of a low-inspired concentration (F_IO_2) increases P_{pa}. This is true for newcomers, for the acclimatized, and for natives.[29] The vasoconstriction is considerable, and in normal people breathing 10 per cent O_2, P_{pa} doubles while pulmonary wedge pressure remains constant.[30] The increased P_{pa} increases perfusion of the apices of the lung (recruitment of previously unused vessels) and results in gas exchange in a region of lung not normally utilized (i.e., zone 1). Thus, with a low F_IO_2, the PaO_2 is greater, and the alveolar-arterial O_2 tension difference and dead space/tidal volume ratio are less than would be expected or predicted on the basis of a normal (sea level) distribution of ventilation and blood flow. High-altitude pulmonary hypertension is an important component in the development of mountain sickness subacutely (hours to days) and cor pulmonale chronically (weeks).[31] In fact, there is now good evidence that in patients with chronic obstructive pulmonary disease, even nocturnal episodes of arterial oxygen desaturation (caused by episodic hypoventilation) are accompanied by elevations in P_{pa} and may account for or lead to sustained pulmonary hypertension and cor pulmonale.[32] Second, hypoventilation (low $\dot{V}_A/\dot{Q}$), atelectasis, or nitrogen ventilation of any region of the lung (one lung, lobe, lobule) generally causes a diversion of blood flow away from the hypoxic to the nonhypoxic lung (40 to 50 per cent, 50 to 60 per cent, 60 to 70 per cent, respectively) (Fig. 3–12).[33, 34] The regional vasoconstriction and blood flow diversion is of great importance in minimizing transpulmonary shunt and normalizing regional $\dot{V}/\dot{Q}$ ratios during disease of one lung, one-lung anesthesia (see chapter 4), and inadvertent intubation of a mainstem bronchus. In regard to one-lung anesthesia in the lateral decubitus position, it is important to note that the strength of the HPV response in humans is sufficient to overcome significant vertical hydrostatic gradients.[35] Third, in patients with chronic obstructive pulmonary disease, asthma, pneumonia, and mitral stenosis who do not have bronchospasm, administration of pulmonary vasodilator drugs such as isoproterenol, sodium nitroprusside, and nitroglycerin cause a decrease is P_aO_2 and pulmonary vascular resistance and an increase in right-to-left transpulmonary shunt.[36] The mechanism for these changes is thought to be deleterious inhibition of pre-existing and, in some of the lesions, geographically widespread HPV without a concomitant and beneficial bronchodilation.[36] In accordance with the latter two lines of evidence (one-lung or regional hypoxia and vasodilator drug effects on whole-lung or generalized disease), HPV is thought to divert blood flow away from hypoxic regions of the lung, thereby serving as an autoregulatory mechanism that protects P_aO_2 by favorably adjusting regional $\dot{V}_A/\dot{Q}$ ratios. Factors that inhibit regional HPV are extensively discussed under physiology and one-lung ventilation in chapter 4.

3. Lung Volume

The functional residual capacity (FRC) is the volume of lung that exists at the end of a normal exhalation after a normal tidal volume and when there is no muscle activity or pressure difference between alveoli and atmosphere. Total pulmonary vascular resistance is increased when lung volume is either increased or decreased from FRC (Fig. 3–13).[37–39] The increase in total pulmonary vascular resistance above FRC is due to alveolar compression of small intra-alveolar vessels, which results in an increase in small vessel pulmonary vascular resis-

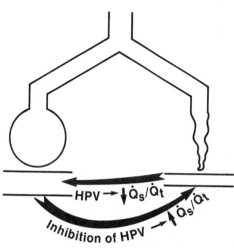

Regional HPV

Figure 3–12. Schematic drawing of regional hypoxic pulmonary vasoconstriction (HPV); one-lung ventilation is a common clinical example of regional HPV. HPV in the hypoxic atelectatic lung causes a redistribution of blood flow away from the hypoxic lung to the normoxic lung, thereby diminishing the amount of shunt flow ($\dot{Q}_s/\dot{Q}_t$) that can occur through the hypoxic lung. Inhibition of hypoxic lung HPV causes an increase in the amount of shunt flow through the hypoxic lung, thereby decreasing Pa_{O_2}.

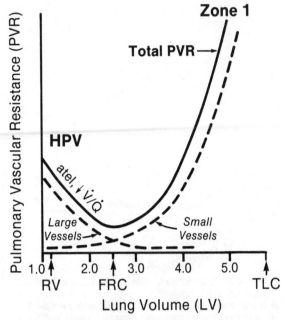

Figure 3–13. An asymmetrical U-shaped curve relates total pulmonary vascular resistance (PVR) to lung volume. The trough of the curve occurs when lung volume equals functional residual capacity (FRC). Total pulmonary resistance is the sum of resistance in small vessels (increased by increasing lung volume) and in large vessels (increased by decreasing lung volume). The endpoint for increasing lung volume (toward total lung capacity [TLC]) is the creation of zone 1 conditions, and the endpoint for decreasing lung volume (toward residual volume [RV]) is the creation of low $\dot{V}/\dot{Q}$ and atelectatic (atel) areas that have hypoxic pulmonary vasoconstriction (HPV). The curve represents a composite of data from references 37 to 39. (Modified with permission from Benumof JL: Respiratory physiology and respiratory function during anesthesia. In Miller RD (ed.): Anesthesia. 2nd ed. Churchill Livingstone, New York, 1983, chapter 32.)

tance (i.e., creation of zones 1 or 2).[40] As a relatively small mitigating or counterbalancing effect to the small vessel compression, the large extra-alveolar vessels may be expanded by the increased negativity of the perivascular pressure at high FRC. The increase in total pulmonary vascular resistance below FRC is due to an increase in pulmonary vascular resistance of large extra-alveolar vessels. The increase in large vessel pulmonary vascular resistance was previously thought to be due to a mechanical tortuosity or kinking of these vessels. However, small or grossly atelectatic lungs are hypoxic, and it has recently been shown that the mechanism of increased large-vessel pulmonary vascular resistance in these lungs is due entirely to hypoxic pulmonary vasoconstriction.[41] This conclusion has been found to be true whether the chest is open or closed and whether venti-

lation is by positive pressure or is spontaneous.[42]

The relationship between lung volume and pulmonary vascular resistance can determine the distribution of pulmonary blood flow within a given single lung if there is a vertical gradient of alveolar volume (Fig. 3–14). At total lung capacity, all alveoli are large, and the small intra-alveolar vessels are homogeneously compressed; there are no low $\dot{V}/\dot{Q}$ or atelectatic areas, and there is no large extra-alveolar vessel vasoconstriction (HPV). Since P_{pa} and P_{pv} increase down the upright lung, blood flow simply increases down the upright lung at total lung capacity (Fig. 3–14A) as it does at FRC (Fig. 3–14B). Near residual volume dependent alveoli are much smaller than nondependent alveoli, and dependent lung may contain hypoxic low $\dot{V}/\dot{Q}$ and atelectatic areas. Consequently, at residual volume, the large extra-alveolar vessels in the dependent lung may be constricted (due to HPV), and blood flow is either uniform[11, 12] or decreases slightly[43] down the upright lung, even though P_{pa} and P_{pv} are increasing (Fig. 3–14C).

4. Alternate (Nonalveolar) Pathways of Blood Flow Through the Lung

Figure 3–15 shows all the possible pathways for blood to travel from the right side to the left side of the heart without being oxygenated and the pathologic conditions during which blood flow through these shunt pathways is significantly increased. Blood flow through poorly ventilated alveoli (low $\dot{V}/\dot{Q}$ regions at F_IO_2 less than 0.3 have a right-to-left shunt effect on oxygenation) and through nonventilated alveoli (atelectatic or consolidated regions) ($\dot{V}/\dot{Q} = 0$ at all F_IO_2) are sources of right-to-left shunt. Low $\dot{V}/\dot{Q}$ and atelectatic lung units occur in conditions in which the functional residual capacity (FRC) is less than the closing capacity (CC) of the lung (see lung volume section below).

There are several right-to-left heart blood flow pathways that do not pass by or involve alveoli at all. The bronchial and pleural circulations originate from systemic arteries and empty into the left side of the heart without being oxygenated, constituting the 1 to 3 per cent true right-to-left shunt normally present. With chronic bronchitis, the bronchial circulation may carry 10 per cent of the cardiac output, and with pleuritis the pleural circulation may carry 5 per cent of the cardiac output. Consequently, there may be as much as a 10 per cent

At TLC

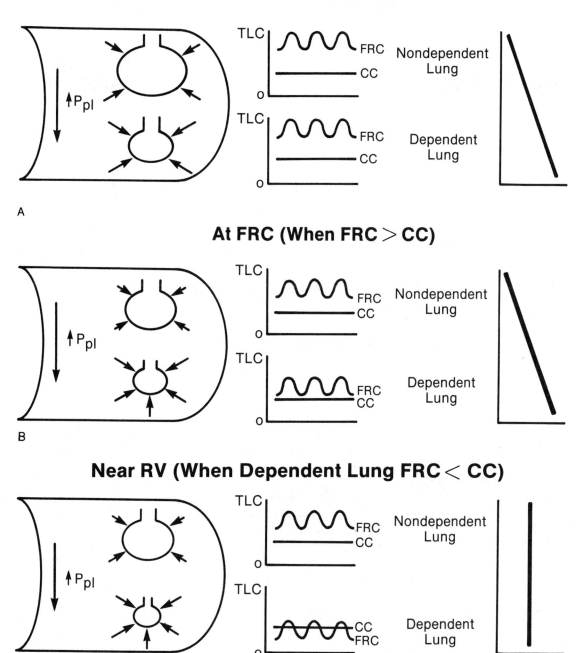

At FRC (When FRC > CC)

Near RV (When Dependent Lung FRC < CC)

Alveolar Volume

FRC-CC
Relationship

Blood
Flow

Figure 3–14. Schematic diagram of how vertical gradients in lung volume may determine the vertical gradient of blood flow. At total lung capacity (TLC) (A) alveoli are almost uniformly large, regional functional residual capacity (FRC) exceeds regional closing capacity (CC) in all parts of the lung, and blood flow distribution is simply a function of gravity. At normal FRC, regional FRC still exceeds CC in all parts of the lung, and blood flow distribution is still a function of gravity (B). At near residual volume (RV) (C), dependent lung FRC may be below dependent lung CC, causing the dependent lung to have either low V̇/Q̇ or atelectatic areas, which may cause dependent lung vasoconstriction. Therefore, the vertical gradient in blood flow is either uniform or decreases with dependency because dependent lung vasoconstriction is able to overcome gravitational effects. (Based on data from reference 43.)

Pulmonary Shunt Pathways

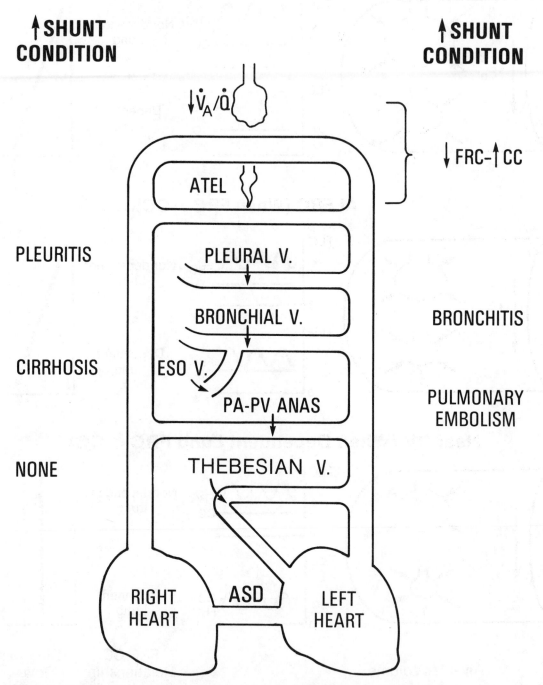

Figure 3–15. Pulmonary shunt pathways. Schematic representation of all possible right to left heart shunt pathways and the pathological conditions during which these shunt pathways are increased. The bronchial and pleural arteries do not arise from the right heart outlet but rather from systemic arteries; therefore, the corresponding bronchial and pleural veins, which empty into the pulmonary veins, contain desaturated blood. Esophageal veins can empty into bronchial veins. ($\dot{V}_A/\dot{Q}$ = ventilation-perfusion ratio; ATEL = atelectasis; FRC = functional residual capacity; CC = closing capacity; V = vein; ESO = esophageal; PA = pulmonary artery; PV = pulmonary vein; ANAS = anastomosis; PUL = pulmonary.) (Modified with permission from Benumof JL: The pulmonary circulation. In Kaplan JA (ed.): Thoracic Anesthesia. New York, Churchill Livingstone, 1983, chapter 7.)

and 5 per cent obligatory right-to-left shunt present, respectively, under these conditions. Intrapulmonary arteriovenous anastomoses are normally closed, but in the face of acute pulmonary hypertension, such as may be caused by a pulmonary embolus, they may open and cause a direct increase in right-to-left shunt. The foramen ovale is patent in 20 to 30 per cent of individuals but normally remains functionally closed because left atrial pressure exceeds right atrial pressure. However, any condition that results in right atrial pressure being greater than left atrial pressure may produce a right-to-left shunt with resultant hypoxemia and possible paradoxic embolization. Such conditions include the use of high levels of PEEP, pulmonary embolization, pulmonary hypertension, chronic obstructive pulmonary disease, pulmonary valvular stenosis, congestive heart failure, and postpneumonectomy states.[44] Esophageal to mediastinal to bronchial to pulmonary vein pathways have been described and may explain in part the hypoxemia associated with portal hypertension and cirrhosis. There are no known conditions that selectively increase Thebesian channel blood flow (Thebesian vessels nourish the left heart myocardium and originate and empty into the left heart).

D. Other (Nongravitational) Important Determinants of Pulmonary Compliance, Resistance, and Lung Volume

1. Pulmonary Compliance

For air to flow into the lungs, a pressure gradient must be developed to overcome the elastic resistance of the lungs and the chest wall to expansion. These structures are arranged concentrically, and their elastic resistances are therefore additive. The relationship between the pressure gradient (ΔP) and the resultant volume increase (ΔV) of the lungs and thorax is independent of time and is known as total compliance (C_T), as expressed below:

$$C_T(L/cm\ H_2O) = \Delta V(L)/\Delta P(cm\ H_2O) \qquad (2)$$

The C_T of lung plus chest wall is related to the individual compliances of lungs (C_L) and chest wall (C_{cw}) according to the following expression:

$$1/C_T = 1/C_L + 1/C_{cw}$$
$$[\text{or } C_T = (C_L)(C_{cw})/C_L + C_{cw}] \qquad (3)$$

Normally, C_L and C_{cw} each equal 0.2 L/cm H_2O; thus $C_T = 0.1$ L/cm H_2O. To determine

C_L, ΔV and the *transpulmonary pressure gradient* ($P_{alveolar}$-$P_{pleural}$, the ΔP for the lung) must be known; to determine C_{cw}, ΔV and the *transmural pressure gradient* ($P_{pleural} - P_{ambient}$, the ΔP for the chest wall) must be known; to determine C_T, ΔV and the *transthoracic pressure gradient* ($P_{alveolar} - P_{ambient}$, the ΔP for the lung and chest wall together) must be known. In clinical practice, only C_T is measured, which can be done dynamically or statically, depending on whether a peak or plateau inspiratory pressure gradient (respectively) is used for the C_T calculation.

During a positive or negative pressure inspiration of sufficient duration, the transthoracic pressure gradient first increases to a peak value and then decreases to a somewhat lower plateau value. The peak transthoracic pressure value is due to pressure required to overcome both elastic and airway resistance (see the following section, Airway Resistance). The transthoracic pressure decreases to a plateau value following the peak value because with time, gas redistributes from stiff alveoli (which expand only a little bit and therefore have only a very short inspiratory period) into more compliant alveoli (which expand a great deal and therefore have a long inspiratory period). Since the gas redistributes into more compliant alveoli, less pressure is required to contain the same amount of gas, and this explains why the pressure decreases. In practical terms, dynamic compliance is the volume change divided by the peak inspiratory transthoracic pressure; static compliance is the volume change divided by the plateau inspiratory transthoracic pressure. Therefore, static C_T is usually greater than dynamic C_T, since the former calculation uses a smaller denominator (lower pressure) than the latter calculation.

The pressure in an alveolus ($P_{alveolar}$) deserves special comment. The alveoli are lined with a layer of liquid. The lining of a curved surface (sphere or cylinder, as are the alveoli, bronchioles, bronchi) with liquid creates a surface tension that tends to make the surface area that is exposed to the atmosphere as small as possible. Simply stated, water molecules crowd much closer together on the surface of a curved layer of water than elsewhere in the fluid. As lung or alveoli size decreases, the degree of curvature and the retractive surface tension force increases.

According to Laplace's equation, the pressure in an alveolus (P, in dyn/cm^2) is above ambient pressure by an amount depending on the surface tension of the lining liquid (T, in dyn/cm)

and the radius of curvature of the alveolus (R, in cm). This is expressed in the following:

$$P = 2T/R \qquad (4)$$

Although surface tension contributes to the elastic resistance and retractive forces of the lung, two difficulties must be resolved. The first problem is that the pressure inside small alveoli should be higher than that for large alveoli, a conclusion that stems directly from Laplace's equation (small R in the denominator). From this reasoning, one would expect a progressive discharge of each small alveolus into a larger one, until eventually only one gigantic alveolus would be left (Fig. 3–16A). The second problem concerns the relationship between lung volume and the transpulmonary pressure gradient ($P_{alveolar} = P_{pleural}$). Theoretically, the retractive forces of the lung should increase as the lung volume decreases. If this were true, lung volume should decrease in a vicious cycle, with the tendency to collapse increasing progressively as the lung volume diminished.

These two problems are resolved by the fact that the surface tension of the fluid lining the alveoli is variable and decreases as its surface area is reduced. The surface tension of alveolar fluid can reach levels that are well below the normal range for body fluids such as water and plasma. When an alveolus decreases in size, the surface tension of the lining fluid falls to a greater extent than the corresponding reduction of radius, so that the transmural pressure gradient (= 2T/R) diminishes. This explains why small alveoli do not discharge their contents into large alveoli (Fig. 3–16B) and why the elastic recoil of small alveoli is less than that of large alveoli.

The substance responsible for the reduction (and variability) of alveolar surface tension is secreted by the intra-alveolar type II pneumocyte and is a lipoprotein called surfactant that floats as a 50-Å thick film on the surface of the alveolar-lining fluid. When the surface film is reduced in area and the concentration of surfactant at the surface is increased, there is an

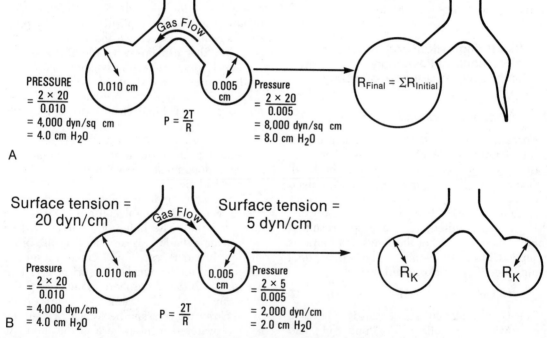

Figure 3–16. A, *Relationship between surface tension (T), alveolar radius (R), and alveolar transmural pressure (P). The diagram shows the pressure relations in two alveoli of different size but with the same surface tension in their lining fluids. The direction of gas flow will be from the higher pressure small alveolus to the lower pressure large alveolus and the result is one large alveolus (R*$_{Final}$ = ΣR$_{Initial}$*). B, The pressure relations of two alveoli of different size when allowance is made for the expected changes in surface tension. The direction of gas flow is from the larger alveolus to the smaller alveolus until the two alveoli are of equal size and are volume stable (R*$_K$*). (ΣR = sum of all individual radii; K = constant.) (Modified with permission from Benumof JL: Respiratory physiology and respiratory function during anesthesia. In Miller RD (ed.): Anesthesia. 2nd ed. Churchill Livingstone, New York, 1983, chapter 32.)*

increased surface-reducing pressure that counteracts the surface tension of the fluid lining the alveoli.

2. Airway Resistance

In order for air to flow into the lungs, a pressure gradient must also be developed to overcome the nonelastic airway resistance of the lungs to air flow. The relationship between the pressure gradient (ΔP) and the rate of air flow ($\dot{V}$) is known as airway resistance (R) and is expressed as follows:

$$R(cm\ H_2O/L/sec) = \frac{\Delta P(cm\ H_2O)}{\Delta \dot{V}(L/sec)} \qquad (5)$$

The pressure gradient (ΔP) along the airway depends on the caliber of the airway and the rate and pattern of air flow. There are three main patterns of air flow; laminar flow occurs when the gas passes down parallel-sided tubes at less than a certain critical velocity. With laminar flow, the pressure drop down the tube is proportional to the flow rate and may be ·calculated from the equation derived by Poiseuille: $P = \dot{V} \times 8\ L \times u/\pi r^4 \times 980$, where P = pressure drop (in cm H_2O), $\dot{V}$ = volume flow rate (in ml/sec), L = length of tube (in cm), r = radius of tube (in cm), and u = viscosity (in poises).

When flow exceeds the critical velocity, it becomes turbulent. The significant feature of turbulent flow is that the pressure drop along the airway is no longer directly proportional to flow rate but is proportional to the square of flow rate according to the equation $P = \dot{V}^2 pfL/4\pi^2 r^5$, where p is a gas or fluid density term and f is a friction factor that depends on the roughness of the tube wall.[45] Thus, with increases in turbulent flow (and/or orifice flow, see immediately below) P increases much more than $\dot{V}$, and therefore R increases (see equation 5).

Orifice flow occurs at severe constrictions, such as a nearly closed larynx. In these situations the pressure drop is also proportional to the square of flow rate, but density replaces viscosity as the important factor in the numerator. This explains why low-density gas such as helium diminishes the resistance to flow (by threefold compared with air) in severe obstructiion of the upper airway.

Since the total cross-sectional area of the airways increases as branching occurs, the velocity of air flow decreases; laminar flow is therefore chiefly confined to the airways below the main bronchi. Orifice flow occurs at the larynx, and flow in the trachea is turbulent during most of the respiratory cycle. Viewing the preceding five equations, one can see that many factors obviously may affect the pressure drop down the airways during respiration. However, variations in diameter of the smaller bronchi and bronchioles are particularly critical (bronchoconstriction may convert laminar flow to turbulent flow), and the pressure drop along the airways may become much more related to flow rate.

3. Different Regional Lung Time Constants

So far, the compliance and airway resistance properties of the chest have been discussed separately. In the following analysis, the pressure at the mouth is assumed to increase suddenly to a fixed positive value (Fig. 3–17)[46] that overcomes both elastic and airway resistance and is maintained at this value during inflation of the lungs. As shown in Figure 3–17, the pressure gradient required to overcome nonelastic airway resistance is the difference between the fixed mouth pressure and the instantaneous height of the dashed line and is proportional to the flow rate during most of the respiratory cycle. Thus, the pressure gradient required to overcome nonelastic airway resistance is maximal initially but then decreases exponentially (Fig. 3–17A, hatched lines). The rate of filling, therefore, also declines in an approximately exponential manner. The remainder of the pressure gradient overcomes the elastic resistance (the instantaneous height of the dashed line in Fig. 3–17A) and is proportional to the change in lung volume. Thus, the pressure gradient required to overcome elastic resistance is minimal initially but then increases exponentially (as does lung volume). Alveolar filling ceases (lung volume remains constant) when the pressure resulting from the retractive elastic forces balances the applied (mouth) pressure (Fig. 3–17A, dashed line).

Since there is only a finite time available for alveolar filling, and alveolar filling occurs in an exponential manner, the degree of filling is obviously dependent on the duration of the inspiration. The rapidity of change in an exponential curve can be described by its time constant Tau (τ). Tau (τ) is the time required to complete 63 per cent of an exponentially changing function if the total time allowed for the function change is unlimited ($2\ \tau = 87$ per

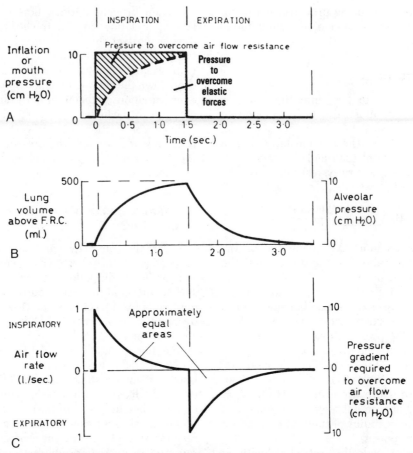

Figure 3–17. Artificial ventilation by intermittent application of a constant pressure (square wave). Expiration is passive. The pressure required to overcome airway resistance (hatched lines, A) and airflow rate (V̇ of equation 5, see panel C), which are proportional to one another, decreases exponentially. The pressure required to overcome elastic resistance (height of dashed line, panel A) and lung volume (see panel B), which are proportional to one another, increases exponentially. Values shown are typical for an anesthetized supine paralyzed patient: total dynamic compliance, 50 ml/cm H_2O; pulmonary resistance, 3 cm H_2O/L/sec; apparatus resistance, 7 cm H_2O/L/sec; total resistance, 10 cm H_2O/L/sec; time constant, 0.5 sec. (Reprinted by permission of the publisher, from Nunn JF: Applied Respiratory Physiology. 2nd ed. London, Butterworths (Publishers) Ltd, 1977.)

cent, $3 \tau = 95$ per cent, and $4 \tau = 99$ per cent). For lung inflation $\tau = C_T \times R$; normally, $C_T = 0.1$ L/cm H_2O, $R = 2.0$ cm H_2O/L/sec, and $\tau = 0.2$ sec and $3 \tau = 0.6$ sec.

Applying this equation to individual alveolar units, the time taken to fill such a unit clearly increases as airway resistance increases. The time to fill an alveolar unit also increases as compliance increases, since a greater volume of air will be transferred into a more compliant alveolus before the retractive force equals the applied pressure. The compliance of individual alveoli differs from the top to bottom of the lung, and the resistance of individual airways will vary widely depending on their length and caliber. Therefore, a wide variety of time constants for inflation exists throughout the lung.

4. The Work of Breathing

The pressure-volume characteristics of the lung also determine the work of breathing. Since

$$\text{Work} = \text{Force} \times \text{Distance}$$
$$\text{and}$$
$$\text{Force} = \text{Pressure} \times \text{Area}$$
$$\text{and}$$
$$\text{Distance} = \text{Volume/Area}$$

$$\text{Work} = (\text{Pressure} \times \text{Area})(\text{Volume/Area}) = \quad (6)$$
$$\text{Pressure} \times \text{Volume}$$

and ventilatory work may be analyzed by plotting pressure against volume.[47]

Two different pressure-volume diagrams are

shown in Figure 3–18. During normal inspiration (left graph) transpulmonary pressure increases from 0 to 5 cm H_2O while 500 ml of air is drawn into the lung. Potential energy is stored by the lung during inspiration and expended during expiration; as a consequence, the entire expiratory cycle is passive. The hatched area plus the triangular area ABC represents pressure multiplied by volume and is the work of breathing. Line AB is a section of the pressure-volume curve of Figure 3–6. The triangular area ABC is the work required to overcome elastic forces (C_T), whereas the hatched area is the work required to overcome air flow or frictional resistance (R). The graph on the right shows an anesthetized patient with diffuse obstructive disease due to the accumulation of mucous secretions. There is a marked increase in both the elastic (triangle AB′C) and airway (hatched area) resistive components of respiratory work. During expiration, only 250 ml of air leave the lungs during the passive

phase when intrathoracic pressure reaches the equilibrium value of 0 cm H_2O. Active effort-producing work is required to force out the remaining 250 ml of air, and intrathoracic pressure actually becomes positive.

For a constant minute volume, the work done against elastic resistance is increased when breathing is deep and slow. On the other hand, the work done against air flow resistance is increased when breathing is rapid and shallow. If the two components are summated and the total work plotted against the respiratory frequency, there is an optimal respiratory frequency at which the total work of breathing is minimal (Fig. 3–19).[48] In patients with diseased lungs, when elastic resistance is high (pulmonary fibrosis, pulmonary edema, infants), the optimum frequency is increased, and rapid shallow breaths are favored. When airway resistance is high (asthma, obstructive lung disease), the optimum frequency is decreased and slow deep breaths are favored.

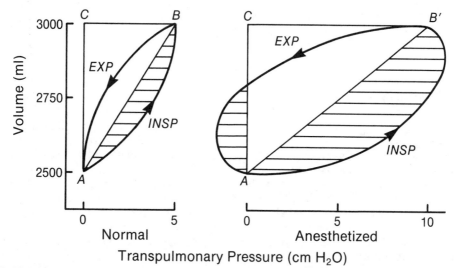

Figure 3–18. *Lung volume is plotted against transpulmonary pressure in a pressure volume diagram for an awake (normal) and an anesthetized patient. The lung compliance of the awake patient (slope of line AB = 100 ml/cm H_2O) equals that shown for the small dependent alveoli in Figure 3–6. The lung compliance of the anesthetized patient (slope of line AB′ = 50 ml/cm H_2O) equals that shown for the medium midlung alveoli in Figure 3–6 and for the anesthetized patient in Figure 3–17. The total area within the oval and triangles has the dimensions of pressure multiplied by volume and represents the total work of breathing. The hatched area to the right of lines AB and AB′ represents active inspiratory work necessary to overcome resistance to airflow during inspiration (INSP). The hatched area to the left of the triangle AB′C represents active expiratory work necessary to overcome resistance to airflow during expiration (EXP). Expiration is passive in the normal subject because sufficient potential energy is stored during inspiration to produce expiratory airflow. The fraction of total inspiratory work necessary to overcome elastic resistance is shown by the triangles ABC and AB′C. The anesthetized patient has a decreased compliance and increased elastic resistance work (triangle AB′C) compared with the normal patient's compliance and elastic resistance work (triangle ABC). The anesthetized patient shown in this figure has an increased airway resistance to both inspiratory and expiratory work. (Reproduced with permission from Benumof JL: Respiratory physiology and respiratory function during anesthesia. In Miller RD (ed.): Anesthesia. 2nd ed. Churchill Livingstone, New York, 1983, chapter 32.)*

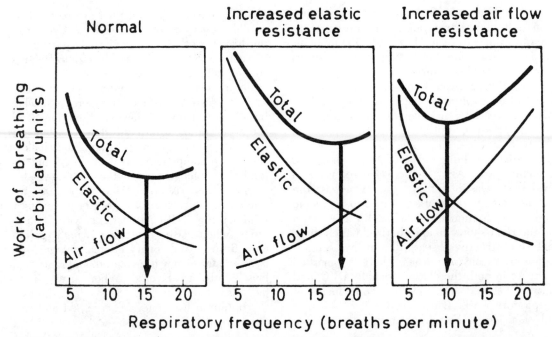

Figure 3–19. *The diagrams show the work done against elastic and airflow resistance separately and are summated to indicate the total work of breathing at different respiratory frequencies. The total work of breathing has a minimum value at about 15 breaths per minute under normal circumstances. For the same minute volume, minimum work is performed at higher frequencies with stiff (less compliant) lungs and at lower frequencies when the airflow resistance is increased. (Reprinted by permission of the publisher, from Nunn JF: Applied Respiratory Physiology. 2nd ed. London, Butterworths (Publishers) Ltd, 1977.)*

5. Lung Volumes, the Functional Residual Capacity, and the Closing Capacity

a. LUNG VOLUMES AND THE FUNCTIONAL RESIDUAL CAPACITY

The functional residual capacity (FRC) is defined as the volume of gas in the lung that exists at the end of a normal expiration when there is no air flow and alveolar pressure equals the ambient pressure. Under these conditions, expansive chest wall elastic forces are exactly balanced by retractive lung tissue elastic forces (Fig. 3–20).[49]

The expiratory reserve volume is part of the FRC and is that additional gas beyond the end-tidal volume that can be consciously exhaled and results in the minimum volume of lung possible, known as the residual volume. Thus, the FRC equals the residual volume plus the expiratory reserve volume (Fig. 3–21). With regard to the other lung volumes shown in Figure 3–21, tidal volume, vital capacity, inspiratory capacity, inspiratory reserve volume, and expiratory reserve volume can all be measured by simple spirometry. Total lung volume, FRC, and residual volume all contain a fraction (the residual volume) that cannot be measured by simple spirometry. However, if one of these three volumes is measured, the others can be easily derived because the other lung volumes, which relate these three volumes to one another, can be meaured by simple spirometry.

FRC can be measured by one of three techniques. The first method is to wash the N_2 out of the lungs by several minutes of O_2 breathing with measurement of the total quantity of N_2 eliminated. Thus, if 2 L of N_2 are eliminated and the initial alveolar N_2 concentration was 80 per cent, it follows that the initial volume of the lung was 2.5 L. The second method uses the wash-in of a tracer gas such as helium. If 50 ml of helium is introduced into the lungs and the helium concentration is then found to be 1 per cent, it follows that the volume of the lung is 5 L. The third method of measurement of FRC uses Boyle's law; namely, PV = K, where P = pressure, V = volume, and K = a constant. The subject is confined within a gas-tight box (plethysmograph) so that changes in the volume of his body may be readily determined as a change in pressure within the box. Disparity between FRC as measured in the body plethysmograph and by the helium

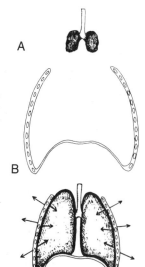

Figure 3–20. A, The resting state of normal lungs when they are removed from the chest cavity; i.e., elastic recoil causes total collapse. B, The resting state of a normal chest wall and diaphragm when the thoracic apex is open to the atmosphere and the thoracic contents are removed. C, The lung volume that exists at the end of expiration—the functional residual capacity. At functional residual capacity the elastic forces of lung and chest walls are equal and in opposite directions. The pleural surfaces link these two opposing forces. (Reproduced with permission from Shapiro BA, Harrison RA, Trout CA: Clinical Application of Respiratory Care. 2nd ed. Copyright 1979 by Year Book Medical Publishers, Inc., Chicago.)

method is often used as a way of detecting large, nonventilating air-trapped blebs.[50] Obviously, there are difficulties in the application of the body plethysmograph to anesthetized patients.

b. AIRWAY CLOSURE AND CLOSING CAPACITY

As discussed in the section Distribution of Ventilation, pleural pressure increases from the top to the bottom of the lung and determines regional alveolar size, complicance, and ventilation. Of even greater importance to the anesthesiologist is the recognition that these gradients in pleural pressure may lead to airway closure and collapse of alveoli.

i. **Airway Closure in Patients with Normal Lungs.** Figure 3–22A illustrates the normal resting end-expiratory (FRC) position of the lung–chest wall combination. The distending

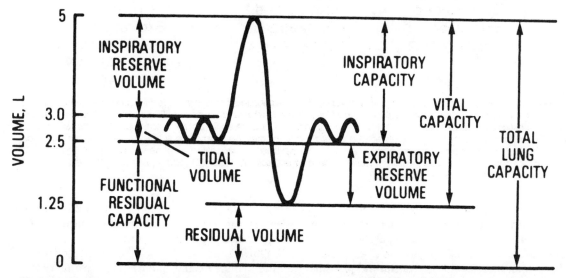

Figure 3–21. The dynamic lung volumes that can be measured by simple spirometry are the tidal volume, inspiratory reserve volume, expiratory reserve volume, inspiratory capacity, and vital capacity. The static lung volumes are the residual volume, functional residual capacity, and total lung capacity. The static lung volumes cannot be measured by observation of a spirometer trace and require separate methods of measurement. (Reproduced with permission from Benumof JL: Respiratory physiology and respiratory function during anesthesia. In Miller RD (ed.): Anesthesia. 2nd ed. Churchill Livingstone, New York, 1983, chapter 32.)

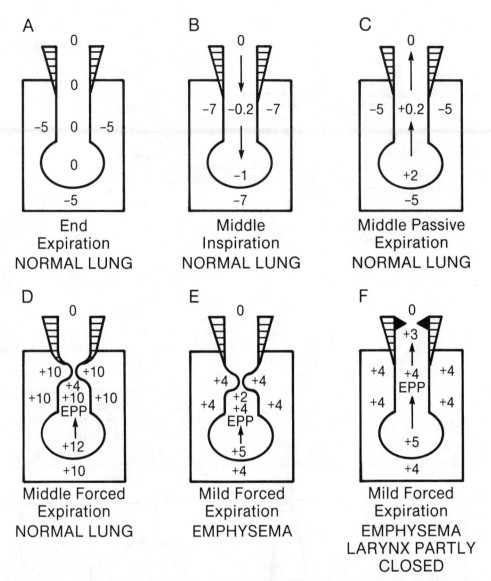

Figure 3–22. Pressure gradients across the airways. The airways consist of a thin-walled intrathoracic portion (near the alveoli) and a more rigid (cartilaginous) intrathoracic and extrathoracic portion. During expiration the pressure due to elastic recoil is assumed to be + 2 cm H_2O in normal lungs (A to D) and + 1 cm H_2O in abnormal lungs (E and F). The total pressure inside the alveolus is pleural pressure plus the elastic recoil. The arrows indicate direction of air flow. (EPP = equal pressure point.) See text for explanation. (Modified with permission from Benumof JL: Respiratory physiology and respiratory function during anesthesia. In Miller RD (ed.): Anesthesia. 2nd ed. Churchill Livingstone, New York, 1983, chapter 32.)

transpulmonary and the intrathoracic air passage transmural pressure gradients are 5 cm H_2O, and the airways remain patent. During the middle of a normal inspiration (Fig. 3–22B), there is an increase in the transmural pressure gradient (to 6.8 cm H_2O), which encourages distention of intrathoracic air passages. During the middle of a normal expiration (Fig. 3–22C), expiration is passive; alveolar pressure is caused only by the elastic recoil of the lung (2 cm

H_2O), and there is a decrease (to 5.2 cm H_2O) but still a favorable (distending) intraluminal transmural pressure gradient.

During the middle of a severe forced expiration (Fig. 3–22D), pleural pressure increases far above atmospheric pressure and is communicated to the alveoli, which have a pressure higher still owing to the elastic recoil of the alveolar septa (an additional 2 cm H_2O). At high gas flow rates, the pressure drop down the air passage is increased, and there will be a point at which intraluminal pressure equals either surrounding parenchymal or pleural pressure; that point is termed the equal pressure point (EPP). If the EPP occurs in small intrathoracic air passages (distal to the eleventh generation the airways have no cartilage and are called bronchioles), they may be held open at that particular point by the tethering effect of the elastic recoil of the immediately adjacent or surrounding lung parenchyma. If the EPP occurs in large extrathoracic air passages (proximal to the eleventh generation the airways are called bronchi), they may be held open at that particular point by their cartilage. Downstream of the EPP (in either small or large airways) the transmural pressure gradient is reversed (-6 cm H_2O) and will result in airway closure. Thus, the patency of airways distal to the eleventh generation is a function of lung volume, and the patency of airways proximal to the eleventh generation is a function of intrathoracic (pleural) pressure. In extrathoracic bronchi with cartilage, the posterior membranous sheath appears to give first by invaginating into the lumen.[51] If lung volume was abnormally decreased (for example, due to splinting) and expiration was still forced, the caliber of the airways would be relatively reduced at all times, causing the equal pressure point and point of collapse to move progressively from larger to smaller air passages (closer to the alveolus).

In patients with normal lungs, airway closure may still occur even if exhalation is not forced, provided residual volume is approached close enough. Even in patients with normal lungs, as lung volume decreases during expiration toward residual volume, the small airways (0.5 to 0.9 mm in diameter) will show a progressive tendency to close, whereas larger airways still remain patent.[52, 53] Airway closure occurs first in the dependent lung regions (as recently directly observed by computed tomography),[54] since the distending transpulmonary pressure is less and the volume change during expiration is greater. The airway closure is most likely to occur in the dependent regions of the lung whether the patient is in the supine or lateral decubitus position.[54]

ii. Airway Closure in Patients with Abnormal Lungs. Airway closure occurs with milder active expiration, lower gas flow rates, and higher lung volumes and occurs closer to the alveolus in patients with emphysema, bronchitis, asthma, and pulmonary interstitial edema. In all four of these conditions airway resistance

is increased, causing a larger pressure decrease from the alveoli to the larger bronchi, thereby creating the potential for negative intrathoracic transmural pressure gradients and narrowed and collapsed airways. In addition, the structural integrity of the conducting airways may be diminished due to inflammation and scarring and, therefore, may close more readily for any given lung volume or transluminal pressure gradient.

In emphysema, the elastic recoil of the lung is reduced (to 1 cm H_2O in Fig. 3–22E), the air passages are poorly supported by the lung parenchyma, the point of airway resistance is close to the alveolus, and the transmural pressure gradient can become negative quickly. Therefore, during only a *mild* forced expiration in an emphysematous patient, the equal pressure point and the point of collapse are near the alveolus (Fig. 3–22E). Use of pursed lip or grunting expiration (the equivalents of partly closing the larynx during expiration), positive end-expiratory pressure, and a continuous positive airway pressure in an emphysematous patient restores a favorable (distending) intrathoracic air pressure transmural gradient (Fig. 3–22F). In bronchitis the airways are structurally weakened and may close when only a small negative transmural pressure gradient is present (as with a mild forced expiration). In asthma, the middle-sized airways are narrowed by bronchospasm, and if expiration is forced, they are further narrowed by a negative transmural pressure gradient. Finally, with pulmonary interstitial edema, perialveolar interstitial edema compresses alveoli and acutely decreases functional residual capacity; the peribronchial edema fluid cuffs (within the connective tissue sheaths around the larger arteries and bronchi) compress the bronchi and acutely increase closing volume.[55-57]

iii. The Measurement of Closing Capacity (CC). Closing capacity is a sensitive test of early small-airway disease and is performed by having the patient exhale to residual volume (Fig. 3–23).[58] An inhalation from residual volume toward total lung capacity is begun and at the beginning of the inhalation a bolus of tracer gas (^{133}Xe, helium) is injected into the inspired gas. During the initial part of this inhalation from residual volume, the first gas to enter the alveolus is the dead space gas and the tracer bolus. The tracer gas will only enter alveoli that are already open (presumably the apices of the lung, hatched lines, Fig. 3–23) and does not enter alveoli that are already closed (presum-

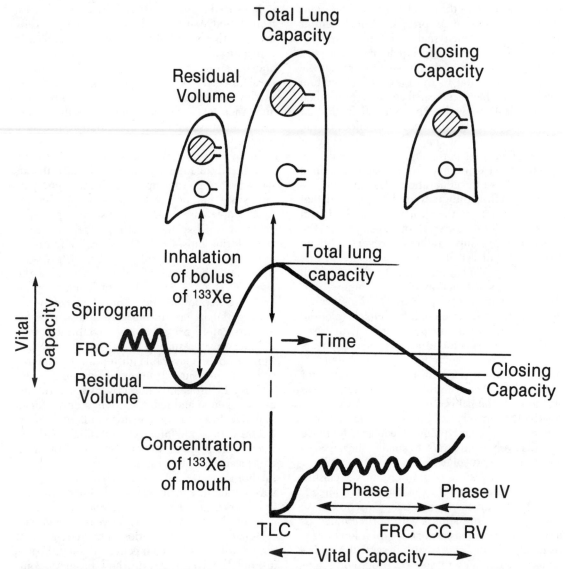

Figure 3–23. Measurement of closing capacity by the use of a tracer gas such as xenon-133 (^{133}Xe). The bolus of tracer gas is inhaled near residual volume and, because of airway closure in the dependent lung, is distributed only to those nondependent alveoli whose air passages are still open (shown hatched in diagram). During expiration, the concentration of the tracer gas becomes constant after the dead space is washed out. This plateau (phase III) gives way to a rising concentration of tracer gas (phase IV) when there is once again closure of the dependent airways because the only contribution made to the expired gas is by the high ^{133}Xe concentration nondependent alveoli. (Reprinted by permission of the publisher, from Nunn JF: Applied Respiratory Physiology. 2nd ed. London, Butterworths (Publishers) Ltd, 1977.)

ably the bases of the lung, no hatched lines, Fig. 3–23). As the inhalation continues, apical alveoli complete filling, and basilar alveoli begin to open and to fill, but with gas that does not contain any tracer gas.

A differential tracer gas concentration is thus established; the gas in the apices has a higher tracer concentration (Fig. 3–23, hatched lines) than that in the bases (Fig. 3–23, no hatched lines). As the subject exhales, and the dia-

phragm ascends, a point is reached at which the small airways just above the diaphragm start to close, limiting air flow from these areas. The air flow now comes more from the upper lung fields, where the alveolar gas has a much higher tracer concentration, thus resulting in a sudden increase in the tracer gas concentration toward the end of exhalation (phase IV).

The closing volume (CV) is the difference between the onset of phase IV and residual volume; since it represents part of a vital capacity maneuver, it is expressed as a per cent of the vital lung capacity. The CV plus the residual volume is known as the closing capacity (CC) and is expressed as a per cent of total lung capacity. Smoking, obesity, aging, and the supine position increase the CC.[59] In healthy individuals at a mean age of 44 years, CC = FRC in the supine position, and at a mean age of 66 years CC = FRC in the upright position.[60]

C. THE RELATIONSHIP BETWEEN THE FUNCTIONAL RESIDUAL CAPACITY AND THE CLOSING CAPACITY

The relationship between FRC and CC is far more important than consideration of the FRC or CC alone because it is the relationship between the two that determines whether a given respiratory unit is normal or atelectatic or has a low V̇/Q̇ ratio. The relationship between FRC and CC is as follows: When the volume of lung at which some airways close is greater than the whole of the tidal volume, then lung volume never increases enough during tidal inspiration to open any of these airways. Thus, these airways stay closed during all of the tidal respiration. Airways that are closed all of the time are equivalent to atelectasis (Fig. 3–24). If the closing volume of some airways lies within the tidal volume, then as lung volume increases during inspiration, some previously closed airways will open for a short period of time until lung volume once again recedes below the closing volume of these airways. Since these opening and closing airways are open for a shorter period of time than normal airways, they have less chance or time to participate in fresh gas exchange, which is a circumstance equivalent to a low ventilation-perfusion region. If the closing volume of the lung is below the whole of tidal respiration, then no airways are closed at any time during tidal respiration; this is a normal circumstance. Anything that decreases FRC relative to CC or increases CC relative to FRC will convert normal areas to low V̇/Q̇ and atelectatic areas. Development of low V̇/Q̇ and atelectatic areas will cause hypoxemia.

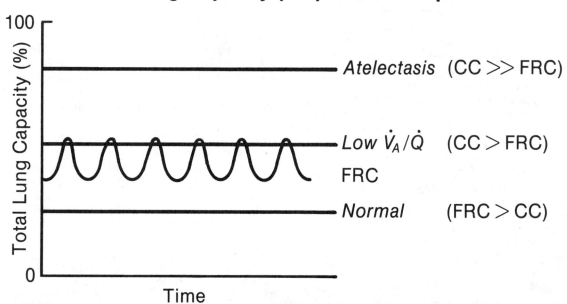

Functional Residual Capacity (FRC) to Closing Capacity (CC) Relationship

Figure 3–24. *The relationship between the functional residual capacity (FRC) (which is the per cent of total lung capacity that exists at the end of the exhalation), shown by the level of each trough of the sine wave tidal volume, and the closing capacity (CC) of the lung (three different closing capacities are indicated by the three different straight lines). The abscissa is time. See text for explanation of why the three different functional residual capacity to closing capacity relationships depicted result in normal, or low ventilation-perfusion ratios (V̇$_A$/Q̇), or atelectasis. (Modified with permission from Benumof JL: The pulmonary circulation. In Kaplan JA (ed.): Thoracic Anesthesia. New York, Churchill Livingstone, 1983, chapter 7.)*

The theory of the $FRC-CC-P_aO_2$ relationship has been quantitatively confirmed in a study in which patients with varying initial FRC-CC relationships were moved from the seated to the supine position (thereby decreasing FRC).[61] In this study,[61] subjects were divided into four groups. In group 1, FRC exceeded CV in both the supine and erect positions. In group 2, FRC exceeded CV only in the seated position. In group 3, CV occurred within the tidal volume in the seated position and exceeded the tidal volume in the supine position. In group 4, CV occurred above the tidal volume in both positions.

Group 1 subjects, whose tidal breathing was above the level of the CV in both postures, showed improved gas exchange in the supine position. This was explained by the presumed improvement in overall uniformity of $\dot{V}_A/\dot{Q}$ and by the observed increase in cardiac output. In group 2 subjects, FRC was greater than CV in the erect position and less than CV in the supine position. The $P(A-a)O_2$ and shunt increased upon changing posture from erect to supine (presumably owing to conversion of normal units to low $\dot{V}/\dot{Q}$ and atelectatic units). In group 3 subjects, CV occurred within the tidal breathing range in the erect position, and the erect $P(A-a)O_2$ and shunt were similar to those of group 2 subjects when supine, while a change to the supine position resulted in a further increase in $P(A-a)O_2$ and shunt fraction (presumably owing to conversion of normal units to low $\dot{V}/\dot{Q}$ and atelectatic units). In group 4 subjects, CV exceeded the whole of tidal respiration in the upright position. Changing to the supine position caused a significant increase in shunt and cardiac output, resulting in no significant change in $P(A-a)O_2$. Thus, the change in cardiac output (and perhaps more uniform lung perfusion) counteracted further airway closure.

The reason mechanical intermittent positive-pressure breathing (IPPB) may be efficacious is that it can take a previously spontaneously breathing patient with a low ventilation-perfusion relationship (where the closing capacity is greater than FRC but still within the tidal volume, as depicted in Fig. 3–25A) and increase the amount of inspiratory time that some previously closed (at end-exhalation) airways spend in fresh gas exchange and thereby increase the ventilation-perfusion relationship (Fig. 3–25B). However, if positive end-expiratory pressure (PEEP) is added to the IPPB, the PEEP increases FRC above or to a lung volume greater than closing capacity and thereby restores a normal FRC-to-closing capacity relationship so that no airways are closed at any time during the tidal respiration, as depicted in Figure 3–25C (IPPB + PEEP). Thus, anesthesia-induced crescent-shaped densities in the dependent regions of patients' lungs have not been reversed with IPPB alone but have been reversed with IPPB + PEEP (5 to 10 cm H_2O).[54]

E. Oxygen and Carbon Dioxide Transport

1. Alveolar and Dead Space Ventilation and Alveolar Gas Tensions

In patients with normal lungs, approximately two thirds of each breath reaches perfused alveoli and thereby takes part in gas exchange. This constitutes the effective or alveolar ventilation. The remaining one third of each breath takes no part in gas exchange and is therefore termed the total (or effective or physiologic) dead space ventilation. The total dead space ventilation may be divided into two components: a volume of gas that ventilates the conducting airways (the anatomic dead space ventilation) and a volume of gas that ventilates unperfused alveoli (e.g., as in zone 1, pulmonary embolus, and destroyed alveolar septae) and therefore does not take part in gas exchange (the alveolar dead space ventilation). Figure 3–26 shows a two-compartment model of the lung in which the anatomic and alveolar dead space compartments have been combined into the total (physiologic) dead space compartment; the other compartment is the alveolar ventilation ($\dot{V}_A$) compartment, whose idealized ventilation-perfusion ratio is 1.0.*

The anatomic dead space varies with lung size and is approximately 2 ml/kg body weight. In the normal patient lying supine, the anatomic and total dead spaces are approximately equal to each other because alveolar dead space is minimal. In the erect posture, the uppermost

---

*Figure 3–26 indicates that in a steady state the volume of CO_2 entering the alveoli ($\dot{V}CO_2$) must equal the volume of CO_2 eliminated in the expired gas ($\dot{V}_E$) ($F_{\bar{E}}CO_2$). Hence: $\dot{V}CO_2 = (\dot{V}_E)$ ($F_{\bar{E}}CO_2$). But the expired gas volume consists of alveolar gas ($\dot{V}_A$) (F_ACO_2) and dead space gas ($\dot{V}_D$) (F_ICO_2). Hence: $\dot{V}CO_2 = (\dot{V}_A)$ (F_ACO_2) + ($\dot{V}_D$) (F_ICO_2). Setting the first equation equal to the second equation and using the relationship $\dot{V}_E = \dot{V}_A + \dot{V}_D$, subsequent algebraic manipulation (including setting $P_ACO_2 = P_aCO_2$) results in the physiologic dead space equation: $\dot{V}_D/\dot{V}_T = (P_aCO_2 - P_{\bar{E}}CO_2)/P_aCO_2$

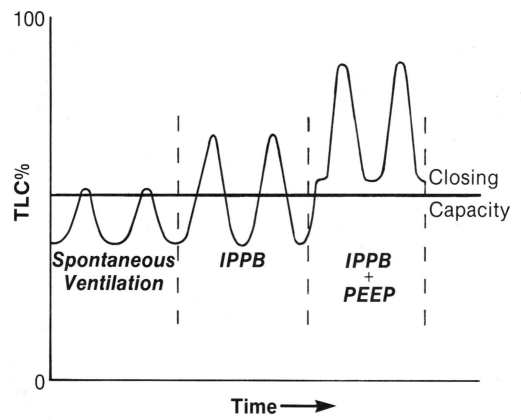

Figure 3–25. *The functional residual capacity to closing capacity relationship during spontaneous ventilation (SPON), intermittent positive pressure breathing (IPPB), and intermittent positive pressure breathing and positive end-expiratory pressure (IPPB and PEEP). See text for explanation of the effect of the two ventilatory maneuvers (IPPB and PEEP) on the functional residual capacity to closing capacity relationship. (TLC = total lung capacity.) (Reproduced with permission from Benumof JL: Respiratory physiology and respiratory function during anesthesia. In Miller RD (ed.): Anesthesia. 2nd ed. Churchill Livingstone, New York, 1983, chapter 32.)*

Figure 3–26. *Two compartment model of lung in which the anatomical and alveolar dead space compartments have been combined onto the total (physiological) dead space ($\dot{V}_D$). $\dot{V}_A$ = alveolar ventilation; $\dot{V}_E$ = expired minute ventilation; $\dot{V}_{CO_2}$ = carbon dioxide production; F_ICO_2 = inspired carbon dioxide fraction; F_ACO_2 = alveolar carbon dioxide fraction; F_ECO_2 = mixed expired carbon dioxide fraction; and $\dot{V}_A/\dot{Q} = 1$, equal ventilation and perfusion in L/min.) Normally, the amount of CO_2 eliminated at the airway ($\dot{V}_E \cdot F_ECO_2$) equals the amount of CO_2 removed by alveolar ventilation ($\dot{V}_A \cdot F_ACO_2$), since there is no CO_2 elimination from alveolar dead space ($F_ICO_2 = 0$). (Modified with permission from Benumof JL: Respiratory physiology and respiratory function during anesthesia. In Miller RD (ed.): Anesthesia. 2nd ed. Churchill Livingstone, New York, 1983, chapter 32.)*

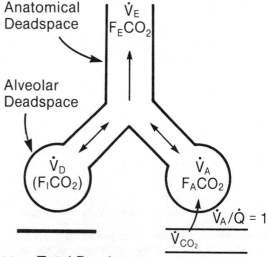

alveoli may not be perfused (zone 1), and alveolar dead space may increase from a negligible amount to 60 to 80 ml.

In severe lung disease, the physiologic dead space–to–tidal volume ratio $\dot{V}_D/\dot{V}_T$ provides a useful expression of the inefficiency of ventilation. In the normal patient, this ratio is usually less than 30 per cent; i.e., ventilation is more than 70 per cent efficient. In the patient with obstructive airway disease, $\dot{V}_D/\dot{V}_T$ may increase to 60 to 70 per cent. Under these conditions, ventilation is obviously grossly inefficient. Figure 3–27 shows the relation between minute ventilation $(\dot{V}_E)$ and $\dot{V}_D/\dot{V}_T$ for several P_aCO_2 values. If $\dot{V}_E$ is constant and $\dot{V}_D/\dot{V}_T$ increases, P_aCO_2 increases. If $\dot{V}_D/\dot{V}_T$ is constant and $\dot{V}_E$ increases, P_aCO_2 decreases. If P_aCO_2 is to remain constant while $\dot{V}_D/\dot{V}_T$ increases, then $\dot{V}_E$ must increase.

The alveolar concentration of a gas is equal to the difference between the inspired concentration of a gas and the ratio of the output (or uptake) of the gas to the $\dot{V}_A$. Thus, for gas X, $P_AX = (P_{dry\ atm})\ [F_IX \pm \dot{V}X\ (\text{output or uptake})]/\dot{V}_A$, where P_AX = alveolar partial pressure of gas X; F_IX = inspired concentration of gas X; $P_{dry\ atm}$ = dry atmospheric pressure = $P_{wet\ atm} - P_{H2O} = 760 - 47 = 713$ torr; $\dot{V}X$ = output or uptake of gas X; $\dot{V}_A$ = alveolar ventilation. For CO_2, $P_ACO_2 = 713\ (F_ICO_2 + \dot{V}CO_2/\dot{V}_A)$. Since $F_ICO_2 = 0$, and using standard conversion factors,

$$P_ACO_2 = 713\ [\dot{V}CO_2\ (\text{ml/min STPD})/\dot{V}_A\ (\text{L/min/BTPS})\ (0.863)]. \tag{7}$$

For example, 36 mm Hg = (713) (200/4000)

For O_2:

$$P_AO_2 = 713\ [F_IO_2 - \dot{V}O_2\ (\text{ml/min})/\dot{V}_A\ (\text{ml/min})] \tag{8}$$

For example, 100 mm Hg = 713 (0.21 − 225/3200)

Figure 3–28 shows the hyperbolic relationships expressed in equations 7 and 8 between P_aCO_2 and $\dot{V}_A$ and between P_AO_2 and $\dot{V}_A$ for different levels of $\dot{V}CO_2$ and $\dot{V}O_2$, respectively. P_aCO_2 is substituted for P_ACO_2, since P_ACO_2 to P_aCO_2 gradients are small (as opposed to P_AO_2 to P_aO_2 gradients, which can be large). Note that as $\dot{V}_A$ increases, the second term of the right-hand side of equations 7 and 8 approaches zero, and the composition of the alveolar gas approaches that of the inspired gas. In addition, it should be noted from Figure 3–27 that since anesthesia is usually administered with an O_2-enriched gas mixture, hypercarbia is a more common result of hypoventilation than hypoxemia.

2. Oxygen Transport

a. THE OXYGEN-HEMOGLOBIN DISSOCIATION CURVE

As a red blood cell (RBC) passes by the alveolus, oxygen diffuses into the plasma, increasing the partial pressure of oxygen (P_aO_2). As P_aO_2 increases, oxygen diffuses into the RBC and combines with hemoglobin. Each hemoglobin molecule consists of four heme molecules attached to a globin molecule. Each heme molecule consists of glycine, α-ketoglutaric acid, and iron (Fe) in the ferrous (Fe^{++}) form. Each ferrous ion has the capacity to bind with one oxygen molecule in a loose reversible combi-

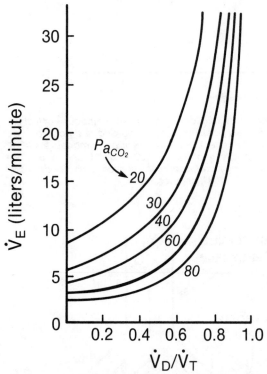

Figure 3–27. The relationship between the total dead space to tidal volume ratio ($\dot{V}_D/\dot{V}_T$) and the minute ventilation ($\dot{V}_E$, L/min) required to maintain P_aCO_2 levels of 20, 30, 40, 60, and 80 torr. These curves are hyperbolic and rise steeply at high $\dot{V}_D/\dot{V}_T$ values. It is apparent from this graph that if a patient with a high $\dot{V}_D/\dot{V}_T$ (for example, 0.65) accepts a P_aCO_2 of 60 torr rather than work to maintain a P_aCO_2 at 40 torr, the patient will save a great deal of $\dot{V}_E$ work (7 L/min in this example). (Reproduced with permission from Benumof JL: Respiratory physiology and respiratory function during anesthesia. In Miller RD (ed.): Anesthesia. 2nd ed. Churchill Livingstone, New York, 1983, chapter 32.)

nation. As the ferrous ions bind to oxygen, the hemoglobin molecule begins to become saturated.

The oxygen-hemoglobin dissociation (oxy-Hb) curve relates the saturation of hemoglobin (y-axis most right in Fig. 3–29) to the P_aO_2. Hemoblogin (Hb) is fully saturated (100 per cent) by a PO_2 of about 700 mm Hg. The normal arterial point on the right side and flat part of the oxy-Hb curve in Figure 3–27 is 95 to 98 per cent saturation by a P_aO_2 of about 90 to 100 mm Hg. When the PO_2 is less than 60 mm Hg (90 per cent saturation), the saturation falls steeply, so that the amount of Hb uncombined with O_2 increases greatly for a given decrease in PO_2. Mixed venous blood has a PO_2 ($P_\bar{v}O_2$) of about 40 mm Hg and is approximately 75 per cent saturation and is indicated by the middle of the three points on the oxy-Hb curve in Figure 3–28.

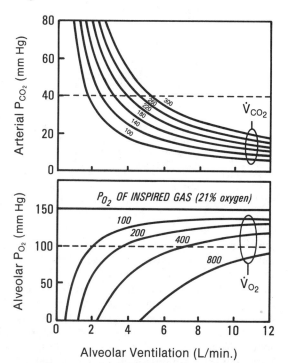

Figure 3–28. *The relationship between alveolar ventilation and alveolar PO_2 and arterial PCO_2 for a family of different O_2 consumption ($\dot{V}O_2$) and CO_2 production ($\dot{V}CO_2$) is derived from equations 7 and 8 in the text and is hyperbolic. Note that as alveolar ventilation increases, the alveolar PO_2 and arterial PCO_2 approach inspired concentrations. Decreases in alveolar ventilation below 4 L/min are accompanied by precipitous decreases in alveolar PO_2 and increases in arterial PCO_2. If the inspired O_2 concentration is increased, then alveolar ventilation must decrease much more to produce hypoxemia. (Reprinted with modification by permission of the publisher, from Nunn JF: Applied Respiratory Physiology. 2nd ed. London, Butterworths (Publishers) Ltd, 1977.)*

The oxy-Hb curve can also relate the O_2 content (CO_2) (vol per cent, ml $O_2/0.1$ L of blood; y-axis second most right in Fig. 3–29) to the PO_2. Oxygen is carried in solution in the plasma, 0.003 ml O_2 per mm Hg $PO_2/0.1$ L, and combined with Hb, 1.39 ml O_2 per g Hb* to the extent (per cent) Hb is saturated. Thus:

$$CO_2 = (1.39)(Hb)(\% \text{ sat}) + 0.003(PO_2) \quad (9)$$

For a patient with a Hb of 15 g/0.1 L, P_aO_2 of 100 mm Hg, and $P_\bar{v}O_2$ of 40 mm Hg, $C_aO_2 = (1.39)(15)(1) + (0.003)(100) = 20.1 + 0.3 = 20.4$ ml $O_2/0.1$ L; $C_\bar{v}O_2 = (1.39)(15)(0.75) + (0.003)(40) = 15.1 + 0.1 = 15.2$ ml $O_2/0.1$ L. Thus, the normal arteriovenous O_2 content difference is approximately 5.2 ml/0.1 L.

The oxy-Hb curve can also relate the O_2 transport (L/min) to the peripheral tissues (y-axis third most right in Fig. 3–29) to the PO_2. This is obtained by multiplying O_2 content by the cardiac output ($\dot{Q}_t$) (O_2 transport = $\dot{Q}_t \times C_aO_2$). In order to do this multiplication one must convert the content unit of ml/0.1 L to ml/L by multiplying the usual O_2 content by 10 (results in ml of O_2/L of blood); subsequent multiplication of ml/L against $\dot{Q}_t$ in L/min yields ml/min. Thus, if $\dot{Q}_t = 5$ L/min and $C_aO_2 = 20.4$ ml $O_2/0.1$ L, then the arterial point corresponds to 1020 ml/min going to the periphery, and the venous point corresponds to 760 ml/min returning to the lungs, with $\dot{V}O_2 = 260$ ml/min.

The oxy-Hb curve can also relate the O_2 actually available to the tissues (y-axis most left in Fig. 3–29) as a function of PO_2. Of the 1000 ml/min of O_2 normally going to the periphery, 200 ml/min of O_2 cannot be extracted because it would lower the PO_2 below the level (rectangular dashed line in Fig. 3–27) at which organs such as the brain can survive; the O_2 available to the tissues is therefore 0.8 L/min. This is approximately three to four times the normal resting $\dot{V}O_2$. When $\dot{Q}_t = 5$ L/min, and the arterial saturation is less than 40 per cent, the total flow of O_2 to the periphery is reduced to 400 ml/min so that the available O_2 is now 200 ml/min and O_2 supply just equals O_2 demand. Consequently, with low arterial saturation, tissue demand can only be met by an increase in cardiac output or, in the longer term, by an increase in Hb concentration.

---

*Controversy exists over the magnitude of this number. Originally 1.34 had been used,[62] but with the determination of the molecular weight of hemoglobin (64,458) the theoretical value of 1.39 has become popular.[63] Following extensive human studies, Gregory observed in 1974 that the applicable value was 1.306 ml/g per cent in human adults.[64] Most of the literature still, however, utilizes 1.39.

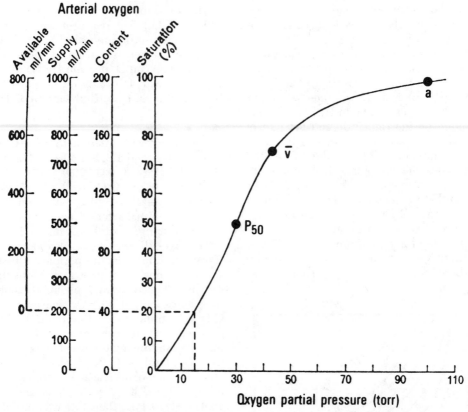

Figure 3–29. The oxygen-hemoglobin dissociation curve. Four different ordinates are shown as a function of oxygen partial pressure (the abscissa). In order of right to left, they are: saturation (%); O_2 content (ml O_2/0.1 L) of blood; O_2 supply to the peripheral tissues (ml/min); and O_2 available to the peripheral tissues (ml/min), which is O_2 supply minus approximately 200 ml/min that cannot be extracted below a partial pressure of 20 mm Hg. Three points are shown on the curve: a = normal arterial; v̄ = normal mixed venous; and P_{50} = the partial pressure (27 mm Hg) at which hemoglobin is 50 per cent saturated. (Reproduced with permission from Benumof JL: Respiratory physiology and respiratory function during anesthesia. In Miller RD (ed.): Anesthesia. 2nd ed. Churchill Livingstone, New York, 1983, chapter 32.)

The position of the oxy-Hb curve is best described by the Po_2 at which Hb is 50 per cent saturated (the P_{50}). The normal adult P_{50}, which is the point on the left side and steep portion of the oxy-Hb curve in Figure 3–29, is 26.7 mm Hg.

The effect of a shift in the position of the oxy-Hb curve on hemoglobin saturation depends greatly on the Po_2. In the region of the normal P_aO_2 (75 to 100 mm Hg), the curve is relatively horizontal, so that shifts of the curve have little effect on saturation. In the region of the mixed venous Po_2 where the curve is relatively steep, a shift of the curve leads to a much greater difference in saturation. A P_{50} of less than (<) 27 mm Hg describes a left-shifted oxy-Hb curve, which means that at any given Po_2, Hb has a higher affinity for O_2 and is therefore more saturated than normal. This may require a higher tissue perfusion than normal to produce the normal amount of O_2 unloading. The

causes of a left-shifted oxy-Hb curve are alkalosis (metabolic and respiratory, called the Bohr effect), hypothermia, abnormal and fetal hemoglobin, CO-Hb, methemoglobin, and decreased red blood cell 2,3-diphosphoglycerate (2,3-DPG) content (which may occur with transfusion of old acid-citrate-dextrose (ACD) stored blood; storage of blood in citrate-phosphate-dextrose (CPD) minimizes changes in 2,3-DPG with time).

A P_{50} of greater than (>) 27 mm Hg describes a right-shifted oxy-Hb curve, which means that at any given Po_2, Hb has a low affinity for O_2 and is less saturated than normal. This may allow a lower tissue perfusion than normal to produce the normal amount of O_2 unloading. The causes of a right-shifted oxy-Hb curve are acidosis (metabolic and respiratory, called the Bohr effect), hyperthermia, abnormal Hb, and increased red blood cell 2,3-DPG content.

Abnormalities in acid-base balance result in

alteration of 2,3-DPG metabolism to shift the oxyhemoglobin dissociation curve to its normal position. This "compensatory" change in 2,3-DPG requires between 24 and 48 hours. Thus, with acute acid-base abnormalities, oxygen affinity and the position of the oxy-Hb curve changes. However, with more prolonged acid-base changes, the altered levels of 2,3-DPG shift the oxy-Hb curve and, therefore, oxygen affinity back toward normal.

b. THE EFFECT OF $\dot{Q}_s/\dot{Q}_t$ ON P_aO_2

Figure 3–30[65] shows the relationship between F_IO_2 and P_aO_2 for a family of right-to-left transpulmonary shunts ($\dot{Q}_s/\dot{Q}_t$); the calculations assume a constant and normal cardiac output and P_aCO_2. With no $\dot{Q}_s/\dot{Q}_t$, a linear increase in F_IO_2 results in a linear increase in P_aO_2 (solid straight line). As shunt is increased, the $\dot{Q}_s/\dot{Q}_t$ lines relating F_IO_2 to P_aO_2 become progressively flatter.[66] With a shunt of 50 per cent of the cardiac output, an increase in F_IO_2 results in almost no

increase in P_aO_2. Thus, it is obvious that the solution to the problem of hypoxemia secondary to a large shunt is not simply increasing the F_IO_2 but rather causing a reduction in shunt (fiberoptic bronchoscopy, PEEP, patient positioning, antibiotics, suctioning, and diuretics).

c. THE EFFECT OF $\dot{Q}_t$ AND $\dot{V}O_2$ ON C_aO_2

In addition to an increased $\dot{Q}_s/\dot{Q}_t$, the C_aO_2 is decreased by a decreased $\dot{Q}_t$ (for a constant $\dot{V}O_2$) and by an increased $\dot{V}O_2$ (for a constant $\dot{Q}_t$). In either case (decreased $\dot{Q}_t$ or increased $\dot{V}O_2$), along with a constant right-to-left shunt, the tissues must extract more O_2 from the blood per unit blood volume, and, therefore, the O_2 content of mixed venous blood ($C_{\bar{v}}O_2$) must primarily decrease (Fig. 3–31). When the blood with lower $C_{\bar{v}}O_2$ passes through whatever shunt that exists in the lung and remains unchanged in its oxygen composition, it must inevitably mix with oxygenated end-pulmonary

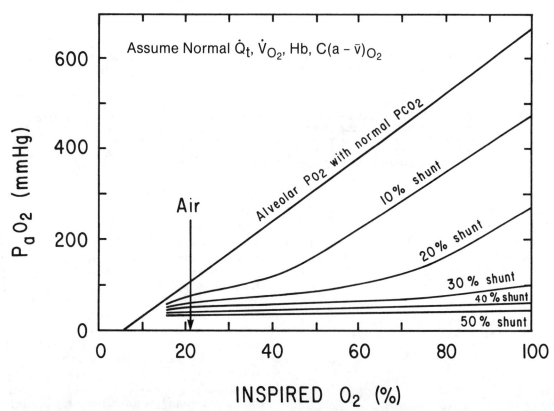

Figure 3–30. Effect of changes in inspired oxygen concentration on arterial Po₂ for various right to left transpulmonary shunts. Cardiac output (Q̇ₜ), hemoglobin (Hb), oxygen consumption (V̇o₂), and arteriovenous oxygen content differences (C[a-v]O₂) were assumed to be normal. (Modified from Nunn JF: Applied Respiratory Physiology. 1st ed. London, Butterworths (Publishers) Ltd, 1977. Reprinted by permission of the publisher, Butterworths.)

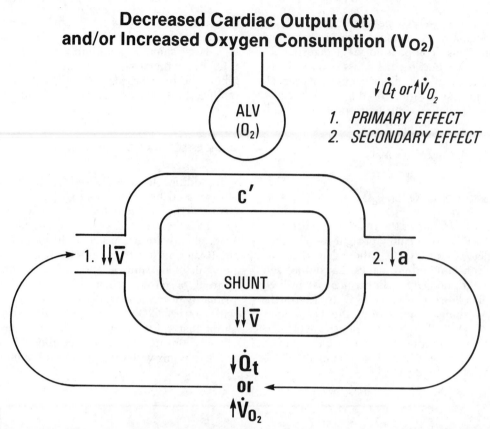

Figure 3–31. *Effect of a decrease in cardiac output or an increase in oxygen consumption on mixed venous and arterial oxygen contents. Mixed venous blood ($\bar{v}$) perfuses either ventilated alveolar (ALV O_2) capillaries and becomes oxygenated end-pulmonary capillary blood (c') or perfuses whatever true shunt pathways exist and remains the same in composition (desaturated). These two pathways must ultimately join together to form mixed arterial (a) blood. If the cardiac output ($\dot{Q}_t$) decreases and/or the oxygen consumption ($\dot{V}o_2$) increases, the tissues must extract more oxygen per unit volume of blood than under normal conditions. Thus, the primary effect of a decrease in $\dot{Q}_t$ or an increase in $\dot{V}o_2$ is a decrease in mixed venous oxygen content. The mixed venous blood with a decreased oxygen content must flow through the shunt pathway as before (which may remain constant in size) and lower the arterial content of oxygen. Thus, the secondary effect of a decrease in $\dot{Q}_t$ or an increase in $\dot{V}o_2$ is a decrease in arterial oxygen content. (Reproduced with permission from Benumof JL: Respiratory physiology and respiratory function during anesthesia. In Miller RD (ed.): Anesthesia. 2nd ed. Churchill Livingstone, New York, 1983, chapter 32.)*

capillary blood (c' flow) and secondarily decrease the C_aO_2 (Fig. 3–31).*

Figure 3–32 shows an example of a patient with a 50 per cent shunt, a normal $C_{\bar{v}}O_2$ of 15 vol per cent, and a moderately low C_aO_2 of 17.5

---

*The amount of O_2 flowing through any given channel per minute in Figure 3–29 is a product of the blood flow times the O_2 content. Hence, from Figure 3–29:

$$\dot{Q}_tC_{\bar{v}}O_2 \nearrow \overset{\dot{Q}_{c'}C_{c'}O_2}{\underset{\dot{Q}_sC_sO_2}{\searrow}} \nearrow \dot{Q}_tC_aO_2$$

$\dot{Q}_tC_aO_2 = \dot{Q}_{c'} \cdot C_{c'}O_2 + \dot{Q}_sC_{\bar{v}}O_2$. With $\dot{Q}_{c'} = \dot{Q}_t - \dot{Q}_s$ and further algebraic manipulation:[69]

$$\dot{Q}_s/\dot{Q}_t = C_{c'}O_2 - C_aO_2/C_{c'}O_2 - C_{\bar{v}}O_2 \quad (10)$$

vol per cent. Decreasing $\dot{Q}_t$ and/or increasing $\dot{V}o_2$ causes a larger primary decrease in $C_{\bar{v}}O_2$ to 10 vol per cent and a smaller, but still significant, secondary decrease in C_aO_2 to 15 vol per cent; the ratio of change in $C_{\bar{v}}O_2$ to C_aO_2 in this example of 50 per cent $\dot{Q}_s/\dot{Q}_t$ is 2:1.

Figure 3–33 shows the quantitative effect of decreasing $\dot{Q}_t$ on C_aO_2 for several different intrapulmonary shunts.[67, 68] The larger the intrapulmonary shunt, the greater is the decrease in C_aO_2 because more venous blood with lower $C_{\bar{v}}O_2$ can admix with end-pulmonary capillary blood.

Thus, the $P(A-a)O_2$ is a function of both the size of the $\dot{Q}_s/\dot{Q}_t$ and what is flowing through the $\dot{Q}_s/\dot{Q}_t$, namely $C_{\bar{v}}O_2$, and is a primary function of $\dot{Q}_t$ and $\dot{V}o_2$.

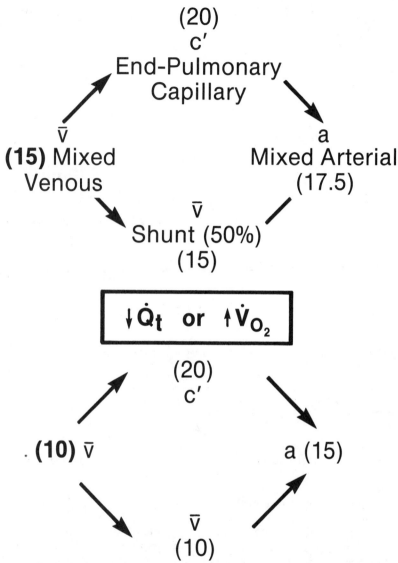

Figure 3–32. The equivalent circuit of the pulmonary circulation in a patient with a 50 per cent right-to-left shunt. Oxygen content is in ml/dl blood (vol %). A decrease in cardiac output ($\dot{Q}_t$) or an increase in O_2 consumption ($\dot{V}_{O_2}$) can cause a decrease in mixed venous oxygen content (from 15 vol % to 10 vol % in this example), which in turn will cause a decrease in the arterial content of oxygen (from 17.5 vol % to 15.0 vol %). In this 50 per cent shunt example, the decrease in mixed venous oxygen content was twice the decrease in arterial oxygen content. (Reproduced with permission from Benumof JL: Respiratory physiology and respiratory function during anesthesia. In Miller RD (ed.): Anesthesia. 2nd ed. Churchill Livingstone, New York, 1983, chapter 32.)

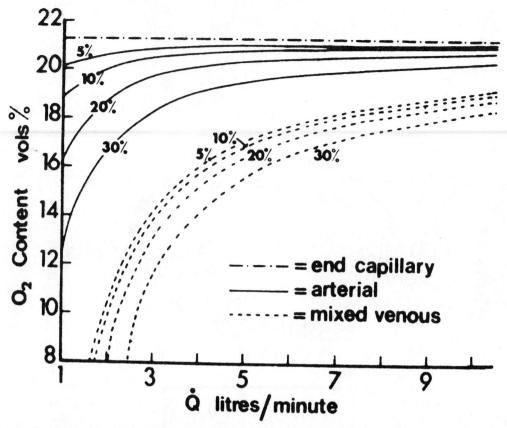

Figure 3–33. Effects of changes in cardiac output (Q̇) on the O_2 content of end-pulmonary capillary, arterial, and mixed venous blood for a family of different transpulmonary right-to-left shunts. The magnitude of the right-to-left shunt is indicated by the various numbered per cent symbols for arterial (solid line) and mixed venous blood (dashed line); the oxygen content of end-capillary blood is unaffected by the degree of shunting. Note that a decrease in Q̇ results in a greater decrease in the arterial content of O_2, the larger the shunt. (Modified with permission from Kelman GF, Nunn JF, Prys-Roberts C, et al: The influence of the cardiac output on arterial oxygenation: A theoretical study. Br J Anaesth 39:450, 1967.)

If a decrease in $\dot{Q}_t$ or an increase in $\dot{V}_{O_2}$ is accompanied by a decrease in $\dot{Q}_s/\dot{Q}_t$, then there may be no change in P_aO_2 (a decreasing effect on P_aO_2 is offset by an increasing effect on P_aO_2) (Table 3–1). These changes sometimes occur in diffuse lung disease. If a decrease in $\dot{Q}_t$ or an increase in $\dot{V}_{O_2}$ is accompanied by an increase in $\dot{Q}_s/\dot{Q}_t$, then P_aO_2 may be greatly decreased (a decreasing effect on P_aO_2 is compounded by another decreasing effect on P_aO_2) (Table 3–1). These changes sometimes occur in regional ARDS and atelectasis.[70]

d. The Fick Principle

The Fick principle allows for calculation of $\dot{V}_{O_2}$ and states that the amount of O_2 consumed by the body ($\dot{V}_{O_2}$ is equal to the amount of O_2 leaving the lungs ($\dot{Q}_t$) (C_aO_2) minus the amount of O_2 returning to the lungs ($\dot{Q}_t$) ($C_{\bar{v}}O_2$). Thus:

$$\dot{V}_{O_2} = (\dot{Q}_t)\,(C_aO_2) - (\dot{Q}_t)\,(C_{\bar{v}}O_2)$$
$$= \dot{Q}_t\,(C_aO_2 - C_{\bar{v}}O_2)$$

Condensing the content symbols yields the usual expression of the Fick equation:

$$\dot{V}_{O_2} = (\dot{Q}_t)\,[C(a - v)O_2] \qquad (11)$$

This equation states that oxygen consumption is equal to the cardiac output times the arteriovenous O_2 content difference. Normally (5 L/min) (5.2 ml)/0.1 L = 0.26 L/min (see section on oxy-Hb curve).

Similarly, the amount of O_2 consumed by the body ($\dot{V}_{O_2}$) is equal to the amount of O_2 brought into the lungs by ventilation ($\dot{V}_I$) (F_IO_2) minus the amount of O_2 leaving the lungs by ventilation ($\dot{V}_{\bar{E}}$) ($F_{\bar{E}}O_2$). Thus, $\dot{V}_{O_2} = (\dot{V}_I)\,(F_IO_2) -$

$(\dot{V}_E)$ $(F_{\bar{E}}O_2)$. Since the difference between $\dot{V}_I$ and $\dot{V}_E$ is due to the difference between $\dot{V}O_2$ (normally, 260 ml/min) and $\dot{V}CO_2$ (normally, 200 ml/min) and is only 60 ml/min (see below), $\dot{V}_I$ essentially equals $\dot{V}_E$; substituting $\dot{V}_E$ for $\dot{V}_I$:

$$\dot{V}O_2 = \dot{V}_E (F_IO_2) - \dot{V}_E (F_{\bar{E}}O_2) = \dot{V}_E (F_IO_2 - F_{\bar{E}}O_2) \quad (12)$$

For example and normally, $\dot{V}O_2 = 5.0$ L/min $(0.21 - 0.16) = 0.25$ L/min. In determining $\dot{V}O_2$ in this way, $\dot{V}_E$ can be measured with a spirometer, F_IO_2 can be measured with an O_2 analyzer or from known fresh gas flows, and $F_{\bar{E}}O_2$ can be measured by collecting expired gas in a bag over the course of a few minutes. A sample of the mixed expired gas is used to measure $P_{\bar{E}}O_2$. To convert $P_{\bar{E}}O_2$ to $F_{\bar{E}}O_2$, simply divide $P_{\bar{E}}O_2$ by dry atmospheric pressure: $P_{\bar{E}}O_2/713 = F_{\bar{E}}O_2$.

Additionally, the Fick equation is useful in understanding the impact of changes in $\dot{Q}_t$ on P_aO_2 and $P_{\bar{v}}O_2$. If $\dot{V}O_2$ remains constant (K) and $\dot{Q}_t$ decreases ($\downarrow$), then the arteriovenous O_2 content difference has to increase ($\uparrow$):

$$\dot{V}O_2 = K = (\downarrow)\dot{Q}_t \times (\uparrow)C(a - \bar{v})O_2.$$

The $C(a - \bar{v})O_2$ difference increases because a decrease in $\dot{Q}_t$ causes a much larger and primary decrease in $C_{\bar{v}}O_2$ compared with a smaller and secondary decrease in C_aO_2:

$$(\uparrow)C(a - \bar{v})O_2 = C(\downarrow a - \downarrow\downarrow\bar{v})O_2.^{67}$$

Thus, the $C_{\bar{v}}O_2$ (and $P_{\bar{v}}O_2$) are much more sensitive indicators of $\dot{Q}_t$, since they change more with the changes in $\dot{Q}_t$ than does C_aO_2 (and P_aO_2).

3. Carbon Dioxide Transport

The amount of CO_2 circulating in the body is a function of both CO_2 elimination and production. Elimination of CO_2 depends on pulmonary blood flow and alveolar ventilation. Production of CO_2 parallels oxygen consumption according to the respiratory quotient (R).

$$R = \frac{\text{Rate of Co}_2 \text{ output}}{\text{Rate of O}_2 \text{ uptake}} \quad (13)$$

Under normal resting conditions R is 0.8; i.e., only 80 per cent as much CO_2 is produced as O_2 is consumed. However, this value changes as the quality of metabolic substrate changes. If only carbohydrate is utilized, the respiratory quotient is 1.0. Conversely, with sole use of fat more O_2 combines with hydrogen to produce water, and the R value drops to 0.7.

Carbon dioxide is transported from the mitochondria to the alveolus in a number of forms. In plasma, CO_2 exists in physical solution and is hydrated to carbonic acid (H_2CO_3) and as bicarbonate (HCO_3^-). In the erythrocyte, CO_2 combines with hemoglobin as carbaminohemoglobin (Hb-CO_2). The approximate relative values of H_2CO_3 ($H_2O + CO_2$), HCO_3^-, and Hb-CO_2 to the total CO_2 transported is 7, 80, and 13 per cent, respectively.

In plasma, CO_2 exists both in physical solution and as H_2CO_3:

$$H_2O + CO_2 \rightleftarrows H_2CO_3 \quad (14)$$

The CO_2 in solution can be related to PCO_2 by use of Henry's law[71]:

$$PCO_2 \times \alpha = [CO_2] \text{ in solution} \quad (15)$$

In this equation, α is the solubility coefficient of CO_2 in plasma (0.03 mmol/L/mm Hg at 37°C). However, the major fraction of CO_2 produced passes into the erythrocyte. As in plasma, CO_2 combines with water to produce carbonic acid. However, unlike in plasma where the reaction is slow and most of the equilibrium is to the left, the reaction in the erythrocyte is catalyzed by the enzyme carbonic anhydrase. This zinc-containing enzyme moves the reaction to the right at a rate 1000 times faster than that in plasma. Further, nearly 99.9 per cent of the carbonic acid dissociates to the bicarbonate and hydrogen ions:

$$H_2O + CO_2 \xrightarrow{\text{carbonic anhydrase}} H_2CO_3$$

$$H_2CO_3 \longrightarrow H^+ + HCO_3^-$$

The hydrogen ion produced from H_2CO_3 in the production of HCO_3^- is buffered by hemo-

Table 3–1. Cardiac Output ($\dot{Q}_t$), Shunt ($\dot{Q}_s/\dot{Q}_t$), and Venous ($P_{\bar{v}}O_2$) and Arterial (P_aO_2) Oxygenation

Changes in $\dot{Q}_t$, $\dot{Q}_s/\dot{Q}_t$, $P_{\bar{v}}O_2$, P_aO_2	Clinical Situation
If $\dot{Q}_t \downarrow \rightarrow \downarrow P_{\bar{v}}O_2$ and $\dot{Q}_s/\dot{Q}_t = K \rightarrow P_aO_2 \downarrow$	Classic theory, normal lung
If $\dot{Q}_t \downarrow \rightarrow \downarrow P_{\bar{v}}O_2$ and $\dot{Q}_s/\dot{Q}_t \downarrow \rightarrow P_aO_2 = K$	Diffuse lung disease
If $\dot{Q}_t \downarrow \rightarrow \downarrow P_{\bar{v}}O_2$ and $\dot{Q}_s/\dot{Q}_t \uparrow \rightarrow P_aO_2 \downarrow\downarrow$	Regional ARDS and atelectasis

K = constant; $\downarrow$ = decrease; $\uparrow$ = increase.

globin (H^+ + Hb $\rightleftarrows$ HHb). The HCO_3^- produced passes out of the erythrocyte into the plasma to perform its function as a buffer. To maintain electrical neutrality within the erythrocyte, the chloride ion moves in as HCO_3^- moves out (chloride shift). Finally, CO_2 can combine with hemoglobin in the erythrocyte (to produce carbaminohemoglobin). Again, as in the HCO_3^- release, an H^+ is formed in the reaction of CO_2 and hemoglobin. This H^+ is also buffered by hemoglobin.

4. The Bohr and Haldane Effects

Just as the per cent saturation of hemoglobin with oxygen is related to Po_2, so is the total CO_2 in blood related to Pco_2. The Bohr effect is the dependence of the position of the oxygen-hemoglobin dissociation curve on Pco_2 and pH; hypercapnia and acidosis shift the curve to the right, and hypocapnia and alkalosis shift the curve to the left. The Haldane effect is the shift in the relationship of Pco_2 to total CO_2 (i.e., the CO_2 dissociation curve) caused by altered levels of oxygen. Low Po_2 shifts the CO_2 dissociation curve to the left so that the blood is able to pick up more CO_2.

F. Pulmonary Vascular Reflexes

Cardiopulmonary receptors, whose afferent fibers course in the cardiac sympathetic nerves, have been described in both of the right-sided cardiac chambers (75 per cent [of total]), both vena cavae (10 per cent), the pulmonary veins (5 per cent), the extrapulmonic portions of the pulmonary artery (5 per cent), and the coronary vessels (5 per cent). The discharge frequency of these cardiopulmonary sympathetic afferent fibers is augmented when the area containing the receptor is stretched by outflow occlusion, volume infusion, or inflation of an intracavity balloon, and it is decreased during an acute hemorrhage.[73-75] However, in contrast to the effect of carotid and aortic baroreceptor function ($\uparrow$ systemic blood pressure $\rightarrow$ $\uparrow$ baroreceptor discharge $\rightarrow$ $\uparrow$ inhibition of medullary cardiovascular center $\rightarrow$ systemic vasodilatation; and conversely, $\downarrow$ systemic blood pressure $\rightarrow$ $\downarrow$ baroreceptor discharge $\rightarrow$ $\downarrow$ inhibition of medullary cardiovascular center $\rightarrow$ systemic vasoconstriction) most studies have shown that stimulation of the central cardiopulmonary sympathetic afferents has a pressor effect on the cardiovascular system.[76-78] Pulmonary vascular

distention causes no change or only mild changes in airway tone.[79]

It has become clear that the pulmonary efferent sympathetic nerves are part of an extensive control system that can be stimulated centrally and reflexively to modify pulmonary vascular tone.[80-82] The effect of sympathetic stimulation is predominantly due to alpha-adrenergic receptor stimulation (alpha receptors predominate both numerically and functionally in the pulmonary circulation) and results in diminished distensibility (stiffening) of the pulmonary arterial tree.[82] The effects of pulmonary sympathetic nerve stimulation on the pulmonary vascular resistance (as opposed to distensibility) are not large, but in special circumstances they can be important. For example, distention of the main pulmonary artery by balloon inflation in the conscious dog reflexively produces constriction of pulmonary arterioles and possibly venules (pressure distal to the balloon increased from 21/6 to 43/14 mm Hg), and this is due to excitation of receptors located in the pulmonary artery or possibly the right side of the heart, or both.[79]

Although the effects of pulmonary sympathetic nerve stimulation are not ordinarily quantitatively large, they are vital for homeostasis during stress and exercise and for maintaining a precise balance between right and left ventricular outputs. An increase in right ventricular output causes an increase in pulmonary sympathetic nerve activity. The resultant increase in stiffness of the large pulmonary arteries increases the rate of transmission of a pulse wave of a given right ventricular beat to a level sufficiently rapid to cause an increase in the stroke volume of the subsequent left ventricular beat.[83]

Without this type of automatic adjustment, the increase in heart rate and cardiac output during exercise or excitement would alter the synchrony of the two ventricles and upset the balance in ventricular outputs. In canine studies, an abrupt onset of exercise (treadmill) without previous warning produces an increase in right ventricular stroke volume, which precedes an increase in left ventricular stroke volume by several beats.[84] Because of this asynchrony between the two ventricles, pulmonary blood volume has to increase (see section H below). However, when dogs are trained to anticipate the start of exercise, and sympathetic nervous activity is presumably heightened, the ventricular outputs change exactly in phase. Direct measurements in humans are consistent with these observations in dogs, since it has been shown that the pulmonary blood volume remains virtually unchanged during exercise.[85] In addition, it is now clear that during experimental excitation of the hypothalmic integrative area, which is necessary in order to produce or stimulate the defense reaction, the pulmonary sympathetic nerves are stimulated to produce moderate pulmonary vasoconstriction, with presumably similar secondary effects on balancing ventricular outputs.[80] On the other hand, there is virtually no effect of vagal stimulation on the pulmonary circulation.

G. Pulmonary Metabolism and Synthesis

It is now well established that the pulmonary circulation has two fundamentally and physiologically important pharmacokinetic functions.[86] First, the pulmonary circulation can inactivate or remove vasoactive substances from the venous blood (5-hydroxytryptamine [5-HT], bradykinin, norepinephrine (NE), prostaglandins [PGE_1, PGE_2, and PGF_2]), whereas other substances, often very closely related to each other as well as to the above substances, are

allowed free passage (epinephrine [E], angiotensin II, oxytocin, and vasopressin) (see Table 3–2). This function seems to be appropriate for the lung because in contrast to all other organs it receives the total venous return and is therefore in an ideal position to regulate the concentration of vasoactive substances in pulmonary capillary blood before they reach the arterial circulation and have profound systemic effects. Consequently, the lung can be thought of as a biochemical or metabolic filter.

The removal of some substances but not of others has led to the classification of vasoactive hormones as local or as circulating, depending upon whether they were removed by the lungs. A local hormone is released at or near the target cells, has its local effect, and is inactivated before reaching the arterial circulation. The inactivation of the hormone occurs either immediately in the tissues, within a few seconds in the venous blood, or within a few more seconds in the pulmonary circulation. It is now apparent that enzymatic degradation (5-HT, NE) and uptake processes (prostaglandins) play a part in the pulmonary inactivation processes for these substances. Defects in this metabolic function of the lung are definitely implicated in

Table 3–2. Handling of Biologically Active Materials in the Pulmonary Capillary Bed

Metabolized at endothelial surface without uptake from plasma
  Bradykinin—Inactivated
  Adenine nucleotides—Inactivated
  Angiotensin I—Activated

Metabolized intracellularly after uptake from plasma
  Serotonin
  Norepinephrine
  Prostaglandins E and F

Unaffected by traversing lungs
  Epinephrine
  Prostaglandin A
  Angiotensin II
  Dopamine
  Vasopressin
  (Acetylcholine)*

Synthesized within lung and released into blood
  Prostaglandins E and F
  Hormones†

Discharged from intrapulmonary stores into blood
  Histamine
  Prostaglandins
  Slow-reacting substance of anaphylaxis
  Kallikreins
  Eosinophil leukocyte chemotactic factor of anaphylaxis

*The ( ) around acetylcholine indicates that normally very little or none reaches the lungs owing to peripheral tissue and blood cholinesterase hydrolysis. However, 90 per cent of what little acetylcholine does reach the lungs is unaffected by passage through the pulmonary circulation.
†See Table 3–3.

the causation of some clinical conditions. For example, potentiation of the cardiovascular effects of NE produced by some drugs (e.g., cocaine, tricyclic antidepressants, some steroids, and certain antihypertensive drugs) may be due to inhibition of pulmonary removal of NE in addition to interference with uptake and storage of NE in peripheral tissues.

The presence of luminal endothelial projections and plasmalemmal cavities, with histochemical verification of the presence of enzymes at these endothelial locations, invites the functional anatomic picture of enzymes in the luminal membrane of the endothelial cell being washed and bathed with substrates that are in a continuously flowing liquid phase.[87-90] The enzyme-substrate interface is enormous at the level of the capillary bed, a condition that favors efficient metabolism by relatively small amounts of enzyme. The presence of intracellular and membrane cavities very likely explains how the metabolic products of some of the substrates (adenine nucleotides and prostaglandins) are returned to the circulation with no apparent delay or uptake by tissue.

The lungs have a number of ways in which they may influence the quantity of endothelial enzymes exposed to circulating substrates. The number of capillaries open at any given time and therefore the amount of endothelial surface exposed to blood flow are complex functions of right-to-left shunting, pulmonary venous pressure, posture, exercise (cardiac output), depth of ventilation, the composition of inhalants, and several other factors, not the least of which is the structural integrity of the lungs themselves. It might be expected that factors that significantly increase or decrease mean transit time of blood through the lungs (e.g., cardiac output, viscosity) could affect the amount of endothelial enzyme-substrate interaction. Changes in inspired oxygen tension have produced somewhat variable and undramatic changes in the amount of lung modification of most vasoactive substances, with angiotensin I conversion being an exception.[91-94]

On the other hand, a circulating hormone is released into the venous blood and then distributed through the arterial circulation without loss of activity on passage through the lungs. By definition, it is not possible for the lung to malfunction in its handling of a circulating hormone. At present there are no known conditions in which the lung begins to inactivate previously unmetabolized hormones.

The second important pharmacokinetic function of the pulmonary circulation is an endocrine one, in that the lung is an organ that can contribute vasoactive hormones to the circulation as well as remove them. It is possible that any substance the lung is capable of synthesizing and/or storing may, under certain conditions, be released into the pulmonary circulation.[95-97] Table 3–3 shows that neoplastic lung disease may produce almost any biologically active polypeptide and the associated characteristic clinical syndrome caused by the polypeptide.[98] Mechanical stimulation of the lung, such as stroking of the lung surface or retraction during surgery, may cause release of various vasoconstrictor and vasodilator substances, respectively.[99, 100] Hyper- or hypoinflation of the lung may cause release of prostaglandins.[99, 101, 102] Chemical stimulation of the lung, such as by alveolar hypoxia, also causes release of prostaglandins, which may then serve to normalize V/Q relationships.[103-105]

In addition, anaphylaxis has been shown to be one of the conditions in which biologically active substances (histamine, slow-reacting substance of anaphylaxis (SRS-A), PGE_1, PGE_2, and PGF_2, and possibly bradykinin) are released from the lungs.[106, 107] Indeed, in humans the lung seems to be the major shock organ of anaphylaxis and the source of mediators. Some of the mediators released during anaphylaxis are also released by damage to lung tissue, such as is caused by overinflation, pulmonary embolism, or physical manipulation. Finally, biologically active substances are also released from the lung when various pharmacologic agents are injected or infused into the pulmonary circulation. Table 3–2 summarizes many of these considerations and the way in which the pulmonary capillary bed handles biologically active materials.

H. Other Special Lung Functions[108-110]

1. Reservoir for Left Ventricle

The pulmonary vessels contain about 750 ml of blood, of which more than half is in readily distensible veins. Since these veins are an extension of the left atrium, they constitute a blood reservoir that supplies blood to fill the left ventricle and to maintain its output, even when the right ventricular pump falls behind for a few beats. Indeed, under experimental conditions the extra-alveolar pulmonary veins can actually be observed changing in volume with each heartbeat, taking up temporary differences between the outputs of the right and

Table 3–3. *Polypeptide Hormone Secretion in Pulmonary Disease:*
Resultant Syndromes and Commonly Associated Lesions

Lung Lesion	Hormones	Syndrome
Oat cell carcinoma, adenoma	ACTH	Hypokalemic, alkalosis, edema, Cushing's syndrome
Oat cell carcinoma, adenoma, tuberculosis, pneumonia, aspergillosis	ADH (arginine vasopressin)	Hyponatremia (SIADH)
Squamous cell, adenocarcinoma, and large-cell undifferentiated carcinoma	PTH or related peptide	Hypercalcemia
Large cell anaplastic carcinoma	Gonadotropins	Gynecomastia (adults), precocious puberty (children)
Squamous, large, or oat cell carcinoma	VIP or related peptide	Watery diarrhea or no symptoms
Squamous cell carcinoma, bronchial adenoma, and oat cell carcinoma	Growth hormone, serotonin, kinins (PGs and other)	Hypertrophic osteoarthropathy, "carcinoid"
Mesenchymal cell tumors	Insulin-like peptide	Hypoglycemia
Fibrosarcoma	Glucagon or related peptide	Hyperglycemia
Anaplastic cell carcinoma	Prolactin	Galactorrhea (or no symptoms)
Anaplastic cell carcinoma	Combinations of above	Multiple syndromes

Abbreviations: ACTH = adrenocorticotrophic hormone; SIADH = syndrome of inappropriate secretion of antidiuretic hormone; PTH = parathyroid hormone; PGs = prostaglandins; VIP = vasoactive intestinal polypeptide.

left ventricles. Thus, the left ventricular stroke volume (output per beat) has been shown to remain unchanged for several beats, even when the pulmonary artery is completely blocked by a balloon. The larger the left atrium and the more distended the pulmonary veins, the more capacious will be the reservoir.

2. Protective Function

The pulmonary vessels act as a filter to trap and prevent emboli from reaching and blocking systemic arteries, arterioles, or capillaries. Although a major amount of pulmonary thromboembolism can be lethal, the lungs can still perform their gas exchange function in the presence of a moderately reduced number of pulmonary arteries, whereas obstruction of a systemic artery is much more likely to lead to tissue necrosis. Thus, concurrent blockage of some pulmonary vessels is far better tolerated than single blockage of most systemic vessels.

3. Nutrition

Blood flow through the alveolar capillaries appears to be essential for the nutrition of the alveoli and alveolar ducts. After unilateral pulmonary artery occlusion, many alveoli become hemorrhagic and collapse within 1 to 3 days, although they recover later and appear almost normal after some months. The early damage

implies that the pulmonary circulation has a nutritive function and that compensation by the bronchial circulation requires several weeks to develop fully.

II. RESPIRATORY FUNCTION DURING ANESTHESIA

A. Introduction

The effect of a given anesthetic on respiratory function will depend on the depth of general anesthesia, the patient's preoperative respiratory condition, and the presence of special intraoperative anesthetic and surgical conditions.

B. Effect of Anesthetic Depth on Respiratory Pattern

The respiratory pattern is altered by the induction and deepening of anesthesia.[111] When the depth of anesthesia is inadequate (less than MAC), the respiratory pattern may vary from excessive hyperventilation and vocalization to breath-holding. As anesthetic depth approaches or equals MAC (light anesthesia), irregular respiration progresses to a more regular pattern, which is associated with a larger than normal tidal volume. However, during light, but deepening anesthesia, the approach to a more regular respiratory pattern may be interrupted by a pause at the end of inspiration (a sort of "hitch" in the inspiration), followed by a relatively prolonged and active expiration in which the patient seems to exhale forcefully, rather than passively. As anesthesia deepens to moderate levels, respiration becomes faster, more regular, but more shallow. The respiratory pattern is a sine wave losing the inspiratory hitch and lengthened expiratory pause. There is little or no inspiratory or expiratory pause, and the inspiratory and expiratory periods are equivalent. Intercostal muscle activity is still present, and there is normal movement of the thoracic cage with lifting of the chest during inspiration. The respiratory rate is generally slower and the tidal volume larger with nitrous oxide–narcotic anesthesia compared with anesthesia with halogenated drugs. During deep anesthesia with halogenated drugs, increasing depression of respiration is manifested by even more rapid, shallow breathing (panting). On the other hand, with deep nitrous oxide–narcotic anesthesia, respirations become slower but may remain deep. With very deep anesthesia with all drugs,

respirations are jerky or gasping in character and irregular in pattern. This results from loss of active intercostal muscle contribution to inspiration. As a result, a "rocking boat" movement occurs in which there is an out-of-phase depression of the chest wall during inspiration, a flaring of the lower chest margins, and a billowing of the abdomen. The reason for this type of movement is that inspiration is dependent solely on diaphragmatic effort. Independent of anesthetic depth, similar chest movements may be simulated by upper and lower airway obstruction and by partial paralysis.

C. Effect of Anesthetic Depth on Spontaneous Minute Ventilation

Despite the variable changes in respiratory pattern and rate as anesthesia deepens, overall spontaneous minute ventilation progressively decreases. The normal awake response to breathing CO_2 (the x-axis in Fig. 3–34 shows increasing end-tidal concentration of CO_2) causes a linear increase in minute ventilation (y-axis in Fig. 3–34). In Figure 3–34 the slope

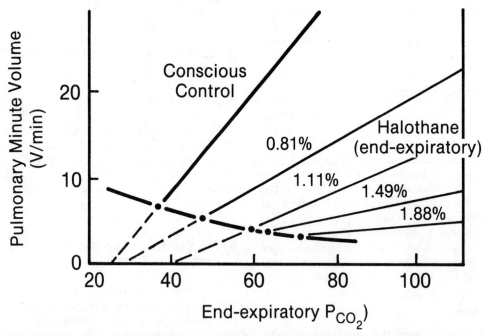

Figure 3–34. In conscious controls (heavy solid line) increasing end-expiratory Pco₂ increases pulmonary minute volume. The dashed line is an extrapolation of the CO₂-response curve to zero ventilation and represents the apneic threshold. An increase in anesthetic (halothane) concentration (end-expiratory concentration) progressively diminishes the slope of the CO₂-response curve and shifts the apneic threshold to a higher Pco₂. The heavy line interrupted by dots shows the decrease in minute ventilation and the increase in Pco₂ that occurs with increasing depth of anesthesia. (Modified with permission from Munson ES, Larson CP Jr, Babad AA, et al: The effects of halothane, fluoroxene and cyclopropane on ventilation: A comparative study in man. Anesthesiology 27:716, 1966.)

of the line relating minute ventilation to end-tidal CO_2 concentration is 2 L/min/mm Hg. Figure 3–34 also shows that increasing halothane concentration displaces the end-tidal CO_2 concentration P_{CO_2}-ventilation response curve progressively to the right (meaning that at any CO_2 concentration ventilation is less than before), decreases the slope of the curve, and shifts the apneic threshold to a higher end-tidal CO_2 concentration level.[112] Similar alterations are observed with other halogenated anesthetics and narcotics. Figure 3–27 shows that decreases in minute ventilation will cause increases in P_aCO_2 and decreases in P_aO_2. In healthy unstimulated spontaneous breathing male volunteers, 1 MAC halothane, isoflurane, and enflurane causes a P_aCO_2 of approximately 46, 48, and 62 mm Hg, respectively.

D. Effect of Pre-existing Respiratory Dysfunction on the Respiratory Effects of Anesthesia

Among the patients that anesthesiologists are frequently required to care for are (1) patients with acute chest disease (pulmonary infection, atelectasis) or systemic diseases (sepsis, cardiac and renal failure, or multiple trauma) that require emergency operations; (2) heavy smokers with subtle pathologic airway and parenchymal conditions and hyperreactive airways; (3) patients with classic emphysematous and bronchitic problems; (4) obese people prone to decreases in functional residual capacity during anesthesia;[113, 114] (5) patients with chest deformities; and (6) very old patients.

The nature and magnitude of these pre-existing respiratory conditions will determine, in part, the effect of a given standard anesthetic on respiratory function. For example, in Figure 3–35 the FRC-CC relationship is depicted for normal, obese, bronchitic, and emphysematous patients. In the normal patient, FRC exceeds CC by approximately 1 L. In the latter three respiratory conditions, CC is 0.5 to 0.75 L less than FRC. If anesthesia causes a 1 L decrease in FRC, then the normal patient will have no change in the qualitative relationship between FRC and CC. In the patient with special respiratory conditions, a 1 L decrease in FRC will cause CC to exceed FRC and change the previously marginally normal FRC-CC relationship to either a grossly low $\dot{V}/\dot{Q}$ relationship or an atelectatic FRC-CC relationship. Similarly, patients with chronic bronchitis, who have copious airway secretions, may suffer more from an anesthetic-induced decrease in mucous velocity flow than other patients. Finally, if an anesthetic drug inhibits HPV, the drug may increase shunting more in patients with pre-existing HPV than in those without pre-existing HPV. Thus, the effect of a standard anesthetic can be expected to produce varying degrees of respiratory change among patients who have different degrees of pre-existing respiratory dysfunction.

E. Effect of Special Intraoperative Conditions on the Respiratory Effects of Anesthesia

Some special intraoperative conditions (such as surgical position, massive blood loss, and surgical retraction on the lung), may cause impaired gas exchange. For example, some of the surgical positions (e.g., the lithotomy, jackknife, and kidney rest positions) and surgical exposure requirements may decrease cardiac output, cause hypoventilation in a spontaneously breathing patient, and reduce the functional residual capacity. The respiratory depressant effects of any anesthetic will be magnified by the type and severity of pre-existing respiratory dysfunction as well as by the number and severity of special intraoperative conditions that can embarrass respiratory function.

F. Mechanisms of Hypoxemia During Anesthesia

1. Malfunction of Equipment

a. MECHANICAL FAILURE OF ANESTHESIA APPARATUS TO DELIVER OXYGEN TO THE PATIENT

Hypoxemia due to mechanical failure of the O_2 supply system or the anesthesia machine is a recognized hazard of anesthesia. Disconnection of the patient from the oxygen supply system (usually at the juncture of the endotracheal tube elbow connector) is by far the most common cause of mechanical failure to deliver oxygen to the patient. Other reported causes of O_2 supply failure during anesthesia include an empty or depleted O_2 cylinder, substitution of an non-O_2 cylinder at the O_2 yoke because of absence or failure of the pin index, an erroneously filled O_2 cylinder, insufficient opening of the O_2 cylinder (which hinders a free flow of gas as pressure decreases), failure of gas pres-

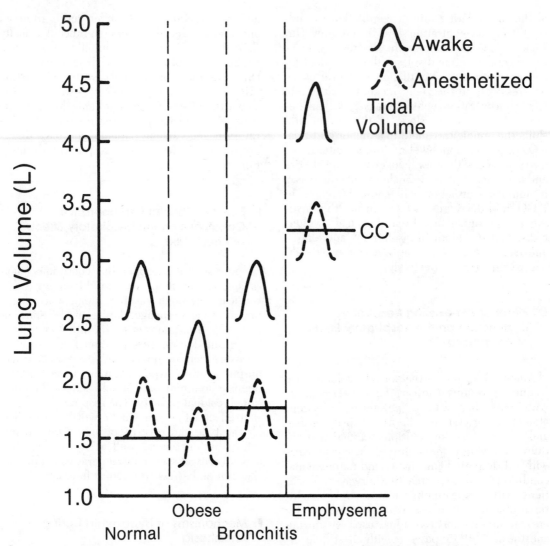

Figure 3–35. The lung volume (ordinate) at which the tidal volume is breathed decreases (by 1 L) from the awake state to the anesthetized state. The functional residual capacity, which is the volume of lung existing at the end of the tidal volume, therefore also decreases (by 1 L) from the awake to the anesthetized state. In normal, obese, bronchitic, and emphysematous patients, the awake functional residual capacity considerably exceeds the closing capacity (CC). In obese, bronchitic, and emphysematous patients, the anesthetized state causes functional residual capacity to be less than closing capacity. In the normal patient, anesthesia causes the functional residual capacity to equal the closing capacity. (Reproduced with permission from Benumof JL: Respiratory physiology and respiratory function during anesthesia. In Miller RD (ed.): Anesthesia. 2nd ed. Churchill Livingstone, New York, 1983, chapter 32.)

sure in a piped O_2 system, faulty locking of the piped O_2 system to the anesthesia machine, inadvertent switching of the Schrader adapters on piped lines, crossing of piped lines during construction, failure of a reducing valve or gas manifold, inadvertent disturbance of the setting of the O_2 flowmeter, employment of the fine O_2 flowmeter instead of the coarse flowmeter, fractured or sticking flowmeters, transposition of rotameter tubes, erroneous filling of a liquid O_2 reservoir with N_2, and fresh gas line disconnection from machine to in-line hosing.[115–119]

b. MECHANICAL FAILURE OF ENDOTRACHEAL TUBE: MAINSTEM BRONCHUS INTUBATION

Esophageal intubation results in almost no ventilation. Virtually all other mechanical problems (except disconnect) with endotracheal tubes (such as kinking, secretion blockage, and herniated or ruptured cuffs) cause an increase in airway resistance and may result in hypoventilation. Intubation of a main stem bronchus results in the absence of ventilation of the contralateral lung. Although potentially minimized by HPV, some perfusion to the contralateral lung will always remain, and shunting will increase while P_aO_2 will decrease. A tube previously well positioned in the trachea may enter a bronchus after the patient or the head of a patient is turned or moved into a new position.[120] Flexion of the head causes caudad movement, and extension of the head causes cephalad movement of an endotracheal tube.[120] A high incidence of main stem bronchus intubation following institution of a 30° Trendelenburg position has been reported.[121] Cephalad shift of the carina during the Trendelenburg position caused the previously "fixed" endotracheal tube to become located in a main stem bronchus.

2. Hypoventilation (Decreased Tidal Volume)

Patients under general anesthesia may have a reduced spontaneous tidal volume for two reasons. First, it may be more difficult to breathe during general anesthesia because of increased airway resistance and decreased lung compliance. Airway resistance may be increased because of reduced FRC, endotracheal intubation, the presence of external breathing apparatus and circuitry, and possible airway obstruction in nonintubated patients (see (Fig. 3–38).[122] Lung compliance is reduced owing to some (or all) of the factors that can decrease FRC (see Decrease in FRC).[123] Second, the patient may be less willing to breathe spontaneously during general anesthesia (decreased chemical control of breathing) (see Fig. 3–34).

There are two ways a decreased tidal volume may cause hypoxemia. First, shallow breathing may promote atelectasis and cause a decrease in FRC (see Ventilation History).[124, 125] Second, decreased minute ventilation decreases the overall $\dot{V}_A/\dot{Q}$ ratio of the lung, which will decrease P_aO_2 (Fig. 3–28). This is likely to occur with spontaneous ventilation during moderate to deep levels of anesthesia in which the chemical control of breathing is significantly altered.

3. Hyperventilation

Hypocapnic alkalosis (hyperventilation) may result in a decreased P_aO_2 via several mechanisms. These mechanisms are decreased cardiac output[67, 68] and increased oxygen consumption[126, 127] (see Decreased Cardiac Output and Increased Oxygen Consumption), a left-shifted oxygen-hemoglobin dissociation curve (see The

Oxygen-Hemoglobin Dissociation Curve), decreased HPV[128] (see Inhibition of Hypoxic Pulmonary Vasoconstriction), and/or increased airway resistance and decreased compliance[129] (see Increased Airway Resistance).

4. Decrease in FRC

Induction of general anesthesia is consistently accompanied by a significant (15 to 20 per cent) decrease in FRC,[54, 61, 130] which usually causes a decrease in compliance.[123] The maximum decrease in FRC appears to occur within the first few minutes of anesthesia[54, 131–133] and, in the absence of any other complicating factor, does not seem to decrease progressively during anesthesia. During anesthesia, the reduction in FRC is of the same order of magnitude whether ventilation is spontaneous or controlled. Conversely, in awake patients, FRC is only slightly reduced during controlled ventilation.[133] The reduction of FRC continues into the postoperative period.[134] For individual patients, the reduction in FRC correlates well with an increase in the alveolar-arterial P_{O_2} gradient during anesthesia with spontaneous breathing,[135] during anesthesia with artificial ventilation,[132] and in the postoperative period.[134] The reduced FRC may be restored to normal or above normal by the application of PEEP.[54, 136] In the following discussion, all possible causes of reduced FRC are considered.

a. Supine Position

Anesthesia and surgery are usually performed with the patient in the supine position. In changing from the upright to the supine position, FRC decreases by 0.5 to 1.0 L[54, 61, 130] because of a 4-cm cephalad displacement of the diaphragm by the abdominal viscera (Fig. 3–36). Pulmonary vascular congestion may also contribute to the decrease in FRC in the supine position, particularly in patients who preoperatively experienced orthopnea.

b. Induction of General Anesthesia—Change in Thoracic Cage Muscle Tone

At the end of a normal (awake state) exhalation, there is slight tension in the inspiratory muscles and no tension in the expiratory muscles. Thus, at the end of a normal exhalation, there is a force tending to maintain lung volume and no force decreasing lung volume (Fig. 3–37). Following the induction of general anes-

Progressive Cephalad Displacement of the Diaphram

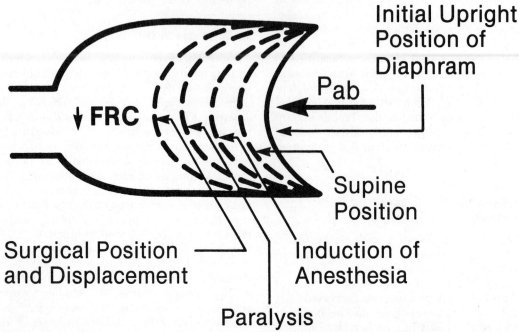

Figure 3–36. Anesthesia and surgery may cause a progressive cephalad displacement of the diaphragm. The sequence of events involves assuming the supine position, induction of anesthesia, causation of paralysis, the assumption of several surgical positions, and displacement by retractors and packs. The cephalad displacement of the diaphragm results in a decreased functional residual capacity ($\downarrow$ FRC). (P_{ab} = pressure of the abdominal contents.)

Spontaneous Ventilation: End Exhalation

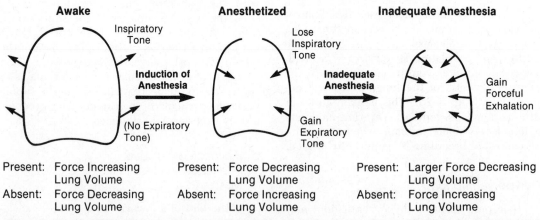

Figure 3–37. Schematic diagram of forces on the chest wall during the awake, anesthetized, and inadequately anesthetized conditions. In the awake state, inspiratory tone is a force increasing lung volume, and there is no force decreasing lung volume. In the anesthetized condition, loss of normally present inspiratory tone results in the absence of a force increasing lung volume, whereas gain of expiratory tone results in the gain of a force decreasing lung volume. In inadequate anesthesia, forceful exhalations result in a larger force tending to decrease lung volume, and the continued loss in inspiratory tone results in a continued absence of a force tending to increase lung volume.

thesia there is a loss of the inspiratory tone and an appearance of end-expiratory tone in the abdominal expiratory muscles at the end of exhalation. The end-expiratory tone in the abdominal expiratory muscles increases intra-abdominal pressure, forces the diaphragm cephalad, and decreases FRC (Fig. 3–36).[131, 137] Thus, following the induction of general anesthesia, there is loss of a force tending to maintain lung volume and gain of a force tending to decrease lung volume. Indeed, Innovar (droperidol and fentanyl citrate) may increase tone in expiratory muscles to such an extent that the reduction in FRC with Innovar anesthesia alone is greater than that with Innovar plus paralysis induced by succinylcholine.[138]

With emphysema, exhalation may be accompanied by pursing the lips or grunting (partially closed larynx). The emphysematous patient exhales in either of these ways because both these maneuvers cause an expiratory retard that produces PEEP in the intrathoracic air passage and decreases the possibility of airway closure and a decrease in FRC (Fig. 3–22F). Endotracheal intubation by-passes the lips and glottis and may abolish normally present pursed-lip or grunting exhalation and in this way contribute to airway closure and a loss in FRC in some spontaneously breathing patients.

c. PARALYSIS

In the upright subject, the FRC and the position of the diaphragm are determined by the balance between the lung elastic recoil pulling the diaphragm cephalad and the weight of the abdominal contents pulling it caudad.[139] There is no transdiaphragmatic pressure gradient.

The situation is more complex in the supine position. The diaphragm separates two compartments of markedly different hydrostatic gradients. On the thoracic side, pressure increases approximately 0.25 cm H_2O/cm lung height[9, 10] and on the abdominal side by 1.0 cm H_2O/cm abdominal height.[139] This means that in horizontal postures, progressively higher transdiaphragmatic pressures must be generated toward dependent parts of the diaphragm to keep the abdominal contents out of the thorax. In the unparalyzed patient, this tension is developed by either passive stretch and shape changes of the diaphragm (causing an increased contractile force), or by neurally mediated active tension. With acute muscle paralysis, neither of these two mechanisms can be operative, and a shift

of the diaphragm to a more cephalad position occurs (Fig. 3–36).[140] The latter position must express the true balance of forces on the diaphragm, unmodified by any passive or active muscle activity.

The cephalad shift in the FRC position of the diaphragm due to expiratory muscle tone during general anesthesia is equal to the shift observed during paralysis (awake or anesthetized patients).[131, 141] The equal shift suggests that the pressure on the diaphragm caused by an increase in expiratory muscle tone during general anesthesia is equal to the pressure on the diaphragm caused by the weight of the abdominal contents during paralysis. It is quite probable that the magnitude of these changes in FRC due to paralysis is also dependent on the body habitus.

d. LIGHT OR INADEQUATE ANESTHESIA AND ACTIVE EXPIRATION

The induction of general anesthesia can result in increased expiratory muscle tone,[137] but the increased expiratory muscle tone is not coordinated and does not contribute to the exhaled volume of gas. In contrast, spontaneous ventilation during light general anesthesia usually results in a coordinated and moderately forceful active exhalation and larger exhaled volumes (Fig. 3–35). Excessively inadequate anesthesia (relative to a given stimulus) results in very forceful active exhalation, which may produce exhaled volumes of gas equal to an awake expiratory vital capacity.

As during an awake expiratory vital capacity maneuver, a forced expiration during anesthesia raises the intrathoracic and alveolar pressures considerably above atmospheric pressure (Fig. 3–22). This results in a rapid outflow of gas, and since part of the expiratory resistance lies in the smaller air passages, a pressure drop will occur between the alveoli and the main bronchi. Under these circumstances, the intrathoracic pressure rises considerably above the pressure within the main bronchi. Collapse will occur if this reversed pressure gradient is sufficiently high to overcome the tethering effect of the surrounding parenchyma on the small intrathoracic bronchioles or the structural rigidity of cartilage in the large extrathoracic bronchi. Such collapse occurs in the normal subject during a maximal forced expiration and it is responsible for the associated wheeze both in awake and anesthetized patients.[142]

In the paralyzed anesthetized patient, the

use of a subatmospheric expiratory pressure phase is analogous to a forced expiration in the conscious subject; the "negative phase" may set up the same adverse pressure gradients that can cause airway closure, gas trapping, and a decrease in FRC. An excessively rapidly descending bellows of a ventilator during expiration has caused a subatmospheric expiratory pressure and has resulted in wheezing.[143]

e. INCREASED AIRWAY RESISTANCE

The overall reduction in all components of lung volume during anesthesia results in a reduced caliber of airway, which increases airway resistance and any tendency toward airway collapse (Fig. 3–38). The relationship between airway resistance and lung volume is well established (Fig. 3–39). The decrease in FRC caused by the supine position (about 0.8 L) and the induction of anesthesia (about 0.4 L) are often sufficient to explain the increased resistance seen in the healthy anesthetized patient.[122]

In addition to this expected increase in airway resistance in anesthetized patients, there are a number of additional special potential sites of increased airway resistance. These consist of the endotracheal tube (if present), the upper and lower airway passages, and the external anesthesia apparatus. Endotracheal intubation reduces the size of the trachea, usually by 30 to 50 per cent (Fig. 3–38). Pharyngeal obstruc-

tion, which can be considered to be a normal feature of unconsciousness, is most common. A minor degree of this type of obstruction occurs in snoring. Laryngospasm and obstructed endotracheal tubes (secretions, kinking, herniated cuffs) are not rare and may be life-threatening.

Respiratory apparatus often causes resistance that is considerably higher than the resistance in the normal human respiratory tract (Fig. 3–38).[58] When a number of resistors such as those shown in Figure 3–38 are joined in a series to form an anesthetic gas circuit, they generally summate to produce a larger resistance (as with resistances in an electrical circuit).

f. THE SUPINE POSITION, IMMOBILITY, AND EXCESSIVE INTRAVENOUS FLUID ADMINISTRATION

Patients undergoing anesthesia and surgery are often kept supine and immobile for long periods of time. Thus, some of the lung may be continually dependent and below the left atrium and therefore in a zone 3 or 4 condition. Being in a dependent position, the lung is predisposed to fluid accumulation. Coupled with excessive fluid administration, conditions sufficient to promote transudation of fluid into the lung are present and will result in pulmonary edema and a decreased FRC. Figure 3–40 shows that when mongrel dogs are placed in a lateral decubitus position and are anesthetized for several hours

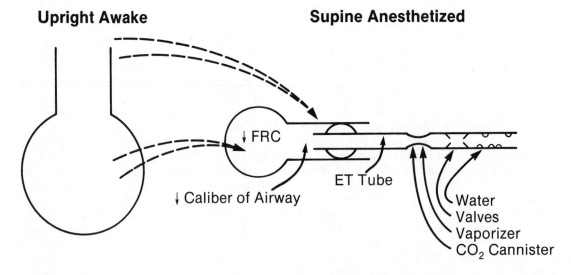

Upright Awake   **Supine Anesthetized**

↓ FRC

ET Tube

↓ Caliber of Airway

Water
Valves
Vaporizer
CO_2 Cannister

Increased Airway Resistance

Figure 3–38. The anesthetized patient in the supine position has an increased airway resistance due to decreased functional residual capacity, decreased caliber of the airways, endotracheal intubation, and connection of the endotracheal tube to external breathing apparatus and circuitry.

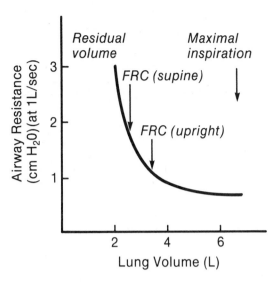

Figure 3–39. Airway resistance is an increasing hyperbolic function of decreasing lung volume. Functional residual capacity (FRC) decreases in changing from the upright to supine position. (Reprinted with modification by permission of the publisher from Nunn JF: Applied Respiratory Physiology. 2nd ed. London, Butterworths (Publishers) Ltd, 1977.)

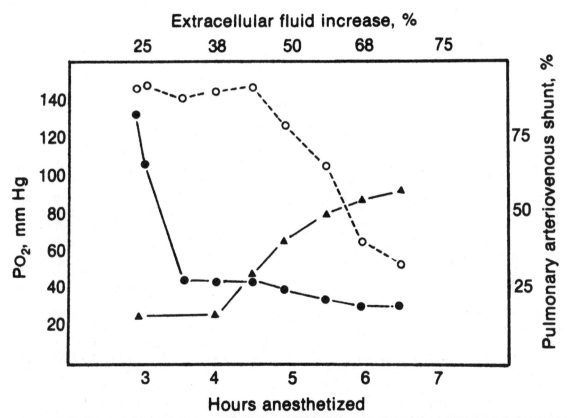

Figure 3–40. Mongrel dogs anesthetized with pentobarbital (bottom axis), placed in a lateral decubitus position, and subjected to progressive extracellular fluid expansion (top axis) have a marked decrease in the Po$_2$ (left vertical axis) of blood draining the dependent lung (solid circles) and a smaller, much slower decrease in Po$_2$ of blood draining the nondependent lung (open circles). The pulmonary arteriovenous shunt (right ventrical axis) rises progressively (triangles). (Modified with permission from Ray JF, Yost L, Moallem S, et al: Immobility, hypoxemia, and pulmonary arteriovenous shunting. Arch Surg 109:537, 1974. Copyright 1974, American Medical Association.)

(bottom horizontal axis), expansion of the extracellular space with fluid (top horizontal axis) causes the P_{O_2} (left-hand axis) of blood draining the dependent lung (closed circles) to decrease precipitously to mixed venous levels (no O_2 uptake).[144] Blood draining the nondependent lung maintains its P_{O_2} for a period of time but in the face of the extracellular fluid expansion also suffers a decline in its P_{O_2} after 5 hours. Transpulmonary shunt (right-hand axis) progressively increases. If the animals were turned every hour (and received the same fluid challenge), only the dependent lung, at the end of each hour period, suffered a decrease in oxygenation. If the animals were turned every half hour and received the same fluid challenge, neither lung suffered a decrease in oxygenation. In patients undergoing pulmonary resection (and therefore have, or will have, a restricted pulmonary vascular bed) in the lateral decubitus position who receive excessive intravenous fluids, the risk of the dependent lung becoming edematous is certainly increased.

g. HIGH INSPIRED OXYGEN CONCENTRATION AND ABSORPTION ATELECTASIS

General anesthesia is usually administered with an increased F_IO_2. In patients who have areas of moderately low $\dot{V}_A/\dot{Q}$ ratios (0.1 to 0.01), the administration of F_IO_2 greater than 0.3 adds enough oxygen into the alveolar space in these areas to eliminate the shunt-like effect that they have, and total measured right-to-left shunt decreases. However, when patients with a significant amount of blood flow perfusing lung units with very low $\dot{V}_A/\dot{Q}$ ratios (0.01 to 0.0001) have a change in F_IO_2 from room air to 1.0, the very low $\dot{V}_A/\dot{Q}$ units virtually disappear and a moderately large right-to-left shunt appears.[19, 20, 145] In these studies, the increase in shunting was equal to the amount of blood flow previously perfusing the low $\dot{V}_A/\dot{Q}$ ratio areas during the breathing of air. Thus, in these studies the effect of breathing O_2 was to convert units that had low $\dot{V}_A/\dot{Q}$ ratios into shunt units. The pathologic basis for this data is the conversion of low $\dot{V}_A/\dot{Q}$ units into atelectatic units.

The cause of the atelectatic shunting during O_2 breathing is presumably due to a large increase in O_2 uptake by the low $\dot{V}_A/\dot{Q}$ ratio lung units.[145, 146] A unit that has a low $\dot{V}_A/\dot{Q}$ ratio during breathing of air will have a low alveolar P_{O_2}. When an enriched O_2 mixture is inspired, alveolar P_{O_2} will rise, and, therefore, the rate at which O_2 moves from the alveolar gas to the capillary blood will greatly increase. The O_2

flux may increase so much that the net flow of gas into the blood exceeds the inspired flow of gas, and the lung unit will begin to become progressively smaller. Collapse is most likely to occur if the F_IO_2 is high, the $\dot{V}_A/\dot{Q}$ ratio is low, the time of exposure of the low $\dot{V}_A/\dot{Q}$ unit to the high F_IO_2 is long, and the content of O_2 in the mixed venous blood is low. Thus, given the right $\dot{V}_A/\dot{Q}$ ratio and time of administration, an F_IO_2 as low as 50 per cent can produce absorption atelectasis.[145, 146] This phenomenon is of considerable significance in the clinical situation for two reasons. First, enriched O_2 mixtures are often used therapeutically, and it is important to know whether this therapy is causing atelectasis. Second, the amount of shunt is often estimated during breathing of 100 per cent O_2, and if this maneuver results in additional shunt, the measurement will be hard to interpret.

h. SURGICAL POSITION

In the supine position the abdominal contents force the diaphragm cephalad and reduce FRC.[61, 131, 137, 141] The Trendelenburg position allows the abdominal contents to push the diaphragm further cephalad, so that the diaphragm must not only ventilate the lungs but must also lift the abdominal contents out of the thorax. The result is a predisposition to decreased FRC and atelectasis.[147] Increased pulmonary blood volume and gravitational force on the mediastinal structures are additional factors that may decrease pulmonary compliance and FRC. In the steep Trendelenburg position, most of the lung may be below the left atrium and, therefore, in a zone 3 or 4 condition. As such, the lung may be prone to develop pulmonary interstitial edema. Thus, patients with elevated pulmonary artery pressure, such as those with mitral stenosis, do not tolerate the Trendelenburg position well.[148]

In the lateral decubitus position, the dependent lung experiences a moderate decrease in FRC and is predisposed to atelectasis (see chapter 4 for a detailed discussion of the physiology of the lateral decubitus position). The kidney and lithotomy positions also cause small decreases in FRC. The prone position may increase FRC.

i. VENTILATORY HISTORY (RAPID SHALLOW BREATHING)

Rapid shallow breathing is often a regular feature of anesthesia. Monotonous shallow breathing may cause a decrease in FRC, pro-

mote atelectasis, and decrease compliance.[124, 125] Initially, these changes may cause hypoxemia with normocarbia and may be reversed by periodic large inspirations and/or PEEP.

j. Decreased Removal of Secretions (Decreased Mucociliary Flow)

Tracheobronchial mucous glands and goblet cells produce mucus, which is swept by cilia up to the larynx where it is swallowed or expectorated. This process clears inhaled organisms and particles from the lungs. The secreted mucus consists of a surface gel layer, which lies on top of a more liquid sol layer in which the cilia beat. The tips of the cilia propel the gel layer toward the larynx (upward) during the forward stroke. As the mucus streams upward and the total cross-sectional area of the airways diminishes, absorption takes place from the sol layer so as to maintain a constant depth of 5 mm.[149]

Poor systemic hydration and low inspired humidity reduce mucociliary flow by increasing the viscosity of secretions and by slowing the ciliary beat.[150-152] Mucociliary flow varies directly with body or mucosal temperature (low inspired temperature) over a range of 32 to 42°C.[153, 154] A high F_IO_2 decreases mucociliary flow.[155] Inflation of an endotracheal tube cuff suppresses tracheal mucous velocity,[156] which occurs within 1 hour, and apparently it does not matter whether a low- or high-compliance cuff is used. Passage of an uncuffed tube through the vocal cords and kept in situ for several hours does not affect tracheal mucous velocity.[156]

The mechanism for endotracheal tube cuff suppression of mucociliary clearance is speculative. In the report of Sackner et al[156] mucous velocity was decreased in the distal trachea, whereas the cuff was inflated in the proximal portion. Thus, the phenomenon cannot be attributed solely to damming of mucus at the cuff site. One possibility is that the endotracheal tube cuff caused a critical increase in the thickness of the layer of mucus proceeding distally from the cuff. Another possibility is that mechanical distention of the trachea by the endotracheal tube cuff initiated a neurogenic reflex arc that altered mucous secretions or frequency of ciliary beating.

Other investigators have recently shown that when all of the preceding factors are controlled, halothane reversibly and progressively decreases, but does not stop, mucous flow over an inspired concentration of 1 to 3 MAC.[157] The halothane-induced depression of mucociliary clearance was likely due to depression of the ciliary beat, an effect that caused slow clearance of mucus from the distal and peripheral airways. In support of this hypothesis is the fact that cilia are morphologically similar throughout the animal kingdom, and in clinical dosages, inhaled anesthetics, including halothane, have been found to cause reversible depression of the ciliary beat of protozoa.[158]

5. Decreased Cardiac Output and Increased Oxygen Consumption

A decreased cardiac output ($\dot{Q}_t$ in the presence of a constant O_2 consumption ($\dot{V}O_2$), or an increased $\dot{V}O_2$ in the presence of a constant $\dot{Q}_t$, or a decreased $\dot{Q}_t$ and an increased $\dot{V}O_2$ must all result in a lower mixed venous O_2 content ($C_{\bar{v}}O_2$). The lowered $C_{\bar{v}}O_2$ will then flow through whichever shunt pathways exist, mix with the oxygenated end-pulmonary capillary blood, and lower the O_2 content of the arterial blood (C_aO_2) (Figs. 3–31, 3–32, and 3–33). Decreased $\dot{Q}_t$ may occur with myocardial failure and hypovolemia; the specific causes of these two conditions is beyond the scope of this chapter. Increased $\dot{V}O_2$ may occur with excessive sympathetic nervous system stimulation, hyperthermia, or shivering and can further contribute to impaired oxygenation of arterial blood.[159]

6. Inhibition of Hypoxic Pulmonary Vasoconstriction (HPV)

Decreased regional alveolar PO_2 causes regional pulmonary vasoconstriction, which diverts blood flow away from hypoxic regions of the lung to better ventilated normoxic regions of the lung. The diversion of blood flow minimizes venous admixture from the underventilated or nonventilated lung regions. Inhibition of regional HPV might impair arterial oxygenation by permitting increased venous admixture from hypoxic or atelectatic areas of the lung (Fig. 3–12). Chapters 4 and 9 discuss in detail the determinants (physiologic variables and anesthetic drugs, respectively) of the amount of HPV during one-lung ventilation. The next paragraph briefly summarizes most of these regional HPV determinants.

Since the pulmonary circulation is poorly endowed with smooth muscle, any condition that increases the pressure against which the vessels must constrict (i.e., the P_{pa}) will decrease HPV. There are numerous clinical conditions that can increase P_{pa} and therefore decrease HPV. Mitral stenosis,[160] volume overload,[160] low (but above room air) F_1O_2 in nondiseased lung,[161] a progressive increase in the amount of diseased lung,[166] thromboembolism,[161] hypothermia,[162] and vasoactive drugs[163] can all increase P_{pa}. Direct vasodilating drugs (such as isoproterenol, nitroglycerin, and nitroprusside),[36, 164] inhaled anesthetics,[165, 166] and hypocapnia[128] can directly decrease HPV. The selective application of PEEP to only the nondiseased lung can selectively increase nondiseased lung PVR and divert blood flow back into the diseased lung.[167]

7. Paralysis

In the supine position, the weight of the abdominal contents pressing against the diaphragm is greatest in the dependent or posterior part of the diaphragm and least in the nondependent or anterior part of the diaphragm (Fig. 3–36). In the awake patient breathing spontaneously, the active tension in the diaphragm is capable of overcoming the weight of the abdominal contents, and the diaphragm moves the most in the posterior portion (because the posterior diaphragm is stretched higher into the chest it has the smallest radius of curvature and therefore it contracts most effectively) and least in the anterior portion. This is a healthy circumstance because the greatest amount of ventilation occurs where there is the most perfusion (posteriorly or dependently), and the least amount of ventilation occurs where there is the least perfusion (anteriorly or nondependently). During paralysis and positive-pressure breathing, the passive diaphragm is displaced by the positive pressure preferentially in the anterior nondependent portion (where there is the least resistance to diaphragmatic movement) and is displaced minimally in the posterior dependent portion (where there is the most resistance to diaphragmatic movement). This is an unhealthy circumstance because the greatest amount of ventilation now occurs where there is the least perfusion, and the least amount of ventilation now occurs where there is the most perfusion.[141]

8. The Involvement of Mechanisms of Hypoxemia in Specific Diseases

In any given pulmonary disease many of the mechanisms of hypoxemia listed above may be involved in producing hypoxemia. Pulmonary embolism (air, fat, thrombi) (Fig. 3–41) and the evolution of the adult respiratory distress syndrome (Fig. 3–42) will be used here to illustrate this point. A significant pulmonary embolus can cause severe increases in pulmonary artery pressure, and these increases can cause right-to-left transpulmonary shunting through opened arteriovenous anastomoses and the foramen ovale (this is possible in 20 per cent of patients), pulmonary edema in nonembolized regions of the lung, and inhibition of HPV. The embolus may cause hypoventilation via increased dead space ventilation. If the embolus contains platelets, serotonin may be released, and this release can cause hypoventilation via bronchoconstriction and pulmonary edema via increased pulmonary capillary permeability. Finally, the pulmonary embolus can increase pulmonary vascular resistance and decrease the cardiac output.

Following major hypotension, shock, or blood loss, respiratory failure often ensues, and this syndrome has been called the adult respiratory distress syndrome (ARDS). This syndrome can evolve during and after anesthesia and has the hallmark characteristics of decreased FRC and compliance and hypoxemia. Following shock and trauma, increased plasma levels of serotonin, histamine, plasmakinins, lysozymes, superoxides, fibrin degradation products, products of complement metabolism, and fatty acids occur. Sepsis and endotoxemia may be present. Increased levels of activated complement activate neutrophils into chemotaxis in patients with trauma and pancreatitis; activated neutrophils can damage endothelial cells. These factors, along with pulmonary contusion (if it occurs), may individually or collectively increase pulmonary capillary permeability. Following shock, it has been shown that acidosis, increased circulating catecholamines and sympathetic nervous system activity, prostaglandin release, histamine release, microembolism (with serotonin release), increased intracranial pressure (with head injury), and alveolar hypoxia may occur and may individually or collectively, particularly postresuscitation, cause a moderate increase in pulmonary artery pressure. Following shock, the normal compensatory response to hypovolemia is movement of a protein-free fluid from the interstitial space into the vascular space in order to restore vascular volume. The dilution of vascular proteins by protein-free interstitial fluid can cause a decreased capillary colloid osmotic pressure. Increased pulmonary capillary permeability and

Pulmonary Embolus: Mechanisms of Hypoxemia

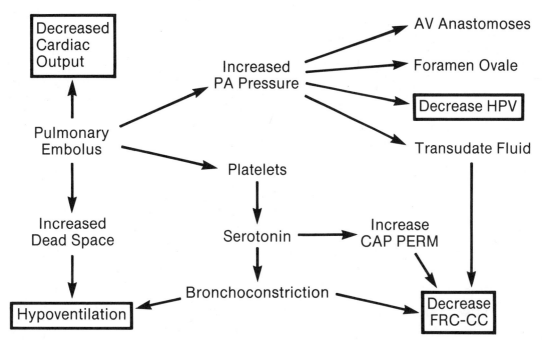

Figure 3–41. Mechanisms of hypoxemia during pulmonary embolism. See text for explanation of the pathophysiologic flow diagram. (CAP PERM = capillary permeability; AV = arterial venous; HPV = hypoxic pulmonary vasoconstriction; PA = pulmonary artery; FRC = functional residual capacity; CC = closing capacity.)

Shock and ARDS: Mechanisms of Hypoxemia

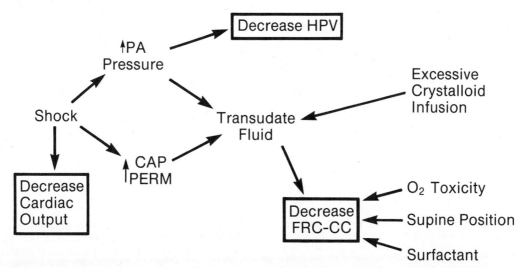

Figure 3–42. Mechanisms of hypoxemia during the adult respiratory distress syndrome (ARDS). See text for explanation of pathophysiologic flow diagram. (PA = pulmonary artery; CAP PERM = capillary permeability; HPV = hypoxic pulmonary vasoconstriction; FRC = functional residual capacity; CC = closing capacity.)

pulmonary artery pressure along with decreased capillary colloid osmotic pressure will cause fluid transudation and pulmonary edema. Additionally, a decreased cardiac output, inhibition of HPV, immobility, supine position, excessive fluid administration, and an excessively high F_IO_2 can contribute to the development of ARDS.

G. Mechanisms of Hypercapnia and Hypocapnia During Anesthesia

1. Hypercapnia (Fig. 3–43)

The following factors can all cause hypercapnia.

a. Hypoventilation

Patients spontaneously hypoventilate during anesthesia because it is more difficult to breathe (abnormal surgical position, increased airway resistance, decreased compliance) and they are less willing to breathe (decreased respiratory drive due to anesthetics). Hypoventilation will result in hypercapnia (Fig. 3–27).

b. Increased Dead Space Ventilation

A decrease in pulmonary artery pressure, as during deliberate hypotension,[168] may cause an increase in zone 1 and alveolar dead space ventilation. An increase in airway pressure (as with PEEP) may cause an increase in zone 1 and alveolar dead space ventilation. Pulmonary embolus, thrombosis, and vascular obliteration (kinking, clamping, blocking of pulmonary artery during surgery) may increase the amount of lung that is ventilated but unperfused. Vascular obliteration may be responsible for the increase in dead space ventilation with age ($\dot{V}_D/\dot{V}_T = 33 + age/3$). Rapid short inspirations may be distributed preferentially to noncompliant (short time constant for inflation) and badly perfused alveoli, while a slow inspiration

Mechanisms of Hypercapnia during Anesthesia

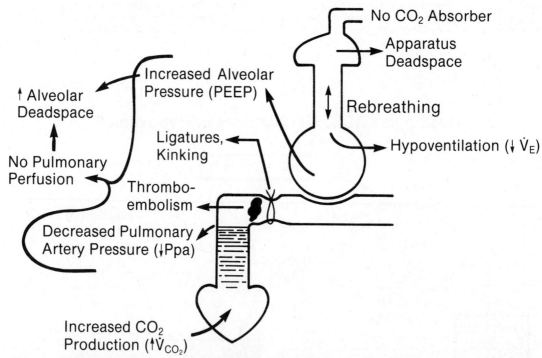

Figure 3–43. Schematic diagram of the causes of hypercapnia during anesthesia. An increase in carbon dioxide production ($\dot{V}co_2$) will increase $Paco_2$ with a constant minute ventilation ($\dot{V}_E$). There are several events that can increase alveolar dead space, and they consist of a decrease in pulmonary artery pressure (P_{pa}), the application of PEEP, thromboembolism, and mechanical interference with pulmonary arterial flow (ligatures and kinking of vessels). A decrease in minute ventilation ($\dot{V}_E$) will cause an increase in $Paco_2$ with a constant $\dot{V}co_2$. It is possible for some anesthesia systems to cause rebreathing of carbon dioxide. Finally, the anesthesia apparatus may increase the anatomical dead space, and inadvertent switching off of the carbon dioxide absorber in the presence of low fresh gas flows can increase $Paco_2$.

allows time for distribution to more compliant (long time constant for inflation) and better perfused alveoli. Thus, rapid short inspirations may have a dead space ventilation effect.

The anesthesia apparatus increases total dead space ($\dot{V}_D/\dot{V}_T$) for two reasons. First, the apparatus simply increases the anatomic dead space. Inclusion of normal apparatus dead space increases the total $\dot{V}_D/\dot{V}_T$ ratio from 33 per cent to about 46 per cent in intubated patients and to about 64 per cent in patients breathing via a mask.[169] Second, anesthesia circuits cause rebreathing of expired gases, which is the equivalent to dead space ventilation. The rebreathing classification by Mapleson is widely accepted.[170] The order of increasing rebreathing (decreasing clinical merit) with spontaneous ventilation with Mapleson circuits is A (Magill), D, C, and B. The order of increasing rebreathing (decreasing clinical merit) with controlled ventilation is D, B, C, and A. There will be no rebreathing in system E (Ayre T-piece) if the patient's respiratory diastole is long enough to permit washout with a given fresh gas flow (common event) or if the fresh gas flow is greater than the peak inspiratory flow rate (uncommon event).

The effects of an increase in dead space can usually be counteracted by a corresponding increase in the respiratory minute volume. If, for example, the minute volume is 10 L/min and the $\dot{V}_D/\dot{V}_T$ ratio is 30 per cent, the alveolar ventilation will be 7 L/min. If a pulmonary embolism occurred resulting in an increase of the $\dot{V}_D/\dot{V}_T$ ratio to 50 per cent, the minute volume would need to be increased to 14 L/min to maintain an alveolar ventilation of 7 L/min (14 L/min × 0.5).

c. Increased Carbon Dioxide Production

All of the causes of increased O_2 consumption will also increase CO_2 production, namely, hyperthermia, shivering, catecholamine release (light anesthesia), hypertension, and thyroid storm. If minute ventilation, total dead space, and ventilation-perfusion relationships are constant, an increase in CO_2 production will result in hypercapnia.

d. Inadvertent Switching Off of a Carbon Dioxide Absorber,

Many factors, such as patient ventilatory responsiveness to CO_2 accumulation, fresh gas flow, circle system design, and CO_2 production, determine whether hypercapnia will result from inadvertent switching off or using up of a circle

CO_2 absorber. However, high fresh gas flows (> 5 L/min) minimize the problem with almost all systems for almost all patients.

2. Hypocapnia

The mechanisms of hypocapnia are the reverse of those that produce hypercapnia. Thus, with all other factors being equal, hyperventilation (spontaneous or controlled ventilation), decreased dead space ventilation (change from mask airway to endotracheal tube airway, decreased PEEP, increased pulmonary artery pressure, or decreased rebreathing), and decreased CO_2 production (hypothermia, deep anesthesia, hypotension) will lead to hypocapnia. By far the most common mechanism of hypocapnia is passive hyperventilation by mechanical means.

H. Physiologic Effects of Abnormalities in the Respiratory Gases

1. Hypoxia

The end-products of aerobic metabolism (oxidative phosphorylation) are carbon dioxide and water, both of which are easily diffusible and lost from the body. The essential feature of hypoxia is the cessation of oxidative phosphorylation when mitochondrial P_{O_2} falls below a critical level. Anaerobic pathways, which produce energy (ATP) inefficiently, are then utilized. The main anaerobic metabolites are hydrogen and lactate ions, which are not easily excreted. They accumulate in the circulation where they may be quantified in terms of the base deficit and the lactate-pyruvate ratio.

Since the various organs have different blood flow and oxygen consumption rates, the presentation and clinical diagnosis of hypoxia is usually related to symptoms arising from the most vulnerable organ. This is usually the brain in an awake patient and the heart in the anesthetized patient (see the following), but in special circumstances it may be the spinal cord (aortic surgery), kidney (acute tubular necrosis), liver (hepatitis), or limb (claudication, gangrene).

The cardiovascular response to hypoxemia[171, 172] is a product of both reflex (neural and humoral) and direct effects (Table 3–4). The reflex effects occur first and are excitory and vasoconstrictive. The neuroreflex effects result from aortic and carotid chemoreceptor, baroreceptor, and central cerebral stimulation, and the hu-

Table 3–4. Cardiovascular Response to Hypoxemia

O₂ Sat	Hemodynamic Variable					Predominant Response
	HR	BP	SV	CO	SVR	
> 80	↑	↑	↑	↑	No Δ	Reflex, excitatory
60 to 80	↑ Baro-receptor	↓	No Δ	No Δ	↓	Local, depressant >
< 60	↓	↓↓	↓	↓	↓↓	Reflex, excitatory / Local, depressant

Abbreviations: O₂ Sat = Oxygen saturation; HR = heart rate; BP = systemic blood pressure; SV = stroke volume; CO = cardiac output; SVR = systemic vascular resistance; Δ = change; ↑ = increase; ↓ = decrease.

moral reflex effects result from catecholamine and renin-angiotensin release. The direct local vascular effects of hypoxia are inhibitory and vasodilatory and occur late. The net response to hypoxia in a subject depends on the severity of the hypoxia; the severity of hypoxia determines the magnitude of and balance between the inhibitory and excitory components; the balance may vary according to the type and depth of anesthesia and the degree of pre-existing cardiovascular disease.

Mild arterial hypoxemia (arterial saturation less than normal but still 80 per cent or higher) causes a general activation of the sympathetic nervous system and release of catecholamines. Consequently, heart rate, stroke volume, cardiac output, and myocardial contractility (as measured by a shortened pre-ejection period, left ventricular ejection time, and a decreased PEP/LVET ratio) are increased. Changes in systemic vascular resistance are usually slight. However, in patients under anesthesia with beta-blockers, hypoxia (and hypercapnia when present) may cause circulating catecholamines to have only an alpha-receptor effect, and the heart may be unstimulated (even depressed by a local hypoxic effect), and systemic vascular resistance may be increased. Consequently, cardiac output may be decreased in these patients. With moderate hypoxemia (arterial oxygen saturation 60 to 80 per cent) local vasodilatation begins to predominate, and systemic vascular resistance and blood pressure decreases, but heart rate may continue to be increased due to a systemic hypotension-induced stimulation of baroreceptors. Finally, with severe hypoxemia (arterial saturation less than 60 per cent), local depressant effects dominate, and blood pressure falls rapidly, the pulse slows, shock develops, and the heart either fibrillates or becomes asystolic. It should be remembered that significant pre-existing hypotension will convert a mild hypoxemia-hemodynamic profile into a moderate hypoxemia-

hemodynamic profile, and a moderate hypoxemia-hemodynamic profile will convert into a severe hypoxemia-hemodynamic profile. Similarly, in well-anesthetized and/or -sedated patients, early sympathetic nervous system reactivity to hypoxemia may be reduced, and the effects of hypoxemia may be expressed only as bradycardia with severe hypotension and, ultimately, circulatory collapse.

Hypoxemia may also cause cardiac arrhythmias, and the cardiac arrhythmias may in turn potentiate the already mentioned deleterious cardiovascular effects. Hypoxemia-induced arrhythmias may be caused by multiple mechanisms; the mechanisms are inter-related by virtue of the fact that they all cause a decrease in the myocardial oxygen supply-demand ratio, which in turn increases myocardial irritability. First, arterial hypoxemia may directly decrease myocardial oxygen supply. Second, early tachycardia may cause an increased myocardial oxygen consumption, and a decreased diastolic filling time may cause a decreased myocardial oxygen supply. Third, early increased systemic blood pressure may cause an increased afterload on the left ventricle, which increases left ventricular oxygen demand. Fourth, late systemic hypotension may decrease myocardial oxygen supply owing to decreased diastolic perfusion pressure. The level of hypoxemia that will cause cardiac arrhythmias cannot be predicted with certainty because the myocardial oxygen supply and demand relationship in a given patient is not known (i.e., the degree of coronary artery atherosclerosis may not be known). However, if a myocardial area (or areas) becomes hypoxic and/or ischemic, unifocal or multifocal premature ventricular contractions, ventricular tachycardia, and ventricular fibrillation may occur.

The cardiovascular response to hypoxia includes a number of other important effects. Cerebral blood flow increases (even if hypocapnic hyperventilation is present). Ventilation will be stimulated no matter why hypoxia exists.

The pulmonary distribution of blood flow is more homogeneous owing to an increased pulmonary artery pressure. Chronic hypoxia will cause an increased hemoglobin concentration and a right-shifted oxygen-hemoglobin dissociation curve (due to either an increase in 2,3-diphosphoglycerate or acidosis), which tend to raise tissue P_{O_2}.

2. Hyperoxia (Oxygen Toxicity)

The dangers associated with the inhalation of excessive O_2 are multiple. Exposure to a high O_2 tension clearly causes pulmonary damage in healthy individuals.[173, 174] A dose-time toxicity curve for humans is available from a number of studies.[173] Since the lungs of normal human volunteers cannot be directly examined to determine the rate of onset and the course of toxicity, indirect measures such as the onset of symptom formation have been employed to construct the dose-time toxicity curves. Examination of the curve indicates that 100 per cent O_2 should not be administered for more than 12 hours, 80 per cent O_2 should not be administered for more than 24 hours, and 60 per cent O_2 should not be administered for more than 36 hours. No measurable changes in pulmonary function or blood-gas exchange occur in man during exposures to less than 50 per cent O_2 or less even for long periods.

The dominant symptom of a toxicity in human volunteers is substernal distress, which begins as a mild irritation in the area of the carina and may be accompanied by occasional coughing. As exposure continues, pain becomes more intense, and the urge to cough and to deep breathe also becomes more intense. These symptoms will progress to severe dyspnea, paroxysmal coughing, and decreased vital capacity when the F_IO_2 has been 1.0 for greater than 12 hours. As toxicity progresses, pulmonary function studies such as compliance and arterial blood gases deteriorate. Pathologically, in animals the lesion progresses from a tracheobronchitis (exposure for 12 hours to a few days), to involvement of the alveolar septae with pulmonary interstitial edema (exposure for a few days to a week), to pulmonary fibrosis of the edema (exposure greater than a week).[175]

Ventilatory depression may occur in those patients who, by reason of drugs or disease, have been ventilating in response to a hypoxic drive. By definition, ventilatory depression resulting from removal of a hypoxic drive by increasing the inspired O_2 concentration will cause hypercapnia but does not necessarily produce hypoxia (due to the increased F_IO_2).

Absorption atelectasis has been previously discussed (see High Inspired Oxygen Concentration and Absorption Atelectasis) and will not be covered here. Retrolental fibroplasia, an abnormal proliferation of the immature retinal vasculature of the prematurely born infant, can occur following exposure to hyperoxia. Very premature infants are most susceptible to retrolental fibroplasia (i.e., those of less than 1.0 kg birth weight and 28 weeks gestation). The risk of retrolental fibroplasia exists whenever an F_IO_2 causes a $P_aO_2 > 80$ mm Hg for more than 3 hours in an infant whose gestational age plus life age is less than 44 weeks. If the ductus arteriosus is patent, arterial blood samples should be drawn from the right radial artery (umbilical or lower extremity P_aO_2 is lower than the P_aO_2 to which the eyes are exposed owing to ductal shunting of unoxygenated blood [see chapter 17]).

The mode of action of toxicity of O_2 in tissues is complex, but interference with metabolism seems to be widespread. Most importantly, there is inactivation of many enzymes, particularly those with sulphydryl groups. The most acute toxic enzyme effect of O_2 in humans is a convulsive effect that occurs during exposure to pressures in excess of 2 atmospheres absolute.

High inspired O_2 concentrations can be of use therapeutically. Clearance of gas loculi in the body may be greatly accelerated by inhalation of 100 per cent O_2. Inhalation of 100 per cent O_2 creates a large N_2 gradient from the gas space to the perfusing blood. As a result, N_2 leaves the gas space, and the space diminishes in size. The technique of using O_2 to remove gas may be employed to ease intestinal gas pressure in patients with intestinal obstruction, to hasten recovery from pneumoencephalography, to decrease the size of an air embolus, and to aid in absorption of pneumoperitoneum and pneumothorax.

3. Hypercapnia

The effects of carbon dioxide on the cardiovascular system are as complex as they are for hypoxia. As with hypoxemia, hypercapnia appears to cause direct depression of both the cardiac muscle and the vascular smooth muscle, but at the same time, it causes reflex stimulation of the sympathoadrenal system, which compensates to a greater or lesser extent for the primary cardiovascular depression. Even in patients under halothane anesthesia, plasma catecholamine levels increase in response to increased CO_2 levels in much the same way as they do in conscious subjects. Thus, hypercapnia, like hypoxemia, may cause increased myocardial oxygen demand (tachycardia, early hypertension) and decreased myocardial oxygen supply (tachycardia, late hypotension).

Table 3–5 summarizes the interaction of anesthesia with hypercapnia in humans; increased cardiac output and decreased systemic vascular resistance should be emphasized.[176] The increase in cardiac output is most marked during anesthesia with drugs that enhance sympathetic activity and is least marked with halothane and nitrous oxide. The decrease in systemic vascular resistance is most marked during anesthesia with enflurane and accompanying hypercapnia.

Arrhythmias have been reported in unanesthetized humans during acute hypercapnia but have seldom been of serious importance. A high P_aCO_2 level, however, is more dangerous during general anesthesia, and with halothane anesthesia arrhythmias will frequently occur above a P_aCO_2 arrhythmic threshold, which is often constant for a particular patient.

The maximal stimulant respiratory effect is attained by a P_aCO_2 of about 100 mm Hg. With a higher P_aCO_2, stimulation is reduced, and at very high levels respiration is depressed and later ceases altogether. The P_{CO_2}/ventilation response curve is generally displaced to the right, and its slope is reduced by anesthetics and other depressant drugs.[177] With profound anesthesia the response curve may be flat, or even sloping downward, and carbon dioxide then acts as a respiratory depressant. In patients with ventilatory failure, carbon dioxide narcosis occurs when the P_aCO_2 rises above 90 to 120 mm Hg. Thirty per cent carbon dioxide is sufficient for the production of anesthesia, and

this concentration causes total but reversible flattening of the electroencephalogram.[178]

Quite apart from the effect of carbon dioxide upon ventilation, it exerts two other important effects that influence the oxygenation of the blood. First, if the concentration of nitrogen (or other "inert" gas) remains constant, the concentration of CO_2 in the alveolar gas can only increase at the expense of O_2, which must be displaced. Thus, P_AO_2 and P_aO_2 may decrease. Second, hypercapnia shifts the oxygen-hemoglobin curve to the right, facilitating tissue oxygenation.

Chronic hypercapnia results in increased resorption of bicarbonate by the kidneys, further raising the plasma bicarbonate level and constituting a secondary or compensatory "metabolic alkalosis." Chronic hypocapnia decreases renal bicarbonate resorption, resulting in further fall of plasma bicarbonate and producing a secondary or compensatory "metabolic acidosis." In each case arterial pH returns toward the normal value, but the bicarbonate ion concentration departs even further from normal.

Hypercapnia is accompanied by a leakage of potassium from the cells into the plasma. A good deal of the potassium comes from the liver, probably from glucose release and mobilization, which occurs in response to the rise in plasma catecholamine levels.[179] Since the plasma potassium level takes an appreciable time to return to normal, repeated bouts of hypercapnia at short intervals result in a stepwise rise in plasma potassium.

4. Hypocapnia

In this section, hypocapnia is considered to be produced by passive hyperventilation (by the anesthesiologist or ventilator).

Table 3–5. Cardiovascular Responses to Hypercapnia (P_aCO_2 = 60 to 83 mm Hg) during Various Types of Anesthesia (1 MAC Equivalent Except for Nitrous Oxide)*

	Heart Rate	Contractility	Cardiac Output	Systemic Vascular Resistance
Conscious	+ +	+ +	+ + +	−
Nitrous oxide	0	+	+ +	− −
Fluroxene	+	+ + +	+ + +	−
Halothane	0	+	+	−
Enflurane	+	+	+ +	− − −
Isoflurane	+ +	+ + +	+ + +	−

Key: + = <10 per cent increase; + + = 10 to 25 per cent increase; + + + = >25 per cent increase; 0 = no change; − = <10 per cent decrease; − − = 10 to 25 per cent decrease; − − − = >25 per cent decrease. MAC = minimum alveolar concentration for adequate anesthesia in 50 per cent of subjects.

*The increase in P_aCO_2 in the conscious subjects was 11.5 mm Hg from a normal level of 38 mm Hg.

Hypocapnia may cause a decrease in the cardiac output by three separate mechanisms. First, if present, an increase in intrathoracic pressure will decrease the cardiac output. Second, hypocapnia is associated with a withdrawal of sympathetic nervous system activity and this can decrease the ionotropic state of the heart. Third, hypocapnia can increase pH, which can in turn decrease ionized Ca^{++}, which may in turn decrease the ionotropic state of the heart. Hypocapnia with an alkalosis will also shift the oxygen-hemoglobin curve to the left, which increases the hemoglobin affinity for O_2, which will impair O_2 unloading at the tissue level. The decrease in peripheral flow and impaired ability to unload oxygen to the tissues is compounded by an increase in whole body oxygen consumption caused by an increased pH-mediated uncoupling of oxidation from phosphorylation;[180] P_aCO_2 of 20 mm Hg will increase tissue O_2 consumption by 30 per cent. Consequently, hypocapnia may simultaneously increase tissue O_2 demand and decrease tissue O_2 supply. Thus, in order to have the same amount of O_2 delivery to the tissues, cardiac output or tissue perfusion has to increase at a time it may not be possible to do so. It has been suggested that the cerebral effects of hypocapnia may be related to a state of cerebral acidosis and hypoxia, since hypocapnia may cause a selective reduction in the cerebral blood flow and also shifts the oxygen-hemoglobin curve to the left.

Hypocapnia may cause $\dot{V}_A/\dot{Q}$ abnormalities by inhibiting HPV or by causing bronchoconstriction and a decreased lung compliance. Finally, passive hypocapnia will produce apnea.

REFERENCES

1. West JB, Dollery CT, Naimark A: Distribution of blood flow in isolated lung: Relation to vascular and alveolar pressures. J Appl Physiol 19:713, 1964.
2. Permutt S, Bramberger-Barnea B, Bane HN: Alveolar pressure, pulmonary venous pressure and the vascular waterfall. Med Thorac 19:239, 1962.
3. Guyton AC: A concept of negative interstitial pressure based on pressures in implanted perforated capsules. Circ Res 12:399, 1963.
4. Smith-Erichsen N, Bo G: Airway closure and fluid filtration in the lung. Br J Anaesth 51:475, 1979.
5. Oswalt CE, Gates GA, Holmstrom EMG: Pulmonary edema as a complication of acute airway obstruction. Rev Surg 34:364, 1977.
6. Staub NC: Pulmonary edema: Physiologic approaches to management. Chest 74:559–564, 1978.
7. Permutt S: Effect of interstitial pressure of the lung on pulmonary circulation. Med Thorac 22:118–131, 1965.
8. Staub NC: "State of the art" review. Pathogenesis of pulmonary edema. Am Rev Resp Dis 109:358–372, 1974.
9. West JB, Dollery CT, Heard BE: Increased pulmonary vascular resistance in the dependent zone of the isolated dog lung caused by perivascular edema. Circ Res 17:191–206, 1965.
10. West JB (ed): Regional Differences in the Lung. New York Academic Press, 1977.
11. Hughes JMB, Glazier JB, Maloney JE, et al: Effect of lung volume on the distribution of pulmonary blood flow in man. Respir Physiol 4:58–72, 1968.
12. Hughes JM, Glazier JB, Maloney JE, et al: Effect of extra-alveolar vessels on the distribution of pulmonary blood flow in the dog. J Appl Physiol 25:701–709, 1968.
13. Permutt S, Caldini P, Maseri A, et al: Recruitment versus distensibility in the pulmonary vascular bed. In Fishman AP, Hecht H (eds): The Pulmonary Circulation and Interstitial Space. Chicago, University of Chicago Press, 1969, pp 375–387.
14. Maseri A, Caldini P, Harward P, et al: Determinants of pulmonary vascular volume. Recruitment versus distensibility. Circ Res 31:218–228, 1972.
15. Hoppin FG Jr, Green ID, Mead J: Distribution of pleural surface pressure. J Appl Physiol 27:863, 1969.
16. Milic-Emili J, Henderson JAM, Dolovich MB, et al: Regional distribution of inspired gas in the lung. J Appl Physiol 21:749, 1966.
17. West JB: Ventilation/Blood Flow and Gas Exchange. 2nd ed. Oxford, Blackwell Scientific Publications, 1970.
18. West JB: Regional differences in gas exchange in the lung of erect man. J Appl Physiol 17:893, 1962.
19. Wagner PD, Saltzman HA, West JB: Measurement of continuous distributions of ventilation-perfusion ratios: Theory. J Appl Physiol 36:588, 1974.
20. West JB: Blood flow to the lung and gas exchange. Anesthesiology 41:124, 1974.
21. Fishman AP: Dynamics of the pulmonary circulation. In Hamilton WF (ed): Handbook of Physiology, Section 2. Circulation. vol 2. Baltimore, Williams & Wilkins Co, 1963, pp 1667–1743.
22. Zapol WM, Snider MT: Pulmonary hypertension in severe acute respiratory failure. N Engl J Med 296:476–480, 1977.
23. Benumof JL: The pulmonary circulation: Relation to ARDS. 1977 Annual Refresher Course Lecture. American Society of Anesthesiologists 132:1–14, 1977.
24. Reid L: Structural and functional reappraisal of the pulmonary arterial system. In The Scientific Basis of Medicine Annual Reviews. London, Athlone Press, 1968.
25. Benumof JL, Mathers JM, Wahrenbrock EA: The pulmonary interstitial compartment and the mediator of hypoxic pulmonary vasoconstriction. Microvasc Res 15:69, 1978.
26. Bohr D: The pulmonary hypoxic response. Chest 71(Suppl):244–246, 1977.
27. Bergofsky EH: Ions and membrane permeability in the regulation of the pulmonary circulation. In Fishman AP and Hecht H (eds): The Pulmonary Circulation and Interstitial Space. Chicago, University of Chicago Press, 1969, pp 269–285.
28. Bergofsky EH: Mechanisms underlying vasomotor regulation of regional pulmonary blood flow in normal and disease states. Am J Med 57:378–391, 1974.
29. Fishman AP: Hypoxia on the pulmonary circulation—how and where it works. Circ Res 38:221–231, 1976.

30. Doyle JT, Wilson JS, Warren JV: The pulmonary vascular responses to short-term hypoxia in human subjects. Circulation 5:263–270, 1952.

31. Fishman AP: State of the art. Chronic cor pulmonale. Am Rev Resp Dis 114:775–794, 1976.

32. Boysen PG, Block AJ, Wynne JW, Hunt LA, Flick MP: Nocturnal pulmonary hypertension in patients with chronic obstructive pulmonary disease. Chest 76:536–542, 1979.

33. Zasslow MA, Benumof JL, Trousdale FR: Hypoxic pulmonary vasoconstriction and the size of the hypoxic compartment. Anesthesiology 55:A379, 1981.

34. Marshall BE, Marshall C: Continuity of response to hypoxic pulmonary vasoconstriction. J Appl Physiol 49:189–196, 1980.

35. Arborelius J Jr, Lilja B, Zauner CW: The relative effect of hypoxia and gravity on pulmonary blood flow. Respiration 31:369–380, 1974.

36. Benumof JL: Hypoxic pulmonary vasoconstriction and sodium nitroprusside perfusion. Anesthesiology 50:481, 1979.

37. Simmons DH, Linde CM, Miller JH, et al: Relation of lung volume and pulmonary vascular resistance. Circ Res 9:465, 1961.

38. Burton AC, Patel DJ: Effect on pulmonary vascular resistance of inflation of the rabbit lungs. J Appl Physiol 12:239, 1958.

39. Wittenberger JL, McGregor M, Berglund E, et al: Influence of state of inflation of the lung on pulmonary vascular resistance. J Appl Physiol 15:878, 1960.

40. Benumof JL, Rogers SN, Moyce PR, et al: Hypoxic pulmonary vasoconstriction and regional and whole lung PEEP in the dog. Anesthesiology 52:503, 1979.

41. Benumof JL: Mechanism of decreased blood flow to the atelectatic lung. J Appl Physiol 46:1047–1048, 1978.

42. Pirlo AF, Benumof JL, Trousdale FR: Atelectatic lobe blood flow: Open vs. closed chest. Positive pressure vs. spontaneous ventilation. J Appl Physiol 50:1022–1026, 1981.

43. Prefaut CH, Engel LA: Vertical distribution of perfusion and inspired gas in supine man. Resp Physiol 43:209–219, 1981.

44. Hagen PT, Scholz DG, Edwards WD: Incidence and size of patent foramen ovale during the first ten decades of life: An autopsy study of 965 normal hearts. Mayo Clin Proc 59:17–20, 1984.

45. Sykes MK: The mechanics of ventilation. In Scurr C, Feldman S (eds): Scientific Foundations of Anesthesia. Philadelphia, FA Davis Co, 1970, pp 174–186.

46. Nunn JF: Mechanisms of pulmonary ventilation. Applied Respiratory Physiology. 2nd ed. London, Butterworths, 1977, pp 139–177.

47. Peters RM: Work of breathing following trauma. J Trauma 8:915, 1968.

48. Nunn JF: The minute volume of pulmonary ventilation. Applied Respiratory Physiology. 2nd ed. London, Butterworths, 1977, pp 178–212.

49. Shapiro BA, Harrison RA, Trout CA: The mechanics of ventilation. In Shapiro BA et al (eds): Clinical Application of Respiratory Care. 2nd ed. Chicago, Year Book Medical Publishers, 1979, pp 57–89.

50. Comroe JH, Forster RE, Dubois AB, et al: In The Lung. 2nd ed. Chicago, Year Book Medical Publishers, 1962.

51. Macklem PT, Fraser RG, Bates DV: Bronchial pressures and dimensions in health and obstructive airway disease. J Appl Physiol 18:699, 1983.

52. Craig DB, Wahba WM, Don HF, et al: "Closing volume" and its relationship to gas exchange in seated and supine positions. J Appl Physiol 31:717, 1971.

53. Burger EJ Jr, Macklem P: Airway closure: Demonstration by breathing 100% O_2 at low lung volumes and by N_2 washout. J Appl Physiol 25:139, 1968.

54. Brismer B, Hedenstierna G, Lundquist H, Strandberg A, Svensson L, Tokics L: Pulmonary densities during anaesthesia with muscular relaxation—A proposal of atelectasis. Anesthesiology 62:422–428, 1985.

55. Hales CA, Kazemi H: Small airways function in myocardial infarction. N Engl J Med 290:761, 1974.

56. Harken AH, O'Connor NE: The influence of clinically undetectable edema on small airway closure in the dog. Ann Surg 184:183, 1976.

57. Biddle TL, Yu PN, Hodges M, et al: Hypoxemia and lung water in acute myocardial infarction. Am Heart J 92:692, 1976.

58. Nunn JF: Resistance to gas flow. Applied Respiratory Physiology. 2nd ed. London, Butterworths, 1977, pp 94–138.

59. Rehder K, Marsh HM, Rodarte JR, et al: Airway closure. Anesthesiology 47:40, 1977.

60. Leblanc P, Ruff F, Milic-Emili J: Effects of age and body position on "airway closure" in man. J Appl Physiol 28:448, 1970.

61. Craig DB, Wahba WM, Don HF, et al: "Closing volume" and its relationship to gas exchange in seated and supine positions. J Appl Physiol 31:717, 1971.

62. Foex P, Prys-Roberts C, Hahn CEW, et al: Comparison of oxygen content of blood measured directly with values derived from measurement of oxygen tension. Br J Anaesth 42:803, 1970.

63. Sykes MK, Adams AP, Finley WEI, et al: The cardiorespiratory effects of hemorrhage and overtransfusion in dogs. Br J Anaesth 42:573, 1970.

64. Gregory IC: The oxygen and carbon monoxide capacities of foetal and adult blood. J Physiol 236:625, 1974.

65. Nunn JF: Oxygen. Applied Respiratory Physiology. 2nd ed. London, Butterworths, 1977, pp 375–444.

66. Lawler PGP, Nunn JF: A re-assessment of the validity of the iso-shunt graph. Br J Anaesth 56:1325–1336, 1984.

67. Kelman GF, Nunn JF, Prys-Roberts C, et al: The influence of the cardiac output on arterial oxygenation: A theoretical study. Br J Anaesth 39:450, 1967.

68. Philbin DM, Sullivan SF, Bowman FO, et al: Postoperative hypoxemia: Contribution of the cardiac output. Anesthesiology 32:136, 1970.

69. Berggren SM: The oxygen deficit of arterial blood caused by non-ventilating parts of the lung. Acta Physiol Scand 4(Supp 11):1, 1942.

70. Cheney FW, Colley PS: The effect of cardiac output on arterial blood oxygenation. Anesthesiology 52:496–503, 1980.

71. Henry W: Experiments on the quantity of gases absorbed by water at different temperatures and under different pressures. Phil Trans Roy Soc 93:29, 1803.

72. Donald DE, Shepherd JT: Reflexes from the heart and lungs: Physiological curiosities or important regulatory mechanisms. Cardiovas Res 12:449–469, 1978.

73. Malliani A, Parks M, Tuckett RP, Brown AM: Reflex increases in heart rate elicited by stimulation of afferent cardiac sympathetic nerve fibers in the cat. Circ Res 32:9–14, 1973.

74. Hess GL, Zuperku EJ, Coon RL, Kampine JP: Sympathetic afferent nerve activity of left ventricular origin. Am J Physiol 227:543–546, 1974.

75. Lombardi F, Malliani A, Pagani M: Nervous activity of afferent sympathetic fibers innervating the pulmonary veins. Brain Res 113:197–200, 1976.

76. Folkow B, Neil E (eds): The pulmonary circulation. In Circulation. Oxford, Oxford University Press, 1971, chapter 18, pp 320–339.

77. Malliani A, Peterson DF, Bishop VS, Brown AM: Spinal sympathetic cardiovascular reflexes. Circ Res 30:158–166, 1972.

78. Malliani A, Recordati G, Schwartz PJ: Nervous activity of afferent cardiac sympathetic fibers with atrial and ventricular endings. J Physiol 229:457–469, 1973.

79. Lloyd TC, Jr: Reflex effects of left heart and pulmonary vascular distention of airways of dogs. J Appl Physiol 49:620–626, 1980.

80. Anderson FL, Brown AM: Pulmonary vasoconstriction elicited by stimulation of the hypothalamic integrative area for the defense reaction. Circ Res 21:747–756, 1967.

81. Laks MM, Juratsch CE, Garner D, Beazell J, Criley JM: Acute pulmonary artery hypertension produced by distention of the main pulmonary artery in the conscious dog. Chest 68:807–813, 1975.

82. Szidon JP, Fishman AP: Autonomic control of the pulmonary circulation. In Fishman AP and Hecht HH (eds): Pulmonary Circulation and Interstitial Space. Chicago, University of Chicago Press, 1969, chapter 17, pp 239–265.

83. Maloney JE, Bergel DH, Glazier JB, Hughes JMB, West JB: Transmission of pulsatile blood pressure and flow through the isolated lung. Circ Res 23:11–24, 1968.

84. Franklin DL, Van Citters RL, Rushmer RF: Balance between right and left ventricular output. Circ Res 10:17–26, 1962.

85. Varnauskas E: The effect of physical exercise on pulmonary blood volume. In Muller C (ed): Conference on Pulmonary Circulation. Oslo, Scandinavian University Book, 1965, pp 105–111.

86. Bakhle YS, Vane JR (eds): Metabolic functions of the lung. vol 4. In Lung Biology in Health and Disease. New York, Marcel Dekker, Inc., 1977.

87. Marchesi VT, Barrnett RJ: The demonstration of enzymatic activity in pinocytotic vesicles of blood capillaries with the electron microscope. J Cell Biol 17:547–556, 1963.

88. Smith U, Ryan JW: Pulmonary endothelial cells and metabolism of adenine nucleotides, kinnins and angiotensin I. In Back N, Sicuteri F (eds): Advances in Experimental Medicine and Biology. vol 21. Vasopeptides. New York, Plenum Press, 1972, pp 267–276.

89. Tierney DF: Lung metabolism and biochemistry. Ann Rev Physiol 36:209–231, 1974.

90. Fishman AP, Pietra GG: Handling of bioactive materials by the lung. N Engl J Med 291:884–890, 1974.

91. Tucker A, Weir KE, Grover RF, Reeves JT: Oxygen-tension-dependent pulmonary vascular responses to vasoactive agents. Canad J Physiol Pharmacol 55:251–257, 1977.

92. Vader CR, Mathias MM, Schatte CL: Pulmonary prostaglandin metabolism during normobaric hyperoxia. Prostaglandins 6:101–110, 1981.

93. Harabin AL, Peake MD, Sylvester JT: Effect of severe hypoxia on the pulmonary vascular response to vasoconstrictor agents. J Appl Physiol 50:561–565, 1981.

94. Leuenberger PJ, Stalcup SA, Mellins RB, Greenbaum LM, Turino GM: Decrease in angiotension I conversion by acute hypoxia in dogs. Proc Soc Exp Biol Med 158:586–592, 1978.

95. Junod AF: Metabolism of vasoactive agents in lung. Am Rev Resp Dis 115:51–57, 1977.

96. Said SI: Endocrine role of the lung in disease. Am J Med 57:453–465, 1974.

97. Junod AF: Metabolism, production and release of hormones and mediators in the lung. Am Rev Resp Dis 112:92–108, 1975.

98. Lipsett MB: Hormonal syndromes associated with neoplasia. Adv Metab Disorders 3:111–152, 1968.

99. Piper PJ, Vane JR: The release of prostaglandins from the lung and other tissues. Ann NY Acad Sci 180:363–385, 1971.

100. Andersen HW, Benumof JL: Intrapulmonary shunting during one-lung ventilation and surgical manipulation. Anesthesiology 55:A377, 1981.

101. Said SI, Kitamura S, Vreim C: Prostaglandins: Release from the lung during mechanical ventilation at large tidal volumes. J Clin Invest 51:83A, 1972.

102. Kitamura S, Preskitt J, Yoshida T, Said SI: Prostaglandin release, respiratory alkalosis and systemic hypertension during mechanical ventilation. Fed Proc 32:341–345, 1973.

103. Said SI, Yoshida T: Release of prostaglandins and other humoral mediators during hypoxic breathing and pulmonary edema. Chest 66:12S, 1974.

104. Said SI, Hara N, Yoshida T: Hypoxic pulmonary vasoconstriction in cats: Modification by aspirin and indomethacin. Fed Proc 34:438–444, 1975.

105. Said SI, Yoshida T, Kitamura S, Vreim C: Pulmonary alveolar hypoxia: Release of prostaglandins and other humoral mediators. Science 185:1181–1185, 1974.

106. Austen KF: Systemic anaphylaxis in the human being. N Engl J Med 291:661–664, 1974.

107. Pavek K: Anaphylactic shock in the monkey: Its hemodynamics and mediators. Acta Anaesth Scand 21:293–307, 1977.

108. Fishman AP: Nonrespiratory functions of the lungs. Chest 72:84–89, 1977.

109. Heinemann HO, Fishman AP: Nonrespiratory functions of the mammalian lung. Physiol Rev 49:1–47, 1969.

110. Mammen EF: Blood coagulation and pulmonary function. In Dal Santo G (ed): Nonrespiratory Functions of the Lung and Anesthesia. vol 15. no 4. Boston, Little, Brown and Company, 1977, pp 91–106.

111. Benumof JL: Monitoring respiratory function during anesthesia. In Saidman LJ, Smith NT (eds): Monitoring in Anesthesia. New York, John Wiley and Sons, 1978, pp 31–51.

112. Munson ES, Larson CP Jr, Babad AA, et al: The effects of halothane, fluroxene and cyclopropane on ventilation: A comparative study in man. Anesthesiology 27:716, 1966.

113. Couture J, Picken J, Trop D, et al: Airway closure in normal, obese, and anesthetized supine subjects. Fed Proc 29:269, 1970.

114. Don HF, Craig DB, Wahba WM, et al: The measurement of gas trapped in the lungs at functional residual capacity and the effects of posture. Anesthesiology 35:582, 1971.

115. Ward CS: The prevention of accidents associated with anesthetic apparatus. Br J Anaesth 40:692, 1968.

116. Mazze RI: Therapeutic misadventures with oxygen delivery systems: The need for continuous in-line oxygen monitors. Anesth Analg 51:787, 1972.

117. Epstein RM, Rackow H, Lee ASJ, et al: Prevention of accidental breathing of anoxic gas mixture during anesthesia. Anesthesiology 23:1, 1962.

118. Sprague DH, Archer GW: Intraoperative hypoxia

from an erroneously filled liquid oxygen reservoir. Anesthesiology 42:360, 1975.

119. Eger EI II, Epstein RM: Hazards of anesthetic equipment. Anesthesiology 25:490, 1964.

120. Martin JT: Positioning in Anesthesia and Surgery. Philadelphia, WB Saunders Co, 1978.

121. Heinonen J, Takki S, Tammisto T: Effect of the Trendelenburg tilt and other procedures on the position of endotracheal tubes. Lancet 1:850, 1969.

122. Mead J, Agostoni E: Dynamics of breathing. In Fenn WO, Rahn H (eds): Handbook of Physiology. Section 3: Respiration. vol 1. Baltimore, Williams & Wilkins Co, 1964, pp 411–427.

123. Don HF, Robson JG: The mechanics of the respiratory system during anesthesia. Anesthesiology 26:168, 1965.

124. Bendixen HH, Hedley-Whyte J, Chir B, et al: Impaired oxygenation in surgical patients during general anesthesia with controlled ventilation. N Engl J Med 269:991, 1963.

125. Bendixen HH, Bullwinkel B, Hedley-Whyte J, et al: Atelectasis and shunting during spontaneous ventilation in anesthetized patients. Anesthesiology 25:297, 1964.

126. Cain SM: Increased oxygen uptake with passive hyperventilation of dogs. J Appl Physiol 28:4, 1970.

127. Karetzky MS, Cain SM: Effect of carbon dioxide on oxygen uptake during hyperventilation in normal man. J Appl Physiol 28:8, 1970.

128. Benumof JL, Mathers JM, Wahrenbrock EA: Cyclic hypoxic pulmonary vasoconstriction induced by concomitant carbon dioxide changes. J Appl Physiol 41:466, 1976.

129. Cutillo A, Omboni E, Perondi R, et al: Effect of hypocapnia on pulmonary mechanics in normal subjects and in patients with chronic obstructive lung disease. Am Rev Resp Dis 110:25, 1974.

130. Don H: The mechanical properties of the respiratory system during anesthesia. In Kafer ER (ed): International Anesthesiology Clinics. vol 15. Anesthesia and Respiratory Function. Boston, Little, Brown and Company, 1977, pp 113–136.

131. Don HF, Wahba M, Cuadrado L, et al: The effects of anesthesia and 100 per cent oxygen on the functional residual capacity of the lungs. Anesthesiology 32:521, 1970.

132. Hewlett AM, Hulands GH, Nunn JF, et al: Functional residual capacity during anaesthesia. III: Artificial ventilation. Br J Anaesth 46:495, 1974.

133. Westbrook PR, Stubbs SE, Sessler AD, et al: Effects of anesthesia and muscle paralysis on respiratory mechanics in normal man. J Appl Physiol 34:81, 1973.

134. Alexander JI, Spence AA, Parikh RK, et al: The role of airway closure in postoperative hypoxemia. Br J Anaesth 45:34, 1973.

135. Hickey RF, Visick W, Fairley HB, et al: Effects of halothane anesthesia on functional residual capacity and alveolar-arterial oxygen tension difference. Anesthesiology 38:20, 1973.

136. Wyche MQ, Teichner RL, Kallos T, et al: Effects of continuous positive-pressure breathing on functional residual capacity and arterial oxygenation during intraabdominal operation. Anesthesiology 38:68, 1973.

137. Freund F, Roos A, Dodd RB: Expiratory activity of the abdominal muscles in man during general anesthesia. J Appl Physiol 19:693, 1964.

138. Kallos T, Wyche MQ, Garman JK: The effect of innovar on functional residual capacity and total chest compliance. Anesthesiology 39:558, 1973.

139. Campbell EJM, Agostini E, David JN: The Respiratory Muscles: Mechanics and Neural Control. 2nd ed. Philadelphia, WB Saunders Co, 1970.

140. Milic-emili J, Mead J, Tanner JM: Topography of esophageal pressure as a function of posture in man. J Appl Physiol 19:212, 1964.

141. Froese AB, Bryan CA: Effects of anesthesia and paralysis on diaphragmatic mechanics in man. Anesthesiology 41:242, 1974.

142. Dekker E, Defares JG, Heemstra H: Direct measurement of intrabronchial pressure. Its application to the location of the check-value mechanism. J Appl Physiol 13:35, 1958.

143. Ward CF, Gagnon RL, Benumof JL: Wheezing after induction of general anesthesia: Negative expiratory pressure revisited. Anesth Analg 58:49, 1979.

144. Ray JF, Yost L, Moallem S, et al: Immobility, hypoxemia, and pulmonary arteriovenous shunting. Arch Surg 109:537, 1974.

145. Wagner PD, Laravuso RB, Uhl RR, et al: Continuous distributions of ventilation-perfusion ratios in normal subjects breathing air and 100% O_2. J Clin Invest 54:54, 1974.

146. Briscoe WA, Cree EM, Filler, et al: Lung volume, alveolar ventilation and perfusion interrelationships in chronic pulmonary emphysema. J Appl Physiol 15:785, 1960.

147. Slocum HC, Hoeflich EA, Allen CR: Circulatory and respiratory distress from extreme positions on the operating table. Surg Gynecol Obstet 84:1065, 1947.

148. Laver MB, Hallowell P, Goldblatt A: Pulmonary dysfunction secondary to heart disease: Aspects relevant to anesthesia and surgery. Anesthesiology 33:161, 1970.

149. Yeaker H: Tracheobronchial secretions. Am J Med 50:493, 1971.

150. Forbes AR: Humidification and mucous flow in the intubated trachea. Br J Anaesth 45:874, 1973.

151. Bang BG, Bang FB: Effect of water deprivation on nasal mucous flow. Proc Soc Exp Biol Med 106:516, 1961.

152. Hirsch JA, Tokayer JL, Robinson MJ, et al: Effects of dry air and subsequent humidification on tracheal mucous velocity in dogs. J Appl Physiol 39:242, 1975.

153. Dalhamn T: Mucous flow and ciliary activity in the tracheas of rats exposed to respiratory irritant gases. Acta Physiol Scand 36(Suppl 123):1, 1956.

154. Hill L: The ciliary movement of the trachea studies in vitro. Lancet 2:802, 1928.

155. Sackner MA, Landa J, Hirsch J, et al: Pulmonary effects of oxygen breathing. Ann Intern Med 82:40, 1975.

156. Sackner MA, Hirsch J, Epstein S: Effect of cuffed endotracheal tubes of tracheal mucous velocity. Chest 68:774, 1975.

157. Forbes AR: Halothane depresses mucociliary flow in the trachea. Anesthesiology 45:59, 1976.

158. Nunn JF, Sturrock JE, Wills EJ, et al: The effect of inhalation anaesthetics on the swimming velocity of *Tetrahymena pyriformis*. J Cell Sci 15:537, 1974.

159. Prys-Roberts C: The metabolic regulation of circulatory transport. In Scurr C, Feldman S (eds): Scientific Foundation of Anesthesia. Philadelphia, FA Davis Co, 1970, pp 87–96.

160. Benumof JL, Wahrenbrock EA: Blunted hypoxic pulmonary vasoconstriction by increased lung vascular pressures. J Appl Physiol 38:846, 1975.

161. Scanlon TS, Benumof JL, Wahrenbrock EA, et al: Hypoxic pulmonary vasoconstriction and the ratio of

hypoxic lung to perfused normoxic lung. Anesthesiology 49:177, 1978.

162. Benumof JL, Wahrenbrock EA: Dependency of hypoxic pulmonary vasoconstriction of temperature. J Appl Physiol 42:56, 1977.

163. Ward CF, Benumof JL, Wahrenbrock EA: Inhibition of hypoxic pulmonary vasoconstriction by vasoactive drugs. Abstracts of Scientific Papers, American Society of Anesthesiology Meeting, 1976, p 333.

164. Johansen I, Benumof JL: Reduction of hypoxia-induced pulmonary artery hypertension by vasodilator drugs. Am Rev Resp Dis 119:375, 1979.

165. Benumof JL, Wahrenbrock EA: The local effect of anesthetics on regional hypoxic pulmonary vasoconstriction. Anesthesiology 43:525, 1975.

166. Mathers JM, Benumof JL, Wahrenbrock EA: General anesthetics and regional hypoxic pulmonary vasoconstriction. Anesthesiology 46:111, 1977.

167. Benumof JL: One lung ventilation: Which lung should be PEEPed? Anesthesiology 56:161, 1982.

168. Eckenhoff JE, Enderby GEH, Larson A, et al: Pulmonary gas exchange during deliberate hypotension. Br J Anaesth 35:750, 1963.

169. Kain ML, Panday J, Nunn JF: The effect of intubation on the dead space during halothane anaesthesia. Br J Anaesth 41:94, 1969.

170. Conway CM: Anesthetic circuits. In Scurr C, Feldman S (eds): Scientific Foundations of Anesthesia. 2nd ed. London, William Heinemann Medical Books, 1974, pp 509–515.

171. Heistad DD, Abboud FM: Circulatory adjustments to hypoxia. Dickinson W. Richards Lecture. Circ 61:463–470, 1980.

172. Roberts JG: The effect of hypoxia on the systemic circulation during anaesthesia. In Prys-Roberts E. (ed): The Circulation in Anaesthesia: Applied Physiology and Pharmacology. London, Blackwell Scientific Publications, 1980, pp 311–326.

173. Winter PM, Smith G: The toxicity of oxygen. Anesthesiology 37:210, 1972.

174. Lambertsen CJ: Effects of oxygen at high partial pressure. Handbook of Physiology. Section 3. Respiration. vol 2. Fenn WO, Rahn H. (eds): Baltimore, Williams & Wilkins Co, 1965, pp 1027–1046.

175. Nash G, Blennerhasset JB, Pontoppidan H: Pulmonary lesions associated with oxygen therapy and artificial ventilation. N Engl J Med 276:368, 1967.

176. Prys-Roberts C: Hypercapnia. In Gray TC, Nunn JF, Utting JE (eds): General Anaesthesia. 4th ed, London, Butterworths, 1980, pp 435–461.

177. Severinghaus JW, Larson CP: Respiration in anesthesia. In Fenn WO, Rahn H (eds): Handbook of Physiology. Section 3. Respiration. vol 2. Baltimore, Williams & Wilkins Co, 1965, pp 1219–1264.

178. Clowes GHA, Hopkins AL, Simeone FA: A comparison of the physiological effects of hypercapnia and hypoxia in the production of cardiac arrest. Ann Surg 142:446, 1955.

179. Fenn WO, Asano T: Effects of carbon dioxide inhalation on potassium liberation from the liver. Am J Physiol 185:567, 1956.

180. Patterson RW: Effect of P_aCO_2 on O_2 consumption during cardiopulmonary bypass in man. Anesth Analg 55:269–273, 1976.

Special Physiology of the Lateral Decubitus Position, the Open Chest, and One-Lung Ventilation

4

I. INTRODUCTION

It is not possible to have adequate gas exchange during spontaneous ventilation with an open chest because of the occurrence of mediastinal shift and paradoxical respiration (see the "pneumothorax problem" discussed in chapter 1). Consequently, intrathoracic surgery cannot be performed with spontaneous ventilation. The first part of this chapter briefly reviews this physiology.

Patients undergoing thoracic surgery are usually in the lateral decubitus position under general anesthesia, have an open chest wall (nondependent hemithorax), are pharmacologically paralyzed, and, of course, have ventilation controlled. Even if both lungs are being ventilated, each of these anesthesia and surgical requirements can cause major alterations in the distribution of perfusion ($\dot{Q}$), and/or ventilation ($\dot{V}$), and ventilation-perfusion relationships ($\dot{V}/\dot{Q}$) (compared with the awake state in the upright position). The second part of this chapter will discuss the physiologic effects of each one of these anesthetic and surgical events on the distribution of $\dot{Q}$, $\dot{V}$, and $\dot{V}/\dot{Q}$ during two-lung ventilation.

In addition, a good deal of thoracic surgery must be performed in the lateral decubitus position with the nondependent lung nonventilated and the dependent lung ventilated (one-lung ventilation). One-lung ventilation imposes a new host of determinants on the distribution of blood flow (and, of course, ventilation), and the third part of this chapter will consider the physiology of one-lung ventilation.

II. PHYSIOLOGY OF SPONTANEOUS VENTILATION WITH AN OPEN CHEST

A. Mediastinal Shift

An examination of the physiology of the open chest during spontaneous ventilation reveals why controlled positive-pressure ventilation is the only practical way to provide adequate gas exchange during thoracotomy. In the spontaneously breathing, closed-chested patient in the lateral decubitus position, gravity causes the pleural pressure in the dependent hemithorax to be less negative than that in the nondependent hemithorax (see Fig. 3–5), but there is still negative pressure in each hemithorax on each side of the mediastinum. In addition, the weight of the mediastinum causes some compression of the lower lung, contributing to the pleural pressure gradient. With the nondependent hemithorax open, atmospheric pressure in that cavity exceeds the negative pleural pressure in the dependent hemithorax; this imbalance of pressure on the two sides of the mediastinum causes a further downward displacement of the mediastinum into the dependent thorax. During inspiration the caudad movement of the dependent-lung diaphragm increases the negative pressure in the dependent lung and causes a still further displacement of the mediastinum into the dependent hemithorax. During expiration, as the dependent-lung diaphragm moves cephalad, the pressure in the dependent hemithorax becomes relatively positive, and the mediastinum is pushed upward out of the dependent hemithorax (Fig. 4–1).[1] Thus, the tidal volume in the dependent lung is decreased by an amount equal to the inspiratory displacement caused by mediastinal movement. This phenomenon is called mediastinal shift and is one mechanism that results in

impaired ventilation in the open-chested spontaneously breathing patient in the lateral decubitus position. The mediastinal shift can also cause circulatory changes (decreased venous return) and reflexes (sympathetic activation) that result in a clinical picture similar to shock: The patient is hypotensive, pale, and cold, with dilated pupils. Local anesthetic infiltration of the pulmonary plexus at the hilum and the vagus nerve can diminish these reflexes. More practically, controlled positive-pressure ventilation abolishes these ventilatory and circulatory changes associated with mediastinal shift.

B. Paradoxical Respiration

When a pleural cavity is exposed to atmospheric pressure, the lung is no longer held open by negative intrapleural pressure, and it tends

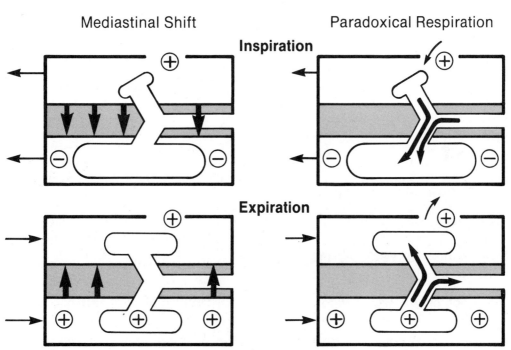

Figure 4–1. Schematic representation of mediastinal shift and paradoxical respiration in the spontaneously ventilating patient with an open chest and placed in the lateral decubitus position. The open chest is always exposed to atmospheric pressure (⊕). During inspiration, negative pressure (⊖) in the intact hemithorax causes the mediastinum to move vertically downward (mediastinal shift). In addition, during inspiration movement of gas from the nondependent lung in the open hemithorax into the dependent lung in the closed hemithorax and movement of air from the environment into the open hemithorax causes the lung in the open hemithorax to collapse (paradoxical respiration). During expiration, relative positive pressure (⊕) in the closed hemithorax causes the mediastinum to move vertically upward (mediastinal shift). In addition, during expiration the gas moves from the dependent lung to the nondependent lung and from the open hemithorax to the environment; consequently, the nondependent lung expands during expiration (paradoxical respiration).

to collapse because of unopposed elastic recoil. Thus, the lung in an open chest is at least partially collapsed. It has long been observed during spontaneous ventilation with an open hemithorax that lung collapse is accentuated during inspiration, and, conversely, the lung expands during expiration. This reversal of lung movement with an open chest during respiration has been termed paradoxical respiration. The mechanism of paradoxical respiration is similar to that of mediastinal shift. During inspiration, the descent of the diaphragm on the side of the open hemithorax causes air from the environment to enter the pleural cavity on that side through the thoracotomy opening and fill the space around the exposed lung. The descent of the hemidiaphragm on the closed-chest side causes gas to enter the closed-chest lung in the normal manner. However, gas also enters the closed-chest lung (which has a relatively negative pressure) from the open-chest lung (which remains at atmospheric pressure); this results in further reduction in the size of the open-chest lung during inspiration. During expiration the reverse occurs, with the collapsed, open-chest lung filling from the intact lung and air moving back out of the exposed hemithorax through the thoracotomy. The phenomenon of paradoxical respiration is illustrated in Figure 4–1.[1] Paradoxical breathing is increased by a large thoracotomy and by increased airway resistance in the intact lung. Paradoxical respiration may be prevented either by manual collapse of the open-chest lung or, more commonly, by controlled positive-pressure ventilation.

III. PHYSIOLOGY OF THE LATERAL DECUBITUS POSITION AND THE OPEN CHEST DURING CONTROLLED TWO-LUNG VENTILATION: DISTRIBUTION OF PERFUSION (Q̇) AND VENTILATION (V̇)

A. Distribution of Q̇, V̇, V̇/Q̇—Lateral Decubitus Position, Awake, Closed Chest

Gravity causes a vertical gradient in the distribution of pulmonary blood flow in the lateral decubitus position for the same reason that it does in the upright position (see Fig. 3–5). Since the vertical hydrostatic gradient is less in the lateral decubitus position than in the upright position, there is ordinarily less zone 1 blood flow (in the nondependent lung) in the

former position compared with the latter position (Fig. 4–2). Nevertheless, blood flow to the dependent lung is still significantly greater than blood flow to the nondependent lung (Fig. 4–2). Thus, when the right lung is nondependent, it should receive approximately 45 per cent of total blood flow, as opposed to the 55 per cent of the total blood flow that it received in the upright and supine positions.[2, 3] When the left lung is nondependent, it should receive approximately 35 per cent of total blood flow, as opposed to the 45 per cent of the total blood flow that it received in the upright and supine positions.[2, 3]

Since gravity also causes a vertical gradient in pleural pressure (P_{pl}) (see Figs. 3–5 and 3–6) in the lateral decubitus position, ventilation is relatively increased in the dependent lung compared with the nondependent lung (Fig. 4–3). In addition, in the lateral decubitus position the dome of the lower diaphragm is pushed higher into the chest than the dome of the upper diaphragm, and therefore the lower diaphragm is more sharply curved than the upper diaphragm. As a result, the lower diaphragm is able to contract more efficiently during spontaneous respiration. Thus, in the lateral decubitus position in the awake patient, the lower lung is normally better ventilated than the upper lung, regardless of the side on which the patient is lying, although there remains a tendency toward greater ventilation of the larger right lung.[4] Since there is greater perfusion to the lower lung, the preferential ventilation to the lower lung is matched by its increased perfusion, so that the distribution of the ventilation-perfusion ratios of the two lungs is not greatly altered when the awake subject assumes the lateral decubitus position. Since the increase in ventilation is less than the increase in perfusion with lung dependency, the V̇/Q̇ ratio decreases from dependent to nondependent lung (just as it does in upright and supine lungs).

B. Distribution of Q̇, V̇—Lateral Decubitus Position, Anesthetized, Closed Chest

Comparing the awake with the anesthetized patient in the lateral decubitus position, there is no difference in the distribution of pulmonary blood flow between the dependent and nondependent lungs. Thus, in the anesthetized patient, the dependent lung continues to receive relatively more perfusion than the nondependent lung. The induction of general anesthesia,

Distribution of Blood Flow
Lateral Decubitus Position

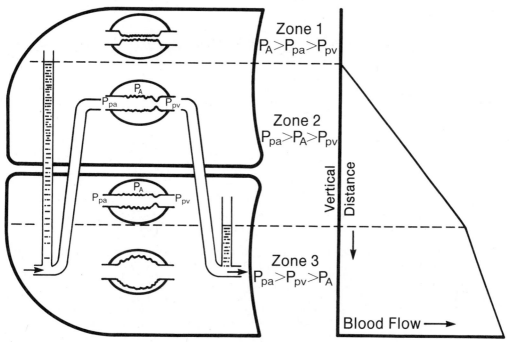

Figure 4–2. Schematic representation of the effects of gravity on the distribution of pulmonary blood flow in the lateral decubitus position. The vertical gradient in the lateral decubitus position is less than that in the upright position (see Fig. 3–1). Consequently, there is less zone 1 and more zone 2 and 3 blood flow in the lateral decubitus position compared with the upright position. Nevertheless, pulmonary blood flow increases with lung dependency and is greater in the dependent lung compared with the nondependent lung. (P$_A$ = alveolar pressure; P$_{pa}$ = pulmonary artery pressure; P$_{pv}$ = pulmonary venous pressure.) (Modified with permission from Benumof JL: Physiology of the open chest and one-lung ventilation. In Kaplan JA (ed.): Thoracic Anesthesia. New York, Churchill Livingstone Inc., 1983, chapter 8.)

however, does cause significant changes in the distribution of ventilation between the two lungs.

In the lateral decubitus position, the majority of ventilation is switched from the dependent lung in the awake subject to the nondependent lung in the anesthetized patient (Fig. 4–4).[5, 6] There are several interrelated reasons for this change in the relative distribution of ventilation between the nondependent and dependent lung. First, the induction of general anesthesia usually causes a decrease in functional residual capacity (FRC), and both lungs share in the loss of lung volume. Since each lung occupies a different initial position on the pulmonary pressure-volume curve while the subject is awake, a general anesthesia-induced reduction in the FRC of each lung causes each lung to move to a lower but still different portion of the pressure-volume curve (Fig. 4–4). The dependent lung moves from an initially steep part of the

curve (with the subject awake) to a lower and flatter part of the curve (after anesthesia is induced), while the nondependent lung moves from an initially flat portion of the pressure-volume curve (with the subject awake) to a lower and steeper part of the curve (after anesthesia is induced). Thus, with the induction of general anesthesia, the lower lung moves to a less favorable (flat, noncompliant) portion and the upper lung to a more favorable (steep, compliant) portion of the pressure-volume curve. Second, if the anesthetized patient in the lateral decubitus position is also paralyzed and artificially ventilated, the high curved diaphragm of the lower lung no longer confers any advantage in ventilation (as it does in the awake state), since it is no longer actively contracting.[7] Third, the mediastinum rests upon the lower lung and physically impedes lower lung expansion, as well as selectively decreasing lower lung FRC. Fourth, the weight of the abdominal

Awake, Closed Chest
Distribution of Ventilation

Upright
Position

Lateral Decubitus
Position

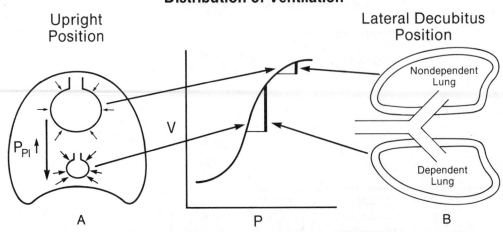

Figure 4–3. Pleural pressure (P_{pl}) in the awake upright patient (A) is most positive in the dependent portion of the lung, and alveoli in this region are therefore most compressed and have the least volume (see Fig. 3–5). Pleural pressure is least positive (most negative) at the apex of the lung, and alveoli in this region are therefore least compressed and have the largest volume. When these regional differences in alveolar volume are translated over to a regional transpulmonary pressure–alveolar volume curve, the small dependent alveoli are on a steep (large-slope) portion of the curve, and the large nondependent alveoli are on a flat (small-slope) portion of the curve (see also Fig. 3–6). In this diagram regional slope equals regional compliance. Thus, for a given and equal change in transpulmonary pressure, the dependent part of the lung receives a much larger share of the tidal volume than the nondependent part of the lung. In the lateral decubitus position (B) gravity also causes pleural pressure gradients and therefore similarly affects the distribution of ventilation. The dependent lung lies on a relatively steep portion, and the upper lung lies on a relatively flat portion of the pressure-volume curve. Thus, in the lateral decubitus position the dependent lung receives the majority of the tidal ventilation. (V = alveolar volume; P = transpulmonary pressure.) (Modified with permission from Benumof JL: Physiology of the open chest and one-lung ventilation. In Kaplan JA (ed.): Thoracic Anesthesia. New York, Churchill Livingstone Inc., 1983, chapter 8.)

Closed Chest, Lateral Decubitus Position
Distribution of Ventilation

Awake

Anesthetized

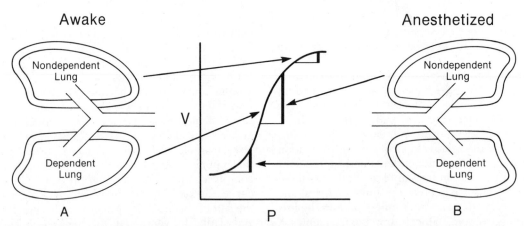

Figure 4–4. This schematic diagram shows the distribution of ventilation in the awake patient in the lateral decubitus position (A) and the distribution of ventilation in the anesthetized patient in the lateral decubitus position (B). The induction of anesthesia has caused a loss in lung volume in both lungs, with the nondependent lung moving from a flat noncompliant portion to a steep compliant portion of the pressure-volume curve and the dependent lung moving from a steep compliant part to a flat, noncompliant part of the pressure-volume curve. Thus, the anesthetized patient in a lateral decubitus position has the majority of the tidal ventilation in the nondependent lung (where there is the least perfusion) and the minority of the tidal ventilation in the dependent lung (where there is the most perfusion). (V = alveolar volume; P = transpulmonary pressure.) (Modified with permission from Benumof JL: Physiology of the open chest and one-lung ventilation. In Kaplan JA (ed.): Thoracic Anesthesia. New York, Churchill Livingstone Inc., 1983, chapter 8.)

contents pushing cephalad against the diaphragm is greatest in the dependent lung, which physically impedes lower lung expansion the most and disproportionately decreases lower lung FRC. Finally, suboptimal positioning, which fails to provide room for lower lung expansion, may considerably compress the dependent lung. Opening the nondependent hemithorax further disproportionately increases ventilation to the nondependent lung (see the following).

In summary, the anesthetized patient, with or without paralysis, in the lateral decubitus position and with a closed chest has a nondependent lung that is well ventilated but poorly perfused and has a dependent lung that is well perfused but poorly ventilated, which results in an increased degree of mismatching of ventilation and perfusion. The application of positive end-expiratory pressure (PEEP) to both lungs restores the majority of ventilation to the lower lung.[3] Presumably, the lower lung returns to a steeper, more favorable part of the pressure-volume curve, and the upper lung resumes its original position on a flat, unfavorable portion of the curve.

C. Distribution of $\dot{Q}$, $\dot{V}$—Lateral Decubitus Position, Anesthetized, Open Chest

Compared with the condition of the anesthetized, closed-chested patient in the lateral decubitus position, opening the chest wall and pleural space alone does not ordinarily cause any significant alteration in the partitioning of pulmonary blood flow between the dependent and nondependent lung; thus, the dependent lung continues to receive relatively more perfusion than the nondependent lung. However, if the compliance of the nondependent lung increases so much (see immediately below) that nondependent lung airway pressure decreases significantly, then nondependent lung blood flow may increase relative to dependent lung blood flow. In addition, the vertical distance between the heart and the nondependent lung may be decreased, which in the face of a constant pulmonary artery pressure might, in theory, result in an increased perfusion of the nondependent lung.[8] Opening the chest wall causes only very minor alterations in pulmonary and systemic vascular pressures and cardiac output.[8]

Opening the chest wall and pleural space, however, does have a significant impact on the distribution of ventilation (which must now be delivered by positive pressure). The change in the distribution of ventilation may result in a further mismatching of ventilation with perfusion (Fig. 4–5).[9]

If the upper lung is no longer restricted by a chest wall and the total effective compliance of that lung is equal to that of the lung parenchyma alone, it will be relatively free to expand and will consequently be overventilated (and remain

Anesthetized, Lateral Decubitus Position
Distribution of Ventilation

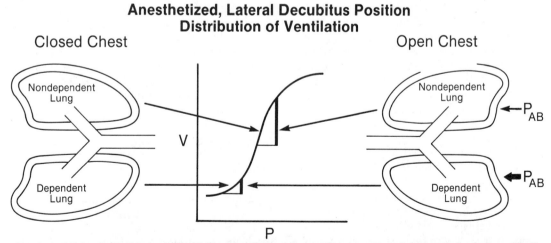

Figure 4–5. *This schematic of a patient in the lateral decubitus position compares the closed-chested anesthetized condition with the open-chested anesthetized and paralyzed condition. Opening the chest increases nondependent lung compliance and reinforces or maintains the larger part of the tidal ventilation going to the nondependent lung. Paralysis also reinforces or maintains the larger part of tidal ventilation going to the nondependent lung because the pressure of the abdominal contents (P_{AB}) pressing against the upper diaphragm is minimal (smaller arrow), and it is therefore easier for positive pressure ventilation to displace this lesser resisting dome of the diaphragm. (V = alveolar volume; P = transpulmonary pressure.) (Modified with permission from Benumof JL: Physiology of the open chest and one-lung ventilation. In Kaplan JA (ed.): Thoracic Anesthesia. New York, Churchill Livingstone Inc., 1983, chapter 8.)*

underperfused). Conversely, the dependent lung may continue to be relatively noncompliant and poorly ventilated and overperfused.[2] From a practical point of view, it is necessary to mention that surgical retraction and compression of the exposed upper lung can provide a partial, although nonphysiologic, solution to this problem in that if expansion of the exposed lung is mechanically or externally restricted, ventilation will be diverted to the dependent, better-perfused lung.[8]

D. Distribution of Q̇, V̇—Lateral Decubitus Position, Anesthetized Open Chest, Paralyzed

In the open-chested anesthetized patient in the lateral decubitus position, the induction of paralysis alone does not cause any significant alteration in the partitioning of pulmonary blood flow between the dependent and nondependent lung. Thus, the dependent lung continues to receive relatively more perfusion than the nondependent lung. There are, however, strong theoretical and experimental considerations that indicate that paralysis might cause significant changes in the distribution of ventilation between the two lungs under these conditions.

In the supine and lateral decubitus positions, the weight of the abdominal contents pressing against the diaphragm is greatest on the dependent part of the diaphragm (posterior lung and lower lung, respectively) and least on the nondependent part of the diaphragm (anterior lung and upper lung, respectively) (Fig. 4–5). In the awake, spontaneously breathing patient, the normally present active tension in the diaphragm overcomes the weight of the abdominal contents, and the diaphragm moves the most (largest excursion) in the dependent portion and least in the nondependent portion. This is a healthy circumstance because this is another factor that maintains the greatest amount of ventilation where there is the most perfusion (dependent lung) and the least amount of ventilation where there is the least perfusion (nondependent lung). During paralysis and positive-pressure breathing, the passive and flaccid diaphragm is displaced preferentially in the nondependent area, where the resistance to passive diaphragmatic movement by the abdominal contents is least; conversely, the diaphragm is displaced minimally in the dependent portion where the resistance to passive diaphragmatic movement by the abdominal contents is great-

est.[10] This is an unhealthy circumstance because the greatest amount of ventilation may occur where there is the least perfusion (nondependent lung), and the least amount of ventilation may occur where there is the most perfusion (dependent lung).[10]

E. Summary of Physiology of Lateral Decubitus Position and the Open Chest

In summary (Fig. 4–6), the preceding section has developed the concept that the anesthetized, paralyzed patient in the lateral decubitus position with an open chest may have a considerable ventilation-perfusion mismatch, consisting of greater ventilation but less perfusion to the nondependent lung and less ventilation but more perfusion to the dependent lung. The blood flow distribution is mainly and simply determined by gravitational effects. The relatively good ventilation of the upper lung is caused, in part, by the open chest and paralysis. The relatively poor ventilation of the dependent lung is caused, in part, by the loss of dependent-lung volume with general anesthesia and by compression of the dependent lung by the mediastinum, abdominal contents, and suboptimal positioning effects. In addition, poor mucociliary clearance and absorption atelectasis with an increased F_IO_2 may cause further dependent-lung volume loss. Consequently, two-lung ventilation under these circumstances may result in an increased alveolar-arterial oxygen tension difference $[P(A-a)O_2]$ and less than optimal oxygenation.

A physiologic solution to the adverse effects of anesthesia and surgery in the lateral decubitus position on the distribution of ventilation and perfusion during two-lung ventilation would be the selective application of PEEP to the dependent lung (via a double-lumen endotracheal tube). Selective PEEP to the lower lung should increase the ventilation to this lung by moving it up to a steeper, more favorable portion of the lung pressure-volume curve. Indeed, this has been done with reasonably good success.[11] A series of 22 mechanically ventilated patients (both lungs) undergoing thoracotomy in the lateral decubitus position was divided into two groups. Group 1 patients had 10 cm H_2O of PEEP applied to the dependent lung while zero end-expiratory pressure (ZEEP) was applied to the nondependent lung. Group 2 (con-

Lateral Decubitus Position
Anesthetized

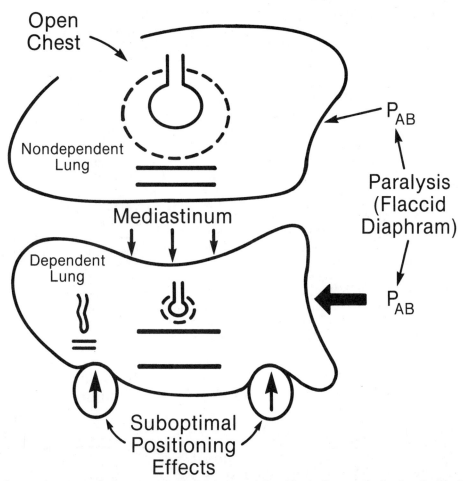

Figure 4–6. *Schematic summary of ventilation-perfusion relationships in the anesthetized patient in the lateral decubitus position who has an open chest and is paralyzed and suboptimally positioned. The nondependent lung is well ventilated (as indicated by the large dashed lines) but poorly perfused (small perfusion vessel), and the dependent lung is poorly ventilated (small dashed lines) but well perfused (large perfusion vessel). In addition, the dependent lung may also develop an atelectatic shunt compartment (indicated on the left side of the lower lung) because of the circumferential compression of this lung. (P_{AB} = pressure of the abdominal contents.) (Modified with permission from Benumof JL: Physiology of the open chest and one-lung ventilation. In Kaplan JA (ed.): Thoracic Anesthesia. New York, Churchill Livingstone Inc., 1983, chapter 8.)*

trol) patients were intubated with a standard endotracheal tube, and both lungs were ventilated with ZEEP. Selective PEEP to the dependent lung in group 1 patients resulted in an adequate P_aO_2 with a lower inspired O_2 concentration during surgery and a smaller $P(A-a)O_2$ at the end of surgery than when both lungs were ventilated with ZEEP. Thus, even if the selective PEEP to the dependent lung in-

creased dependent lung pulmonary vascular resistance and diverted some blood flow to the nondependent lung, the diverted blood flow could still participate in gas exchange with the ZEEP-ventilated nondependent lung.[12] However, it should be noted that this technique requires that the nondependent (and operative) lung be ventilated, and this may impede the performance of surgery.

IV. PHYSIOLOGY OF ONE-LUNG VENTILATION

A. Comparison of Arterial Oxygenation and CO_2 Elimination During Two-Lung Versus One-Lung Ventilation

As discussed previously, the matching of ventilation and perfusion is impaired during two-lung ventilation in an anesthetized, paralyzed, open-chested patient in the lateral decubitus position. The reason for the mismatching of ventilation and perfusion is relatively good ventilation but poor perfusion of the nondependent lung and poor ventilation and good perfusion of the dependent lung (Figs. 4–6 and 4–7A). The blood flow distribution was seen to be mainly and simply determined by gravitational effects. The relatively good ventilation of the nondependent lung was seen to be caused, in part, by the open chest and paralysis. The relatively poor ventilation of the dependent lung was seen to be caused, in part, by the loss of dependent lung volume with general anesthesia and by circumferential compression of the dependent lung by the mediastinum, abdominal contents, and suboptimal positioning effect. The compression of the dependent lung may cause the development of a shunt compartment in the dependent lung (Figs. 4–6 and 4–7A). Consequently, two-lung ventilation under these circumstances may result in an increased $P(A-a)O_2$ and impaired oxygenation.

However, if the nondependent lung is nonventilated, as during one-lung ventilation, then any blood flow to the nonventilated lung becomes shunt flow, in addition to whatever shunt flow might exist in the dependent lung (Fig. 4–7B). (Table 4–1 and discussion on page 115 show a quantitative analysis of the two-lung ventilation to the one-lung ventilation conversion process.) Thus, one-lung ventilation creates an obligatory right-to-left transpulmonary shunt through the nonventilated nondependent lung, which is not present during two-lung ventilation. Consequently, it is not surprising to find that, given the same inspired oxygen concentration (F_IO_2) and hemodynamic and metabolic status, one-lung ventilation results in a much larger alveolar-to-arterial oxygen tension difference $P(A-a)O_2$ and lower P_aO_2 than does two-lung ventilation. This contention is best supported by studies that compare arterial oxygenation during two-lung with one-lung ventilation, wherein each patient serves as their own control.[13]

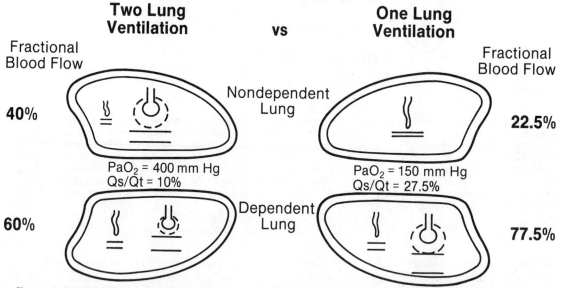

Figure 4–7. *Schematic representation of two-lung ventilation versus one-lung ventilation. Typical values for fractional blood flow to the nondependent and dependent lungs as well as P_aO_2 and $\dot{Q}_s/\dot{Q}_t$ for the two conditions are shown. The $\dot{Q}_s/\dot{Q}_t$ during two-lung ventilation is assumed to be distributed equally between the two lungs (5 per cent to each lung). The essential difference between two-lung and one-lung ventilation is that during one-lung ventilation the nonventilated lung has some blood flow and, therefore, an obligatory shunt, which is not present during two-lung ventilation. The 35 per cent of total flow perfusing the nondependent lung, which was not shunt flow, was assumed to be able to reduce its blood flow by 50 per cent by hypoxic pulmonary vasoconstriction.[21] The increase in $\dot{Q}_s/\dot{Q}_t$ from two-lung to one-lung ventilation is assumed to be solely due to the increase in blood flow through the nonventilated nondependent lung during one-lung ventilation.*

Table 4-1. Model of Converting Two-Lung to One-Lung Ventilation

Lung	Two-Lung Ventilation			One-Lung Ventilation		
	Fractional Normal Flow	Total Shunt Flow	Fractional Shunt Flow	Fractional Normal Flow	Total Shunt Flow*	Fractional Shunt Flow
ND	0.400		0	0		0.200† (0.200 + 0)
		0			0.200	
D	0.600		0	0.800		0
ND	0.350		0.050	0		0.225† (0.175 + 0.050)
		0.100			0.275	
D	0.550		0.050	0.725		0.050
ND	0.300		0.100	0		0.250† (0.150 + 0.100)
		0.200			0.350	
D	0.500		0.100	0.650		0.100
ND	0.200		0.200	0		0.300† (0.100 + 0.200)
		0.400			0.500	
D	0.400		0.200	0.500		0.200
ND	0.100		0.300	0		0.350† (0.050 + 0.300)
		0.600			0.650	
D	0.300		0.300	0.350		0.300

*Sum of ND and D lung fractional shunt flows.

†Half of two-lung ventilation fractional normal flow (due to hypoxic pulmonary vasoconstriction) plus all of two-lung ventilation fractional shunt flow [see ( ) immediately below figure]

ND = nondependent lung

D = dependent lung

One-lung ventilation has much less of an effect on P_aCO_2 in comparison with its effect on P_aO_2. Blood passing through underventilated alveoli retains more than a normal amount of CO_2 and does not take up a normal amount of O_2; blood traversing overventilated alveoli gives off more than a normal amount of CO_2 but cannot take up a proportionately increased amount of O_2 owing to the flatness of the top end of the oxygen-hemoglobin dissociation curve (see Fig. 3–29). Thus, during one-lung ventilation, the ventilated lung can eliminate enough CO_2 to compensate for the nonventilated lung, and P_ACO_2 to P_aCO_2 gradients are small; however, the ventilated lung cannot take up enough O_2 to compensate for the nonventilated lung, and P_AO_2 to P_aO_2 gradients are usually large.

B. Blood Flow Distribution During One-Lung Ventilation

1. Blood Flow to the Nondependent, Nonventilated Lung

Fortunately, there are both passive mechanical and active vasoconstrictor mechanisms that are usually operant during one-lung ventilation that minimize the blood flow to the nondependent nonventilated lung and thereby prevent the P_aO_2 from decreasing as much as might be expected on the basis of the distribution of blood flow during two-lung ventilation. The passive mechanical mechanisms that decrease blood flow to nondependent lung consist of gravity, surgical interference with blood flow, and perhaps the amount of pre-existing disease in the nondependent lung (Fig. 4–8). Gravity causes a vertical gradient in the distribution of pulmonary blood flow in the lateral decubitus position for the same reason that it does in the upright position (see Figs. 3–5 and 4–2). Consequently, blood flow to the nondependent lung is less than blood flow to the dependent lung. The gravity component of blood flow reduction to the nondependent lung should be constant with respect to both time and magnitude.

Severe surgical compression (directly compressing lung vessels) and retraction (causing kinking and tortuosity of lung vessels) of the nondependent lung may further passively reduce nondependent lung blood flow. In addition, ligation of pulmonary vessels for pulmonary resection will greatly decrease nondependent lung

One Lung Ventilation: Determinents
Of Blood Flow Distribution

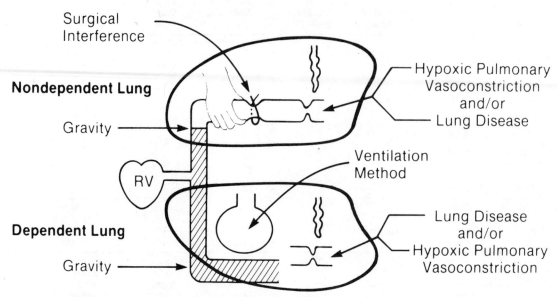

Figure 4–8. *Schematic diagram of the determinants of blood flow distribution during one-lung ventilation. The major determinants of blood flow to the nondependent lung are gravity, surgical interference with blood flow, the amount of nondependent lung disease, and the magnitude of nondependent lung hypoxic pulmonary vasconstriction. The determinants of dependent lung blood flow are gravity, amount of dependent lung disease, and dependent lung hypoxic pulmonary vasoconstriction. (RV = right ventricle.)*

blood flow. The surgical interference component of blood flow reduction to the nondependent lung should be variable with respect to both time and magnitude.

However, it should be noted that recent evidence indicates that some physical stimuli, such as the stroking of pulmonary tissue, may cause local release of vasodilator prostaglandins.[14] Indeed, one study has shown that the shunt fraction increases significantly when the nonventilated lung is exposed to mild-to-moderate degrees of surgical manipulation.[15] Thus, it appears that the effect of surgical manipulation on arterial oxygenation may depend on the exact nature of the physical stimulus.

The amount of disease in the nondependent lung should also be a significant determinant of the amount of blood flow to the nondependent lung. If the nondependent lung is severely diseased, then there may be a fixed reduction in blood flow to this lung preoperatively, and collapse of such a diseased lung may not cause much of an increase in shunt (see Table 4–1). The notion that a diseased pulmonary vasculature might be incapable of HPV is supported by the observation that administration of sodium nitroprusside and nitroglycerin (which should abolish any pre-existing HPV) to chronic obstructive pulmonary disease patients (who have a fixed reduction in the cross-sectional area of their pulmonary vascular bed) does not cause an increase in shunt,[16] whereas these drugs do increase shunt in patients with acute regional lung disease who have an otherwise normal pulmonary vascular bed.[17] If the nondependent lung is normal and has a normal amount of blood flow, then collapse of such a normal lung may be associated with a higher nonventilated nondependent lung blood flow and shunt. A higher one-lung ventilation shunt through the nondependent lung is much more likely to occur in patients who require thoracotomy for nonpulmonary disease.[18] However, this theoretical relationship between the amount of nondependent lung disease and shunt during one-lung ventilation has not been systematically studied to the author's knowledge.

The most significant reduction in blood flow to the nondependent lung is caused by an active vasoconstrictor mechanism. The normal response of the pulmonary vasculature to atelectasis is an increase in pulmonary vascular resistance (in just the atelectatic lung), and the increase in atelectatic lung pulmonary vascular resistance is thought to be due almost entirely to hypoxic pulmonary vasoconstriction (HPV).[19, 20] The selective increase in atelectatic lung pulmonary vascular resistance diverts blood flow away from the atelectatic lung toward the remaining normoxic or hyperoxic ventilated lung. The diversion of blood flow minimizes the amount of shunt flow that occurs through hypoxic lung. Figure 4–9 shows the theoretically expected effect of HPV on arterial oxygen tension (P_aO_2) as the amount of lung that becomes hypoxic increases.[21] When very little of the lung is hypoxic (near 0 per cent), it does not matter, in terms of P_aO_2, whether the small amount of lung has HPV or not because in either case the shunt will be small. When most of the lung is hypoxic (near 100 per cent), there is no significant normoxic region to which the hypoxic region can divert flow, and, again, it does not matter, in terms of P_aO_2, whether the hypoxic region has HPV or not. When the percentage of lung that is hypoxic is intermediate (between 30 and 70 per cent), which is the amount of

Effect of HPV on PaO2

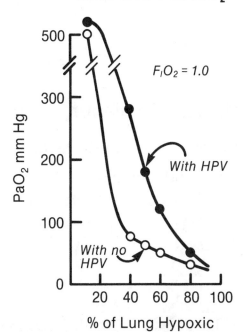

Figure 4–9. The graph is a model of the effect of hypoxic pulmonary vasoconstriction (HPV) on P_aO_2 as a function of the per cent of lung that is hypoxic. The model assumes an F_IO_2 of 1.0, a normal hemoglobin, cardiac output, and oxygen consumption. In the range of 30 to 70 per cent of the lung being hypoxic, the normal expected amount of HPV can increase P_aO_2 significantly.

lung that is hypoxic during the one-lung ventilation/anesthesia condition, there is a large difference between the P_aO_2 expected with a normal amount of HPV (which is a 50 per cent blood flow reduction for a single lung)[21] compared with when there is no HPV. In fact, in this range of hypoxic lung, HPV can increase P_aO_2 from hypoxemic levels to much higher and safer values. It is not surprising, then, that numerous clinical studies on one-lung ventilation[13, 18, 22–28] have found that the shunt through the nonventilated lung is usually 20 to 30 per cent of the cardiac output as opposed to the 40 to 50 per cent shunt that might be expected if there was no HPV in the nonventilated lung. Thus, HPV is an autoregulatory mechanism that protects the P_aO_2 by decreasing the amount of shunt flow that can occur through hypoxic lung.

It is possible to model the two-lung ventilation conversion process for various initial two-lung ventilation shunts; the model shown in Table 4–1 makes several assumptions. First, the initial two-lung ventilation shunt flow is equally distributed between the nondependent and dependent lung. Second, the remaining normal blood flow to the nondependent lung can decrease its blood flow by 50 per cent owing to HPV,[21] and any initial shunt flow (i.e., during two-lung ventilation) does not participate in an HPV response. Third, the total one-lung ventilation shunt flow is a sum of half the normal flow to the nondependent lung when it was ventilated plus the original nondependent and dependent lung shunt flows. Table 4–1 shows that as the two-lung ventilation shunt increases, the amount of nondependent lung flow that is able to participate in an HPV response decreases; therefore, the amount of blood flow diversion due to nondependent lung HPV decreases, and, thus, the total one-lung ventilation shunt increases.

Figure 4–10 outlines the major determinants of the amount of atelectatic lung HPV that might occur during anesthesia. In the following discussion, the HPV issues or considerations are numbered as they appear in Figure 4–10.

1. The distribution of the alveolar hypoxia is probably not a determinant of the amount of HPV; all regions of the lung (either the basilar or dependent parts of the lungs [supine or upright] or discrete anatomic units such as a lobe or single lung) respond to alveolar hypoxia with vasoconstriction.[29] However, recent evidence suggests that on a sublobar level, collateral ventilation may be the first line and HPV the second line of defense against the develop-

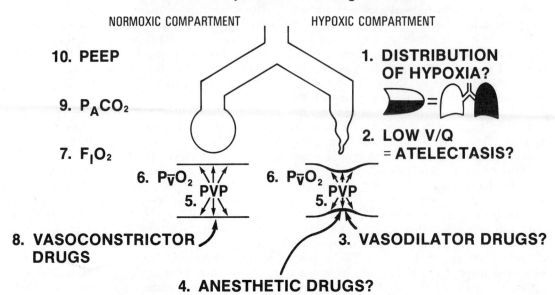

Anesthetic Experience and Regional HPV

NORMOXIC COMPARTMENT   HYPOXIC COMPARTMENT

10. PEEP

9. P_ACO_2

7. F_IO_2

6. $P_{\bar{V}}O_2$ 6. $P_{\bar{V}}O_2$
5. PVP   5. PVP

8. VASOCONSTRICTOR DRUGS

1. DISTRIBUTION OF HYPOXIA?

2. LOW V/Q = ATELECTASIS?

3. VASODILATOR DRUGS?

4. ANESTHETIC DRUGS?

Figure 4–10. This figure lists many of the components of the anesthetic experience that might determine the amount of regional hypoxic pulmonary vasoconstriction (HPV). The clockwise numbering of considerations corresponds to the order in which these considerations are discussed in the text. (PVP = pulmonary vascular pressure.)

ment of arterial hypoxemia (Fig. 4–11).[30] In species with extensive collateral ventilation, such as canines, the development of sublobar atelectasis or low $\dot{V}/\dot{Q}$ areas does not cause as much sublobar HPV because collateral ventilation prevents the sublobar area in question from becoming very hypoxic. This protective phenomenon seems reasonable when one considers that air (O_2) is less dense than blood and therefore easier to redistribute. On the other hand, in consolidated lesions and in species with no collateral ventilation, such as the coatimundi, cattle, and swine, the development of sublobar atelectasis and low $\dot{V}/\dot{Q}$ areas does elicit a great deal of sublobar HPV, which minimizes decreases in P_aO_2.

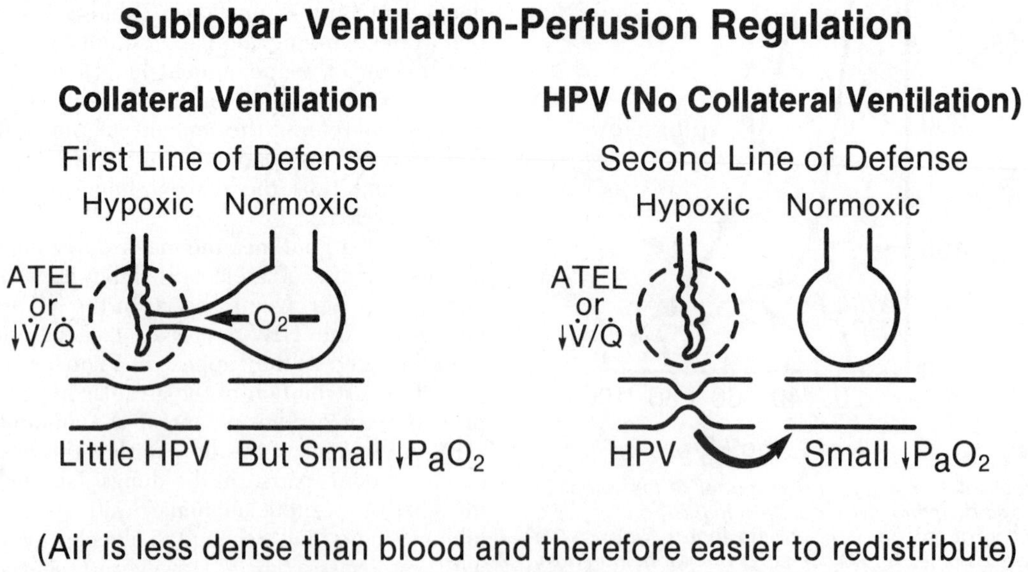

Sublobar Ventilation-Perfusion Regulation

Collateral Ventilation
First Line of Defense
Hypoxic Normoxic
ATEL or $\downarrow\dot{V}/\dot{Q}$ ←O_2—
Little HPV But Small $\downarrow P_aO_2$

HPV (No Collateral Ventilation)
Second Line of Defense
Hypoxic Normoxic
ATEL or $\downarrow\dot{V}/\dot{Q}$
HPV Small $\downarrow P_aO_2$

(Air is less dense than blood and therefore easier to redistribute)

Figure 4–11. Since gas is much less dense than blood and, therefore, easier to redistribute, collateral ventilation may be the first line of defense and HPV the second line of defense against the development of arterial hypoxemia due to sublobar atelectasis (ATEL) or low $\dot{V}/\dot{Q}$ areas. (HPV = hypoxic pulmonary vasoconstriction.)

2. As with low $\dot{V}/\dot{Q}$ and nitrogen-ventilated lungs, it appears that the vast majority of blood flow reduction in acutely atelectatic lung is due to HPV, and none of the blood flow reduction is due to passive mechanical factors (such as vessel tortuosity).[19, 20] This conclusion is based on the observation that re-expansion and ventilation of a collapsed lung with nitrogen (removing any mechanical factor) does not increase the blood flow to the lung, whereas ventilation with oxygen restores all of the blood flow back to precollapse values. This conclusion applies whether ventilation is spontaneous or with positive pressure, and whether the chest is open or closed.[31] In canines, a slight amount of further subacute (greater than 30 minutes) decrease in blood flow to atelectatic lung may have been due to some mechanical effect of the atelectasis on lung blood vessels.[32] However, in humans a prolonged unilateral hypoxic challenge during anesthesia results in an immediate vasoconstrictor response with no further potentiation or diminution of the response.[33]

3. Most systemic vasodilator drugs have been shown either to inhibit regional HPV directly or to have an effect in a clinical situation that is consistent with inhibition of regional HPV (i.e., decreasing P_aO_2 and increasing shunt in patients with acute respiratory disease). The vasodilator drugs that have been shown to inhibit HPV or to have a clinical effect consistent with inhibition of HPV are nitroglycerin,[17, 34–40] nitroprusside,[17, 41–47] dobutamine,[48, 49] several calcium antagonists,[50–55] and many B_2-agonists (isoproterenol, ritodrine, orciprenaline, salbutamol, ATP, and glucagon).[49, 56–62] Aminophylline and hydrazaline may not decrease HPV.[63, 64]

4. The effect of anesthetic drugs on regional HPV will be covered extensively in chapter 8, Choice of Anesthesia.

5. The HPV response is maximal when pulmonary vascular pressure is normal and is decreased by either high or low pulmonary vascular pressure (Fig. 4–12). The mechanism for high pulmonary vascular pressure inhibition of HPV is simple; the pulmonary circulation is poorly endowed with smooth muscle and cannot constrict against an increased vascular pressure.[65–67] The mechanism for low pulmonary vascular pressure inhibition of HPV is more complex. In order for this to occur, the hypoxic compartment must be atelectatic. Under these circumstances, when pulmonary vascular pressure decreases, it is possible for part of the ventilated lung (but not the atelectatic lung) to be in a zone 1 condition (alveolar pressure increases relative to pulmonary artery pressure)

and experience a disproportionate increase in pulmonary vascular resistance, which would divert blood flow back over to the atelectatic lung, thereby inhibiting atelectatic lung HPV.[68] Figures 4–12 and 4–15 summarize these mechanisms.

6. The HPV response is also maximal when the mixed venous P_{O_2} ($P_{\bar{v}}O_2$) is normal and is decreased by either high or low $P_{\bar{v}}O_2$ (Fig. 4–13). The mechanism for high $P_{\bar{v}}O_2$ inhibition of HPV is presumably due to reverse diffusion of oxygen, causing the oxygen tension of either the vessels or interstitial or alveolar spaces or all of these to be increased above the HPV threshold.[69] That is, if enough oxygen can get to some receptor in the small arteriole-capillary-alveolar area, then the vessels will not vasoconstrict. The mechanism for low $P_{\bar{v}}O_2$ inhibition of HPV is a result of the low $P_{\bar{v}}O_2$ decreasing alveolar oxygen tension in the normoxic compartment down to a level sufficient to induce HPV in the supposedly "normoxic" lung.[70, 71] The HPV in the "normoxic" lung competes against and offsets the HPV in the originally hypoxic lung and results in no blood flow diversion away from the more obviously hypoxic lung. Figures 4–13 and 4–15 summarize these mechanisms.

7. Selectively decreasing the F_IO_2 in the normoxic compartment (from 1.0 to 0.5 to 0.3) will cause an increase in normoxic lung vascular tone, thereby decreasing blood flow diversion from hypoxic to normoxic lung.[67, 71]

8. Vasoconstrictor drugs (dopamine, epinephrine, phenylephrine) seem to constrict normoxic lung vessels preferentially, thereby disproportionately increasing normoxic lung pulmonary vascular resistance.[48, 49, 59, 65] The increase in normoxic lung vascular resistance will decrease normoxic lung blood flow and increase atelectatic lung blood flow. The HPV-inhibiting effect of vasoconstrictor drugs is similar to decreasing normoxic lung F_IO_2 (see previous discussion).

9. Hypocapnia has been thought to inhibit directly regional HPV and hypercapnia to enhance regional HPV directly.[66, 72] In addition, during one-lung ventilation conditions, hypocapnia can only be produced by hyperventilation of the one lung. The hyperventilation requires an increased ventilated lung airway pressure, which may cause increased ventilated lung pulmonary vascular resistance, which in turn may divert blood flow back into the hypoxic lung. Hypercapnia during one-lung ventilation seems to act as a vasoconstrictor drug by selectively increasing ventilated lung pulmonary vas-

Pulmonary Vascular Pressure (PVP) and HPV:
One Lung Ventilation Conditions

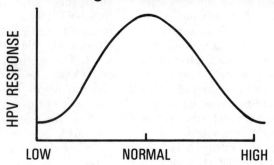

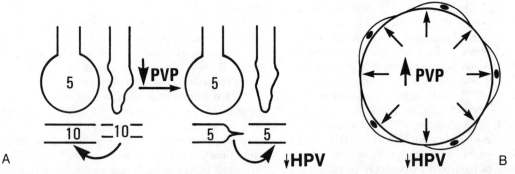

Figure 4–12. A schematic diagram of the effect of changes in pulmonary vascular pressure (PVP) on regional hypoxic pulmonary vasoconstriction (HPV). Both high and low pulmonary vascular pressures inhibit the HPV response. A shows an average PVP of 10 mm Hg and an average ventilated lung alveolar pressure of 5 mm Hg. Since vascular resistance is greater in the nonventilated lung, blood flow is diverted to the ventilated lung (arrow, the HPV response). When PVP decreases to 5 mm Hg, it is possible for zone 1 to develop in the ventilated lung (i.e., collapse of pulmonary vessels due to alveolar pressure). The collapse of pulmonary vessels increases vascular resistance in the ventilated lung and diverts blood flow to the nonventilated lung (arrow, inhibition of the HPV response [↓HPV]). With increased pulmonary vascular pressure (B) the poorly muscled pulmonary arteries cannot constrict as effectively as with a normal PVP, and the HPV response is decreased.

P$\bar{v}$O$_2$ and HPV: One Lung Ventilation Conditions

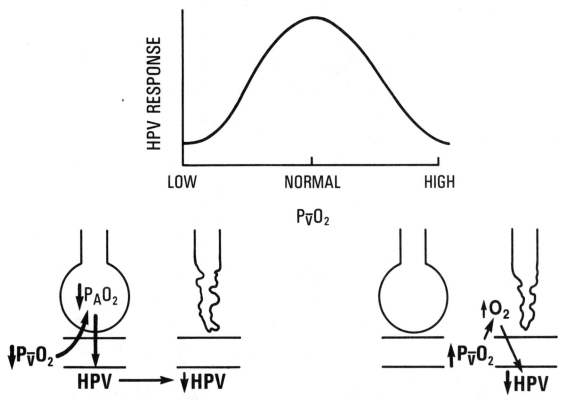

Figure 4-13. Schematic diagram of the effect of changes in mixed venous oxygen tension (P$_\bar{v}$O$_2$) on regional hypoxic pulmonary vasoconstriction (HPV). Both high and low P$_\bar{v}$O$_2$ inhibit the HPV response. Low P$_\bar{v}$O$_2$ lowers the alveolar P$_{O_2}$ (P$_A$O$_2$) in the ventilated lung, causing offsetting and competing HPV in the ventilated lung. Increased P$_\bar{v}$O$_2$ causes the oxygen tension to increase in the nonventilated lung (perhaps in the pulmonary arteries, interstitium, alveolar space, and/or veins), thereby inhibiting nonventilated lung HPV.

cular resistance (which would divert blood flow back to the nonventilated lung). In addition, hypercapnia is ordinarily caused by hypoventilation of the ventilated lung, which greatly increases the risk of developing low $\dot{V}/\dot{Q}$ and atelectatic regions in the dependent lung. However, it should be noted as a theoretical possibility that if hypoventilation of the dependent lung is associated with decreased ventilated lung airway pressure, ventilated lung pulmonary vascular resistance may be decreased, which in turn would promote or enhance HPV in the nonventilated lung. Figures 4-14 and 4-15 summarize these mechanisms.

10. The effects of changes in airway pressure due to end-expiratory pressure and tidal volume changes will be discussed in detail in chapter 11. In brief, selective application of PEEP to just normoxic ventilated lung will selectively increase pulmonary vascular resistance in the ventilated lung and shunt blood flow back into the hypoxic nonventilated lung (i.e., decrease nonventilated lung HPV).[12, 73] On the other hand, high-frequency ventilation of the gas-exchanging lung is associated with a low airway pressure and an enhancement of HPV in the collapsed lung.[74]

There is some evidence that certain types of infections (which may cause atelectasis), particularly granulomatous and pneumococcal infections, may inhibit HPV.[75, 76]

2. Blood Flow to the Dependent Ventilated Lung

The dependent lung usually has an increased amount of blood flow owing to both passive gravitational effects and active nondependent lung vasoconstrictor effects (Fig. 4-8, lower panel). However, the dependent lung may also have a hypoxic compartment (areas of low ventilation-perfusion ratio and atelectasis) that was

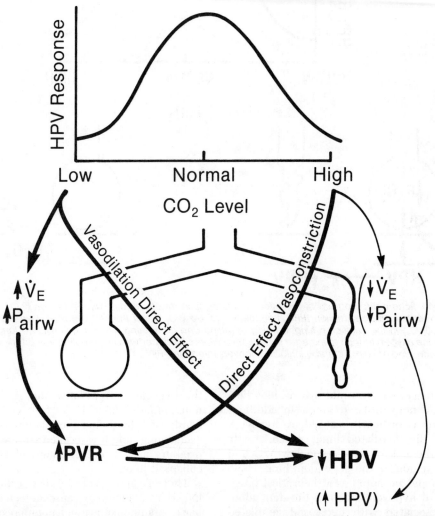

Figure 4–14. Schematic diagram of the effect of changes in CO_2 and regional hypoxic pulmonary vasoconstriction (HPV). Both hypocapnia and hypercapnia inhibit the HPV response. Hypocapnia can directly pharmacologically dilate the hypoxic lung. In addition, hypocapnia must be achieved by increasing minute ventilation ($\dot{V}_E$) and airway pressure (P_{airw}) in the ventilated lung. The increased airway pressure in the ventilated lung may selectively increase ventilated lung pulmonary vascular resistance (PVR), thereby inhibiting nonventilated lung HPV. Hypercapnia may directly vasoconstrict the ventilated lung, thereby increasing ventilated lung pulmonary vascular resistance, which will inhibit nonventilated lung HPV. In addition, hypercapnia may possibly be achieved by decreasing minute ventilation, which would decrease airway pressure in the ventilated lung, which would decrease ventilated lung pulmonary vascular resistance, which would enhance nonventilated lung pulmonary vascular resistance. This latter offsetting mechanism to inhibition of nonventilated lung HPV is in brackets on the right-hand side of the figure.

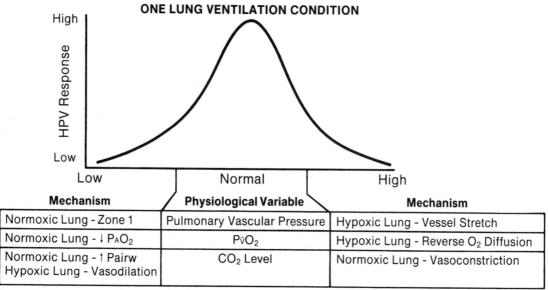

Mechanism	Physiological Variable	Mechanism
Normoxic Lung - Zone 1	Pulmonary Vascular Pressure	Hypoxic Lung - Vessel Stretch
Normoxic Lung - ↓ P_AO_2	$P\bar{v}O_2$	Hypoxic Lung - Reverse O_2 Diffusion
Normoxic Lung - ↑ Pairw Hypoxic Lung - Vasodilation	CO_2 Level	Normoxic Lung - Vasoconstriction

Figure 4–15. Summary of the mechanisms of change in the hypoxic pulmonary vasoconstriction (HPV) response in Figures 4–12, 4–13, and 4–14 caused by the changes in the physiologic variables of pulmonary vascular pressure, $P\bar{v}O_2$ and CO_2 level.

present preoperatively or that developed intra-operatively. The dependent lung hypoxic compartment may develop intraoperatively for several reasons. First, in the lateral decubitus position, the ventilated dependent lung usually has a reduced lung volume owing to the combined factors of induction of general anesthesia and circumferential (and perhaps severe) compression by the mediastinum from above, by the abdominal contents pressing against the diaphragm from the caudad side, and by suboptimal positioning effects (rolls, packs, shoulder supports) pushing in from the dependent side and axilla (Fig. 4–6).[3, 7, 10, 77] Second, absorption atelectasis can also occur in regions of the dependent lung that have low ventilation-perfusion ratios when they are exposed to high inspired oxygen concentration.[78, 79] Third, difficulty in secretion removal may also cause the development of poorly ventilated and atelectatic areas in the dependent lung. Finally, maintaining the lateral decubitus position for prolonged periods of time may cause fluid to transudate into the dependent lung (which may be vertically below the left atrium) and cause further decreased lung volume and increased airway closure in the dependent lung.[80] A decrease in lung volume and an increase in airway closure in the dependent lung will create areas that have a low ventilation-perfusion ratio or atelectasis (see chapter 3).[78]

The development of low ventilation-perfusion ratio and/or atelectatic areas in the dependent lung will increase vascular resistance in the dependent lung[77, 81] (due to dependent lung HPV),[29] thereby decreasing dependent lung blood flow and increasing nondependent lung blood flow.[82] Stated differently, the pulmonary vascular resistance in the ventilated compartment of the lung determines the ability of the ventilated, and supposedly normoxic, lung to accept redistributed blood flow from the hypoxic lung. Clinical conditions that are independent of specific dependent lung disease, but which may still increase dependent lung vascular resistance in a dose dependent manner, are a decreasing inspired oxygen tension in the dependent lung (from 1.0 to 0.5 to 0.3[67, 71, 82] and a decreasing temperature (from 40 to 30°C).[83]

In view of the factors just listed, which can affect dependent and nondependent lung vascular resistance and blood flow, it is obvious that the method used to ventilate the dependent lung is an extremely important determinant of blood flow distribution during one-lung ventilation (see chapters 11 and 12). For example, if the dependent lung is hyperventilated, then the resultant hypocapnia may inhibit HPV. If the method of ventilation involves an excessive amount of airway pressure, due either to use of high PEEP levels or to very large tidal volumes, the deleterious effects of increased dependent lung airway pressure, namely increasing dependent lung vascular resistance (which would increase nondependent lung blood flow), may outweigh the beneficial effects of the opening of atelectatic and low $\dot{V}/\dot{Q}$ areas in the dependent lung. Finally, a high inspired oxygen concentration to the dependent lung may cause vasodilation in it, enhancing nondependent lung HPV; however, absorption atelectasis is promoted by a high inspired oxygen concentration to low $\dot{V}/\dot{Q}$ areas in the dependent lung.[78, 79, 82]

3. Miscellaneous Causes of Hypoxemia During One-Lung Ventilation

Still other factors may contribute to hypoxemia during one-lung ventilation (see chapter 3). Hypoxemia due to mechanical failure of the O_2 supply system or of the anesthesia machine is a recognized hazard of any kind of anesthesia.[84-87] Gross hypoventilation of the dependent lung can be a major cause of hypoxemia. Malfunction of the dependent lung airway lumen (blockage by secretions) and malposition of the double-lumen endotracheal tube are other common causes of an increased $P(A-a)O_2$ and hypoxemia. Resorption of residual oxygen from the clamped nonventilated lung is time-dependent and may account for a gradual increase in shunt and decrease in P_aO_2 after one-lung ventilation is initiated.[81] With all other anesthetic and surgical factors constant, anything that decreases the mixed venous partial pressure of oxygen ($P_{\bar{v}}O_2$ (decreased cardiac output, increased oxygen consumption [excessive sympathetic nervous system stimulation, hyperthermia, shivering]) will cause an increased $P(A-a)O_2$.[88, 89]

REFERENCES

1. Tarhan S, Moffitt EA: Principles of thoracic anesthesia. Surg Clin North Am 53:813–826, 1973.
2. Wulff KE, Aulin I: The regional lung function in the lateral decubitus position during anesthesia and operation. Acta Anesthesiol Scand; 16:195–205, 1972.
3. Rehder K, Wenthe FM, Sessler AD: Function of each lung during mechanical ventilation with ZEEP and with PEEP in man anesthetized with thiopental-meperidine. Anesthesiology 39:597–606, 1973.
4. Svanberg L: Influence of posture on lung volumes, ventilation and circulation in normals. Scand J Clin Lab Invest (Suppl 25) 9:1–95, 1957.
5. Rehder K, Sessler AD: Function of each lung in spontaneously breathing man anesthetized with thiopental-meperidine. Anesthesiology 38:320–327, 1973.
6. Potgieter SV: Atelectasis: Its evolution during upper urinary tract surgery. Br J Anaesth 31:472–483, 1959.
7. Rehder K, Hatch DJ, Sessler AD, Fowler WS: The function of each lung of anesthetized and paralyzed man during mechanical ventilation. Anesthesiology 37:16–26, 1972.
8. Werner O, Malmkvist G, Beckman A, Stahle S, Nordstrom L: Gas exchange and haemodynamics during thoracotomy. Br J Anaesth 56:1343–1349, 1984.
9. Nunn JF: The distribution of inspired gas during thoracic surgery. Ann R Coll Surg Engl 28:223–237, 1961.
10. Froese AB, Bryan CA: Effects of anesthesia and paralysis on diaphragmatic mechanics in man. Anesthesiology 41:242–255, 1974.
11. Brown DR, Kafer ER, Roberson VO, et al: Improved oxygenation during thoracotomy with selective PEEP to the dependent lung. Anesth Analg 56:26–31, 1977.
12. Benumof JL, Rogers SN, Moyce PR, Berryhill RE, Wahrenbrock EA: Hypoxic pulmonary vasoconstriction and regional and whole-lung PEEP in the dog. Anesthesiology 51:503–507, 1979.
13. Tarhan S, Lundborg RO: Carlens endobronchial catheter versus regular endotracheal tube during thoracic surgery: A comparison of blood gas and pulmonary shunting. Can Anaesth Soc J 18:594–599, 1971.
14. Piper P, Vane J: The release of prostaglandins from lung and other tissues. Ann NY Acad Sci 180:363–385, 1971.
15. Anderson HW, Benumof JL: Intrapulmonary shunting during one-lung ventilation and surgical manipulation. Anesthesiology 55:A377, 1981.
16. Casthely PA, Lear F, Cottrell JE, Lear E: Intrapulmonary shunting during induced hypotension. Anesth Analg 61:231–235, 1982.
17. Benumof JL: Hypoxic pulmonary vasoconstriction and sodium nitroprusside infusion. Anesthesiology 50:481–483, 1979.
18. Kerr JH, Smith AC, Prys-Roberts C, Meloche R, Foex P: Observations during endobronchial anesthesia II. Oxygenation. Br J Anaesth 46:84–92, 1974.
19. Benumof JL: Mechanism of decreased blood flow to atelectatic lung. J Appl Physiol 46:1047–1048, 1978.
20. Bjertnaes LJ, Mundal R, Hauge A, Nicolaysen A: Vascular resistance in atelectatic lungs: Effect of inhalation anesthetics. Acta Anaesth Scand 24:109–118, 1980.
21. Marshall BE, Marshall C: Continuity of response to hypoxic pulmonary vasoconstriction. J Appl Physiol 1980;59:189–196.
22. Rogers SN, Benumof JL: Halothane and isoflurane do not impair arterial oxygenation during one-lung ventilation in patients undergoing thoracotomy. Anesth Analg 64:946–954, 1985.
23. Torda TA, McCulloch CH, O'Brien HD, Wright JS, Horton DA: Pulmonary venous admixture during one-lung anesthesia. The effect of inhaled oxygen tension and respiration rate. Anaesthesia 29:272–279, 1974.
24. Khanom T, Branthwaite MA: Arterial oxygenation during one-lung anaesthesia (1): A study in man. Anaesthesia 28:132–138, 1973.
25. Flacke JW, Thompson DS, Read RC: Influence of tidal volume and pulmonary artery occlusion on arterial oxygenation during endobronchial anesthesia. South Med J 69:619–626, 1976.
26. Tarhan S, Lundborg RO: Blood gas and pH studies during use of Carlens catheter. Can Anaesth Soc J 15:458–467, 1968.
27. Tarhan S, Lundborg RO: Effects of increased expiratory pressure on blood gas tensions and pulmonary shunting during thoracotomy with use of the Carlens Catheter. Can Anaesth Soc J 17:4–11, 1970.

28. Fiser WP, Friday CD, Read RC: Changes in arterial oxygenation and pulmonary shunt during thoracotomy with endobronchial anesthesia. J Thorac Cardiovasc Surg 83:523–531, 1982.
29. Prefaut CH, Engel LA: Vertical distribution of perfusion and inspired gas in supine man. Resp Physiol 43:209–219, 1981.
30. Kuriyama T, Wagner WW Jr: Collateral ventilation may protect against high-altitude pulmonary hypertension. J Appl Physiol 51:1251, 1981.
31. Pirlo AF, Benumof JL, Trousdale FR: Atelectatic lung lobe blood flow: Open vs. closed chest, positive-pressure vs. spontaneous ventilation. J Appl Physiol 50:1022–1026, 1981.
32. Glasser SA, Domino KB, Lindgren L, et al: Pulmonary pressure and flow during atelectasis. Anesthesiology 57:A504, 1982.
33. Carlsson AJ, Bindslev L, Santesson J, et al: Hypoxic pulmonary vasoconstriction in the human lung: The effect of prolonged unilateral hypoxic challenge during anesthesia. Acta Anaesth Scand 29:346–351, 1985.
34. Hill NS, Antman EM, Green LH, Alpert JS: Intravenous nitroglycerin. A review of pharmacology, indications, therapeutic effects and indications. Chest 79:69–76, 1981.
35. Colley PS, Cheney FW, Hlastala MP: Pulmonary gas exchange effects of nitroglycerin in canine edematous lungs. Anesthesiology 55:114–119, 1981.
36. Chick TW, Kochukoshy KN, Matsumoto S, Leach JK: The effect of nitroglycerin on gas exchange, hemodynamics and oxygen transport in patients with chronic obstructive pulmonary disease. Am J Med Sci 276:105–111, 1978.
37. Kadowitz PJ, Nandiwada P, Grueter CA, Ignarro LJ, Hyman AL: Pulmonary vasodilator responses to nitroprusside and nitroglycerin in the dog. J Clin Invest 67:893–902, 1981.
38. Anjou-Lindskog E, Broman L, Holmgren A: Effects of nitroglycerin on central hemodynamics and V̇A/Q̇ distribution early after coronary bypass surgery. Acta Anesth Scand 26:489–497, 1982.
39. Kochukoshy KN, Chick TW, Jenne JW: The effect of nitroglycerin in gas exchange on chronic obstructive pulmonary disease. Am Rev Resp Dis 111:177–183, 1975.
40. Holmgren A, Anjou E, Broman L, Lundberg S: Influence of nitroglycerin on central hemodynamics and V̇A/Q̇c of the lungs in the postoperative period after coronary bypass surgery. Acta Med Scand S562:135–142, 1982.
41. Parsons GH, Leventhal JP, Hansen MM, Goldstein JD: Effect of sodium nitroprusside on hypoxic pulmonary vasoconstriction in the dog. J Appl Physiol 51:288–292, 1981.
42. Sivak ED, Gray BA, McCurdy TH, Phillips AK: Pulmonary vascular response to nitroprusside in dogs. Circ Res 45:360–365, 1979.
43. Hill AB, Sykes MK, Reyes A: Hypoxic pulmonary vasoconstrictor response in dogs during and after sodium nitroprusside infusion. Anesthesiology 50:484–488, 1979.
44. Colley PS, Cheney FW, Hlastala MP: Ventilation-perfusion and gas exchange effects of nitroprusside in dogs with normal and edematous lungs. Anesthesiology 50:489–495, 1979.
45. Colley PS, Cheney FW: Sodium nitroprusside increases Q̇s/Q̇t in dogs with regional atelectasis. Anesthesiology 47:338–341, 1977.
46. Wildsmith JAW, Drummond GB, Macrae WR: Blood gas changes during induced hypotension with sodium nitroprusside. Br J Anaesth 47:1205–1211, 1975.
47. Veltzer JL, Doto JO, Jacoby J: Depressed arterial oxygenation during sodium nitroprusside administration for intraoperative hypertension. Anesth Analg 55:880–881, 1976.
48. McFarlane PA, Mortimer AJ, Ryder WA, Madgwick RJ, Gardaz JP, Harrison BJ, Sykes MK: Effects of dopamine and dobutamine on the distribution of pulmonary blood flow during lobar ventilation hypoxia and lobar collapse in dogs. Europ J Clin Invest 15:53–59, 1985.
49. Furman WR, Summer WR, Kennedy PP, Silvester JT: Comparison of the effects of dobutamine, dopamine and isoproterenol on hypoxic pulmonary vasoconstriction in the pig. Crit Care Med 10:371–374, 1982.
50. Bishop MJ, Cheney FW: Minoxidil and nifedipine inhibit hypoxic pulmonary vasoconstriction. J Cardiovasc Pharmacol 5:184–189, 1983.
51. Tucker A, McMurtry IF, Grover RF, et al: Attenuation of hypoxic pulmonary vasoconstriction by verapamil in intact dogs. Proc Soc Exp Biol Med 151:611–614, 1976.
52. Simonneau J, Escourrou P, Duroux P, Lockhart A: Inhibition of hypoxic pulmonary vasoconstriction by nifedipine. N Engl J Med 304:1582–1585, 1981.
53. Redding GJ, Tuck R, Escourrou P: Nifedipine attenuates hypoxic pulmonary vasoconstriction in awake piglets. Am Rev Respir Dis 129:785–789, 1984.
54. McMurtry IF, Davidson AB, Reeves TJ, Grover RF: Inhibition of hypoxic pulmonary vasoconstriction by calcium antagonists in isolated rat lungs. Circ Res 38:99–104, 1976.
55. Brown SE, Linden GS, King RR, Blair GP, Stansbury DW, Light RW: Effect of verapamil on pulmonary haemodynamics during hypoxaemia at rest, and during exercise in patients with chronic obstructive pulmonary disease. Thorax 38:840–844, 1983.
56. Ward CF, Benumof JL, Wahrenbrock EA: Inhibition of hypoxic pulmonary vasoconstriction by vasoactive drugs. Abstracts of Scientific Papers, 1976 Annual Meeting, American Society of Anesthesiology, 1976, pp 333–334.
57. Johansen I, Benumof JL: Reduction of hypoxia-induced pulmonary artery hypertension by vasodilator drugs. Am Rev Respir Dis 199:375, 1979.
58. Conover WB, Benumof JL, Key TC: Ritodrine inhibition of hypoxic pulmonary vasoconstriction. Am J Ob Gyn 146:652–656, 1983.
59. Marin JLB, Orchard C, Chakrabarti MK, Sykes MK: Depression of hypoxic pulmonary vasoconstriction in the dog by dopamine and isoprenaline. Br J Anaesth 51:303–312, 1979.
60. Reyes A, Sykes MK, Chakrabarti MK, Carruthers B, Petrie A: Effect of orciprenaline on hypoxic pulmonary vasoconstriction in dogs. Respiration 38:185–193, 1979.
61. Reyes A, Sykes MK, Charkrabarti MK, Tait A, Petrie A: The effect of salbutamol on hypoxic pulmonary vasoconstriction in dogs. Bull Europ Physiopath Resp 14:741–753, 1978.
62. Rubin LJ, Lazar JD: Nonadrenergic effects of isoproterenol in dogs with hypoxic pulmonary vasoconstriction: Possible role of prostaglandins. J Clin Invest 71:1366–1374, 1983.
63. Benumof JL, Trousdale FR: Aminophylline does not inhibit canine hypoxic pulmonary vasoconstriction. Am Rev Respir Dis 126:1017–1019, 1982.

64. Bishop MJ, Kennard S, Artman LD, Cheney FW: Hydralazine does not inhibit canine hypoxic pulmonary vasoconstriction. Am Rev Resp Dis 128:998–1001, 1983.

65. Gardaz JP, McFarlane PA, Madgwick RG, Ryder WA, Sykes MK: Effect of dopamine, increased cardiac output and increased pulmonary artery pressure on hypoxic pulmonary vasoconstriction. Br J Anaesth 55:238P–239P, 1983.

66. Benumof JL, Wahrenbrock EA: Blunted hypoxic pulmonary vasoconstriction by increased lung vascular pressures. J Appl Physiol 38:846–850, 1975.

67. Scanlon TS, Benumof JL, Wahrenbrock EA, Nelson WL: Hypoxic pulmonary vasoconstriction and the ratio of hypoxic lung to perfused normoxic lung. Anesthesiology 49:177–181, 1978.

68. Colley PS, Cheney FW, Butler J: Mechanism of change in pulmonary shunt flow with hemorrhage. J Appl Physiol 42:196–201, 1977.

69. Domino KB, Glasser SA, Wetstein L, et al: Influence of P_vO_2 on blood flow to atelectatic lung. Anesthesiology 57:A471, 1982.

70. Benumof JL, Pirlo AF, Trousdale FR: Inhibition of hypoxic pulmonary vasoconstriction by decreased P_vO_2: A new indirect mechanism. J Appl Physiol 51:871–874, 1981.

71. Pease RD, Benumof JL: P_AO_2 and P_vO_2 interaction on hypoxic pulmonary vasoconstriction. J Appl Physiol 53:134–139, 1982.

72. Benumof JL, Mathers JM, Wahrenbrock EA: Cyclic hypoxic pulmonary vasoconstriction induced by concomitant carbon dioxide changes. J Appl Physiol 41:466–469, 1976.

73. Benumof JL: One-lung ventilation and hypoxic pulmonary vasoconstriction: Implications for anesthetic management. Anesth Analg 64:821–833, 1985.

74. Hall SM, Chapleau M, Cairo J, et al: Effect of high-frequency positive-pressure ventilation on halothane ablation of hypoxic pulmonary vasoconstriction. Crit Care Med 13:641–645, 1985.

75. Irwin RS, Martinez-Gonzalez-Rio H, Thomas HM III, Fritts HW Jr: The effect of granulomatous pulmonary disease in dogs on the response of the pulmonary circulation to hypoxia. J Clin Invest 60:1258–1265, 1977.

76. Light RB, Mink SN, Wood LDH: Pathophysiology of gas exchange and pulmonary perfusion in pneumococcal lobar pneumonia in dogs. J Appl Physiol 50:524–530, 1981.

77. Craig JOC, Bromley LL, Williams R: Thoracotomy and contralateral lung. A study of the changes occurring in the dependent and contralateral lung during and after thoracotomy in the lateral decubitus position. Thorax 17:9–15, 1962.

78. Benumof JL: Respiratory physiology and respiratory function during anesthesia. In Miller R (ed): Anesthesia. New York, Churchill-Livingstone, 1986, chapter 32, pp 1115–1162.

79. Dantzker DR, Wagner PD, West JB: Instability of lung units with low $\dot{V}/\dot{Q}$ ratios during O_2 breathing. J Appl Physiol 38:886–895, 1975.

80. Ray JF III, Yost L, Moallem S, Sanodos GM, Villamena P, Paredes RM, Clauss RH: Immobility, hypoxemia and pulmonary arteriovenous shunting. Arch Surg 109:537–541, 1974.

81. Kerr JH: Physiological aspects of one lung (endobronchial) anesthesia. Int Anesth Clin 10:61–78, 1972.

82. Johansen I, Benumof JL: Flow distribution in abnormal lung as a function of F_IO_2 (Abstr). Anesthesiology 51:369, 1979.

83. Benumof JL, Wahrenbrock EA: Dependency of hypoxic pulmonary vasoconstriction on temperature. J Appl Physiol 72:56–58, 1977.

84. Benumof JL: Monitoring respiratory function during anesthesia. In Saidman LJ, Smith NT (eds): Monitoring in Anesthesia. New York, John Wiley and Sons, Inc, 1984.

85. Mazze RI: Therapeutic misadventures of oxygen delivery systems: The need for continuous in-line oxygen monitors. Anesth Analg 51:787–792, 1972.

86. Ward CS: The prevention of accidents associated with anesthetic apparatus. Br J Anaesth 40:692–701, 1968.

87. Epstein RM, Rackow H, Lee ASJ, et al: Prevention of accidental breathing of anoxic gas mixture during anesthesia. Anesthesiology 23:1–4, 1962.

88. Kelman GF, Nunn JF, Prys-Roberts C, et al: The influence of the cardiac output on arterial oxygenation: A theoretical study. Br J Anaesth 39:450–458, 1967.

89. Prys-Roberts C: The metabolic regulation of circulatory transport. In Scurr C, Feldman S (eds): Scientific Foundations of Anesthesia. Chicago, Yearbook Medical Publishers, 1982.

PREOPERATIVE CONSIDERATIONS

Preoperative Cardiopulmonary Evaluation

5

I. INTRODUCTION

The vast majority of noncardiac, noncardio-pulmonary bypass thoracic surgery consists of resectional or repair procedures for cancer and other masses of the lung and bronchi (including infectious processes such as tuberculosis, fungal diseases, bronchiectasis, lung abscess and empyema, and anomalies such as arteriovenous malformations and pulmonary sequestration), mediastinal masses (including thoracic aortic aneurysms), and esophageal lesions. Consequently, this chapter is divided into these three basic preoperative evaluation categories: lung and bronchial masses, mediastinal masses, and esophageal lesions. However, since broncho-genic carcinoma of the lung is by far the most common indication for thoracic surgery (see reference 6 of chapter 1) this chapter places special emphasis on the evaluation of this type of lesion.

II. TUMORS AND OTHER MASSES OF THE LUNG AND BRONCHI

Figure 5–1 shows the overall preoperative evaluation logic plan for patients with lung and/or bronchial masses. The plan involves three basic steps: First, is lung cancer present (diagnosis of mass lesion) and if so what is the cell type? Second, has the lung cancer spread (is the lung cancer resectable based on T, N, M staging)? Third, can the patient tolerate the planned procedure (is the lung mass operable based on physiologic assessment of the patient)? The following text discusses these three steps, and each step has its own logic tree.

A. History[1–4]

The history often raises suspicion of the diagnosis of lung cancer. The average patient with

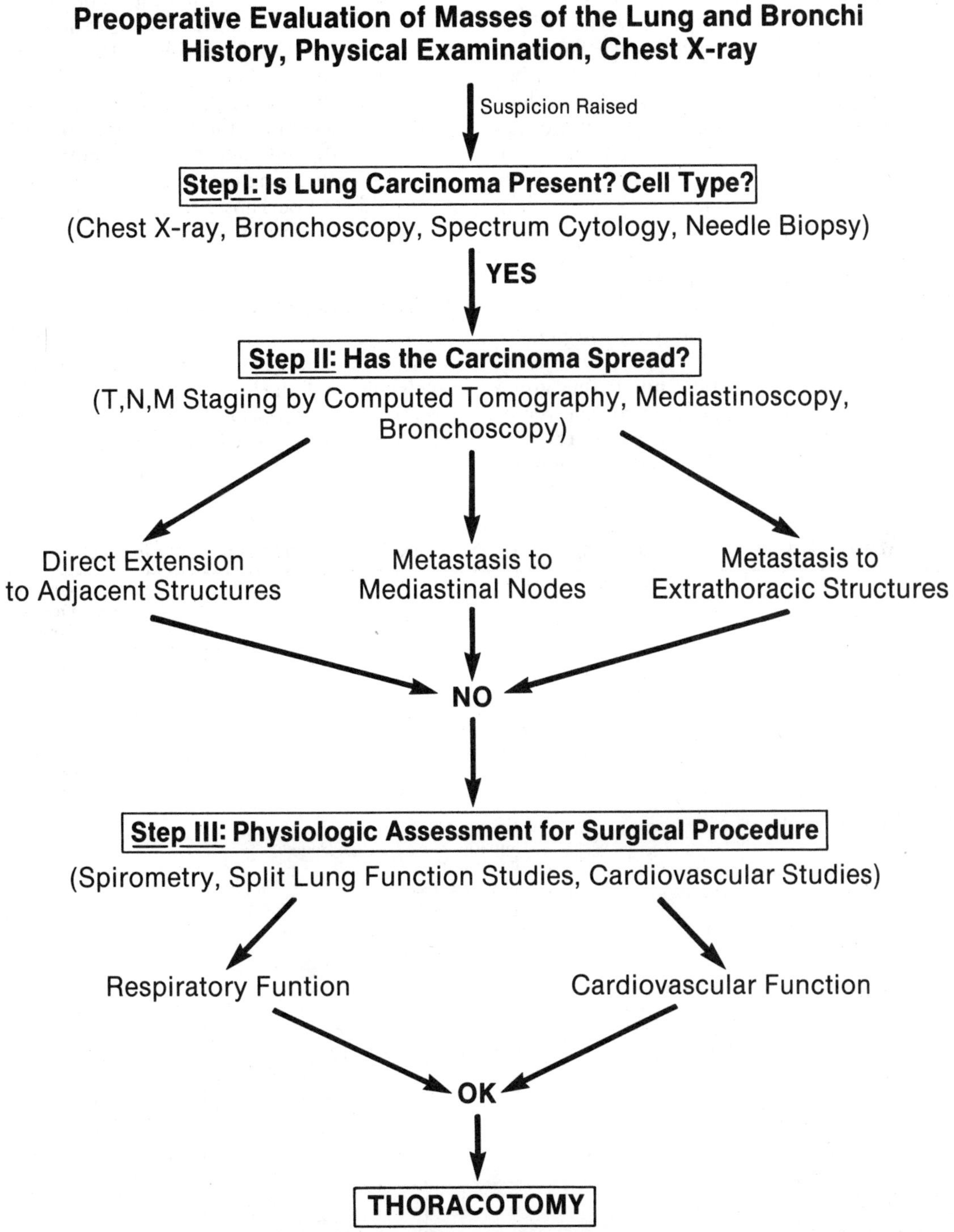

**Preoperative Evaluation of Masses of the Lung and Bronchi
History, Physical Examination, Chest X-ray**

Suspicion Raised

Step I: Is Lung Carcinoma Present? Cell Type?

(Chest X-ray, Bronchoscopy, Spectrum Cytology, Needle Biopsy)

YES

Step II: Has the Carcinoma Spread?

(T,N,M Staging by Computed Tomography, Mediastinoscopy,
Bronchoscopy)

Direct Extension   Metastasis to   Metastasis to
to Adjacent Structures   Mediastinal Nodes   Extrathoracic Structures

NO

Step III: Physiologic Assessment for Surgical Procedure

(Spirometry, Split Lung Function Studies, Cardiovascular Studies)

Respiratory Funtion   Cardiovascular Function

OK

THORACOTOMY

Figure 5-1. *The preoperative evaluation of masses of the lung and bronchi involves three basic steps. Step 1 consists of determining whether lung carcinoma is present, and if so, the cell type. Step 2 consists of determining whether the carcinoma has spread beyond its local confines. Step 3 involves physiologic assessment of the patient for the planned surgical procedure. This preoperative evaluation diagram displays the logic necessary for a patient to arrive at thoracotomy.*

cancer of the lung (carcinoma comprises approximately 90 per cent, adenomas 8 to 10 per cent, and benign masses 1 per cent of lung cancer) is in the sixth or seventh decade of life, has a history of heavy cigarette smoking and recent weight loss, and resides in an urban area. However, a small percentage of lung carcinomas occur in nonsmokers (< 10 per cent), and lung carcinoma has a higher incidence of occurrence in workers in some chemical industries (such as asbestos, arsenic, chromates, and nickel) than in the general population. Uranium miners have a greatly increased risk for the development of lung carcinoma, especially if they smoke. All age groups are affected, but the disease is rare in persons under 30 years of age. Five per cent of the patients are asymptomatic, and in this group the tumor is discovered only on routine roentgenographic examination of the chest. The vast majority of patients, however, have one or more symptoms related to the presence of the tumor. The symptoms may be designated as bronchopulmonary, extrapulmonary intrathoracic, extrathoracic metastatic, extrathoracic nonmetastatic, and nonspecific (Table 5–1).[1-4] On the average, symptoms have been present for 6 to 7 months prior to the time the patient seeks medical advice; since the first chest x-ray findings frequently antedate the first symptoms by several months, lung carcinoma will be at least a year old (and perhaps 2 to 5 years old) by the time of clinical presentation.

1. Bronchopulmonary Symptoms

Bronchopulmonary symptoms arising from involvement of the lung are due to bronchial irritation, ulceration, obstruction, infection distal to the obstruction, or a combination of these processes.

Table 5–1. Frequency of Symptom Occurrence in Bronchogenic Carcinoma[1-4]

Symptom		Frequency of Occurrence (Per Cent)
Asymptomatic		5
Bronchopulmonary	Cough	75
	Hemoptysis	57
	Chest pain	40
	Dyspnea	30
	Wheeze	10
Extrapulmonary intrathoracic symptoms	Hoarseness	5
	Superior vena cava syndrome	4
	Chest wall pain	< 5
	Pain down the arm	< 5
	Horner's syndrome	< 5
	Dysphagia	1
	Pleural effusion	10
Extrathoracic metastatic manifestation (See text)	Brain / Skeletal / Liver / Adrenals / Gastrointestinal tract / Kidneys / Pancreas	3 to 6
Extrathoracic nonmetastatic symptoms (See text)	Endocrine / Neuromuscular / Skeletal / Dermatologic / Hematologic	2
Nonspecific (See text)	Weight loss / Weakness / Anorexia / Lethargy / Malaise / Fever	10 to 22

a. Cough

In a large series of patients with carcinoma of the lung, 75 per cent had cough as one of the major symptoms, and this symptom was severe in 40 per cent of the patients. However, cough is possibly the most common manifestation of respiratory disease in general. It is so common among cigarette smokers that many of them regard a morning cough as "normal." The commonest stimulus to cough is the formation of sputum in the respiratory tract (see the following), and the cough process is an essential element in keeping the tract clear.

b. Sputum

The normal adult produces about 100 ml of mucus from the respiratory tract in a day. When excess mucus is formed it may accumulate, stimulate the mucus membrane, and be coughed up as sputum. Sputum in patients with bronchogenic carcinoma may be formed in response to physical, chemical, or infective insult to the mucus membrane of the airways.

Mucoid sputum is clear or white. Black sputum is due to the detritus of cigarette or atmospheric smoke. Purulent sputum contains pus mixed with mucus. Purulent sputum is usually yellow, but if it has been stagnant it may be green, owing to the action of verdoperoxidase, derived from neutrophils. Failure to clear a recent change in the quality and quantity of sputum within a few days of initiating antibiotic therapy should raise suspicion of a neoplasm. Blood-stained sputum can vary from small streaks to gross hemoptysis (see the following), and always warrants investigation for carcinoma. Hemoptysis, generally episodic blood streaking of the sputum, is present in 57 per cent of patients with bronchogenic carcinoma and is the first symptom in many.

c. Chest Pain

Chest pain is present in 40 per cent of patients presenting with a new carcinoma. It is usually a mild, constant, dull ache on the side of the tumor. Another important form of chest pain with lung carcinoma is pleuritic pain. It is due to direct tumor extension and is characteristically worse on breathing and coughing and can usually be accurately localized by the patient.

d. Dyspnea

Dyspnea is a common complaint in both patients with chronic lung disease and lung carcinoma (30 per cent). In chronic diseases it is common to find that the patient begins to complain of dyspnea only after his respiratory reserve is quite severely impaired, whereas in patients with lung carcinoma dyspnea occurs more abruptly and with less objective functional impairment.

e. Wheeze

This is described by 10 per cent of patients and is frequently localized to one side. It is due to airway obstruction and, if located in the trachea, severe dyspnea and stridor may develop.

2. Extrapulmonary Intrathoracic Symptoms

Other symptoms of chest disease occur as a result of growth of the tumor beyond the confines of the lung. These symptoms are due to involvement of the pleura, chest wall, diaphragm, mediastinal structures, and contiguous nerves. Approximately 15 per cent of patients with carcinoma of the lung have these kinds of extrapulmonary intrathoracic symptoms.

Pleural effusion is due to either metastatic involvement of the pleura (blood stained) or obstruction of lymphatic drainage (clear color). Chest wall pain is due to direct involvement of the chest wall by tumor. Dysphagia is due to partial obstruction of the esophagus by tumor in the paraesophageal lymph nodes. The superior vena cava syndrome is due to obstruction of the superior vena cava by paratracheal lymphadenopathy. Pain down the arm is due to involvement of the branches of the brachial plexus from tumors located in the superior sulcus. Horner's syndrome will often be present in patients who have pain down the arm. Hoarseness is due to paralysis of the vocal cord as the result of involvement of the left recurrent laryngeal nerve (at the left hilum) or, rarely, of the right recurrent laryngeal nerve.

3. Extrathoracic Metastatic Symptoms

Symptoms resulting from metastatic spread of the tumor outside the thorax account for a small percentage of the presenting or major complaints of patients with carcinoma of the lung. These extrathoracic metastatic symptoms can be referable, in order of general decreasing frequency, to brain, skeleton, liver, adrenals, gastrointestinal tract, kidneys, and pancreas. In these cases the history is extremely important because any positive history referable to these organs requires specific organ work-up for metastatic disease (see staging below) and, if found, precludes surgery.

4. Extrathoracic Nonmetastatic Symptoms

The extrathoracic nonmetastatic symptoms are usually due to paraneoplastic syndrome caused by secretion of endocrine or endocrine-like substances by the tumor (see chapter 3, Table 3–3). The endocrine-like manifestations include Cushing's syndrome, excessive antidiuretic hormone secretion, carcinoid syndrome, hypercalcemia, ectopic gonadotropin secretion, and hypoglycemia. The neuromuscular manifestations consist of carcinomatous myopathies and various myopathies related to brain dysfunction. Other manifestations can be skeletal (clubbing, pulmonary hypertrophic osteoarthropathy), dermatologic (scleroderma, acanthosis nigricans), vascular (thrombophlebitis), and hematologic.

5. Nonspecific Symptoms

Weight loss, weakness, anorexia, lethargy, and malaise occur in a large number of patients. Vague febrile respiratory syndromes (coldlike) may be present in 22 per cent of these patients. In 10 to 15 per cent, these symptoms instigate the initial visit to the physician.

B. Physical Examination

The basic tools of observation, inspection, palpation, and percussion should allow the physician to assess, in a gross way, the overall severity of chronic lung disease, whether major consolidation, atelectasis, or pleural effusion is present, and whether there is any obvious extrathoracic complication of thoracic carcinoma (Table 5–2). However, it should be noted that the most common manifestation of lung cancer upon physical examination is the presence of palpable supraclavicular lymph nodes. The reason for this is that lung carcinoma is most often in an advanced, inoperable stage at the time of presentation. Since it is mandatory subsequently to use much more sensitive radiologic means of determining resectability, further discussion of physical examination methods for making these determinations will not be continued here. Similarly, the questions of overall severity of chronic lung disease and whether

the patient can tolerate the planned procedure (operability) can be much more quantitatively answered by pulmonary function testing than by the findings of the physical examination (see Physiologic Assessment of the Patient for Surgery).

C. Common Laboratory Tests

Some of the routine laboratory tests that are performed on all patients are especially relevant to the preoperative evaluation of the patient with a lung or bronchial mass. These tests can be divided into those that help establish the diagnosis of lung cancer (e.g., chest x-ray and sputum for cytology), those that help establish the diagnosis of metastatic lung cancer (e.g., liver and bone enzymes, blood urea nitrogen and creatinine, and the urinalysis), and those that help physiologic assessment (e.g., hemoglobin concentration). Each of these three diagnostic areas is fully discussed in the following pages (along with the role of the common laboratory test in the work-up logic).

D. Diagnosis of Lung Cancer

1. The Carcinomas of the Lung[1, 2, 5, 6]

In order to understand fully the diagnosis and the staging of lung carcinoma it is necessary to have some appreciation of the natural history of each of the lung carcinoma cell types. Carcinoma of the lung may spread by direct extension, by lymphatic metastasis to lymph nodes, and by hematogenous metastasis to distant organs (Fig. 5–2). Direct extension can be in any direction and can involve any structure within the chest (pleura, chest wall, diaphragm, all mediastinal structures). Blockage of a bronchus can cause distal atelectasis and infection. Cavitation may be due either to necrosis within the tumor mass or to abscess formation distal to an obstructed bronchus. Lymphatic metastasis follows the lymph sump pathway of hilar and mediastinal nodal stations to the venous outlets (see chapter 2). All mediastinal structures can be potentially affected by lymph node enlargement and erosion. Hematogenous spread is due to invasion of the pulmonary veins by tumor cells. The blood-transported tumor cells are most frequently deposited and grow in brain, bone, liver, adrenal glands, and kidney.

The most common carcinomas of the lung (epidermoid, small cell, adeno, large cell), their

Table 5–2. Physical Findings That Occur with Pulmonary Pathology

Condition	Inspection and Palpation	Percussion	Fremitus	Breath Sounds	Adventitious Sounds	Other
Normal	Equal rib and diaphragm movement	Resonant	Present	Vesicular	None	"Bronchophony" in normal spoken voice
Consolidation	Slight restriction of motion on side affected	Dull	Increased	Bronchial	Rales	"Egophony" (E to A) and whispered pectoriloquy
Major atelectasis	Slightly small and restricted on side affected	Dull	Normal	Diminished	Rales after deep breath or cough	Tracheal and mediastinal shift toward
Pleural effusion or empyema	Reduced movement on side affected	Dull or flat	Absent	Diminished or absent	Friction rub early	Mediastinal shift away
Cavitation	Normal	Usually normal	Usually present	Amphoric	Coarse rales	Coin sign
Diffuse pulmonary fibrosis; interstitial lung disease	Symmetrically diminished	Normal	Normal	Harsh vesicular with prolonged expiration	Coarse rales uninfluenced by coughing	—
Emphysema	Enlarged and restricted bilaterally	Hyper-resonant	Normal or reduced	Diminished with prolonged expiratory phase	Occasional rhonchi; fine rales late in inspiration	Hoover's sign; high clavicle; muscular wasting (pink puffer)
Bronchitis	Normal	Normal	Normal	Vesicular with prolonged expiratory phase	Rhonchi with coarse rales	Cyanotic (blue bloater)
Bronchial asthma	Normal or enlarged	Hyper-resonant	Reduced	Diminished with prolonged expiratory phase	Wheezes	Distress
Pulmonary edema	Normal	Normal	Normal	Bronchial if interstitial; vesicular if alveolar	Moist rales	Distress
Pneumothorax	Slightly enlarged and restricted movement	Hyper-resonant	Absent	Diminished or absent	None	Mediastinal shift away
Fibrothorax	Small and very restricted movement	Dull	Present	Reduced to absent	None	Mediastinal shift toward

Spread of Carcinoma of the Lung

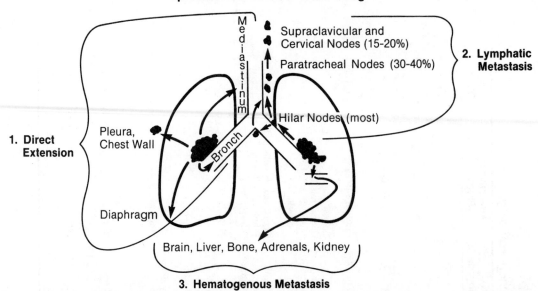

Figure 5–2. *Carcinoma of the lung spreads in three ways: first, by direct extension to the mediastinum, pleura and chest wall, diaphragm, and bronchi; second, by lymphatic metastasis to hilar, paratracheal and superclavicular, and cervicle nodes (proceeding from the distal to the proximal nodes, the incidence of involvement of the nodes decreases); third, by hematogenous metastasis to brain, liver, bone, adrenals, and kidney.*

relative incidence of occurrence, and most usual growth rate characteristics are listed in Table 5–3. However, it should be realized that all of these carcinomas are capable of a wide range of growth characteristics. Other very rare malignant pulmonary neoplasms (not listed in Table 5–3) are combined epidermoid-adenocarcinoma, carcinoid tumors, bronchial gland tumors, papillary tumors, sarcomas, and melanomas.

2. The Diagnosis of the Presence of Lung Cancer (Is Lung Carcinoma Present? Cell Type?)[1–6]

The diagnosis of the presence of lung cancer is made most often by use of the chest roentgenogram, bronchoscopy, sputum cytology, and percutaneous needle biopsy (Fig. 5–3). Although clearly positive results from any of these four tests establishes the diagnosis of lung car-

Table 5–3. The Carcinomas of the Lung

Carcinoma	Per Cent of All Carcinomas	Growth Rate	Metastatic Characteristics	Most Common Location	Cellular Characteristics	Prognosis
Epidermoid (squamous cell)	50 to 60	Slow	Slow, late	2/3 central*	Polygonal or prickle type cells with keratin	Fair
Undifferentiated small cell	15 to 35	Fast	Extensive, early	4/5 central	Anaplastic	Very poor to fatal
Adeno	1 to 10	Moderate	Infrequent	Peripheral†	Well differentiated	Good
Undifferentiated large cell	5 to 15 (1 per cent giant cell)	Rapid	Extensive, early	Central and peripheral	Anaplastic (giant cell)	Poor (rapidly fatal)

*Central = Inner two thirds of lung or proximal to third to fourth bronchial generation and usually visualized with a fiberoptic bronchoscope.
†Peripheral = Outer one third of lung or distal to third to fourth bronchial generation and not usually visualized with a fiberoptic bronchoscope.

Preoperative Evaluation of Masses of the Lung and Bronchi
Step I: Is Lung Carcinoma Present? Cell Type?

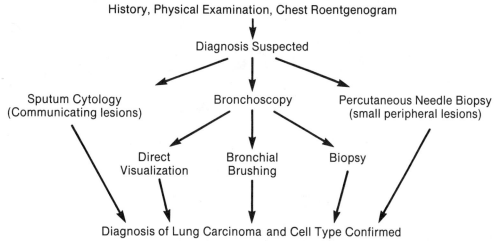

Figure 5–3. *Preoperative evaluation logic of step 1 for determining the presence of lung carcinoma and its cell type. See text for full explanation.*

cinoma, the diagnosis is most often established by a combination of chest roentgenogram consistent with the diagnosis along with a positive result from one of the other three tests. The latter three tests permit diagnosis of cell type in 75 per cent of cases.

a. THE CHEST ROENTGENOGRAM

It has been estimated that when a tumor of the lung is first detected on a chest roentgenogram, it has completed three fourths of its natural history,[7] and this first roentgenographic abnormality frequently antedates the first symptoms or signs of the disease by 7 or more months.[8] By the time bronchial carcinoma becomes symptomatic, the chest roentgenogram is abnormal in 98 per cent and the abnormality is most suggestive of tumor in over four fifths of all these patients.

The roentgenographic findings present due to carcinoma of the lung (Fig. 5–4) may be the result of the presence of the tumor itself within the lung (70 per cent are centrally located), of changes in the pulmonary parenchyma distal to a bronchus obstructed by the tumor (atelectasis, infection, and cavitation), and of spread of the tumor to extrapulmonary intrathoracic sites (hilar and mediastinal lymph nodes, pleura, chest wall, and diaphragm).

The early roentgenographic features are, unfortunately, subtle in nature and often are appreciated only in retrospect.[8] The earliest signs

visible in the roentgenogram of the chest are locally produced by the tumor itself. These signs may include any abnormal density within the lung parenchyma (most common), segmental atelectasis, a cavitation within the lung, and a mediastinal mass (uncommon). A newly appreciated pulmonary density must be compared with old films to establish how long it has been present. Malignant pulmonary lesions usually have doubling times of less than 1 year. A lesion that remains the same size for at least 2 years can be presumed to be benign.

The usual roentgenographic manifestations of lung carcinoma more frequently include the hilar and extrapulmonary intrathoracic manifestations in addition to the pulmonary parenchymal manifestations. In a review of the roentgenograms of the chest of 600 patients with carcinoma of the lung,[9] the average lung cancer mass at radiologic presentation was 3 to 4 cm in diameter. A larger parenchymal mass was present in 22 per cent and a smaller mass in 20 per cent; multiple masses were present in only 1 per cent. Obstructive pneumonitis, collapse, or consolidation was present in 41 per cent. A hilar abnormality, either alone or associated with other abnormalities, was present in 41 per cent of the patients. The various extrapulmonary intrathoracic manifestations, with mediastinal widening, pleural effusion, and raised hemidiaphragm being the most common of these, were present in 11 per cent.

Certain roentgenographic patterns are char-

Chest Roentgenographic Findings Due to Lung Carcinoma

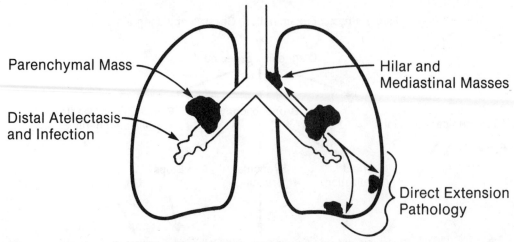

Figure 5–4. *In patients with lung carcinoma the chest roentgenographic findings result from the presence of the tumor itself within the lung (parenchymal mass), changes in the pulmonary parenchyma distal to a bronchus obstructed by the tumor (atelectasis and infection), and spread of the tumor to extrapulmonary intrathoracic sites (hilar and mediastinal masses and other direct extension pathology).*

acteristic of the various cell types.[9] Calcification is the most reliable sign of benign disease, especially if the lesion is a peripheral nodule. Since squamous cell carcinoma has a propensity to obstruct a bronchus, squamous cell carcinoma most often presents the picture of obstructive pneumonitis, collapse, consolidation, or cavitation. A hilar abnormality is also usually present with a squamous cell carcinoma. Adenocarcinomas are most often peripheral masses, and two thirds of these are larger than 4 cm. Hilar abnormalities, obstructive parenchymal lesions (atelectasis, abscess), and cavitation are infrequent to rare. Large cell undifferentiated carcinomas are most likely to be peripheral lesions and are larger than 4 cm. Cavitation is infrequent, and hilar abnormalities and parenchymal changes are present in approximately 30 per cent of cases. Small cell undifferentiated tumors appear primarily as hilar abnormalities (80 per cent), and a parenchymal obstructive lesion occurs in approximately 40 per cent.

b. Bronchoscopy

The examination of the tracheobronchial tree with either flexible fiberoptic (by far most common) or rigid bronchoscope should be done in almost all patients suspected of having a tumor of the lung. An exception may be made in patients with a very small peripheral lesion with no evidence of hilar or mediastinal lymph adenopathy. Direct visualization of the tumor, positive biopsy findings, or positive bronchial brushing or trap suction specimens or some combination of these three findings is obtained in a high percentage of the patients. Cell type influences the rate of positive findings; small cell tumors are identified proportionately more often than are squamous cell or large cell undifferentiated tumors, and adenocarcinomas are identified least frequently of all.

In addition to actual assessment of the tumor, other valuable information may be obtained at bronchoscopy. For example, the length of normal bronchus proximal to the tumor and the status of the carina (subcarinal nodes) may be determined, both of which are determinants of the exact surgical procedure to be performed (lobectomy, pneumonectomy, sleeve resection, or inoperable). In addition, bronchoscopy may reveal the presence of a second central tumor that was not visible on chest x-ray.

c. Sputum Cytology

Cytologic examination of sputum has been found to be positive in approximately half of patients suspected of having carcinoma of the lung. With appropriate cytologic study of several sputum specimens, tumor cells may be found in a higher percentage of patients. In one study, one or two sputum samples yielded a 59 per cent positive result, three sputa a 69 per cent, and four sputa a 90 per cent positive result.[10] A false-positive incidence of only 1 per cent was found, although in most laboratories this incidence is reported to be in the range of 2 to 3 per cent. Cell type as determined by cytologic study agrees with that of the final histologic diagnosis in approximately 85 per cent of the patients. Well-differentiated epidermoid carcinomas, undifferentiated small cell carcinomas, and adenocarcinomas can all be effectively typed by cytology. The undifferentiated large cell carcinomas, the poorly differentiated epidermoid carcinomas, and combined carcinomas are more difficult to type correctly. Cytologic studies are most often positive in patients with large tumors that communicate with the main bronchi. Parenchymal lesions frequently do not communicate with a bronchus, and cytologic studies in patients with such lesions are less rewarding.

d. Needle Biopsy

Percutaneous, transthoracic needle biopsy (with either fluoroscopic or computed tomographic guidance) has been suggested as a routine procedure for indeterminate (and noncommunicating) solitary peripheral lesions. With these lesions, this procedure has been found to be more accurate than the use of flexible fiberoptic bronchoscopy. The procedure can be performed on central lesions as well. Percutaneous needle biopsy causes a significant incidence of a small pneumothorax, which fortunately does not require drainage; however, the anesthesiologist must be aware of the history of a recent needle biopsy because of the possibility of the development of a tension pneumothorax with the commencement of positive-pressure ventilation.

e. Summary of Diagnosis of Lung Carcinoma

The diagnosis of lung carcinoma is almost always certain, but in 20 to 25 per cent of patients a histologic cell type diagnosis is not known preoperatively. For these patients, the findings at surgery (which often begins with an open lung biopsy) complete the first step in the work-up.

E. The Staging of Lung Cancer (Has the Carcinoma Spread?)[1, 2, 11–16]

Simply making the diagnosis of lung cancer alone is a grossly inadequate preoperative evaluation. In order to devise a rational approach to treatment, it is absolutely essential to determine the nature and extent of the disease in terms of any direct extension of the tumor to adjacent structures, metastasis of the tumor to the thoracic lymph node system, and extension of the tumor to extrathoracic structures. Any of these three forms of tumor extension may render the tumor inoperable, and the preoperative diagnosis of such extension will greatly decrease the incidence of unnecessary thoracotomy and surgical morbidity and mortality. The need for precise classification of the anatomic extent or stage of lung cancers led to the application of the size of tumor–nodal involvement–metastasis (TNM) system to this disease in 1973 (Table 5–4).

In brief, the T (for tumor) classification describes the size of the tumor and any direct extension of the tumor into surrounding tissues. T_0 indicates no evidence of a primary tumor; T_X indicates malignant cytology, but tumor is not seen roentgenographically or bronchoscopically; and T_1, T_2, and T_3 represent increasing size of the lesion (to greater than 3.0 cm) and/or direct extension of the primary tumor into adjacent tissues (visceral or parietal pleura, chest wall, diaphragm, mediastinum, mainstem bronchus), causation of atelectasis or obstructive pneumonitis of an entire lung, or pleural effusion. The classification of N (for nodes) describes intrathoracic nodal metastases. N_0 indicates no evidence of regional-node metastasis; N_1, metastasis to the lymph nodes of the ipsilateral hilar region; and N_2, metastasis to the mediastinal lymph nodes. The classification of M (for metastasis) describes extrathoracic metastases. M_0 indicates no known distant metastasis, and M_1 indicates distant extrathoracic metastasis (anywhere).

The basic T, N, and M classifications have been grouped into three main stages, indicating progressive extension of the carcinoma (bottom of Table 5–4). The breakdown of stages into three groups serves three purposes. First, the stage of the disease closely correlates with survival rate (Tables 5–5 and 5–6) except for small cell carcinoma (see Staging in Small Cell Lung Cancer).[17] Small cell carcinoma is thought to have metastatic spread by the time of diagnosis, and, therefore, its natural history and behavior are independent of (and much more lethal than) the TNM system predictions (Fig. 5–5).[17] The diagnosis of small cell carcinoma should be made from the bronchoscopic procedures (brushings, biopsy), or sputum cytology or needle biopsy (see preceding). Second, the

Table 5–4. Staging of Lung Cancer

Primary Tumor

T_X Malignant cell in cytology; site undetermined.
T_0 No evidence of primary tumor.
T_1 Tumor $\leq$ 3 cm in size; surrounded by lung tissue.
T_2 Tumor > 3 cm in size.
T_3 Tumor of any size with extension to chest wall, parietal pleura, diaphragm, mediastinum, or within 2 cm of carina.

Nodal Involvement

N_0 No lymph node involvement.
N_1 Metastasis to peribronchial or ipsilateral hilar region only.
N_2 Mediastinal lymph node metastasis.

Distant Metastasis

M_0 No distant metastasis.
M_1 Distant metastasis present.

Stage Grouping

Stage I $T_1N_0M_0$
          $T_1N_1M_0$
          $T_2N_0M_0$
Stage II $T_2N_1M_0$
Stage III T_3 with any N or M
          N_2 with any T or M
          M_1 with any T or N

Table 5–5. Two-Year Survival Rates According to Bronchogenic Carcinoma Cell Type[17]

Cell Type	Stage (in per cent)		
	1	2	3
Squamous	46.6	39.8	11.5
Adeno	45.9	14.3	7.9
Large	42.8	12.9	12.9
Small	6.0	5.0	3.8

stage of the disease (I and II, approximately 30 to 35 per cent of all patients) usually dictates the surgical procedure of choice (see Surgical Procedures as Dictated by Staging). Third, the diagnosis of stage III (approximately 60 to 65 per cent of all patients) may preclude surgery, and, therefore, staging tests are most vitally concerned with determining T_3, N_2, or M_1 disease. However, it should be noted that outstanding 5-year survival results (30 per cent) have recently been obtained with some stage III subsets (T_3, N_0–N_2, M_0).[18]

In summary, the introduction of the TNM staging system has encouraged an orderly assessment for selecting those cases most suitable for surgery and the type of surgery that should be performed. As a corollary to the above, appropriate staging should reduce the incidence of unnecessary thoracotomy to less than 20 per cent.[19, 20] As a consequence of these improvements, the staging should result in an overall improvement in the present postsurgery 5- and 10-year survival rates of approximately 30 and 16 to 18 per cent, respectively. Although T, N, and M staging are really done in parallel, for the sake of clarity they will be discussed separately in the following sections (Fig. 5–6).

1. T Staging (Tumor Size and Direct Extension)

The advent of computed tomographic scans of the thorax (lung parenchyma, pleura, and mediastinum) has had a profound and simplifying effect on the T staging of lung cancer (Fig. 5–6). Computed tomographic scans of the thorax have been shown to provide a clear delineation of the tumor mass and can suggest direct tumor extension (particularly direct spread to the pleura with or without an accompanying effusion and direct spread to the mediastinal structures) in many patients in whom the more conventional diagnostic radiologic methods fail to do so. For example, computed

Table 5–6. Five-Year Postsurgical Survival Rates According to Stage[31]

Stage	Five-Year Survival Rate (per cent)
I	40
II	20 to 25
III	10

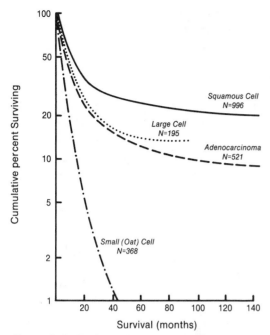

Figure 5–5. Survival of patients with lung cancer according to histologic type. (Oat) cell carcinoma is very lethal, whereas the percentage of patients surviving after 5 years with squamous cell, large cell, and adenocarcinoma of the lung levels off between 10 and 20 per cent after 5 years. (Redrawn with permission from Mountain CF, Carr DT, Anderson WAD: A system for the clinical staging of lung cancer. Am J Roentgenol Radium Ther Nucl Med 120:130–138, 1974.)

tomographic scanning in non–small cell cancer when compared with conventional chest radiology, tomography, and bronchoscopy increases the T stage in 40 per cent of cases[21] and in small cell cancer increases the T stage from 1 or 2 to 3 in anywhere from 30 to 84 per cent of cases.[22] These T stage changes were due to direct tumor extension into the mediastinum, pleura, or diaphragm.

The results of and extra information gained from computed tomographic T staging have to be interpreted carefully with regard to pulmonary nodules. Computed tomography detects 50 per cent more pulmonary nodules than whole lung tomograms.[23] Most of these nodules are small, less than 6 mm, and serial follow-up shows that the majority (60 per cent) are benign. Thus, an additional intrapulmonary nodule (other than the primary) seen only with computed tomography does not necessarily represent an intrapulmonary metastasis and is not necessarily a contraindiction to surgery.

Several other roentgenographic studies may demonstrate direct extension involvement of thoracic structures, which may preclude resec-

tion. Cardiac angiocardiography may demonstrate mainstem pulmonary artery invasion (at least 1 to 2 cm of a mainstem pulmonry artery that is free of tumor is required for pneumonectomy). Pulmonary artery angiography may be necessary to demonstrate pulmonary arteriovenous malformations and aortography to demonstrate pulmonary sequestrations. A barium swallow may demonstrate fixation and/or distortion of the esophagus. Bronchography may be necessary for defining bronchopleural and bronchoesophageal fistulas. Azygography may reveal mediastinal lymph node involvement as well as involvement of the vena cava by tumor.

2. N Staging (Metastasis to Lymph Nodes)

There are 13 node stations, with station 13 being most distal (peripheral) and station 1 being most proximal (central).[24] N_1 nodes are segmental (#13), lobar (#12), interlobar (#11), and hilar (#10). N_2 nodes are inferior mediastinal (#7 to #9), aortic (#5 and #6), and superior mediastinal (#1 to #4). The final precise enumeration of nodal involvement often requires staging at the time of operation (see section on postsurgery staging).

The preoperative assignment of N classification involves the use of computed tomography of the thorax (lung parenchyma, hilum, and mediastinum) and mediastinoscopy (Fig. 5–6). As with T staging, use of computed tomography has also had a profound and simplifying effect on tumor staging. Although paratracheal and hilar lymph node adenopathy can usually be adequately identified by conventional radiology, computed tomographic scans are clearly superior in detecting subcarinal node enlargement. Computed tomography compared with conventional radiology causes an upstaging of N status in 32 per cent of cases of lung carcinoma.[21]

The results of and extra information gained from computed tomographic scanning for nodes also have to be interpreted carefully. The demonstration of enlarged mediastinal glands should not automatically lead to the conclusion that they are infiltrated by tumor. Glands are frequently enlarged and fleshy and may be subsequently found to be free of disease, and the false-positive rate of computed tomography mediastinal lymphadenopathy is about 25 per cent of cases.[25] Consequently, a positive computed tomographic scan still requires mediastinoscopy. On the other hand, the predictive value of a negative computed tomographic scan is on

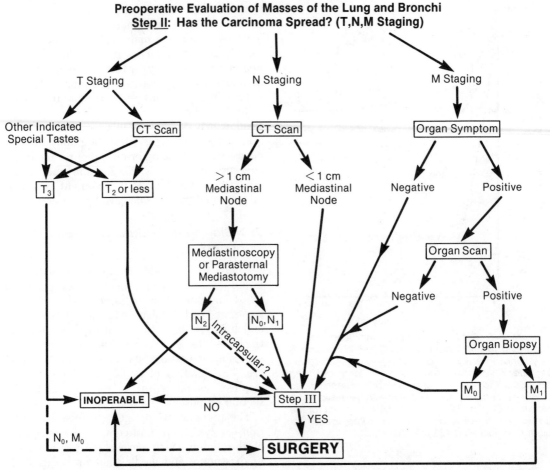

Preoperative Evaluation of Masses of the Lung and Bronchi
Step II: Has the Carcinoma Spread? (T,N,M Staging)

Figure 5–6. Preoperative evaluation logic of step II to determine whether lung carcinoma has spread beyond its local confines. Definition of T, N, and M staging and the various T, N, and M subsets are described in Table 5–4. The dashed lines indicate that surgery has recently been performed with an encouraging degree of success.[18] Step III is physiologic assessment of the patients for the planned surgical procedure.

the order of 90 to 95 per cent, and in such cases mediastinoscopy (see the following) may be omitted before thoracotomy.[25] However, it should be noted that for the remaining 5 to 10 per cent a normal-sized mediastinal gland does not mean that it is tumor free, and the results of studies comparing computed tomography findings in the mediastinum with histologic evaluation show that there is a definite small false-negative rate.[25, 26] Thus, the main advantage of computed tomography is that it can save unnecessary mediastinoscopies. Since, however, it tends to "overstage" tumors, thoracic surgical units without computed tomographic scanners will achieve equally good N staging results with routine preoperative mediastinal exploration.

Mediastinoscopy or mediastinotomy (anterior resection of a costosternal cartilage) should be carried out as the final procedure to assess N

staging whenever computed tomography is positive or computed tomography is not available. Mediastinoscopy or mediastinotomy should be performed even if the mediastinum looks normal with conventional radiologic techniques, since almost 50 per cent of patients with mediastinal nodal involvement do not have mediastinal widening on chest x-ray.[27] Mediastinotomy is particularly important for left upper lobe lesions because it can provide better access to the left anterior mediastinal lymph nodes. If glands resected at mediastinoscopy or mediastinotomy are found to contain tumor (N_2), most would classify the case as inoperable.

3. M (Metastasis) Staging

M staging begins with a complete history and physical examination that covers the function of all organ systems, with particular emphasis on brain, bone, and liver (Fig. 5–6). If the history or physical is positive for any given organ system, then that particular organ system should be further investigated for metastases. The investigation should first involve an organ scan of some type (radioisotopic, computed tomographic). If the organ scan is negative, then metastases can be considered to have been ruled out. If the organ scan is positive, then biopsy of the particular organ in question is generally indicated. A positive biopsy establishes the diagnosis of M_1 disease.

4. Postsurgical Staging

Microscopic analysis of specimens resected at surgery allows further postsurgical pathologic staging. Meaningful postsurgical staging requires routine sampling and labeling of all mediastinal gland stations at thoracotomy (as recommended by the American Joint Committee for Cancer Staging and End-Results Reporting: Staging of Lung Cancer, 1979. Chicago, 1979; and reference 24). The pathology reports should include comments on the cell type and its differentiation, homogeneity of cell type, presence of pleural disease in cases of peripheral tumors, status of resection margins and bronchial stump, and the extent of glandular extension and whether such extension is intracapsular or locally invasive.

5. Staging in Small Cell Lung Cancer

The particularly high incidence of mediastinal lymph node disease in small cell lung cancer and the coexisting evidence of extrathoracic dissemination at the time of presentation mean that the T, N, and M classifications have no bearing on prognosis. Thus, for most patients with small cell tumors, staging is somewhat academic. However, there are a few patients for whom small cell carcinoma staging is relevant and who should have surgery. In the few cases in which the primary tumor is peripheral and is truly stage 1 (no nodes are affected) survival rates are more favorable. For example, a 60 per cent 5-year survival rate has been reported in 26 patients with T_1, N_0 disease.[28] Recently, further attempts to improve survival have been made by "debulking" surgery for patients with T_1 or T_2, N_0 lesions followed by a combination of cytotoxic chemotherapy and radiotherapy.[29]

6. Surgical Procedure as Dictated by Staging

Segmental resection is indicated for small (< 3 cm in diameter) stage I (T_1, N_0, M_0) peripheral lesions and for patients with severely compromised cardiopulmonary status. Relative contraindications to segmental resection are T_2 lesions or a lesion that crosses an intersegmental plane. Mortality for segmental resection is < 0.5 per cent.[30]

At the present time, lobectomy is the operation of choice for carcinoma of the lung. It is indicated when technically feasible for all stage I and II disease and some stage III lesions. It has a mortality of 1.3 per cent.[30]

Pneumonectomy is indicated with more extensive disease, generally T_2, N_0, M_0 or T_2, N_1, M_0 with hilar involvement. The mortality for pneumonectomy is about 5 per cent.[30]

With few exceptions[18] patients with stage III disease are not candidates for definitive surgical resection. The exceptions may include certain patients with central lesions and only hilar node involvement, Pancoast's tumors, or certain lesions with chest wall involvement. Patients who are not candidates for surgical resection may receive radiation therapy, chemotherapy, and/or immunotherapy. Unfortunately, none of these latter therapeutic modalities have significantly impacted on survival rates for bronchogenic carcinoma. Surgery, when it can be performed, is still a patient's only hope for cure of bronchogenic carcinoma.

7. Summary of Results of Diagnosis and Staging of Lung Cancer

The fate of a "typical" 100 consecutive cases of non–small cell lung carcinoma is shown schematically in Figure 5–7. Approximately 65 per cent of the patients would be considered inoperable at presentation because of intrathoracic spread, the detection of extrathoracic metastases, or extremely poor lung function. The remaining 35 per cent would undergo a thoracotomy, although the figure may be nearer 20 to 30 per cent if mediastinoscopy was routinely performed prior to definitive surgery. At thoracotomy, 15 per cent of the original 100 cases would be found to be inoperable because of previously unrecognized tumor spread. The remaining 20 per cent would undergo "curative" resection. The 5- and 10-year survival rates for all persons undergoing resection would be 30 per cent and 16 to 18 per cent, respectively (6

Fate of 100 'Typical' Patients with Non-Small Cell Lung Carcinoma

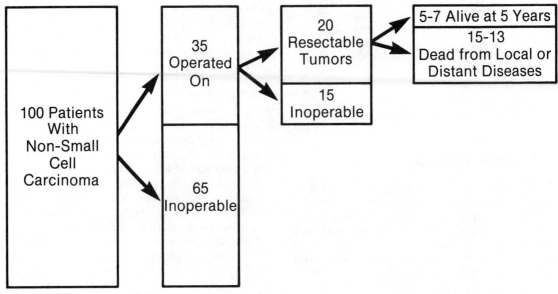

Figure 5–7. The fate of 100 "typical" patients with non–small cell lung carcinoma.

and 3 to 4 patients, respectively, of the original 100 patients). The 5-year postsurgical survival rates according to stage I, II, and III are 40, 20 to 25, and 10 per cent, respectively (Table 5–6).[31] The reason "curative" resection may fail so often in the lower stages is due to the inability to detect small asymptomatic metastases prior to operation.

F. Physiologic Assessment of the Patient for Surgery

1. History and Physical Examination

Aside from smoking/stopping smoking, there are three other aspects of poor lung function that can be diagnosed by history and/or physical examination and can be treated or improved preoperatively; therefore, the patient should always be questioned about these areas. If the patient reports a significant departure from his or her usual state of health with regard to any of the following, then a preoperative pulmonary preparation regimen should be instituted (see chapter 6). First, all patients should be questioned about bronchospasm. Most patients who have bronchospasm (or wheezing) are very aware of varying degrees of airway resistance and chest tightness and of which medications

relieve these symptoms. Auscultation of the chest for bronchospasm should also always be performed. If the amount of bronchospasm as reported by the patient, or heard by auscultation, is more than usual, then therapeutic levels of bronchodilator drugs should be achieved (see chapter 6). Second, all patients should be questioned about the amount of their secretions. If secretions are much more copious than usual, a few days of secretion removal (see chapter 6) may be of great benefit. Third, if the color of the sputum has recently changed from mucoid to yellow or green, a sputum culture and sensitivity test should be performed and appropriate antibiotic therapy instituted.

2. Pulmonary Function Tests

Within the context of the proposed operation, the purpose of pulmonary function testing is to identify those patients who are at high risk for postoperative respiratory complications (atelectasis, infection, unacceptable degree of dyspnea, or development of cor pulmonale or acute respiratory failure). In this section the various individual whole lung and regional lung function tests will be described first, and then the sequence in which these tests should be performed is detailed.

Table 5–7. Minimal Pulmonary Function Test Criteria for Various-Sized Pulmonary Resections[5, 33]

Test	Unit	Normal	Pneumonectomy	Lobectomy	Biopsy or Segmental
MBC	Liters/min	> 100	> 70	40 to 70	40
MBC	Per cent predicted	100	> 55	> 40	> 35
FEV_1	Liters	> 2	> 2	> 1	> 0.6
FEV_1	Per cent predicted	> 100	> 55	40 to 50	> 40
FEV_{25-75}	Liters	2	> 1.6	> 0.6 to 1.6	> 0.6

MBC = maximum breathing capacity; FEV = forced expired volume.

a. WHOLE LUNG FUNCTION TESTS[32]

All patients undergoing resectional thoracic surgery should have a timed expiratory spirogram (spirometry); those undergoing a pneumonectomy should also have a maximum breathing capacity and a lung volume determination. The minimal pulmonary function criteria indicating increased risk to performing various-sized pulmonary resectional surgery are shown in Table 5–7.[5, 33] Values below the ones listed in Table 5–7 are associated with a greatly increased incidence of postoperative respiratory complications.[5, 33]

i. Spirometry. The simplest spirometry test is measuring vital capacity. To measure vital capacity, the patient inspires maximally to total lung capacity (TLC) and then exhales either slowly (slow vital capacity) or forcefully (forced vital capacity, FVC) and completely, and the exhaled volume is recorded. With regard to the lung volumes shown in Figure 3–21, inspiratory capacity, inspiratory reserve volume, and expiratory reserve volume can all be measured directly from the vital capacity spirogram.

The volume exhaled rapidly from one breath has been quantified in many ways; the most commonly used value is the volume of gas exhaled in the first second and is usually expressed as a percentage of the FVC (forced expired volume in 1 sec/FVC or $FEV_1\%$) (Fig. 5–8). Normally, an individual can exhale 70 to 80 per cent of the VC in 1 second; the remainder may take 2 additional seconds (FEV_3). Patients with significant airway obstruction are able to exhale much less volume in the first second and require a much longer time to deliver the entire volume.

The measurement of the maximum instantaneous "peak" expiratory flow rate (PEFR) is measured with an automated device such as the Wright peak flow meter. The PEFR is defined as the highest expiratory flow rate sustained for at least 10 msec. Since flow rate at any given lung volume or moment is equal to the slope

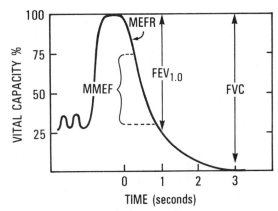

Figure 5–8. Spirogram of a patient taking two small tidal volume breaths, then an inspiration to total lung capacity, and then a forced exhaled breath to residual volume cycle. (MEFR = maximum expiratory flow rate—the average rate of flow (slope) over a 1 L segment of the early portion of the expiratory spirogram trace. $FEV_{1.0}$ = forced expired volume in 1 sec. FVC = forced vital capacity, which equals 100 per cent of the y-axis. MMEF = maximum midexpiratory flow rate, which is measured on the timed expiratory spirogram between 25 and 75 per cent of the FVC curve.)

of the tangent line to the timed expiratory spirogram curve (such as the one shown in Fig. 5–8), and it is difficult to pick out accurately the steepest slope, the PEFR cannot be measured easily or with precision by hand from a recorded spirogram. However, a comparable, albeit slightly lower value, the maximum expiratory flow rate (MEFR), can be derived by taking the average rate of flow (slope) over a 1-liter segment of the early portion of the spirogram trace (Fig. 5–8). Usually, the segment between 200 and 1200 ml of expired volume is chosen; hence, the measurement is often referred to as $FEF_{200-1200}$, the subscript designating the volume segment used.

FEV_1, PEFR, and MEFR are easily measured indices of airflow obstruction and correlate well with gross functional impairment. Nevertheless, they are relatively insensitive to increases in the frictional resistance in small airways, which are important at low lung volumes near the terminal portion of the FVC maneuver. Rather, FEV_1, PEFR, and MEFR represent measurements of flow occurring within the first second of the FVC maneuver and at relatively high lung volumes. These measurements are highly dependent on patient effort (and therefore variable) as well as on the resistance of the larger airways. The value of FEV_1, PEFR, and MEFR as screening tests is thus limited by the extent to which disease involves the larger airways. This helps to explain the relative lack of sensitivity that these measurements have in detecting early mild (small airway) obstructive disease. However, these effort-dependent large airway pulmonary function tests are the ones most responsive to and capable of detecting bronchodilator drug effects; they are, therefore, the most useful tests in the assessment of the presence of bronchospasm and the therapeutic benefit of these drugs.

The maximum midexpiratory flow rate (MMEF, or MMRF) is measured on the timed expiratory spirogram during the middle half of the FVC curve between 25 and 75 per cent Fig. 5–8). However, it is not truly the "maximum" flow (the PEFR), since the latter occurs at a point much closer to the TLC. For this reason, use of "forced midexpiratory flow" has been advocated, with the more precise symbol of $FEV_{25-75\%}$. The MMEF, by considering only the middle segment of the FVC, eliminates the initial highly effort-dependent and more variable segment of the trace. The flow rate during this segment has been shown to be largely independent of patient effort and is slowed by obstruction of smaller airways. Because of this, the MMEF is accepted as an indirect measure of small airway resistance and has been advocated as a sensitive test for the early detection of small-airway disease.[34]

ii. Maximum Breathing Capacity. The maximum breathing capacity (MBC) is the maximum amount of air that can be breathed in 1 minute. It is expiratory effort–dependent and reflects the total function of the entire cardiorespiratory apparatus. However, the maximal breathing capacity may have unique value in that it also depends on the intangible variables of cooperation, motivation, and stamina in addition to cardiorespiratory function. Thus, the predictive value of maximal breathing capacity should be similar to an exercise test, such as bicycle ergometry.[35]

iii. Lung Volume. The functional residual capacity (FRC) is defined as the volume of gas in the lung that exists at the end of a normal expiration when there is no airflow and alveolar pressure equals the ambient pressure. The expiratory reserve volume is additional gas below FRC that can be consciously exhaled and results in the minimum volume of lung possible, known as the residual volume (RV). Thus, the FRC equals the residual volume plus the expiratory reserve volume (Fig. 3–21). Total lung volume, FRC, and residual volume all contain a fraction (the residual volume) that cannot be measured by simple spirometry. However, since FRC is usually measured (by N_2 washout, He dilution, or plethysmographically; see chapter 3), total lung capacity and residual volume can be easily derived by using the other lung volumes that are measured by simple spirometry.

b. REGIONAL LUNG FUNCTION TESTS[29]

When a tumor completely occludes a mainstem bronchus, then tests of whole lung function evaluate the function of the nonaffected side; in other words, physiologically the patient has already had a pneumonectomy. However, in the large majority of cases, tests of whole lung function do not separate out the relative contribution made by the lung tissue to be resected from the contribution made by the lung tissue that would remain after resection to the total preoperative ventilation and gas exchange. In fact, ventilation-perfusion scans have shown that, apparently, small tumors may greatly distort the distribution of ventilation or perfusion or both, and this may result in a misleading interpretation of whole lung function, especially if there is coexistent underlying generalized disease such as chronic bronchitis.[36] Thus, tests of whole lung function may fail to resolve whether the patient would survive a resection without being left unduly dyspneic in cor pulmonale. The regional lung function tests consist of radioisotope studies (radiospirometry) (which is the most important one) and somewhat less important nonradioisotope studies (the lateral position test, bronchial blockade, mainstem pulmonary artery blockade).

i. Radioisotope Regional Perfusion, Ventilation-Perfusion Studies (Radiospirometry).[37–39] In the past, regional lung function was measured by differential bronchospirometry. The procedure involved considerable patient discomfort due to double-lumen endotracheal tube insertion (usually into an awake patient) and technical and physiologic uncertainties related to the required use of the Fick principle. Presently, right-left split pulmonary functions are obtained with easily performed noninvasive ^{133}Xe radiospirometry and ^{133}Xe and macroaggregate ([99]Te) perfusion scanning.

Usually, three studies are performed to determine right-left split pulmonary function (regional ventilation, regional perfusion, regional lung volume [and regional ventilation/perfusion, ventilation/volume, perfusion/volume relationships by appropriate division of the primary three numbers], Fig. 5–9). First, [133]Xe (or [99]Te or ^{131}I-MAA)[33] is infused as a bolus intravenously (Fig. 5–9A). Since ^{133}Xe is a very insoluble gas, almost all of the [133]Xe (95 per cent) evolves out of the blood into the alveoli, and this is respired out of the body into an open system. Regional external chest scintillation counters record these events as a time (x-axis) versus activity (y-axis) curve. The time versus activity curve shows a rapid vascular-to-alveolar washin peak and then an exponential alveolar-to-environment washout. Since ^{133}Xe appears in the air space only in proportion to the perfusion of the region, the regional perfusion washin peak count divided by the total count equals the regional fractional perfusion. Since [99]Te and ^{131}I-MAA simply lodge in the pulmonary microcirculation, the regional activity count divided by the total chest count with these isotopes more directly yields the regional fractional perfusion.

In the second study, a vital capacity breath of a bolus of ^{133}Xe results in a ventilation washin peak (environment-to-alveolar) followed by an exponential alveolar-to-environment washout of [133]Xe (Fig. 5–9B). Regional ventilation washin peak counts divided by the total chest count yield the regional fractional ventilation.

In the third study, ^{133}Xe is again administered as an intravenous bolus, but after the ^{133}Xe evolves into the alveoli from the vascular space, it is respired into a closed system (Fig. 5–9C). After 10 to 15 minutes of equilibration, the ^{133}Xe should have reached all gas spaces within the lungs (slow and fast time constants), and the concentration of ^{133}Xe should be uniform throughout the lungs and the attached closed system. The regional radioactive counts/unit time then is proportional to the regional volume of lung.

Radioactive-scanning radiospirometry therefore yields regional perfusion, ventilation, and lung volume. Dividing regional perfusion and ventilation by regional lung volume results in regional perfusion and ventilation per unit lung volume. Finally, dividing regional ventilation by regional perfusion results in the regional ventilation/perfusion ratio.

Regional Lung Function

Regional Perfusion

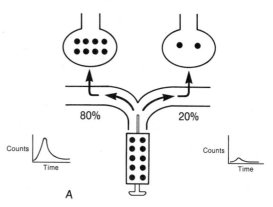

Regional Ventilation

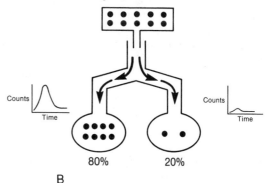

Regional Volume

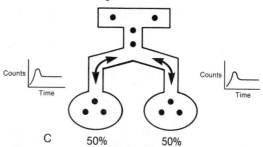

Figure 5–9. Three studies are usually performed to determine regional lung function. Regional perfusion (A) is determined by intravenous injection of an insoluble radioisotope, which distributes to the two lungs according to the blood flow to each lung. Peak radioactivity over each lung (peak counts with time) is proportional to each lung blood flow. Regional ventilation (B) is determined by having the patient inhale an insoluble gaseous radioisotope. Peak radioactivity over each lung (peak counts with time) is proportional to each lung ventilation. Regional volume (C) is determined by equilibrating radioactive material within the lungs with a connected closed space. The plateau radioactivity of each lung (plateau count with time) is then proportional to the volume of each lung. See text for fuller explanation.

Conventional whole lung function tests (VC, FEV_1, maximal breathing capacity) cannot predict postpneumonectomy lung function, since the amount of lung function to be removed is otherwise unknown. However, multiplication of preoperative whole lung pulmonary function tests by the percentage of lung to be removed, as determined by radioactive-scanning radiospirometry, should theoretically predict postoperative pulmonary function testing.[33] For example, if the preoperative vital capacity and FEV_1 was 2.00 L and 1.40 L, respectively, and the ventilation of the lung to be removed was 40 per cent of the total ventilation, then the predicted postoperative vital capacity and FEV_1 would be 1.20 L and 0.84 L, respectively. Indeed, combining radiospirometry with conventional pulmonary function tests has in fact resulted in a fair degree of correlation between predicted and measured postpneumonectomy pulmonary function testing.[40-44] The literature suggests that a predicted postoperative FEV_1 of 0.8 or greater yields an "acceptable" incidence of postoperative morbidity and mortality.[33, 37-40, 44] The availability of lung scanning in most hospitals, the high degree of accuracy of prediction of postoperative pulmonary function, and the ready acceptance of the test by patients make the quantitative lung scan the most useful preoperative regional lung function test.

ii. The Lateral Position Test. The lateral position test has had some success in approximating individual lung ventilation. When a patient with normal lungs turns from the supine position to the lateral decubitus position, there is an increase in total lung functional residual capacity because the increase in nondependent lung functional residual capacity (due to less exposure of the nondependent lung to the weight of the mediastinum and pressure of the abdominal contents) exceeds the decrease in dependent lung functional residual capacity (due to greater exposure of the dependent lung to the weight of the mediastinum and the pressure of the abdominal contents). Thus, the procedure is thought to be a test of the expansile and ventilatory capability of the nondependent lung.

The test is performed by having the patient breathe continuously into a spirometer while sequentially turning from the supine position to one of the lateral decubitus positions, back to the supine position, then into the other lateral decubitus position, and finally back into the supine position. The increase in total lung functional residual capacity is easily and non-invasively determined by noting the rise in the end-expiratory level of the continuously recorded spirogram; that is, the sine wave tidal ventilation on the spirogram first shows a gradual slope upward and then a plateau at a new stable level. The results are expressed as the increase in functional residual capacity in one lateral decubitus position divided by the increase in functional residual capacity in both lateral decubitus positions.

The relative increase in functional residual capacity in each lung has correlated well with oxygen consumption and minute ventilation determined bronchospirometrically[45] in each lung and with radionuclide ventilation-perfusion studies when the lung disease was symmetrical,[46] and moderately well when the lung disease was asymmetrical,[47] but predicts postpneumonectomy FEV_1 only fairly well.[48] The lateral position test is most likely to give false information whenever the disease process has little effect on the compliance of the lung in question. It should be stressed that since radionuclide ventilation-perfusion studies are well tolerated, safe, and simple to perform and provide exquisitely detailed information about both regional ventilation and perfusion, they must be considered the tests of choice of regional lung function. However, radionuclide studies require the use of sophisticated equipment, which may not be available in all hospitals, and it would seem that the lateral position test might be a useful alternative in this situation.

iii. Regional Bronchial Balloon Occlusion. Postpneumonectomy (or after any resection) ventilatory function can also be simulated preoperatively by passing, with the aid of a fiberoptic bronchoscope, a balloon occlusion catheter, which can occlude either lung (or any lobe), and then measuring spirometry of the remaining lung tissue (after careful withdrawal of the bronchoscope). Supplemental oxygen must be administered during bronchial blockade because the blocked segment would still be perfused, and all of this perfusion would be right-to-left shunt flow, which would create a risk of hypoxemia.

The regional bronchial balloon occlusion method of predicting postpneumonectomy ventilatory function has been studied during cycling exercise with a steady state load equivalent to walking at a brisk pace for that patient.[49] The effects on minute ventilation and oxygen uptake were observed during occlusion of the bronchus to the diseased lobe. If the patient was able to continue cycling and maintain the same workload during occlusion, this was regarded as evidence that they would withstand resection of the occluded lung tissue. All patients who could maintain the workload during preoperative bronchial occlusion were able to do so postoperatively.

iv. Regional Pulmonary Artery Balloon Occlusion. Postpneumonectomy pulmonary circulatory and right ventricular function can be simulated preoperatively by passing into the main pulmonary artery on the side to be resected a pulmonary artery catheter (using fluoroscopy) that has a 5-ml balloon at the tip of the catheter and a port for measuring pressure that is proximal to the balloon. Inflation of the distal balloon functionally resects the vasculature distal to the balloon; the pulmonary artery balloon inflation can be done with and without exercise. Under these conditions, all the pulmonary blood flow is diverted to the lung that will remain after the pneumonectomy, and the distensibility and compliance of the remaining pulmonary vascular bed are therefore tested. However, the test is unphysiologic in the sense that the blocked lung would still be ventilated, and all the ventilation to this lung would be dead space ventilation, which would not be present postpneumonectomy. If the mean pulmonary artery pressure increases above 40 mm Hg, the P_aCO_2 increases above 60 mm Hg, or the P_aO_2 decreases below 45 mm Hg, it is likely that the patient will not be able to tolerate resection of that amount of pulmonary vascular bed without development of right ventricular failure and cor pulmonale.[33, 41, 50-54] Since this test is highly invasive, requires special equipment, and is technically difficult, it is rarely clinically used today.

Simultaneous balloon occlusion of both a mainstem pulmonary artery and bronchus should completely simulate the physiologic effects of pneumonectomy and provide the most realistic assessment of total postpneumonectomy lung function; there would be no acute increase in shunt and/or dead space. However, since this potentially very accurate simulation of the postresection condition is so invasive and complicated, it can only be regarded as a research tool; the combined blockade test has not yet been reported in humans.

C. Sequence of Tests for Lung Resection Surgery

With special reference to the performance of a pneumonectomy, there is a consensus that pulmonary function testing should proceed in three phases (Fig. 5-10).[33, 41, 50, 55-57] The first phase evaluates total lung (both, bilateral lung) function and consists of arterial blood gas measurements, simple spirometry, and lung volume determination. Increased risk is present when hypercapnia is found on a room air blood gas sample, the forced expired volume in 1 second (FEV_1) and/or the maximum breathing capacity (MBC) is less than 50 per cent of that predicted, and/or the residual volume–to–total lung capacity ratio (RV/TLC) is greater than 50 per cent. If any of these whole lung pulmonary function values are worse than these stated limits, testing should proceed to the second phase, which evaluates the function of each lung separately (single, unilateral lung function) and consists of measurement of the ventilation and perfusion of each individual lung (as a fraction of the total) by radioisotopic (^{133}Xe, ^{99}Te) scanning. Combining right-left fractional lung function tests with conventional spirometry should yield a predicted postoperative FEV_1 that is greater than 0.8 L.[33, 37-40, 44] If this second level criterion cannot be met and surgery is still contemplated or desired, the postoperative condition of the patient can be simulated (the third phase of testing; see also next section on pulmonary vascular function testing) by functionally resecting the vascular bed of the lung to be taken out by temporary balloon occlusion of the major pulmonary artery on that side, with and without exercise. An increase in mean pulmonary artery pressure above 40 mm Hg (or an increase in P_aCO_2 above 60 mm Hg, or a decrease in P_aO_2 below 45 mm Hg) indicates an inability to tolerate the removal of this amount of lung.[33, 41, 50-54] This pulmonary function test cascade is logical because it starts out with simple, inexpensive, and noninvasive tests and only increases the degree of difficulty, expense, and invasiveness as necessary; thus, in practice, the third phase of testing is rarely performed. In interpreting the results of this preoperative pulmonary function test cascade, physicians should always ask themselves what is an acceptable surgical mortality risk in a disease that has close to a 100 per cent natural history 5-year mortality rate.

Although less restrictive pulmonary function test criteria for operability for pulmonary resections less than pneumonectomy have been published (see Table 5-7),[58] there are several reasons why in some patients it may be prudent to think of a lobectomy (and lesser procedures) as a functional pneumonectomy.[59] First, in the

Preoperative Evaluation of Masses of the Lung and Bronchi
Step III: Respiratory Function

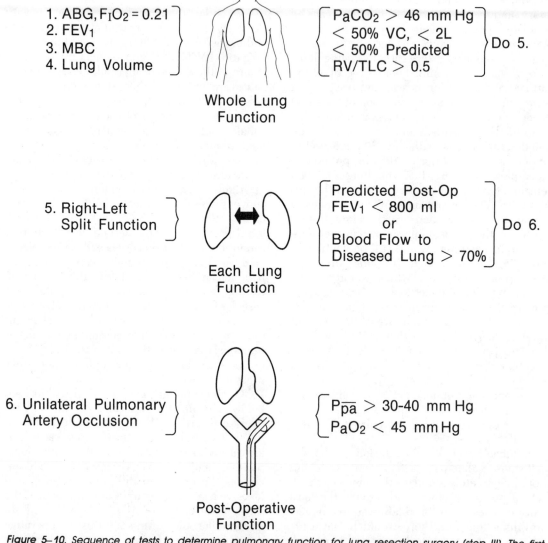

1. ABG, $F_IO_2 = 0.21$
2. FEV_1
3. MBC
4. Lung Volume

Whole Lung Function

$PaCO_2 > 46$ mm Hg
< 50% VC, < 2L
< 50% Predicted
RV/TLC > 0.5

Do 5.

5. Right-Left Split Function

Each Lung Function

Predicted Post-Op
FEV_1 < 800 ml
or
Blood Flow to
Diseased Lung > 70%

Do 6.

6. Unilateral Pulmonary Artery Occlusion

Post-Operative Function

$P\overline{pa} > 30-40$ mm Hg
$PaO_2 < 45$ mm Hg

Figure 5–10. Sequence of tests to determine pulmonary function for lung resection surgery (step III). The first group of tests determines whole lung function, the second test determines regional lung function, and the third test mimics postoperative lung function. See text for full explanation and definition of abbreviations.

immediate postoperative period, the function of the lung tissue remaining on the operative side may be significantly impaired by atelectasis and perhaps infection, and consequently, these patients may experience significant transient postoperative functional impairment.[60] Patients who are most likely to have a stormy postop-

erative course with minor resections are those in whom the surgeon had intraoperative exposure problems that required severe and prolonged lung handling, retraction, compression, and packing. Intraoperative exposure problems are more likely to occur when the lung under operation is large and moving (large tidal volume positive-pressure ventilation). Second, at the time of thoracotomy, more accurate staging of the disease is possible, and it may become apparent that it is necessary to do a pneumonectomy.[55] Third, the function of the lung on the nonoperated side may be impaired preoperatively[60] and may acutely deteriorate further intraoperatively (aspiration and/or spillage of blood and/or pus from the operated to the nonoperated lung, inability of the nonoperated lung to tolerate dependency and compression in the lateral decubitus position). Finally, postoperative studies have shown that although the ventilation and perfusion of the lung remaining on the operated side increases significantly during the long-term interval (3 to 51 months) after lobectomy, the volume of the remaining lung increases even more, so that the ventilation and perfusion per unit volume of the remaining lung decreases; this is equivalent to hyperinflation.[43] The compensatory hyperinflation represents dilatation of the pre-existing respiratory units without disruption or fragmentation of the elastic tissue as seen in pathologic emphysema; however, the pulmonary hyperinflation decreases the compliance and therefore the ventilation per unit volume of the ipsilateral remaining pulmonary tissue. In addition, the hyperinflated lung stretches and thins out the capillaries in the alveolar walls, which decreases the perfusion per unit volume of the remaining pulmonary tissue on the ipsilateral side.

d. PULMONARY VASCULAR AND RIGHT VENTRICULAR (RV) FUNCTION AND TESTING

The vast majority of patients with pulmonary tumors have had a long history of smoking, and consequently, they have varying degrees of chronic obstructive pulmonary disease (COPD). The cardiovascular response to the pathologic alveolar and airway changes in COPD consists of the development of pulmonary hypertension and increased pulmonary vascular resistance (PVR), followed by right ventricular (RV) hypertrophy and dilatation.

Increased pulmonary vascular resistance has very important implications for patients undergoing pulmonary resection. Whereas a normal pulmonary vasculature is distensible and capable of accommodating large increases in pulmonary blood flow (to approximately 2 to 2.5 times greater than normal, as would occur through the remaining lung following a pneumonectomy) with only minor increases in pulmonary artery pressure (Fig. 5–11), the rela-

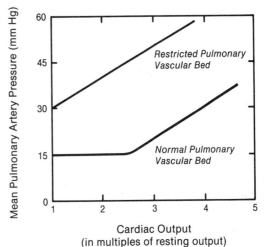

Figure 5–11. Mean pulmonary artery pressure (y-axis) does not increase until cardiac output (x-axis) has been increased to 2 to 2.5 times when the pulmonary vascular bed is normal, whereas mean pulmonary artery pressure increases linearly when cardiac output is increased when the pulmonary vascular bed is restricted.[61]

tively rigid and restricted pulmonary vascular bed of patients with chronic lung disease cannot accommodate even small increases in pulmonary blood flow without concomitant increases in pulmonary vascular pressure.[61] The inability to tolerate increases in blood flow occurs over the entire range of physiologic cardiac output and may be an important contributing factor to the development of postpneumonectomy pulmonary edema when it occurs.[62]

The preoperative pulmonary function testing cascade as outlined in phases one and two in the section Sequence of Tests for Lung Resection Surgery (which, in reality, is the extent to which the large majority of patients are studied preoperatively) does not allow for diagnosis of increased PVR and RV disease. Increased PVR may be noninvasively suspected preoperatively by the presence of the auscultatory and radiographic signs of pulmonary hypertension and by electrocardiographic evidence of right atrial and ventricular hypertrophy (Table 5–8). The development of a positive hepatojugular reflex, ascites, and peripheral edema indicates the onset of cor pulmonale.

Measurements of pulmonary vascular resistance (PVR) have been directly made by determining mean pulmonary artery and pulmonary wedge pressures at various levels of cardiac output produced by varying treadmill exercises. Thus, using the patient's own cardiac output, pulmonary vascular compliance can be deter-

Table 5–8. Noninvasive Diagnosis of Pulmonary Hypertension (↑ PAP),
Increased Pulmonary Vascular Resistance (↑ PVR),
Right Atrial and Ventricular Hypertrophy (↑ RA and ↑ RV), and Cor Pulmonale (CP)

Auscultatory Signs of ↑ PAP and ↑ PVR	Radiographic Signs of ↑ PAP and ↑ PVR	Electrocardiographic Signs of ↑ RA and ↑ RV	Additional Signs of CP
		↑ RV	
↑ Pulmonary component of second heart sound.	Dilation of main pulmonary artery.	Clockwise vector rotation	All of those of ↑ PAP, ↑ PVR, ↑ RA, ↑ RV
Loss of normally present split in second heart sound.	Fullness of apical pulmonary vessels.	Right axis deviation	Pulmonary diastolic murmur
Presence of fourth heart sound.	Counterclockwise cardiac rotation: Globular shape on P-A film (RV comprises left heart border, aortic knob).	↑ R and ↑ ing S wave V_2–V_6	Third heart sound
Appearance of high pitched early systolic ejection click.		Inverted T V_1–V_6	Prominent right sternal border pulsation plus retraction over left chest → rocking motion synchronous with heart beat.
		↑ RA	
		↓ ST segment V_2–V_6	
		↑ P II and III diphasic P V_1	Chronic dependent edema, large tender liver, ascites, distention neck veins, (large A waves).

mined. PVR measurements, made in this way, have been good indicators of risk for pneumonectomy.[63, 64] Operative risk was considered to be increased if pulmonary vascular resistance was greater than 190 dynes/sec/cm^{-5}. However, if the risk, expense, and time have been taken to insert a pulmonary artery catheter, then it is logical to take one further step and measure pulmonary vascular pressures during temporary unilateral pulmonary artery balloon occlusion in states of rest and exercise. This specifically tests the compliance of just the pulmonary vascular bed that will remain after pneumonectomy.

Temporary unilateral pulmonary artery balloon occlusion simulates the pulmonary vascular conditions to be expected after pneumonectomy. If significant pulmonary hypertension ($P_{\overline{pa}}$ > 40 mm Hg) or arterial hypoxemia ensues, pneumonectomy will likely not be tolerated because of the high risk of causing cor pulmonale, pulmonary edema, and low ventilation-perfusion relationships. Performing this procedure during exercise is the most realistic preoperative approximation of pulmonary vascular and right ventricular function that can be expected in the ambulatory postpneumonectomy patient.[41, 50–54]

e. LEFT VENTRICULAR AND CORONARY ARTERY FUNCTION AND TESTING

Considering the usual age, the long and heavy smoking history, and the frequently sedentary lifestyle of patients undergoing thoracic surgery, it is not surprising that coronary artery disease is by far the most likely independent cause of left ventricular (LV) dysfunction. If a history of angina is suggestive, then further preoperative evaluation of coronary artery function is necessary (Fig. 5–12). The first step should be noninvasive exercise testing. Electrocardiography and thallium scans (in that order) appear to be the best such exercise tests at this time. An exercise study provides information about the functional level of the patient. Unfortunately, the degre of exercise stress may be limited by low ventilatory reserve as well as by low cardiac reserve. If the exercise electrocardiogram is normal, then surgery should proceed; if the exercise electrocardiogram indicates ischemia, then a thallium exercise test is indicated.[65] If the thallium exercise test is negative, then the planned pulmonary resection should proceed. If the thallium exercise scan is positive for ischemia, then coronary angiography should be done.[66] However, if for any reason there is a strong suspicion that the patient is indeed having significant angina, even though exercise testing is negative or equivocal, coronary angiography is indicated. Consideration should always be given to coronary angiography in the patient with proven previous myocardial infarction, especially if the patient currently has angina.

If significant coronary artery disease is present, the patient needs coronary artery by-pass grafting before or at the time of pulmonary resection. For lesser degrees of coronary artery disease, pulmonary resection for carcinoma of the lung should be done after appropriate medical therapy for coronary insufficiency has been initiated. If the patient needs coronary artery by-pass grafting, and a limited resection can encompass the cancer, both procedures can be done under the same anesthetic, but the coronary artery by-pass grafting should be done

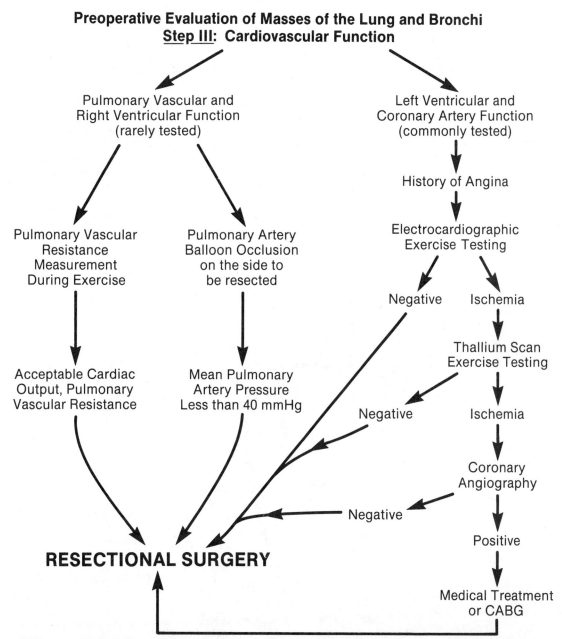

Preoperative Evaluation of Masses of the Lung and Bronchi
Step III: Cardiovascular Function

Figure 5–12. Preoperative evaluation logic to determine cardiovascular function in patients with lung and bronchial carcinoma (step III). (CABG = coronary artery bypass grafting.) See text for full explanation.

before pulmonary resection.[67, 68] After by-pass, if the patient is stable with good myocardial function and not bleeding, a pulmonary wedge resection can be done. For patients who require coronary artery by-pass grafting and have pulmonary lesions that require segmentectomy, lobectomy, or pneumonectomy, there is a good possibility that the prolonged nature of the pulmonary procedure will increase the operative mortality (and therefore should not be done), although a small number of successful combined procedures have been reported.[68, 69] In cases that require large resections in compromised patients, coronary artery by-pass grafting should be done first, and pulmonary resection should be delayed until the patient has gained weight and muscle mass (usually 4 to 6 weeks). The risk of general anesthesia for a noncardiac operation in the patient with previous coronary artery by-pass grafting is similar to that in patients without proven coronary artery disease.[70, 71] Although it is not possible to estimate the true effects of delay in pulmonary resection, in terms of tumor spread in a possibly immunocompromised patient (especially after general anesthesia[72]), it seems reasonable that in the latter group (those requiring by-pass grafting and major pulmonary resection) the operative risk of combined procedures probably exceeds the risk of tumor spread.

III. MEDIASTINAL MASSES

A. History

The anatomy of the mediastinum is complex and contains many structures (see chapter 2) and cell types (see Fig. 2–27). The most common tumors by location are as follows (Fig. 5–13): In the anterior mediastinum are thymoma, dermoid cysts, thyroid tumors, and lymphoma; in the middle mediastinum are pericardial cysts, bronchogenic cysts, and lymphomas; and in the posterior mediastinum are neurogenic tumors and cysts.[5] The most common tumors by cell type are neurogenic (24 per cent), cysts (pericardial bronchogenic, enteric,

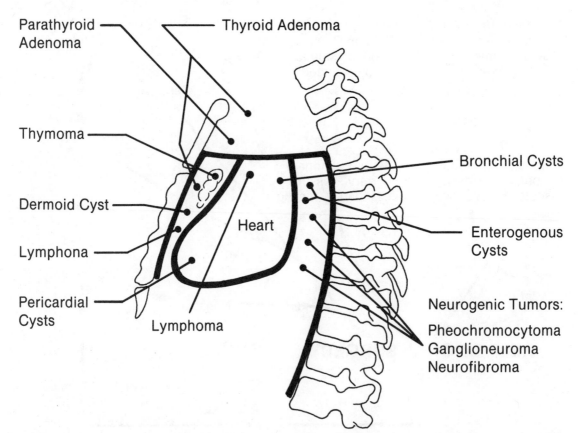

Figure 5–13. The location of commonly occurring mediastinal tumors. See Figure 2–27 for the division of the mediastinum into conventional compartments.

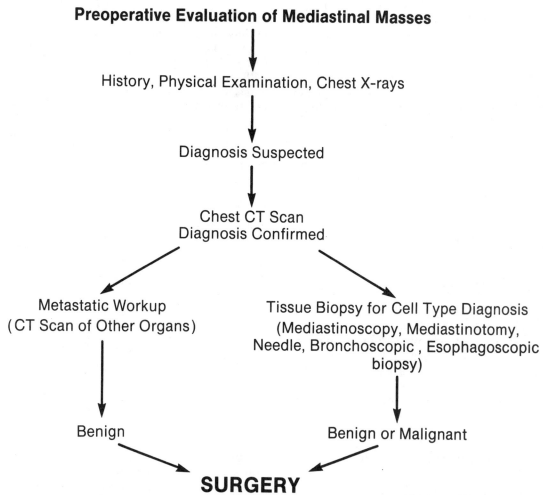

Preoperative Evaluation of Mediastinal Masses

History, Physical Examination, Chest X-rays

Diagnosis Suspected

Chest CT Scan
Diagnosis Confirmed

Metastatic Workup
(CT Scan of Other Organs)

Tissue Biopsy for Cell Type Diagnosis
(Mediastinoscopy, Mediastinotomy,
Needle, Bronchoscopic , Esophagoscopic
biopsy)

Benign

Benign or Malignant

SURGERY

Figure 5–14. *Preoperative evaluation logic of mediastinal masses. (CT = computed tomography.) See text for full explanation.*

and nonspecific, totaling 21 per cent), and teratodermoids, thymomas, lymphomas, and others (each 13–17 per cent). Signs and symptoms of mediastinal masses can be referable to any of several of the many organs within the mediastinum (heart, great vessels, the airway, esophagus, vertebral column). In one large series, the symptoms consisted of cough (40 per cent), pain (40 per cent), dyspnea (20 per cent), dysphagia (20 per cent), and hoarseness (3 per cent). The signs consisted of weight loss (24 per cent), fever (24 per cent), superior vena cava obstruction (16 per cent), tracheal deviation (12 per cent), Horner's syndrome (7 per cent), spinal cord compression (5 per cent), cyanosis (3 per cent), and mediastinal widening (3 per cent). Symptoms were absent in 22 per cent, signs were absent in 30 per cent, and both signs and symptoms were absent in 20 per cent.[73] Usually, mediastinal masses are suggested by a combination of clinical signs and symptoms and standard anteroposterior and lateral chest roentgenograms.

B. Diagnostic Work-up Logic for Mediastinal Masses

Once a mediastinal mass is suggested, computed tomography is the single best test to perform in a stable patient to identify the nature and the location of the mass (Fig. 5–14). Computed tomography can determine more accurately than other diagnostic procedures whether the mass is primarily vascular, fatty, cystic, or soft tissue in nature. For example, fluoroscopy, conventional tomography, barium esophagogram, radionuclide angiography and thyroid imaging, angiography, bronchoscopy, scalene node biopsy, and mediastinoscopy will all be normal in patients with mediastinal lipomatosis.[74, 75] Once a soft tissue mass is identified in the mediastinum, the next logical question is whether the process is benign or malignant. Approximately 32 per cent of mediastinal masses are malignant.[73] Unfortunately, computed tomography cannot distinguish benign from malignant masses based on any intrinsic appearance of the mass itself. However, computed tomography may demonstrate invasion of the pulmonary arteries, airway, pericardium, or myocardium or may demonstrate pleural or parenchymal metastases. In each of these instances, the malignant nature of the mediastinal mass is more apparent. More commonly, the diagnosis of benign versus malignant will depend on a diagnosis of cell type, and this must come from more invasive procedures such as mediastinoscopy, mediastinotomy, needle biopsy, bronchoscopy, or esophagoscopy. If the lesion may potentially involve the aorta or any of its branches, this is best demonstrated by intraarterial digital or conventional angiographic examinations.[76] The evaluation of acute traumatic injuries of the thorax is still best accomplished using conventional arteriography and angiography (especially if the diagnosis of dissection of the aorta or its major branches is suspected). The assessment of physiologic function of the patient with a mediastinal mass is similar to that for a patient with lung cancer.

IV. ESOPHAGEAL LESIONS

A. History[77]

The most common symptom of esophageal disease is difficulty in swallowing, which is termed dysphagia. The difficulty may be characterized as various degrees of obstruction and/or pain during swallowing. Dysphagia that has been present for any significant length of time is almost always accompanied by significant weight loss and is often accompanied by dehydration, prerenal failure, hypoalbuminemia, decreased plasma oncotic pressure, anemia, electrolyte abnormalities, and depressed immune mechanisms and muscle power (see section V of chapter 13). Heartburn is also a common sympton and is due to reflux of gastric contents into the esophagus. Heartburn is often a postprandial symptom brought on by recumbency, leaning forward, belching, and severe exercise. In addition, many patients with esophageal disease (those with a significant pouch proximal to an obstruction and those with hiatal hernia) are prone to chronic regurgitation and aspiration and may have chronic lung disease (see section V of chapter 13). Finally, patients with esophageal cancer are often treated with anticancer drugs that may cause considerable organ toxicity; doxorubicin (Adriamycin) can cause a very severe refractory left ventricular myopathy, bleomycin can cause respiratory failure, and mitomycin can cause both pulmonary and nephrotoxicity (see section V of chapter 13).

B. Diagnostic Work-up Logic for Esophageal Lesions[78]

There are numerous esophageal lesions and disorders. In order of decreasing frequency of occurrence, they are tumors (squamous cell carcinomas and adenocarcinomas are most common), hiatal hernia, benign strictures (ingestion of caustic fluids causes strictures in the cervical esophagus, whereas reflux esophagitis causes strictures in the lower third of the esophagus), foreign bodies, diverticula, achalasia, esophageal-respiratory tract fistula, traumatic perforations, and various motility disorders (such as scleroderma).

Following routine screening chest x-rays, a barium swallow (esophagogram) under cinefluoroscopy should be performed (Fig. 5–15). The only contraindication to obtaining an esophagogram is if a fistula to the trachea or bronchus is suspected. The barium swallow in a very high percentage of cases gives a strong indication of diagnosis. The esophagogram should be followed by esophagoscopy. Esophagoscopy should be performed with a flexible fiberoptic instrument in the majority of cases except when difficulty with obtaining an adequate biopsy specimen is encountered; in this situation a rigid esophagoscope may provide improved conditions for taking a biopsy. Rigid esophagoscopy should be avoided as the first diagnostic test whenever possible because of the risk of inadvertent perforation of an esophageal tumor. Rarely, following an esophago gram that shows that dysphagia is not due to any organic obstruction, manometric motility studies and pH studies are indicated. If the sequence of esophagogram and esophagoscopy has not made possible a diagnosis, a thoracotomy rarely will be required for diagnosis. If the diagnosis of carcinoma of the esophagus is being entertained, strong consideration should be given to examination of the mediastinum (mediastinoscopy or

Preoperative Evaluation of Esophageal Lesions

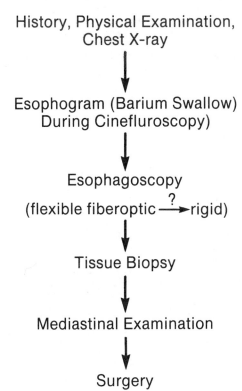

History, Physical Examination,
Chest X-ray

⬇

Esophogram (Barium Swallow)
During Cinefluroscopy)

⬇

Esophagoscopy
(flexible fiberoptic —?→ rigid)

⬇

Tissue Biopsy

⬇

Mediastinal Examination

⬇

Surgery

Figure 5–15. *Preoperative evaluation logic of esophageal lesions. See text for full explanation.*

computed tomographic scanning), since 80 per cent of esophageal tumors may involve the mediastinum by the time surgery is performed. The physiologic assessment of overall cardiorespiratory function of the patient requiring esophageal surgery is similar to that of a patient with lung cancer.

REFERENCES

1. Shields TW: Carcinoma of the lung. General Thoracic Surgery. Philadelphia, Lea & Febiger, 1983, chapter 54, pp 729–769.
2. Spiro SG: The diagnosis and staging of lung cancer. In Smyth JF (ed): The Management of Lung Cancer. Edward Arnold, Ltd., 1984, chapter 3, pp 36–52.
3. Le Roux BT: Bronchial Carcinoma. London, E. & F. Livingstone, Ltd., 1968.
4. Jones DP: Diagnostic work-up of chest disease. In symposium on noncardiac thoracic surgery. Surg Clin North Am 60:743–755, 1980.
5. Miller JI: Thoracic surgery. In Kaplan J (ed): Thoracic Anesthesia. New York, Churchill Livingstone, 1983, chapter 2, pp 9–32.
6. Holmes EC: Lung cancer. In Simmons DH (ed): Current Pulmonology. Vol. 1. Boston, Houghton Mifflin Co, 1979, chapter 8, pp 239–250.
7. Garland LH: The rate of growth and natural duration of primary bronchial cancer. Am J Roentgenol 96:604, 1966.
8. Rigler LG: The earliest roentgenographic signs of carcinoma of the lung. JAMA 195:655, 1966.
9. Byrd RB, Carr DT, Miller WE, et al: Radiographic abnormalities in carcinoma of the lung as related to histological cell type. Thorax 24:573, 1969.
10. Oswald NC, Hinson KF, Canti G, Miller AB: The diagnosis of primary lung cancer with special reference to sputum cytology. Thorax 26:623, 1971.
11. Spiro SG, Goldstraw P: The staging of lung cancer. Thorax 39:401–407, 1984.
12. Moore AV, Putnam CE: Radiologic diagnosis of chest disease. Symposium on noncardiac thoracic surgery. Surg Clin North Am 60:715–742, 1980.
13. Lillimoe K, Lipford E: Staging of bronchial carcinoma. Surg Gyn & Obst 158:566–568, 1984.
14. Lawrence GH: Current management of carcinoma of the lung. J Thorac Cardiovasc Surg 88:858–862, 1984.
15. Tisi GH, Friedman PJ, Peters RN, et al: Clinical staging of primary lung cancer. Am Rev Resp Dis 127:1–6, 1983.
16. Newell JD: Evaluation of pulmonary and mediastinal masses. Symposium on radiology. Med Clin North Am 68:1463–1480, 1984.
17. Mountain CF, Carr DT, Anderson WAD: A system for the clinical staging of lung cancer. Am J Roentgenol Rad Ther Nuc Med 120:130, 1974.
18. Mountain CF: The biological operability of Stage III non-small cell lung carcinoma. Ann Thorac Surg 40:60–64, 1985.
19. Miller JI, Mansour KA, Hatcher CR: Carcinoma of the lung: 5-year experience in a university hospital. Am Surg 46:147–150, 1980.
20. Sarin CL, Nohl-Oser HC: Mediastinoscopy: A clinical evaluation of 400 consecutive cases. Thorax 24:585, 1969.
21. Emami B, Melo A, Carter BL, Munzenrider JE, Piro AJ: Value of computed tomography in radiotherapy of lung cancer. Am J Roentgenol 131:63, 1978.
22. Harper PG, Houang N, Spiro SG, Geddes DM, Hodson ME, Souhami RL: Computerized axial tomography in the pre-treatment assessment of small cell carcinoma of the bronchus. Cancer 47:1775, 1981.
23. Schaner EG, Chang AE, Doppman JL, Conkie DM, Flye MW, Rosenberg SA: Comparison of computed and conventional whole lung tomography in detecting pulmonary nodules: A prospective radiologic pathologic study. Am J Roentgenol 131:37, 1978.
24. The American Thoracic Society. Clinical staging of primary lung cancer. Am Rev Resp Dis 127:659–664, 1983.
25. Richey HM, Matthews JI, Helsel RA, Cable H: Thoracic CT scanning in the staging of bronchogenic carcinoma. Chest 85:218–221, 1984.
26. Underwood GH, Hooper RG, Axelbaum SP, Goodwin BW: Computed tomography scanning of the thorax in the staging of bronchogenic carcinoma. N Engl J Med 300:777, 1979.
27. Whitcomb ME, Barham E, Goldman AL, Green VC: Indications for pneumonectomy in bronchogenic carcinoma. Am Rev Resp Dis 113:189, 1976.
28. Shields TW, Higgins GA, Matthews NJ, Keehn RJ: Surgical resection in the management of small cell

carcinoma of the lung. J Thorac Cardiovasc Surg 84:481–488, 1982.

29. Meyer JA, Comis RL, Ginsberg SJ, et al: Phase II trial of expended indications for resection in small cell carcinoma of the lung. J Thorax Cardiovasc Surg 83:12, 1982.

30. Miller JI, Grossman G, Hatcher CR: Pulmonary function test criteria for operability and pulmonary resection. Surg Gynecol Obstet 153:893–895, 1981.

31. Benfield JR, Yellin A: New Horizons for lung cancer. Surg Rounds April:26–52, 1985.

32. Benumof JL, Alfery DD: Pulmonary Function Testing. In Miller R (ed): Anesthesia. New York, Churchill Livingstone, 1981, chapter 42, pp 1363–1378.

33. Gass GD, Olsen GN: Clinical significance of pulmonary function tests. Preoperative pulmonary function testing to predict postoperative morbidity and mortality. Chest 89:127–135, 1986.

34. McFadden ER, Linden DA: A reduction in maximum midexpiratory flow rate, a thorough graphic manifestation of small airway disease. Am J Med 57:171, 1974.

35. Berggren H, Ekroth R, Malmberg R, Naucler J, William-Olsson G: Hospital mortality and long-term survival in relation to preoperative function in elderly patients with bronchogenic carcinoma. Ann Thorac Surg 38:633–636, 1984.

36. Sorensen PG, Groth F, Hansen SW, Hansen F, Dirksen H: Patterns of perfusion and ventilation of the lungs in patients with small cell lung cancer before and after combination chemotherapy. Clin Physiol 5(Suppl. 3):99–104, 1985.

37. DeMeester TR, Van Heertum RL, Karas JR, et al: Preoperative evaluation with differential pulmonary function. Ann Thorac Surg 18:61–71, 1974.

38. Boysen PG, Block AJ, Olsen GN, et al: Prospective evaluation for pneumonectomy using the ^{99}Technetium quantitative perfusion lung scan. Chest 72:422–425, 1977.

39. Boysen PG, Harris JO, Block AJ, et al: Prospective evaluation for pneumonectomy using perfusion scanning. Chest 80:163–166, 1981.

40. Kristersson S, Lindel SE, Svanberg L: Prediction of pulmonary function loss due to pneumonectomy using ^{133}Xe-radiospirometry. Chest 62:694, 1972.

41. Olsen GE, Block AJ, Swenson EW, et al: Pulmonary function evaluation of the lung resection candidate: A prospective study. Am Rev Resp Dis 111:379–387, 1975.

42. Ali MK, Mountain C, Miller JM, Johnston DA, Shullenberger CC: Regional pulmonary function before and after pneumonectomy using ^{133}Xe. Chest 68:288, 1975.

43. Ali MK, Mountain CF, Ewer MS, et al: Predicting loss of pulmonary function after pulmonary resection for bronchogenic carcinoma. Chest 77:337–342, 1980.

44. Olsen GN, Block AJ, Tobias JA: Prediction of postpneumonectomy function using quantitative macroaggregate lung scanning. Chest 66:13–16, 1974.

45. Hazlett DR, Watson RL: Lateral position test: A simple, inexpensive, yet accurate method of studying the separate functions of the lungs. Chest 59:276–279, 1970.

46. Marion JM, Alderson PO, Lefrak SS, Siniorr RM, Jacobs MH: Unilateral lung function: Comparison of the lateral position test with radionuclide ventilation-perfusion studies. Chest 69:5–9, 1976.

47. Walkup RH, Vossel LF, Griffin JP, Proctor RJ: Prediction of postoperative pulmonary function with the lateral position test. Chest 77:224–226, 1980.

48. Schoonover JA, Olsen GN, McLain WC, Habibian MR, Edwards DG, Spurrier T: Lateral position test and quantitative lung scan in the preoperative evaluation for lung resection. Chest 86:854–859, 1984.

49. Pierce RJ, Pretto JJ, Rochford, PD, et al: Lobar occlusion in the preoperative assessment of patients with lung cancer. Br J Dis Chest 80:27–36, 1986.

50. Tisi GM: Preoperative evaluation of pulmonary function. Am. Rev Respir Dis 119:293–310, 1979.

51. Uggla LG: Indications for and results of thoracic surgery with regard to respiratory and circulatory function tests. Acta Chir Scand 111:197–212, 1956.

52. Laros CD, Swierengo J: Temporary unilateral pulmonary artery occlusion in the preoperative evaluation of patients with bronchial carcinoma. Med Thorac 24:269, 1967.

53. Sloan H, Morris JD, Figley M, Lee R: Temporary unilateral occlusion of the pulmonary artery in the preoperative evaluation of thoracic patients. J Thorac Surg 30:591, 1955.

54. Soderholm B: The hemodynamics of the lesser circulation in pulmonary tuberculosis. Effect of exercise, temporary unilateral pulmonary artery occlusion and operation. Scand J Clin Lab Invest Suppl. 26, 1957.

55. Brindley GV Jr, Walsh RE, Schnarr WT, et al: Pulmonary resection in patients with impaired pulmonary function. Surg Clin North Am 62:199–214, 1982.

56. Harman E, Lillington G: Pulmonary risk factors in surgery. Med Clin North Am 63:1289–1298, 1979.

57. Block AJ, Olsen GN. Preoperative pulmonary function testing. JAMA 235:257–258, 1976.

58. Miller JI, Grossman GD, Hatcher CR. Pulmonary function test criteria for operability and pulmonary resection. Surg Gyn Obstet 153:893–895, 1981.

59. Boysen PG: Pulmonary resection and postoperative pulmonary function. Chest 77:718–719, 1980.

60. Boysen PG, Block AG, Moulder PV: Relationship between preoperative pulmonary function tests and complications after thoracotomy. Surg Gyn Obstet 152:813–815, 1981.

61. Robin ED, Gaudio R: Cor Pulmonale. Disease-A-Month May:138, 1970.

62. Zeldin RA, Normandin D, Landtwing D, et al: Postpneumonectomy pulmonary edema. J Thorac Cardiovasc Surg 87:359–365, 1984.

63. Fee HJ, Holmes EC, Gewirltz HS, et al: Role of pulmonary vascular resistance measurements in preoperative evaluation of candidates for pulmonary resection. J Thorac Cardiovasc Surg 75:519, 1978.

64. Pecora DV, Hohenberger M: Effects of postpneumonectomy distention on pulmonary compliance and vascular resistance. Am Surg 45:797–801, 1979.

65. Peters RM, Swain JA: Management of the patient with emphysema, coronary artery disease and lung cancer. Am J Surg 143:701–705, 1982.

66. Chaitman BR, Bourassa MG, Davis K, et al: Angiographic prevalence of high risk coronary artery disease in patient subsets (CASS). Circulation 64:360–367, 1981.

67. Peters RM: The role of limited resection in carcinoma of the lung. Am J Surg 143:706–710, 1982.

68. Piehler JM, Trastek VF, Pairolero PC, et al: Concomitant cardiac and pulmonary operations. J Thorac Cardiovasc Surg 90:662–667, 1985.

69. Dalton ML Jr, Parker TM, Mistrot J, et al: Concomitant coronary artery bypass and major noncardiac surgery. J Thorac Cardiovasc Surg 85:621–631, 1978.

70. Crawford ES, Morris GC Jr, Howell JF, et al: Operative risk in patients with previous coronary artery bypass. Ann Thorac Surg 26:215–221, 1978.

71. McCollum CJ, Garcia-Rinaldi R, Graham JM, et al: Myocardial revascularization prior to subsequent major surgery in patients with coronary artery disease. Surgery 81:302–304, 1977.

72. Shapiro J, Jersky J, Katzav S, et al: Anesthetic drugs accelerate the progression of postoperative metastases of mouse tumors. J Clin Invest 68:678–685, 1981.

73. Adkins RB Jr, Maples MD, Hainsworth JD: Primary malignant mediastinal tumors. Ann Thorac Surg 38:648–659, 1984.

74. Newell JD: Evaluation of pulmonary and mediastinal masses. Med Clin North Am 68:1463–1480, 1984.

75. Homer MJ, Wechsler RJ, Carter BL: Mediastinal lipomatosis: CT confirmation of a normal variant. Radiology 128:657–661, 1978.

76. Heitzman ER: Computed tomography of the thorax: Current perspectives. Am J Roentgenol 136:2–12, 1981.

77. Hardy JD: Diseases of the esophagus: An overview. In Hardy JD (ed): Textbook of Surgery. Philadelphia, JB Lippincott Co, chapter 37, 1977.

78. Hardy JD, Conn JH: Disease of the esophagus: An analysis of 308 consecutive cases. Ann Surg 155:971, 1962.

79. Gatzinsky P, Berglin E, Dernevik L, et al: Resectional operations and long-term results in carcinoma of the esophagus. J Thorac Cardiovasc Surg 89:71–76, 1985.

Preoperative Respiratory Preparation

6

I. INTRODUCTION

Thoracic surgical patients are at high risk for the development of postoperative pulmonary complications. In most of the literature, "postoperative complications" refers to the development of atelectasis and/or pneumonia.[1] The incidence of pneumonia usually parallels the incidence of atelectasis, and the onset of pneumonia lags behind the onset of atelectasis because atelectasis provides the ventilatory and mucociliary stasis condition necessary for the development and culture of pneumonia.[2, 3]

There are three major reasons why thoracic surgery promotes postoperative pulmonary complications; these reasons originate in the preoperative, intraoperative, and postoperative period (Fig. 6–1). First, the incidence of postoperative respiratory complications following any surgery is positively correlated with the degree of preoperative respiratory dysfunction, and most thoracic surgical patients come to surgery with some degree of preoperative lung dysfunction. Preoperative pulmonary function testing will identify the patients at high risk due to poor preoperative lung function. Second, the performance of thoracic surgery can impair lung function in any patient. During surgery, nondependent lung function may be impaired by resection of functional lung and/or by trauma to the remaining nondependent lung (due to various nondependent lung manipulations), and dependent lung function may be impaired due to the development of atelectasis and edema

formation. Third, thoracotomy incisions are painful and cause patients to resist deep breathing and coughing in the postoperative period, leading to retained secretions, atelectasis, and pneumonia. The second factor (impaired lung function due to the performance of thoracic surgery) can be minimized by appropriate intraoperative management (such as one-lung ventilation, positive end-expiratory pressure, continuous positive airway pressure) (see chapter 8). The third factor can be minimized by appropriate postoperative pain management (e.g., epidural narcotics) (see chapter 20). The impact of the first factor (presence of preoperative respiratory dysfunction) can be significantly reduced by preoperative prophylactic respiratory preparation measures.

This chapter first documents the correlation between degree of pre-existing respiratory disease and incidence of postoperative respiratory complications. Next, the correlation between thoracic surgery and the increased incidence of postoperative respiratory complications will be discussed. Proof is then offered that preoperative respiratory preparation decreases the incidence of postoperative respiratory complications, and the main body of the chapter details a full preoperative respiratory preparation regimen. The mechanism by which preoperative respiratory preparation decreases the incidence of postoperative repiratory complications is considered. Finally, premedication, as part of a preoperative respiratory preparation plan, is discussed.

Thoracic Surgery Impairs Postoperative Lung Function

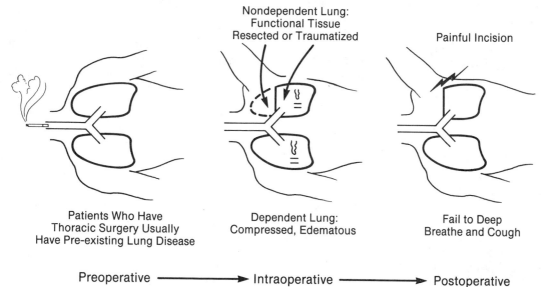

Figure 6–1. There are preoperative, intraoperative, and postoperative reasons why thoracic surgery impairs postoperative lung function.

II. CORRELATION OF RESPIRATORY COMPLICATIONS WITH DEGREE OF PRE-EXISTING LUNG DISEASE

The relationship between lack of preoperative pulmonary reserve and postoperative respiratory morbidity and mortality is very well recognized and may be very dramatic. Compared with nonsmokers, smokers have a sixfold increase in the incidence of postoperative pulmonary complications after major operative procedures.[4, 5] Three major mechanisms appear to be responsible for the adverse smoking/surgery interaction, and they are small airway disease (spasm, collapse), hypersecretion of mucus, and impairment of tracheobronchial tree clearance. In patients with chronic lung disease, compared with normal healthy patients, there is a 20-fold increase in the incidence of postoperative pulmonary complications.[6] Thus, it is not surprising to find widespread agreement that the risk of postoperative pulmonary complications progressively increases as preoperative pulmonary function progressively decreases.

Preoperative pulmonary function is best quantitated by preoperative pulmonary function tests, and patients with a vital capacity, maximum breathing capacity, FEV_1 or $FEF_{25-75}\%$ of less than 50 per cent of predicted capacity and/or grossly hypercapnic patients are at very high risk (see chapter 5 references and reference 7 for extensive substantiation of this contention). However, even if pulmonary function tests are not available, it should be remembered that gross observations such as the production of a great deal of sputum by the patient (more than 2 ounces per day),[8] minimal exercise tolerance capability, severe cardiac disease, obesity, sepsis, and very advanced age also indicate great risk for developing postoperative pulmonary complications.[7, 9]

III. CORRELATION OF RESPIRATORY COMPLICATIONS WITH SITE OF OPERATION

The correlation between postoperative pulmonary complications in both patients with and without respiratory disease and the site and type of operation has long been known, with the highest incidence of complications following major thoracic and upper abdominal procedures.[7-11] In a series of 1500 surgical patients with a wide variety of respiratory diseases treated over a 30-year period, the incidence of respiratory complications averaged 63 per cent following thoracic and gastric operations, 15 to 19 per cent following mid-abdominal operations, and 9 per cent following lower abdominal procedures.[12] In a group of 464 patients with chronic respiratory disease who did not have any preoperative respiratory preparation, the highest risk of pulmonary complications involved patients with thoracotomy or abdominal operations (compared with surgery on other parts of the body).[13] Even when the patient population was specifically defined as those with chronic obstructive pulmonary disease who underwent preoperative respiratory preparation, the incidence of respiratory complications was still highest for thoracic and abdominal operations compared with surgery on other parts of the body.[8] Similarly, other patients with severe chronic obstructive pulmonary disease who had operations on the thorax or upper abdomen were found to have twice the mortality compared with those with a similar amount of respiratory impairment and who were subjected to operations on other body regions.[14] The mechanisms by which thoracic surgery (and abdominal surgery) especially predisposes patients to postoperative respiratory complications include resection of, or trauma to, functional lung, and the degree to which the bellows function of the lung is affected (Fig. 6–1). It is painful for patients who have incisions in these areas to deep breathe and to stretch either the chest or abdominal wall (i.e., the incision); consequently, they fail to cough (which requires a deep breath), and they retain secretions (which promotes the development of atelectasis and infection).

IV. PROOF THAT PREOPERATIVE PULMONARY PREPARATION DECREASES INCIDENCE OF POSTOPERATIVE RESPIRATORY COMPLICATIONS

Considerable evidence has accumulated over the last three decades to demonstrate that vigorous preoperative pulmonary preparation can significantly reduce postoperative pulmonary complications. Several decades ago, it was demonstrated that simple preoperative physical therapy instruction, as opposed to the same instruction given postoperatively or not at all, decreased the incidence of atelectasis from 42 per cent (no instruction), to 27 per cent (postoperative instruction), to 12 per cent (preoperative instruction).[15] About the same time, it was demonstrated that the use of nebulized isoproterenol three times daily before and after surgery, in conjunction with postural drainage and chest physiotherapy, reduced the incidence of postoperative atelectasis from 43 to 9 per cent.[16]

Patients with chronic obstructive pulmonary disease are the ones most likely to benefit from preoperative respiratory preparation. In 1959 it was impressively shown in a group of 250 surgical patients with obstructive pulmonary disease that when an intensive pulmonary preparation was utilized, consisting of oral therapy with a bronchodilator drug, IPPV with nebulized bronchodilator therapy, use of an expectorant, postural drainage, cough training, and antibiotic treatment for purulent sputum, only two patients (1 per cent) developed atelectasis.[17] In 1970 randomly selected "poor risk" patients were treated preoperatively and postoperatively with a very comprehensive respiratory care regimen (bronchodilators, antibiotics, inhalation of humidified gas, segmental postural drainage, and chest physical therapy). When the treated patients were compared with the nontreated patients, the treated patients had a pulmonary complication rate of only 22 per cent (all mild), whereas the untreated patients had a pulmonary complication rate of 60 per cent (of which 60 per cent were severe).[18] Similarly, in a retrospective study of patients with chronic obstructive pulmonary disease who underwent various surgical procedures under inhalation anesthesia, the incidence of postoperative respiratory complications was only 24 per cent in those given preoperative pulmonary preparation compared with 43 per cent in a control nonprepared group.[13]

Since preoperative pulmonary preparation can significantly reduce postoperative pulmonary complications, especially in patients with lung disease, it is not surprising to find that a high risk group of patients with moderate to severe respiratory dysfunction who required thoracic surgery also greatly benefited from preoperative pulmonary preparation.[19] This high risk group was managed with vigorous prophylactic measures and suffered less pulmonary complications than did a more normal respiratory function group that had not been exposed to the same preoperative regimen. Similarly, in another study the differences in pulmonary complication rate were insignificant between untreated young "good risk" and treated "poor risk" patients.[18] Thus, the frequency and severity of pulmonary complications may not increase in going from nontreated young "good risk" patients to treated "poor risk" patients (implying that the preoperative treatments corrected, at least in part, the preoperative respiratory dysfunction), but the respiratory complication rate definitely increases in going from treated "poor risk" patients to untreated "poor risk" patients.[13, 17-19]

More recently (1979), a very careful, meticulous prospective report has described the effect of a standardized preoperative pulmonary regimen on preoperative pulmonary function tests in a series of 157 patients with chronic obstructive pulmonary disease.[8] The pulmonary regimen consisted of 48 to 72 hours of aerosolized isoproterenol in saline given four times a day, oral therapy with theophylline, guaiacol glyceryl ether, hydration, and chest physiotherapy. In addition, most of the patients discontinued smoking. The preoperative respiratory preparation regimen improved preoperative pulmonary function tests but not in a predictable or consistent way. The rate of complications was highest in those patients who had upper or long abdominal incisions or thoracotomy, although the incidence of respiratory complications was significantly reduced as a result of the preoperative preparation. The authors were unable to determine which patients would develop significant pulmonary complications not requiring mechanical ventilation, but those requiring respiratory support were predictable on the basis of the severity of their pulmonary functional impairment and minimal response to the pulmonary preparation used (i.e., those who had irreversible disease).

V. THE PREOPERATIVE RESPIRATORY PREPARATION MANEUVERS

The preceding data indicate that patients undergoing thoracic surgery are particularly susceptible to postoperative respiratory complications[4-14] and that prophylactic measures do decrease postoperative respiratory complications.[8, 14-19] Consequently, preoperative evaluation should be followed by preoperative preparation efforts directed toward optimally managing any pre-existing pulmonary disease.[20] In general, a full preoperative respiratory preparation regimen involves a five-pronged attack on airway disease. The five elements of the preoperative regimen are stopping smoking, dilating airways, loosening and removing secretions, and taking measures to increase motivation and education and to facilitate postoperative care (Table 6-1 and Fig. 6-2).

The five treatment modalities are instituted and proceed in parallel fashion. Before discussing each element separately, it is important to

Table 6-1. Preoperative Respiratory Care Regimen

1. Stop smoking
2. Dilate the airways
   a. Beta$_2$ agonists
   b. Theophylline
   c. Steroids
   d. Cromolyn sodium
3. Loosen the secretions
   a. Airway hydration (humidifier/nebulizer)
   b. Systemic hydration
   c. ? Mucolytic and expectorant drugs
   d. Antibiotics
4. Remove the secretions
   a. Postural drainage
   b. Coughing
   c. Chest physiotherapy (percussion and vibration)
5. Increased education, motivation, and facilitation of postoperative care
   a. Psychologic preparation
   b. Incentive spirometry
   c. Exposure to secretion removal maneuvers
   d. Exercise
   e. Weight loss/gain
   f. Stabilize other medical problems

point out that the desirable results of these maneuvers should be, for the purpose of understanding their interaction, achieved in a sequential manner (Fig. 6-2). The logic behind this concept is as follows. First, stopping smoking eliminates the stimulation for the production of airway secretions and bronchoconstriction. Next, the airways should be dilated to facilitate secretion removal. Similarly, thick, tenacious, and adherent secretions must be loosened in order to be removed. Once the airways are dilated and the secretions loosened, it makes sense to use physical maneuvers to remove the secretions. Finally, the patients should assist, as much as possible, in their preoperative preparation and postoperative respiratory care. The studies cited below indicate that using the maneuvers in this sequence (dilating the airways, loosening the secretions, removing the secretions) allows the maneuvers to complement one another in improving mucociliary transport function. The following section discusses each of these five preoperative preparation maneuvers in the order and context of the above conceptual approach. Of course, it is recognized that patients who do not have bronchospasm will not benefit from bronchodilator treatment and that patients who do not have secretions will not benefit from measures to enhance secretion removal.[21]

Preoperative Respiratory Preparation Regimen

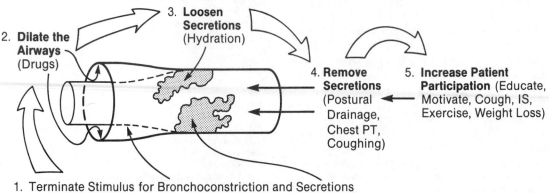

Figure 6–2. A full, aggressive, preoperative respiratory preparation regimen consists of a five-pronged attack: (1) require the patient to stop smoking, (2) dilate the airways, (3) loosen secretions, (4) remove secretions, and (5) increase patient participation. Using these five maneuvers in the numbered sequence allows them to complement one another in improving secretion removal.

A. Discontinue Smoking

An improvement in mucociliary transport and small airway function and a decrease in airway secretions and reactivity occur over several weeks following cessation of smoking.[22, 23] Consequently, preoperative cessation of smoking for greater than 4 to 8 weeks is associated with a decrease in the incidence of postoperative respiratory complications.[22, 23] Although stopping smoking for only 24 hours will do nothing to decrease the amount of secretions (at least 1 to 2 weeks are required),[23, 24] airway irritability, and incidence of postoperative respiratory complications, there are still a number of important benefits that accrue in the first 1 to 2 days of abstinence.[22–24] Cessation of smoking for as short a time as 12 to 48 hours has been shown to decrease carboxyhemoglobin levels significantly (increase hemoglobin available for oxygen transport), to shift the oxyhemoglobin dissociation curve to the right (increase the availability of O_2 to the tissues),[25] and to reduce nicotine-induced tachycardia,[23–24] and cessation of smoking for a few days may greatly improve ciliary beating.[23, 24] All these very acute effects may confer a critical benefit to the marginal patient. Indeed, the association between cigarettes with a high yield of carbon monoxide and an increase of symptoms of ischemia in susceptible people, both at rest and during exercise, underscores the importance of these effects.[24]

There are a few select patients in whom the risks of stopping smoking for a day or two may outweigh the benefits. First, although stopping smoking will cause some anxiety in many patients, cessation of smoking may induce a great deal of anxiety in some patients (due in part to acute nicotine withdrawal in nicotine-addicted patients).[26] In patients with significant coronary artery disease the large increase in anxiety preoperatively may lead to a critical ischemic event. Second, sudden cessation in smoking can occasionally induce a hypersecretory and bronchospastic state. In patients who have difficulty with secretions, a preoperative increase in secretions may lead to airways that are more obstructed preoperatively.[22] Third, there are some experimental data to indicate that continued smoking may result in a decreased incidence of postoperative deep vein thrombosis.[23, 24] Nevertheless, a good argument can be made that these potential benefits of continuing smoking during the day or two prior to surgery can just as easily be accomplished with anxiolytics, bronchodilators, and anticoagulants. Thus, the potential benefits do not provide sufficient reason to continue smoking.

B. Dilating the Airways

The next step should be to dilate the airways. Beta$_2$ sympathomimetic drugs, such as albuterol, terbutaline, and metaproterenol, are administered to patients who have a demonstrable reversible bronchospastic airway component to their respiratory disease.[27, 28] The sympathomimetics (so-called "first messengers") are believed to act on their target cells in the lungs by increasing the activity of adenyl cyclase, an enzyme in the cell membrane that catalyzes the formation of cyclic adenosine 3', 5'-monophosphate (c'AMP) from adenosine triphosphate (ATP). c'AMP acts as a "second messenger" in the cell, where it acts upon smooth muscle to decrease tension and motility. In addition, adrenergic compounds (epinephrine, ephedrine, isopropyl, norepinephrine) can also increase ciliary activity, which may help in removing secretions.[29, 30]

c'AMP is broken down by a cytoplasmic enzyme, phosphodiesterase, whose activity can be inhibited by methylxanthines, such as theophylline and aminophylline. Thus, the methylxanthines also increase c'AMP but by a mechanism different from that of the beta$_2$ agonists. Because the methylxanthines and beta$_2$ agonists act by different mechanisms, theophylline is often added to patients with bronchospasm already receiving beta adrenergics, and thus they work in synergy to increase intracellular concentrations of c'AMP.[31, 32] In addition, aminophylline improves diaphragmatic contractility and renders it less susceptible to fatigue.[33] Recently, however, there has been considerable concern regarding the short-term toxicity of inhaled beta-adrenergic agents when used in the presence of methylxanthines; specifically, myocardial ischemia might occur as a result of the drugs' combined effect on the heart with resultant (and possibly fatal) ventricular arrhythmias.[34, 35] Thus, appropriate caution should be exercised when combining inhaled beta$_2$ agonists with methylxanthines.[36] Optimal therapeutic levels of theophylline can be assured and toxicity avoided if an intravenous loading dose (5 to 7 mg/kg) is given, followed by continuous infusion (0.2 to 0.8 mg/kg/hr; dose decreases with increasing age) and measuring of serum levels.[39] Although the patient's subjective feeling of relief is an important endpoint (see chapter 5), the effect of bronchodilator drug treatment should be quantitated by pulmonary function tests.

Cromolyn sodium, a drug that inhibits the release of bronchoconstricting mediators, is of value in the chronic treatment of severe asthmatics; it has no value in the treatment of acute asthma. In addition, it is of little help in most patients with chronic obstructive pulmonary disease, although it may be useful if a patient has a history suggestive of atopy. Adrenocorticosteroids may also be given, orally, parenterally, or by aerosol, to the subgroup of patients with chronic obstructive pulmonary disease having especially reactive airways.[38] Steroids are not considered to be bronchodilators but probably act by decreasing mucosal edema and preventing the release of bronchoconstricting substances.

C. Loosening the Secretions

The next step should be to thin and to loosen thick adherent secretions. The most efficacious method is hydration. When tracheal mucus transport velocity is quantitatively measured by radioactive tracer methods, it can clearly be shown that dehydration decreases and rehydration increases, respectively, tracheal transport velocity.[39] The most common method of hydrating secretions is by use of a jet humidifier or ultrasonic nebulizer to produce a heated, sterile water aerosol that is delivered by a close-fitting mask for 20 minutes to a deeply spontaneously breathing patient. Concurrently, continuous systemic hydration must be assured per os or intravenously.

Very occasionally, administration of mucolytic agents (such as acetylcysteine [Mucomyst]) by a nebulizer and/or oral expectorants (such as guaifenesin, potassium iodide, iodinated glycerol) may be of limited benefit in patients with very viscous secretions, but both of these treatments (mucolytic agents, oral expectorants) have side effects that would obviate their use in most patients. The benefit of mucolytic agents is that they decrease the viscosity of secretions (by depolymerizing mucopolysaccharides),[40] but at the same time they may induce irritability of the airways and bronchospasm. The benefit of oral expectorants is that they increase the amount of secretions removed, but at the same time they increase the absolute amount of secretions (and may cause gastrointestinal upset and skin lesions).[26, 40]

Pulmonary infection, if present, is treated according to the results of culture and sensitivity tests; broad spectrum antibiotics such as ampicillin or a cephalosporin frequently have the required specificity and potency. If the antibiotic treatment clears the infection to any extent, it may also decrease the tenacity, viscosity, and volume of secretions.

D. Removing the Secretions

The next preoperative respiratory preparation step is the actual removal of secretions, and this is accomplished by a combination of postural drainage (several different positions may be required), coughing, and chest percussion and vibration (common methods include tapping with cupped hands and electric vibrators) for a period of 15 to 20 minutes several times a day.[26, 41, 42] Consequently, therapy to remove secretions utilizes gravity, patient-generated expiratory airflow, and mechanical measures to dislodge and to propel the secretions proximally.

When removal of tracheobronchial secretions is quantitatively measured with radioactive tracer methods in patients with chronic obstructive lung disease, chest physiotherapy (chest percussion and vibration along with postural drainage) with cough is effective in increasing both central and peripheral airway clearance and sputum yield, whereas cough alone is effective in increasing only central airway clearance and sputum yield.[43] Thus, chest physiotherapy moves peripheral bronchial secretions to more central airways for expectoration by coughing. The reason cough alone cannot clear peripheral airways is that an effective cough must attain a high enough airflow rate so as to shear secretions away from the airway wall. In patients with chronic lung disease, flow rates are low (especially peripherally), and the shearing of secretions by cough may well be limited to the trachea and perhaps the first two airway generations.[44] Obviously, with either chest physiotherapy or cough it will be much easier to expel the secretions if the airways have already been dilated and the secretions loosened.

Chest physical therapy is relatively contraindicated in patients with lung abscesses, bone metastases, and a history of significant hemoptysis and inability to tolerate the postural drainage positions. It is generally agreed that intermittent positive-pressure breathing regimens do not have sufficient efficacy to warrant the excessive cost ($60 per treatment) of routine use.[45–48]

E. Measures to Increase Motivation and Education and to Facilitate Postoperative Respiratory Care

The last step consists of general measures designed to increase motivation and education and to facilitate postoperative respiratory care. Preoperative psychologic preparation (i.e., positive suggestion and encouragement), including orientation to the intensive care environment, can reduce fear and improve patient outlook and cooperation. Still, patients should be given realistic expectations about postoperative pain and how it will be handled. With this type of positive but realistic approach, patients will have a diminished postoperative narcotic analgesic requirement and a shorter period of hospitalization.[50]

Preoperative patient education in the procedures that will be used for respiratory care postoperatively and explaining why these procedures are going to be used will greatly help to assure optimal postoperative compliance with and performance of the respiratory care maneuvers. There is no question that a critical factor in treating patients is to preserve and to enhance an individual's ability to do things for him- or herself.[51] In this regard, preoperative practice with an incentive spirometer prepares the patient to participate in restoring lung volume and coughing postoperatively. Controlled studies have shown that incentive spirometry is superior to intermittent positive-pressure breathing in terms of both effectiveness and cost.[52, 53] Several incentive spirometers are available, with the more popular ones being Triflo II (which is a relatively inexpensive, small, and easily carried flow-sensitive device), the original volume-sensitive Bartlett-Edwards Incentive Spirometer, and Spirocare, a relatively expensive, nondisposable, volume-sensitive device that must be plugged into an electric outlet.[54] There does not appear to be any significant difference in effectiveness among these three different devices.[9] However, it has become eminently clear that the most effective use of these devices depends very heavily upon an effective bedside coach (nurse, respiratory therapist, family member, or friend) who provides frequent verbal encouragement designed to maximize patient compliance with the incentive of the device[9] (the devices use either visual or auditory cues to signal achievement of either the volume or flow endpoint). Other deep breathing maneuvers, such as blow bottles and blow gloves, really depend on the inspiratory maneuver that must precede the emphasized expiratory maneuver and, therefore, must be regarded as mild, short-duration forms of incentive spirometry. Carbon dioxide breathing devices had a short period of popularity until it was shown that the resulting increase in minute ventilation was due to an increase in respiratory rate rather than depth of breathing.

Preoperative exposure to chest physiotherapy (percussion and vibration), postural drainage, and deep breathing exercises facilitates use of these maneuvers postoperatively and thereby reduces the incidence of atelectasis.[15] Graded activity programs may provide considerable preoperative subjective improvement. If obese patients will cooperate, preoperative weight loss should be strived for. Malnutrition, sometimes present in patients with carcinoma or advanced pulmonary disease, may require preoperative treatment (by nasogastric or intravenous feeding).[55] Any other concurrent medical problems (e.g., diabetes) should be stabilized. Oxygen supplementation by nasal cannula at flows of 1 to 2 L/min may be helpful for patients with severe hypoxemia and manifesting secondary polycythemia, cor pulmonale, or impaired mentation. The mainstays of therapy for cor pulmonale are a vigorous pulmonary toilet regimen, oxygen supplementation to relieve hypoxic pulmonary vasoconstriction, diuretics, and possibly digitalis (see the following).

The preoperative use of digitalis in the thoracic surgical patient deserves special comment. Resection of pulmonary tissue reduces the available pulmonary vascular bed for perfusion and can cause postoperative right ventricular and right atrial enlargement. Thus, it is not surprising that the incidence of postoperative arrhythmias (due to atrial stretching) increases progressively with age and amount of lung resected. In addition, there is a higher incidence of atrial arrhythmias following left pneumonectomy than right pneumonectomy because a greater degree of manipulation of the atrium occurs during the former operation. Although the postoperative incidence of arrhythmias has provided the basis for the prophylactic use of digitalis in thoracic surgical patients without evidence of congestive heart failure, this practice is still controversial.[56–59] Widely accepted indications for preoperative digitalization in patients without cor pulmonale undergoing thoracic surgery include congestive (left-sided) heart failure and supraventricular arrhythmias with a rapid ventricular response.[60]

The indications for preoperative digitalization are more straightforward in patients with cor pulmonale. However, it is important to note that these patients have a propensity to develop hypoxemia, hypercarbia, and acidosis, and they are therefore at an increased risk of developing digitalis toxicity; the drug should therefore be used with caution.[61, 62] If these patients do receive digitalis preoperatively, it is important to normalize the serum potassium in order to decrease the risk of rhythmias. Digitalis should probably be withheld on the day of surgery to

help avoid confusion with digitalis intoxication if arrhythmias occur postoperatively.[63]

VI. MECHANISM OF PREOPERATIVE RESPIRATORY PREPARATION BENEFIT

There are several possible mechanisms to explain why preoperative respiratory care preparation maneuvers benefit the patient and result in a decreased incidence of postoperative respiratory complications. Preoperative removal of secretions from the airways is probably the main beneficial result of such intensive preparations for surgery. The removal of secretions is accomplished by the therapeutic cascade of dilating the airways, loosening the secretions, and then removing the secretions. Second, the patients may respond nonspecifically to the attention given them, and because of an improved psychologic and motivational status, they may have improved compliance with postoperative respiratory care maneuvers and may ambulate earlier. Third, preoperative instructions in deep breathing exercises, incentive spirometry and coughing maneuvers, and exposure to chest physiotherapy probably improve the efficaciousness of these maneuvers in the postoperative period. Fourth, there is evidence that many of the techniques used (aminophylline, the various exercises) improve respiratory muscle strength and endurance; however, it is not clear whether the usual 1- to 2-day preoperative regimen is capable of producing significant muscular conditioning as compared with the 5-week period allowed for in more carefully controlled situations.[8] Finally, the preoperative respiratory care regimen may actually improve pulmonary function and pulmonary function testing, although this does not occur in every prepared patient even though the incidence of respiratory complications decreases in prepared patients versus nonprepared patients.[8] It is likely that some or all of these mechanisms contribute in part to the ability of preoperative respiratory care preparatory maneuvers to decrease the incidence of postoperative respiratory complications.

VII. PREMEDICATION

Premedication is individualized according to the psychologic needs of the patient, the severity of pre-existing pulmonary disease, and the anticipated operation. An explanation of the need for various vascular catheters, specific monitoring devices, and use of the face mask for oxygenation (and possibly for inhalation induction of anesthesia) helps alleviate anxiety and promotes patient cooperation in the operating room. For most patients with reasonably good preoperative pulmonary function a combination of a narcotic analgesic with a benzodiazepine (diazepam, lorazepam) in moderate dosage provides sedation, perioperative analgesia, reduction of anesthetic requirements, and amnesia without concern of predisposing the patient to preoperative respiratory depression. Depression of spontaneous ventilation during anesthesia caused by this type of premedication is rarely a concern because the vast majority of these patients will have their ventilation controlled intraoperatively. Excessively long-acting drugs or very heavy sedation are to be avoided if the operative procedure is short and early postoperative mobilization is desired.

The use of anticholinergic drugs in most normal patients and in patients with mild to moderate chronic obstructive pulmonary disease often causes a fairly uncomfortable feeling due to excessive drying; the drying may theoretically cause difficulty in removing secretions. Consequently, anticholinergic drugs are not ordinarily employed preoperatively. However, since there is good evidence that atropine does not increase the viscosity of secretions but merely decreases the volume of secretions,[64] these drugs should be considered for patients with copious and troublesome amounts of secretions. Although anticholinergic drugs do increase the dead space to tidal volume ratio, the increase is small.

For patients in whom histamine release might be a problem (patients with chronic obstructive lung disease and reactive airways, asthmatics) premedication with Benadryl would seem to be a logical choice. For patients who are thought to have, or may develop, predominance of vagal tone that could induce bronchospasm, atropine is relatively indicated. For patients with a predominance of alpha adrenergic activity that might result in bronchospasm and hypertension, use of droperidol for premedication is relatively indicated.

Patients who are hypoxemic on room air (P_aO_2 < 60 mm Hg) or hypercarbic (P_aCO_2 > 45 mm Hg) are given little or no premedicants that might further depress gas exchange. Patients who are already on supplemental oxygen preoperatively must be transported to the operat-

ing room with the same oxygen flow as previously administered, along with appropriate personnel in constant attendance. Patients who experience orthopnea need to be transported in a semiupright position.

REFERENCES

1. Ford GT, Guenta CA: Toward prevention of postoperative pulmonary complications. Am Rev Respir Dis 130:4–5, 1984.
2. Lansing AM, Jamilson WG: Mechanisms of fever in atelectasis. Arch Surg 87:168, 1963.
3. Harris JD, Johanson WG, Jr, Pierce AK: Bacterial lung clearance in hypoxic mice. Am Rev Respir Dis 111:910, 1975.
4. Latimer G, Dickman M, Clinton DW, Gunn MI, DuWayne SC: Ventilatory patterns and pulmonary complications after upper abdominal surgery determined by preoperative and postoperative computerized spirometry and blood gas analysis. Am J Surg 122:622, 1971.
5. Morton HJV, Camb DA: Tobacco smoking and pulmonary complications after operation. Lancet 1:368, 1944.
6. Stein M, Koota GM, Simon M, et al: Pulmonary evaluation of surgical patients. JAMA 181:765–770, 1962.
7. Tisi GM: Preoperative evaluation of pulmonary function. Am Rev Respir Dis 119:293–310, 1979.
8. Gracey DR, Divertie MB, Didier EP: Preoperative pulmonary preparation of patients with chronic obstructive pulmonary disease. Chest 76:123–129, 1979.
9. Van De Water JM: Preoperative and postoperative techniques in the prevention of pulmonary complications. Surg Clin North Am 60:1339–1348, 1980.
10. Johnson WC: Postoperative ventilatory performance. Dependence upon surgical incision. Am J Surg 41:615–619, 1967.
11. Ali J, Weisel RD, Layng AB, Kripke BJ, Hechtman HB: Consequences of postoperative alterations and respiratory mechanics. Am J Surg 128:376–382, 1974.
12. Anderson WH, Dosett BE Jr, Hamilton GE: Prevention of postoperative pulmonary complications. JAMA 186:763–766, 1963.
13. Tarhan S, Moffitt EA, Sessler AD, et al: Risk of anesthesia and surgery in patients with chronic bronchitis and chronic obstructive pulmonary disease. Surgery 74:720–726, 1973.
14. Harmon E, Lillington G: Pulmonary risk factors in surgery. Med Clin North Am 63:1289–1298, 1979.
15. Thoren L: Postoperative pulmonary complications: Observations on their prevention by means of physiotherapy. Acta Chir Scan 107:193–205, 1954.
16. Palmer KN, Sellick BA: The prevention of postoperative pulmonary atelectasis. Lancet 1:164–168, 1953.
17. Veith FJ, Rocco AG: Evaluation of respiratory function in surgical patients: Importance of preoperative preparation and in the prediction of pulmonary complications. Surgery 45:905–911, 1959.
18. Stein M, Cassara EL: Preoperative pulmonary evaluation and therapy for surgical patients. JAMA 211:787–790, 1970.
19. Swenson EW, Stallberg-Stenhagen S, Beck M: Arterial oxygen, carbon dioxide, and pH levels in patients

undergoing pulmonary resection. J Thorac Cardiovasc Surg 42:179–192, 1961.

20. Gaensler EA, Weisel RD: The risks of abdominal and thoracic surgery in COPD. Postgrad Med 54:183–192, 1973.

21. Kirilloff LH, Owens GR, Rogers RM, et al: Does chest physical therapy work? Chest 88:436–444, 1985.

22. Warner MA, Tinker JH, Divertie MB: Preoperative cessation of smoking and pulmonary complications in pulmonary dysfunction. Anesthesiology 59:A60, 1983.

23. Pearce AC, Jones RM: Smoking and anesthesia: Preoperative abstinence and perioperative morbidity. Anesthesiology 61:576–584, 1984.

24. Jones RM: Smoking before surgery: The case for stopping smoking. Br Med J 290:1763–1764, 1985.

25. Davies JM, Latto IP, Jones JG, et al: Effects of stopping smoking for 48 hours on oxygen availability from the blood: A study on pregnant women. Br Med J 2:355–356, 1979.

26. Haas A, Peneda H, Haas F, Axen K: Therapeutic modalities. In: Pulmonary Therapy and Rehabilitation: Principles and Practice. Baltimore, Williams & Wilkins Co, 1979, Chapter 12, p. 110–142.

27. Lertzman MM, Cherniack RM: Rehabilitation of patients with chronic obstructive pulmonary disease. Am Rev Respir Dis 114:1145–1165, 1976.

28. Snider GL: Control of bronchospasm in patients with chronic obstructive disease. Chest 73(Suppl):927–934, 1978.

29. Melville GN, Horstmann G, Irvani J: Adrenergic compounds and the respiratory tract. A physiological and electronic microscopal study. Respiration 33:261, 1976.

30. Foster WM, Bergofsky EH, Bohning DE, Lippman M, Albert RE: Effect of adrenergic agents and their modes of action of mucociliary clearance in man. J Appl Physiol 41:146, 1976.

31. Webb-Johnson DC, Chir B, Andrews JL: Bronchodilator therapy. N Engl J Med 297:476–482, 1977.

32. Isles AF, Newth CJL: Combined beta agonists and methylxanthines in asthma. N Engl J Med 309:432, 1983.

33. Aubier M, De Troyer A, Sampson M, et al: Aminophylline improves diaphragmatic contractility. N Engl J Med 305:249–252, 1981.

34. Jackson RT, Beaglehold R, Rea HH, et al: Mortality from asthma: A new epidemic in New Zealand. Br Med J 285:771–776, 1982.

35. Wilson JD, Sutherland DC: Combined beta agonists and methylxanthines in asthma. N Engl J Med 307:1707, 1982.

36. Lehr D, Guideri G: More on combined beta agonists and methylxanthines in asthma. N Engl J Med 309:1581–1582, 1983.

37. Mitkenko PA, Ogilvie RI: Rational intravenous dose of theophylline. N Engl J Med 289:600–603, 1973.

38. Petty TL, Brink GA, Miller MW, et al: Objective functional improvement in chronic airway obstruction. Chest 57:216–223, 1970.

39. Chopra SK, Taplin GV, Simmons DH, Robinson GD, Jr, Elam D, Coulson A: Effects of hydration and physical therapy on tracheal transport velocity. Am Rev Respir Dis 115:1009–1014, 1977.

40. Scheffner AL: The mucolytic activity and mechanism of action and metabolism of acetylcysteine. Pharmaco Ther 1:47, 1964.

41. May DB, Munt PW: Physiologic effects of chest percussion and postural drainage in patients with stable chronic bronchitis. Chest 75:29–32, 1979.

42. Oldenburg FA Jr, Dolovich MB, Montgomery JM, et al: Effects of postural drainage, exercise, and cough on mucus clearance in chronic bronchitis. Am Rev Respir Dis 120:739–745, 1979.

43. Bateman, JRM, Newman ST, Daunt KM, Sheahan NF, Pavia D, Clarke FW: Is cough as effective as chest physiotherapy in the removal of excessive tracheobronchial secretions? Thorax 36:683–687, 1981.

44. Harris RS, Lawson TV: The relative mechanical effectiveness and efficiency of successive voluntary coughs in healthy young adults. Clin Sci 34:569–577, 1968.

45. Cherniack RM, Sanvhill E: Long-term use of intermittent positive-pressure breathing (IPPB) in chronic obstructive pulmonary disease. Am Rev Respir Dis 113:721–727, 1976.

46. Gold MI: The present status of IPPB therapy. Chest 67:469–471, 1975.

47. Loren M, Chai H, Miklich D, et al: Comparison between simple nebulization and intermittent positive-pressure in asthmatic children with severe bronchospasm. Chest 72:145–147, 1977.

48. Gold MI: Is intermittent positive-pressure breathing therapy (IPPB Rx) necessary in the surgical patient? Ann Surg 184:122–123, 1976.

49. Petty TL: A critical look at IPPB. Chest 66:1–3, 1974.

50. Egbert LD, Battit GE, Welch CE, et al: Reduction of postoperative pain by encouragement and instruction of patients. N Engl J Med 270:825, 1964.

51. Peters RM: Pulmonary physiologic studies of the perioperative period. Chest 76:576, 1979.

52. Dohi S, Gold MI: Comparison of two methods of postoperative respiratory care. Chest 73:592, 1978.

53. Van De Water JM, Watring WG, Linton LA, et al: Prevention of postoperative pulmonary complications. Surg Gynecol Obstet 135:229, 1972.

54. Lederer DH, Van De Water JM, Indech RB: Incentive spirometry: A comparative study of selected patient aids. Chest 77:610, 1980.

55. Williams CD, Brenowitz JB: "Prohibitive" lung function and major surgical procedures. Am J Surg 132:763, 1976.

56. Shields TW, Ujiki GT: Digitalization for prevention of arrhythmias following pulmonary surgery. Surg Gynecol Obstet 126:743–746, 1968.

57. Juler GL, Stemmer EA, Connolly JE: Complications of prophylactic digitalization in thoracic surgical patients. J Thorac Cardiovasc Surg 58:352–360, 1969.

58. Burman SO: The prophylactic use of digitalis before thoracotomy. Ann Thorac Surg 14:359–368, 1972.

59. Wheat MW, Burford TH: Digitalis in surgery: Extension of classical indications. J Thorac Cardiovasc Surg 41:162–168, 1961.

60. Deutsch S, Dalen JE: Indications for prophylactic digitalization. Anesthesiology 30:648–656, 1969.

61. Green LH, Smith TW: The use of digitalis in patients with pulmonary disease. Ann Intern Med 87:459–465, 1977.

62. Mason DT, Zelis R, Lee G, et al: Current concepts and treatments of digitalis toxicity. Am J Cardiol 27:546–559, 1971.

63. Dreifus LS, Rabbino MD, Watanabe Y, et al: Arrhythmias in the postoperative period. Am J Cardiol 12:431–435, 1963.

64. Aviado DM: Regulation of bronchomotor tone during anesthesia. Anesthesiology 42:68–80, 1975.

III

INTRAOPERATIVE CONSIDERATIONS FOR ALL THORACIC SURGERY

Monitoring

7

I. INTRODUCTION

Although thoracic surgery may affect both pulmonary and cardiovascular function, it more commonly threatens respiratory much more so than cardiovascular function. Consequently this chapter will emphasize the monitoring of respiratory function more than cardiovascular function for the routine thoracic surgery patient. In addition, for the very ill patient or for very physiologically intrusive and demanding thoracic surgery cases, advanced cardiovascular function monitoring techniques are equally and fully discussed.

Patients undergoing thoracic surgery are most prone to impaired gas exchange because with either one- or two-lung ventilation both nondependent and dependent lung function (with reference to lateral decubitus position) will be impaired (see chapter 4). The consequences of both inadequate oxygenation and carbon dioxide elimination are serious. Even slight decreases in the content of oxygen in

arterial blood from a marginally normal level may alter a delicate balance of supply and demand to certain tissues and also have widespread effects due to activation of the sympathetic nervous system. Similarly, changes in blood carbon dioxide content can alter sympathetic nervous system activity, and, in addition, concomitant changes in pH may impair the function of several vital organs. The heart, especially in patients with coronary artery disease, may be the first organ to dramatically show the occurrence of hypoxemia and hypercapnia with the development of ischemia and arrhythmias (see chapter 3). Thus, the need to monitor respiratory function during thoracic anesthesia is a critical and continuous responsibility.

The monitoring responsibility can be fulfilled in various ways with various degrees of sophistication depending on a particular patient's preoperative condition and intraoperative requirements. The philosophy espoused by this approach is based upon the concept that there are two considerations that dictate the type of monitoring used. First, patients undergoing thoracic operations have varying degrees of pre-existing cardiorespiratory disease (see chapter 5). Second, the very nature of thoracic procedures causes further derangements in cardiorespiratory function during the perioperative period (see chapter 4). Thus, based on these two considerations and their interactions, individual patients can and should be categorized into a progressively sophisticated and complex tier system with regard to what monitoring is necessary to make possible accurate and rapid diagnosis and therapy during anesthesia (Table 7–1).[1]

A. Special Intraoperative Conditions

Patients undergoing thoracic surgery may experience several hazardous intraoperative conditions. First, most thoracic surgical procedures are performed in the lateral decubitus position, which may compromise gas exchange (with either one- or two-lung ventilation, but especially with one-lung ventilation; see chapter 4). Second, the surgical procedure may adversely affect the function of mediastinal organs (e.g., irritate the heart, obstruct the vena cava). Third, some thoracic procedures may require massive transfusion (such as excision of some arteriovenous malformations); hypotension and massive transfusion are associated with the development of the adult respiratory distress syndrome. Fourth, operations necessitating deliberate hypotension increase monitoring requirements because of changes in pulmonary vascular autoregulation (HPV), in V_D/V_T, and perhaps in oxygen transport. Fifth, operations of excessive duration will promote transudation of fluid into dependent regions of the lung and thereby cause progressive oxygenation difficul-

ties. Lastly, operations involving the airway, such as laryngoscopy, which frequently necessitates apnea, or bronchoscopy, which frequently imposes restrictions on positive-pressure ventilation, require increased respiratory function monitoring.

B. Pre-existing Lung Disease

Patients undergoing thoracic surgery often have significant pre-existing cardiopulmonary disease (see chapter 5). Most of these patients have a long history of heavy smoking and therefore have chronic lung disease with reactive airways and excessive secretions. Due to the lifestyle associated with smoking, many may have coronary artery disease and some may be very obese (with a propensity for decreases in functional residual capacity during anesthesia; see chapter 3). Some patients presenting for emergency thoracic surgery will have acute chest disease (pulmonary infection, hemorrhage, contusion, infarction) or acute systemic diseases (sepsis, renal, cardiac, or liver failure or multiple trauma). Some patients requiring thoracic surgery may be very old.

C. Tiered Monitoring System

Based on the presence of special intraoperative conditions and the degree of pre-existing lung disease, and the interaction between these two factors, a progressively sophisticated three-tiered monitoring system should be used (Table 7–1). The first tier (tier I) includes healthy young patients without special intraoperative conditions, such as a young patient undergoing pleurodesis. This tier contains the minimal, yet essential, monitoring that is required for any patient undergoing a thoracic procedure. The

Table 7–1. *Derivation of a Tiered Monitoring System for Anesthesia for Thoracic Surgery*

Pre-existing Lung Disease	And/Or	Special Intraoperative Conditions	Risk of Respiratory Morbidity and Mortality	Tiered Monitoring System
None		None	Very low	I. Essential monitoring
None		Moderate	Moderate	II. Special intermittent
Moderate		None	Moderate	and/or continuous
Moderate		Moderate	High moderate	monitoring
None		Severe	High	III. Advanced monitoring
Severe		None	High	
Severe		Severe	Very high	

second tier (tier II) represents an increase in risk, caused by either the presence of special unfavorable intraoperative conditions for relatively healthy patients or by the presence of significant pre-existing cardiopulmonary disease in patients who will not experience special unfavorable intraoperative conditions. An example of the former circumstance is a patient with mild lung disease having a lobectomy. An example of the latter circumstance is a patient with moderate interstitial lung disease who requires an open lung biopsy. Anyone with some lung disease undergoing one-lung ventilation for a major thoracic procedure must be considered to be in a high tier II category, which really represents a transition category between the tier II and tier III continuum. Finally, a third tier (tier III) of monitoring requirements is constructed for patients with significant pre-existing cardiopulmonary disease and/or for those who will experience major compromising intraoperative conditions. An example of such a patient is one with cor pulmonale undergoing lobectomy or pneumonectomy. Thus, it should be apparent from this monitoring approach that an individual with severe pulmonary disease who is to undergo a minor surgical procedure may well require as extensive a monitoring system as a patient with normal lungs who is to have extensive thoracic surgery.

II. TIER I: THE ESSENTIAL MONITORING SYSTEM

An essential monitoring system is used for healthy patients undergoing simple physiologically nonintrusive thoracic procedures (Table 7–2). Patients belonging exclusively to this monitoring tier comprise relatively few of the patients undergoing thoracic surgery. However, since the system represents the minimum amount of monitoring, it is a component of all levels of monitoring for all patients and should allow one to anticipate incipient ventilatory failure as well as to recognize ventilatory failure when it does occur. Although superficially this system may seem unsophisticated, an alert anesthesiologist uses the senses of sight, sound, and touch to gather automatically and reflexly a great deal of information about the well-being of the patient. In view of the many possible mechanical mishaps described in chapter 3 that can impair respiratory function, monitoring respiratory function during anesthesia begins prior to the induction of anesthesia with checking the anesthesia machine.

A. Checking the Anesthesia Machine

Failure to check equipment properly before the induction of anesthesia is responsible for 22 per cent of critical incidents that occur during anesthesia.[2] Accordingly, preanesthesia checklists have been written to help fulfill this responsibility completely.[3] Inspect the machine to ensure that component parts are connected in the proper order. Vaporizers should be filled, and the caps and drains closed. The central gas supply lines should be properly seated in the appropriate pin-indexed wall or ceiling outlets. The tanks should have a wrench, be color coded, be on the proper yokes, and be pin indexed. The tanks should be opened serially, and adequately pressurized, and the flow of gas observed through the appropriate flowmeter. The carbon dioxide absorber cannister should be full, functional as indicated by color, and fastened securely. The breathing circuit should be tested for leaks under pressure, but the circuit should only be partially filled, and the pressure should be released slowly to avoid depositing soda lime in the inspiratory limb.[4] Competence of unidirectional valves should be tested for by breathing into the circuit and by noting any undue resistance, presence of irritating gas, and motion (sticking) of the directional valves. A head strap should be available.

For the vast majority of thoracic surgery cases, the function of the anesthesia machine ventilator needs to be assessed preoperatively. This can be done easily for both pressure- and volume-limited ventilators by serially attaching a rebreathing bag to the patient connection, closing the anesthesia machine overflow valve, turning on the ventilator to either a high pressure or a volume limit, and observing the movements of the bag. The bag, serving as a test lung, should expand smoothly and easily and deflate in a similar way through the ventilator overflow valve.

B. Continuous Monitoring of the Oxygen-Delivery System

Since some of the causes of failure of the oxygen delivery system listed in chapter 3 can occur even when the anesthesia machine appeared to function properly preoperatively (for example, wrong gas in central storage tanks, crossed pipe lines, failure of fail-safe mechanism), the oxygen concentration in the inspired gas should be continuously monitored.[5] Numerous paramagnetic, polarographic, and fuel-

Table 7-2. Tiered Monitoring System Based on Amount of Pre-existing Lung Disease and Presence of Special Intraoperative Conditions

Patient Category	Tiered Monitoring System	Required Monitoring Related to Respiratory Function								
		A Anesthesia Machine	B Oxygen Delivery	C Apnea	D Minute Ventilation	E Gas Exchange	F Airway Mechanics	G Cardiovascular Functions	H Muscle Relaxation	I Temp
Routine healthy patients without special intraoperative conditions	Tier I. Essential (used in all patients)	Complete check plus ventilator	Inspired O_2 monitor	Stethoscope, alarm system, observation	Respiratory rate, bag and chest movements	Color of shed blood, cyanosis, capillary and venous blood gas tensions, oximetry	Stethoscope, feel of breathing bag	Heart rate, blood pressure, EKG	Simple motor tests, blockade monitor	Probe
Routine healthy patients with special intraoperative conditions and/or patients with moderate pre-existing lung disease without special intraoperative conditions	Tier II. Special intermittent and/or continuous monitoring	As above	As above	As above plus D, E, G, and F	As above plus respirometer spirometer	As above plus arterial blood gas tensions and end-tidal CO_2 measurement, oximetry or transcutaneous gases	Whole lung and individual lung compliance, vital capacity, peak inspiratory force (postoperative)	As above plus accurate input vs output, and central venous pressures	As above	As above
Patients with severe pre-existing respiratory disease with special intraoperative conditions	Tier III. Advanced monitoring	As above	As above	As above	As above	As above plus $\dot{Q}_s/\dot{Q}_t$, V_D/V_T, $\dot{Q}_t$, $\dot{V}O_2$ mass spectrometry	As above plus airway resistance	As above plus pulmonary vascular pressures, cardiac output, lung water measurements	As above	As above

cell analyzers are available. Ideally, the oxygen analyzer should have a fast response time, high and low alarm setting capabilities, which when exceeded, trigger audio and visual alarm signals. A model for the study of commercially available oxygen monitors has recently been published.[6] It should be noted that a mass spectrometer can function as a most elegant in-line oxygen analyzer.

If the oxygen sensor is placed on the expiratory side of the anesthesia circle system (between the corrugated tubing and the expiratory unidirectional valve), then the oxygen sensor will detect the minimum oxygen concentration in the circuit (usually the fraction of oxygen in expired gas is 0.05 less than the fraction in the inspired gas). However, in this position the oxygen monitor can also double as a circuit disconnection alarm (in addition to continuous chest auscultation, chest observation, and low-pressure alarms) if a falling bellows ventilator (which is the most common type) is in use. The falling bellows of the ventilator draws room air

past the oxygen probe, and within one or two breaths following circuit disconnection the alarm will sound if the low limit is set above 20 per cent oxygen.[7]

C. Continuous Monitoring of Apnea
(Fig. 7–1)

Precordial and esophageal stethoscopes enable essential and continuous monitoring of breath sounds. Additionally, the anesthesiologist should frequently (every minute) scan the chest, the breathing bag, the ventilator bellows, and the pressure manometers on the anesthesia machine for appropriate movement. The anesthesia machine–mechanical ventilator system should have a low and high positive-pressure audiovisual alarm system. This latter monitoring aid must now be viewed as essential in view of the fact that most accidental anesthesia-caused or -related deaths (brain and/or whole body) have been, and presently are, due to ventilator

Monitoring of Only Apnea and Minute Ventilation

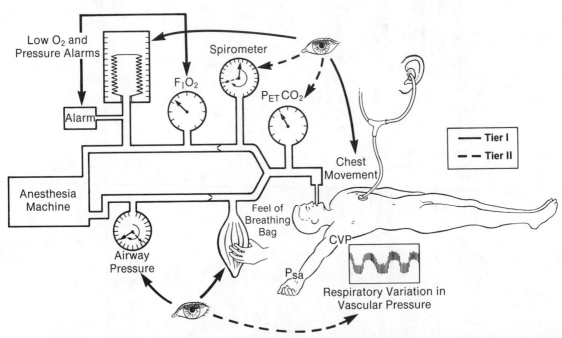

Figure 7–1. *The number of things that an anesthesiologist does to monitor minute ventilation and to detect continuously the onset of apnea is considerable. Most of the monitoring utilizes the basic senses of sight, sound, and touch and is done reflexively and automatically by an experienced anesthesiologist. These automatic monitoring efforts, for the most part, make up the tier I monitoring level (solid arrows). Additional tier I monitoring modalities include use of an in-line F_IO_2 monitor and low and high airway pressure alarm systems. Tier II monitoring efforts include use of end tidal CO_2 concentration, movement of in-line spirometer, and observation of respiratory variation in vascular pressures (dashed arrows). Both tier I and tier II monitoring efforts should be continuously conducted in a systematic and frequently recurring circular pattern (cockpit analogy).*

disconnects in otherwise healthy patients. As just discussed, oxygen sensors can serve as disconnect alarms if placed on the expiratory limb of an anesthesia circle system and if a falling bellows ventilator is in use.

D. Minute Ventilation (Fig. 7–1)

For the healthy patient having a physiologically nonintrusive thoracic procedure, only a crude assessment of minute ventilation is necessary. Minute ventilation is the product of respiratory rate per minute and tidal volume. Counting respiratory rate with either spontaneous, assisted, or mechanically controlled respiration presents no difficulties. However, the limitation in measuring minute ventilation precisely without instrumentation is in accurately measuring the tidal volume. When a tier I patient is mechanically ventilated, the setting of ventilator bellows (10 to 15 ml/kg) and patient chest movement usually suffices to gauge the tidal volume. However, it should be realized that the movement of ventilator bellows may be in error by 50 per cent, depending on respiratory rate, inspiratory-to-expiratory ratio, gas flow rates, and patient compliance and resistance (M. Scheller, personal communication). In addition, it should also be realized that with spontaneous ventilation, visual or "educated" hand assessments of chest or anesthesia reservoir bag movements in questionable or marginal cases may be misleading,[8] especially with inexperienced observers.[9] In any patient, an unusually strong respiratory drive in the presence of high doses of inhaled or intravenously administered anesthetics may be the consequence of hypercapnia and hypoxia.

E. Gas Exchange

The simplest and perhaps most common signs of hypoxemia are purple or dark shed blood and/or the appearance of cyanosis. Most of the blood in skin and mucous membranes is venous and is related to the C_aO_2 as follows (rearranged Fick equation; see equation 11 in chapter 3):

$$C_vO_2 = C_aO_2 - C(a\text{-}v)O_2 = C_aO_2 - \frac{\text{tissue } \dot{V}O_2}{\text{tissue } \dot{Q}}$$

The oxygen consumption by skin ($\dot{V}O_2$) is very low in relation to its circulation ($\dot{Q}$) so that the quantity in the far right term is generally small. Therefore skin C_vO_2 is close to C_aO_2. Cyanosis

can be detected by experienced observers in 95 per cent of patients with an arterial saturation (S_aO_2) of 89 per cent,[10] which would correspond with an unacceptably low P_aO_2 of 55 mm Hg. However, when skin circulation is reduced in relation to skin oxygen consumption, as may occur in hypovolemia (vasoconstriction) and in the Trendelenburg position (stagnant flow), cyanosis may occur in the presence of normal C_aO_2 (peripheral cyanosis). Alternatively, in cases of anemia in which it is not possible to obtain the level of 5 g/100 ml of reduced hemoglobin, which is generally accepted to be required for the appearance of cyanosis, cyanosis may not occur in the presence of abnormal C_aO_2 ("central cyanosis").[11] Clearly, cyanosis could never occur if the hemoglobin concentration was only 5 g/100 ml. Thus, cyanosis should always be looked for, but since it can be falsely positive, it should be regarded as a warning sign requiring further investigation. Since the absence of cyanosis can be falsely negative, the anesthesiologist should not be lulled into a sense of complacency. In addition, recognition of cyanosis depends upon the quality of lighting, reflection from drapes, and the observers themselves.

Frequently, it may be desirable to obtain a rough approximation of arterial blood gas tensions in tier I patients by measuring gas tensions in compartments that are in some sort of equilibrium with arterial blood. Because pulse oximetry (see detailed discussion of this monitor in Gas Exchange) is so simple and easy to apply, is accurate for continuous oxygen saturation, and carries no risk for the patient (because it is noninvasive) a reasonable case can be made for using this monitor in every case. However, if a serious question arises about the adequacy of arterial oxygenation while the pulse oximeter is being used, then arterial blood gases should be drawn; thus, pulse oximetry should not be regarded as a substitute for arterial blood gases. Venous blood from the back of a warmed hand or large neck vein obtained with no or a short-time low-pressure tourniquet has a P_{CO_2} near enough to that of arterial blood (usually 4 to 8 mm Hg) to be useful for most clinical purposes.[12, 13] In addition, under these sampling conditions a sufficiently high oxygen tension and saturation of venous blood (greater than 40 mm Hg and 75 per cent, respectively) provides a good indication that arterial hypoxemia is most probably absent. As an alternative sampling site, capillary ear lobe blood (obtained by needle prick or cut) is usually acceptable for clinical management, since this blood has a $P_aCO_2 \pm 2.0$ per cent of simultaneous arterial samples.[14] The ear lobe vascular bed is more accurate than fingertip or heel vascular beds with respect to PCO_2 determinations.[15] Finally, P_aCO_2 can be very roughly approximated by sampling gas from an endotracheal tube cuff after 1 hour of cuff inflation at patient diastolic blood pressure.[16]

Lastly, the CO_2 absorber cannister should be felt for warmth and the color observed, particularly during induction of anesthesia. The temperature and color of the cannister are proportional to the patient's production of CO_2. When the dreaded complication of malignant hyperpyrexia occurs, an early indication of what is happening is an increase in cannister warmth and perhaps changes in color. This situation demands special monitoring and urgent treatment.

F. Airway Mechanics

Maintenance of a clear, compliant, low resistance tracheobronchial tree is of paramount importance to the anesthesiologist, and in monitoring this aspect of respiratory function, the stethoscope and the feel of the breathing bag are again essential monitoring tools. The stethoscope allows detection of adventitious breath sound (rales, rhonchi, and especially bronchospasm). The breathing bag indicates bronchospasm by classically emptying and refilling slowly, and changes in the feel of the reservoir bag when squeezed indicate changes in compliance. During the induction of anesthesia, the anesthesiologist should continuously listen for air movement with a stethoscope over the chest or trachea and, during the maintenance of anesthesia, with an esophageal stethoscope (preferable) or with a stethoscope taped over the lateral aspect of the dependent lung.

Lastly, the volume of air used to inflate the endotracheal tube cuff needs to be adjusted to a just-seal volume. This maneuver is important prophylactically in preventing postoperative upper airway obstruction secondary to tracheal mucosal edema (reactive hyperemia) caused by excessive cuff pressures. This maneuver will also avoid herniation of the balloon cuff into an obstructing position as well as invagination of compression of the lumen of the tube. If nitrous oxide anesthesia is being used, the just-seal volume needs to be assessed periodically, since

nitrous oxide will diffuse into the cuff and increase cuff volume and pressure.[17]

G. Cardiovascular Parameters

Since cardiovascular function can affect respiratory function and vice versa, monitoring cardiovascular function has important respiratory function implications. Essential monitoring of the cardiovascular system consists of heart rate, noninvasive systemic blood pressure, and electrocardiogram. As previously mentioned, use of pulse oximetry may be considered as a routine oxygenation monitor and, consequently, may also serve as an independent heart rate monitor.

H. Muscle Relaxation

In order to determine the depth of neuromuscular blockade and the adequacy of reversal of neuromuscular blockade, neuromuscular transmission must be monitored quantitatively. There are numerous neuromuscular blockade monitors available, and many provide all or some combination of simple twitch, tetanus, and train of four capability. At the tier I level it is not important to make a priority distinction between these various indices of neuromuscular blockade. However, for the sake of brevity and efficiency, these indices are listed in order of increasing ability to detect neuromuscular blockade. More crude methods of assessment of neuromuscular function, especially postoperatively, include presence of intercostal muscle activity with spontaneous ventilation, grip strength, and ability to lift the head. Ability to sustain head lifting for 5 seconds has been correlated with 83 per cent of preparalysis vital capacity.[18]

I. Temperature

Monitoring temperature is an essential aspect of monitoring respiratory function because of the large changes in oxygen consumption and carbon dioxide production that can be caused by hyperthermia and shivering. Hyperthermia right shifts and hypothermia left shifts the oxygen-hemoglobin dissociation curve, causing facilitated and impaired oxygen unloading to the tissues, respectively.

III. TIER II: SPECIAL INTERMITTENT AND/ OR CONTINUOUS MONITORING

In addition to the essential monitoring of respiratory function of all patients previously described, patients with pre-existing lung disease and healthy patients who have special intraoperative conditions should have special measurements made that are either intermittent or continuous. This monitoring tier comprises the majority of patients undergoing thoracic surgery. These measurements should increase the rapidity and accuracy of diagnostic and therapeutic judgment. Monitoring techniques for respiratory functions A, B, H, and I are the same as those described for tier I essential monitoring.

C. Continuous Monitoring of Apnea
(Fig. 7–1)

In addition to the essential monitors of observation of the chest, breathing bag, ventilator bellows, and in-line airway pressure gauge movement and the alarms signaling abnormal pressure or oxygen concentration in the breathing circuit, the anesthesiologist should regularly observe movement of an in-line spirometer (see Minute Ventilation), changes in on-line end-tidal CO_2 and O_2 concentration readouts (see Gas Exchange), and changes in the paper write-out of vascular pressures with respiration (at this tier II monitoring level an arterial line will be in situ in most cases, and a central venous pressure will be in situ in many cases; see Cardiovascular Parameters).

D. Minute Ventilation (Fig. 7–1)

Essential monitoring yields only a rough estimate of minute ventilation because tidal volume can be assessed only either visually or by touch. Fairly precise measurement of the tidal volume can be made by placing on the expiratory limb an in-line respirometer which works by a vane anemometer principle (e.g., the Wright or Boehringer spirometer). As indicated above, there are a number of situations in which the calibrated plastic cylinder around the bellow of the ventilator can be quite inaccurate (50 per cent error possible depending on fresh gas flow rates, I:E ratio, and patient mechanics). Since the anemometer respirometer is much more accurate than the ventilator bellows, the former

may be used to check the latter. Both can be used continuously, but the anemometer respirometers become less accurate after exposure to moisture for a long period of time and are therefore better preserved by intermittent use.

E. Gas Exchange

Essential monitoring of gas exchange consists of observing the color of the skin, mucous membranes, and shed blood for a very gross estimate of the presence of hypoxemia. Much more precise information can be obtained about gas exchange by measuring the arterial partial pressure of oxygen (P_aO_2) and carbon dioxide (P_aCO_2). If there is any suspicion about the adequacy of respiratory function, as there may often be in patients with pre-existing lung disease and special intraoperative conditions, it is mandatory that blood-gas measurements be made. Without blood gas analysis no anesthesiologist can unequivocally accurately assess the degree of respiratory impairment. Trying to diagnose and to treat respiratory impairment without making blood-gas measurements is comparable to treating diabetic coma without measuring blood or urine sugar. The P_aO_2 precisely defines and quantitates hypoxemia, and the P_aCO_2 precisely defines and quantitates carbon dioxide retention. When dealing with the lower and simpler tier II cases, it is reasonable to sample arterial blood gases by a few intermittent punctures if a peripheral systemic artery (usually radial artery, occasionally dorsalis pedis) is conveniently available, whereas for all other cases (middle and high level tier II situations, including almost all one-lung ventilation cases) arterial blood gases should be sampled from an indwelling peripheral arterial catheter. An indwelling peripheral arterial catheter guarantees immediate, frequent, and certain arterial blood samples.

Although blood gas analysis defines the efficiency and quantity of ventilation, the usefulness of the information is diminished by the fact that the results are static intermittent values that existed several minutes ago (see Table 7–3). In addition, the method suffers from being invasive. On the other hand, there are three new techniques of measuring oxygen gas exchange—transcutaneous oxygen tension, ear and conjunctival oximetry (oxygen saturation), and pulse oximetry (oxygen saturation); and two techniques of measuring carbon dioxide exchange—transcutaneous CO_2 tension and end-

Table 7–3. Comparison of Three Types of Continuous Noninvasive Monitors of Gas Exchange with Arterial Blood Gases

Gas Exchange Monitor	Blood Compartment	Blood Flow Dependency	Response Time	Comparison to Arterial Value	Overall Ease of Use
Arterial blood gases	Arterial	None	Several minutes	Identical	Invasive, requires time
Pulse oximeter	Arterial	Little	None	Excellent (saturation)	Very easy
Ear oximeter	Capillary	Moderate	Seconds	Good (saturation)	Moderately easy
Transcutaneous gas tensions	Capillary, venous	Large	1 to 2 minutes	Fair (tension)	Requires time and ?ABGs

tidal CO_2 analysis—that allow noninvasive and continuous monitoring of these gases. However, since each of these continuous noninvasive monitoring techniques depends, to a varying extent, on the blood flow to the region over which the oxygen sensor is located (see Table 7–3), each has the monitoring cost, especially in low-flow states, of only approximating P_aO_2 or S_aO_2 and P_aCO_2 (for discussion of each of these continuous monitoring techniques and references, see the following text). In addition, each of these continuous monitoring techniques may suffer from external mechanical difficulties and interference (poor application, physical bumping, electrocautery, lighting, and humidity). Thus, on the one hand, arterial blood gases are accurately measured by intermittent and invasive methods, whereas transcutaneous gas tensions and oximetry only approximate arterial oxygen tension/saturation (pulse oximetry is most accurate and reliable; see below), but on a continuous and noninvasive basis.

Since peripheral oximetry and transcutaneous measurements are continuous, one would expect that these continuous methods would be able to diagnose many more periods of hypoxemia in patients who have medical problems or who are in situations in which P_aO_2 may vary rapidly and significantly, compared with intermittent blood gas analysis.[19, 20] Indeed, in neonates who require mechanical ventilation and elevated F_IO_2, continuous oxygen monitoring by the transcutaneous method detected significantly more hypoxia than intermittent blood gas samples (237 minutes/24 hours versus 136 minutes/24 hours, $P < 0.01$).[21] No instance in this study had an arterial P_aO_2 of < 30 mm Hg by blood gas analysis, whereas this low value was noted for 32 minutes/24 hours by the continuous transcutaneous oxygen monitoring method. These extremely low oxygenation values were most frequently observed in association with airway suctioning or spontaneous crying or during chest physiotherapy.

In view of the extensive experience with continuous arterial oxygen monitoring in critically ill patients,[19, 20] such as the neonatal experience just described,[21] it is not surprising that continuous oxygen monitoring methods were quickly used for patients undergoing one-lung ventilation. Indeed, in the last 2 years six different reports (four utilizing transcutaneous monitoring,[22–25] and two utilizing pulse oximetry[26, 27] have documented that continuous arterial oxygenation monitoring during one-lung ventilation revealed dangerous fluctuations in arterial oxygenation that might have been missed by only sampling arterial blood gases intermittently.

Of the three noninvasive continuous methods of following arterial oxygenation, pulse oximetry is the most accurate and non–blood flow dependent method. Pulse oximetry requires no heat source or warm-up period and is ready for immediate use. The pulse oximeter works by placing a pulsating arteriovascular bed between a light source and a detector. The pulsating vascular bed, by expanding and contracting, creates a change in the light path that modifies the amount of light detected. Nonpulsatile substances, such as skin, bone, and venous blood, are not detected. In order to determine the per cent of arterial hemoglobin saturated with oxygen, the oximeter measures the ratio of a transmitted red light (660 nm) to infrared light (940 nm) during one arterial pulsation. The ratio of red light to infrared light varies depending upon the relative fraction of saturated to unsaturated hemoglobin in the arterial blood and therefore the ratio allows calculation of the saturation of arterial blood with oxygen. Pulse oximetry is accurate over S_aO_2 values from 100 to 70 per cent over a wide range of hemodynamic conditions as long as a pulse is present beneath the sensor (r = 0.93).[26, 28] There is virtually no lag time between changes in arterial oxygen saturation and changes in the pulse oximetry readout. It is not necessary to calibrate a peripheral pulse oximeter with arterial blood gases. However, it should be understood from the oxygen-hemoglobin dissociation curve that decreases in P_aO_2 from values higher than 80 mm Hg to values near 80 mm Hg will produce relatively minor changes in S_aO_2.

Ear oximetry is similar to pulse oximetry. However, the ear oximeter probes are large and bulky and for infants, older children, and patients in the lateral decubitus position the device is often difficult to fix in place for an appreciable length of time, which greatly reduces its applicability for use during anesthesia. Aside from this drawback, the ear oximeter, like the pulse oximeter, is easy to operate and is accurate (under normotensive conditions r = 0.96 compared with simultaneous arterial blood oxygen saturation).[29, 30] However, ear oximeters are more flow dependent than pulse oximeters, and the correlation with arterial blood oxygen saturation is not as good during low-flow conditions.

Transcutaneous blood gas tension measurements are probably the most inaccurate and blood flow dependent of the three noninvasive continuous gas exchange monitoring methods. When the skin is made sufficiently hyperemic (to 44°C by the transcutaneous probe), the skin O_2 consumption and CO_2 production become insignificant relative to O_2 supply and CO_2 washout, the right hand term in the equation on page 173 becomes insignificant, and the tissue and transcutaneous Po_2 and Pco_2 ($P_{tc}O_2$ and $P_{tc}CO_2$, respectively) approach the P_aO_2 and P_aCO_2, respectively.[19, 20, 22] In general, in normal patients, $P_{tc}O_2$ should be expected to be 80 per cent of P_aO_2, and $P_{tc}CO_2$ should be expected to be 25 per cent greater than (1.3 ×) P_aCO_2.[19, 20, 22] However, when cardiac index decreases below 2.2 L/min/m², $P_{tc}O_2$ values decrease further relative to P_aO_2, and $P_{tc}O_2$ becomes linearly related to cardiac output and regional oxygen transport (which is the product of oxygen content and regional blood flow). Thus, when either skin blood flow or P_aO_2 is reduced, $P_{tc}O_2$ is decreased. In addition, the transcutaneous monitors require a 10 minute warm-up period and involve significant calibration procedures, usually including blood gas analysis. In addition, the response times of

transcutaneous electrodes are moderately slow during decreases in P_aO_2 (50 per cent response = 45 to 54 sec), increases in P_aO_2 (50 per cent response = 78 to 84 sec),[31] and changes in P_aCO_2 (50 per cent response time = 3 min).[32, 33] Response times of this magnitude are better than those of intermittent arterial blood gases but much slower than those from a pulse oximeter. With these constraints in mind, several studies have documented these transcutaneous blood–respiratory gas tension relationships when measured and studied in adult patients in the intensive care unit,[32, 34] in patients undergoing thoracic surgery,[22–25, 35] and in those undergoing PEEP-response titration.[36] The correlation coefficient comparing $P_{tc}O_2$ and P_aO_2 and $P_{tc}CO_2$ and P_aCO_2 in all of the above studies was consistently high, with r values usually near 0.9.

Lastly, the end-tidal carbon dioxide tension has found wide clinical application as an alternative to frequent arterial sampling for Pco_2[37, 38] during changes in ventilatory pattern. End-tidal–to–arterial CO_2 gradients are normally small, and therefore changes in ventilation are reflected early and continuously by end-tidal CO_2 measurements. The rising Pco_2 of a patient with a step decrease in minute ventilation can be noted almost immediately during continuous end-tidal CO_2 analysis. Conversely, significant loss of pulmonary perfusion (kinking or compression of vessels, particulate embolization) causes an easily detected immediate decrease in the end-tidal CO_2 concentration. It should be understood by the user of end-tidal CO_2 analysis that with severe lung disease, large end-tidal–to–arterial CO_2 gradients may exist, and P_aCO_2 should be measured early to quantify the gradient.

In summary, of the three noninvasive continuous monitors of arterial oxygenation, pulse oximeters are the most reliable, accurate, rapidly responding, and non–blood flow dependent. Ear oximeters are reasonably accurate and temporally responsive but are cumbersome and awkward to use in most anesthesia situations. Transcutaneous monitors are relatively slow responding and somewhat uncertain (especially whenever cardiovascular function is suspect) approximations of P_aO_2. Thus, of the three noninvasive continuous monitors of arterial oxygenation that are relevant to tier II patients, the pulse oximeter is clearly the most desirable monitor. Of the two noninvasive continuous monitors of carbon dioxide elimination that are relevant to tier II patients, end-tidal CO_2 measurement is more accurate and easier to use (with either a dedicated meter or as part of mass spectrometry; see the following) than transcutaneous CO_2 monitoring.

For low-level tier II type cases gas exchange may be adequately monitored by intermittent arterial blood gases (drawn either from single punctures or from an indwelling catheter). At the present time there is an insufficient amount of evidence to support the contention that gas exchange may be adequately monitored at this low tier II level with only one of the noninvasive continuous monitors of gas exchange.[22-27] The absolute values from continuous arterial oxygenation monitors should be regarded as the minimum P_aO_2 and S_aO_2 possible, and a downward trend in the continuous arterial oxygenation monitor value should be regarded as an early warning sign of impending hypoxemia; both a low absolute value and a downward trend should be documented by arterial blood gas analysis. For middle level tier II patients, arterial blood gases should be monitored from an indwelling peripheral arterial catheter. At this middle tier II level a continuous oxygen monitor should be used as supplementary early indicators of gas exchange problems (usually the continuous monitor decreases the number of arterial blood gases required).[26] For high-level tier II cases arterial blood gases should be regularly monitored from an indwelling arterial catheter (i.e., sampling should not be based on the data from a continuous monitor), although the continuous monitors of gas exchange can certainly still be used to indicate any interval problems.

The P_aO_2 alone does not describe the efficiency of oxygenation of the blood in terms of wasted perfusion ($\dot{Q}_s/\dot{Q}_t$), nor does the P_aCO_2 alone describe the efficiency of ventilation in terms of wasted ventilation ($\dot{V}_D/\dot{V}_T$). More complex steps (see the following), such as actually measuring $\dot{V}_D/\dot{V}_T$ and $\dot{Q}_s/\dot{Q}_t$, cardiac output, and $C_{\bar{v}}O_2$, are necessary to do this with precision. However, given a cardiac output and oxygen consumption in the normal range, a reasonably close approximation of $\dot{Q}_s/\dot{Q}_t$ can be made if the P_aO_2 is known in relation to the inspired oxygen concentration (F_IO_2) (see Fig. 3–6). Likewise, a reasonably close approximation of $\dot{V}_D/\dot{V}_T$ can be made if the P_aCO_2 is known in relation to the minute ventilation.[39] For example, a 70 kg patient whose minute ventilation is twice normal (e.g., 10 L/min) and whose $P_aCO_2 = 40$ mm Hg will have twice normal wasted ventilation (60 per cent). A simplified, but relatively accurate, equation for $\dot{V}_D/\dot{V}_T$ requiring only the patient's minute ventilation, expected ventilation (Radford nomogram), and P_aCO_2 has been described.[39]

F. Airway Mechanics

In addition to detecting airway obstruction, adventitious sounds, and bronchospasm by listening to breath sounds, airway mechanics can be monitored in more quantitative terms. The anesthesia machine and ventilator have pressure gauges. Dividing the peak and/or plateau (if present) pressure during inspiration into the tidal volume (as measured by a spirometer) allows one to calculate dynamic and static lung compliance, respectively. At the mid- to higher-tier II level, whole lung and individual lung airway pressures and tidal volumes should be measured separately, so that the compliance of the whole lung and each individual lung can be calculated separately. Knowledge of individual lung compliance allows the anesthesiologist to know what compliance each lung should have after any thoracic procedure (but especially after unilateral lung lavage); this number should serve as the end point for postoperative individual lung PEEP and sighing maneuvers.

In patients who have undergone long operations, have experienced many physiological interventions, or have received large amounts of anesthetic drugs, it is both reasonable and wise to question whether they will be able to breathe adequately spontaneously following such an anesthetic and surgical experience. In an attempt to identify those few variables that singly or in combination best predict the outcome of the first trial of spontaneous respiration following cardiac surgery, a stepwise linear discriminant analysis of over 50 physiologic and clinical predictors of postoperative respiratory adequacy indicated that postoperative vital capacity per kilogram and maximum inspiratory force were the most useful variables. The difference between extubation successes and failures is represented by a vital capacity of 15 ml/kg and a maximum inspiratory force of 28 cm H_2O.[40] Measurements of passive pulmonary mechanics, cardiac function, and arterial blood gases were surprisingly poor predictors (however, see use of $P_{\bar{v}}O_2$ and $S_{\bar{v}}O_2$ in section E of Tier III).

G. Cardiovascular Parameters

Since both hypovolemia and hypervolemia have important implications for gas exchange, increased monitoring efforts should be directed toward monitoring the blood pressure and blood volume. Systemic arterial blood pressure and central venous pressure can be accurately measured by direct catheter monitoring and can be displayed on an oscilloscope. Insertion of an indwelling peripheral arterial catheter is sufficiently justified for hemodynamic monitoring in patients who have moderate cardiovascular compromise or in patients who will undergo moderately physiologically intrusive operations. When used with a paper read-out, the trend in arterial pressure is readily demonstrated and frequently reveals changes in hemodynamic status that might not otherwise be appreciated. An electrical mean pressure can be calculated, allowing for a more precise measurement of perfusion pressure. Finally, a rough estimate of myocardial contractility can be made by observing the steepness of the upstroke of the arterial pressure waveform. The combined hemodynamic and blood gas measurement indications for arterial line insertion at the tier II level virtually guarantees that almost all patients at the tier II level should have an indwelling arterial catheter placed. In patients without significant cardiovascular disease, central venous pressure monitoring will track intravascular volume satisfactorily (see Cardiovascular Parameters under Tier III: Advanced Monitoring Techniques).

Input and output balance can be followed more closely by weighing all sponges and by measuring the urine output from a Foley catheter every half hour. Hematocrit values, osmolality, and serum electrolytes can be measured intermittently. These measurements, in addition to essential monitoring, will reflect the contribution of the cardiovascular system to respiratory function.

IV. TIER III: ADVANCED MONITORING TECHNIQUES

Patients who have severe pre-existing respiratory disease and/or especially severe special intraoperative conditions are a challenge because the potential for respiratory function to deteriorate is great. For example, an elderly patient with severe chronic obstructive pulmonary disease undergoing a major pulmonary resection or esophagogastrectomy is a likely candidate for having some degree of postoperative respiratory failure. Similarly, some patients are so critically ill preoperatively (e.g.,

thoracic trauma, bleeding, sepsis) that anesthetic requirements are minimal and the anesthesiologist's main concerns reside in resuscitation and monitoring. Under these circumstances maximum monitoring of cardiopulmonary function is necessary to keep those physiologic variables related to respiratory function as near to normal as possible. The following sections discuss advanced monitoring techniques for respiratory functions E to G in Table 7–2 that further increase the degree of accuracy and rapidity of diagnosis and treatment of cardiac and/or pulmonary failure. Monitoring techniques for respiratory functions A to D, H, and I in Table 7–2 are the same as those described in previous sections.

E. Gas Exchange

The amount of total venous admixture ($\dot{Q}_s/\dot{Q}_t$) can be measured accurately in the clinical setting, provided a pulmonary artery catheter is in situ. To determine $\dot{Q}_s/\dot{Q}_t$ properly, the partial pressure of oxygen in the pulmonary artery mixed venous and systemic arterial blood ($P_{\bar{v}}O_2$ and P_aO_2, respectively), the partial pressure of carbon dioxide in arterial blood (P_aCO_2), hemoglobin concentration, and the inspired oxygen concentration need to be measured. From these data the content of oxygen in mixed venous ($C_{\bar{v}}O_2$), arterial (C_aO_2), and end-pulmonary capillary blood ($C_{c'}O_2$) can be calculated (see chapter 3). Knowing these various oxygen contents enables calculation of $\dot{Q}_s/\dot{Q}_t$:

$$\frac{\dot{Q}_s}{\dot{Q}_t} = \frac{C_{c'}O_2 - C_aO_2}{C_{c'}O_2 - C_{\bar{v}}O_2}$$

In addition, if the cardiac output is known (which should be the case if a pulmonary artery catheter is in situ; see Cardiovascular Parameters, following), V_{O_2} can be calculated by the Fick principle:

$$\dot{V}_{O_2} = \dot{Q}_t \times C(a-\bar{v})O_2$$

The normal arteriovenous oxygen content difference [$C(a-\bar{v})O_2$] is 5 vol per cent. It is important that the $P_{\bar{v}}O_2$ be measured directly. If the content of mixed venous blood is simply assumed to be 5 vol per cent less than arterial blood, rather than actually measured, large errors in the $\dot{Q}_s/\dot{Q}_t$ determination may be encountered.[41] For example, if the $C(a-\bar{v})O_2$ is really only half or twice normal, then the $\dot{Q}_s/\dot{Q}_t$ determined by assuming 5 vol per cent will be

50 per cent lower and 100 per cent higher, respectively, than it really is. Similarly, large errors in the shunt determination will be encountered if superior vena cava blood samples are substituted for pulmonary artery samples in the calculation of $C_{\bar{v}}O_2$.[42]

In addition, direct measurement of $P_{\bar{v}}O_2$ can serve as an indirect monitor of P_aO_2, oxygen consumption, and cardiac output (see Cardiovascular Parameters, following); a decrease in $P_{\bar{v}}O_2$ may reflect either a decrease in P_aO_2 or cardiac output or an increase in oxygen consumption. Therefore, the $P_{\bar{v}}O_2$ should not be regarded as having much specificity as a monitor of arterial oxygenation. Since the best use of $P_{\bar{v}}O_2$ and $S_{\bar{v}}O_2$ may be as a monitor of global well-being, it is not surprising that an $S_{\bar{v}}O_2$ of less than 60 per cent ($P_{\bar{v}}O_2$ of approximately 30 mm Hg) has been found to be an extremely important criterion for the need for mechanical ventilation following cardiac surgery.[43]

Measurement of the inspired and expired concentration of respiratory gases by mass spectrometry is now extremely accurate, rapid, and commercially available and as such has been in progressively widespread clinical use over the past 10 years. A mass spectrometer causes the inspired and expired respiratory gases that will be measured to pass through a magnetic field that differentiates between and quantifies the different gases by deflecting the gases in an amount that is inversely proportional to the molecular weight of the gas.

End-tidal and inspired concentrations of eight gases (O_2, N_2, CO_2, N_2O, argon, halothane, enflurane, and isoflurane) can be measured from each patient. Continuous monitoring of the inspired oxygen concentration at the mouth or endotracheal tube confirms that a gas mixture of the required composition is being delivered and that rebreathing is not occurring. An alarm system can be included to detect any deviation of the gas mixture outside preset, adjustable limits, which can be selected appropriately for each patient. The most important breath-by-breath monitoring functions of a mass spectrometer are end-tidal carbon dioxide tension (to follow ventilation patterns), inspired oxygen concentrations (which are now a standard of anesthesia practice in all cases), and inspired and end-tidal anesthetic drug concentrations (for both clinical management and safety concerns).

The cost of a mass spectrometer alone (approximately $35,000) inhibits its use for single-patient monitoring. However, the monitoring cost per operating room can be reduced significantly by using one mass spectrometer that can rapidly sample many operating rooms on a rotating basis. The total equipment and installation cost of a single mass spectrometer designed to serve an entire operating room suite ($60,000) is competitive with the summed cost of individual CO_2, O_2, and halogenated drug analyzers for 5 to 10 operating rooms (Puritan Corp., personal communication). However, the mass spectrometer is proving so far to be a fairly delicate machine, and most users have experienced considerable amounts of time in which it is unavailable because of equipment malfunction.

Finally, progress has been made toward measuring S_aO_2 and P_aO_2 directly and continuously. This is an important step forward because presently used indirect estimates of P_aO_2 and P_aCO_2 (i.e., $P_{tc}O_2$ and $P_{tc}CO_2$) do not eliminate the need for arterial blood gas analysis, especially in unstable patients, and intermittent arterial blood samples only document what has occurred in the recent past, which is obviously of less value than present observation. Unfortunately, presently available indwelling intra-arterial continuous S_aO_2 electrodes are for single patient, short-term use only and are expensive ($200). These catheters usually require recalibration once every 12 to 24 hours, and they therefore do not replace the need for blood gas analysis. Although when functioning properly, they may greatly reduce the number of arterial blood gas samples required. However, and fortunately, electrode systems for continuously measuring arterial oxygen tension that are easy to calibrate, small (20 gauge), and inexpensive ($50) may be available in the next 2 years (American Bentley Co., personal communication). Pulmonary artery catheter systems for the continuous monitoring of mixed venous oxygen saturation are now available; $S_{\bar{v}}O_2$ and $P_{\bar{v}}O_2$ are necessary for the $\dot{Q}_s/\dot{Q}_t$ calculation. Since $S_{\bar{v}}O_2$ and $P_{\bar{v}}O_2$ are determined by the P_aO_2, cardiac output, and oxygen consumption, the absolute value and trend in mixed venous oxygenation can be considered as a monitor of total or global well-being. A decrease in $S_{\bar{v}}O_2$ and $P_{\bar{v}}O_2$ below normal values is never good and requires investigation of lung shunting, cardiac output, and oxygen consumption. Progress has also been made in the continuous direct measurement of P_aCO_2 (American Bentley Co., personal communication), since miniature intravascular Pco_2 sensors were first introduced several years ago.[44]

F. Airway Mechanics

Determination of compliance is simple because the measurements required are pressure and volume. Determination of airway resistance is more difficult because the measurements required are pressure and flow. Airway resistance is calculated as follows:

$$\text{Airway resistance} = \frac{\text{Pressure, cm } H_2O}{\text{Flow, L/min}}$$

Airflow can be measured with a pneumotachograph, which is a rapid-response measuring device based on a form of constant-orifice flowmeter. It consists of an airflow resistance, across which a pressure drop occurs, a differential pressure transducer, and a means of recording the output (the differential pressure translated into airflow rate). The useful range of airflow resistances is limited at low flow by a small pressure difference and at high flows by nonlinearity due to turbulence. If airway pressure is recorded as relative to atmospheric, then total (lung and chest wall) resistance is calculated. If airway pressure is relative to pleural pressure, then lung resistance is calculated. There does exist a clinically applicable technique for direct measurement of intrapleural pressure.[45] The monitoring of resistance allows for detection of subtle degrees of bronchospasm not possible by other means. However, at the present time, airway resistance measurements are largely a research technique.

The determination of functional residual capacity (FRC) during mechanical ventilation has become important in clinical investigation in anesthesiology and for diagnostic and therapeutic evaluation of patients in acute respiratory failure. Most previous methods used a closed-circuit helium dilution technique,[46-48] but a new sulfahexafluride method appears most promising.[49] Measurement of other lung volumes such as closing volume and volume of trapped gas are research tools.

G. Cardiovascular Parameters

Normally, and at the tier I and tier II levels, the central venous pressure (CVP) is an adequate index of intravascular volume (see the following discussion of use of CVP in normal hearts). However, in patients with abnormal hearts, and at the high tier II and tier III levels, central venous pressure may be an inadequate

and misleading index of intravascular volume, and the more sensitive method of pulmonary vascular pressure monitoring may be necessary to follow intravascular volume status. In addition, the cardiovascular status of the patient may be so precarious that it is also necessary to know other indices of cardiovascular function such as $P_{\bar{v}}O_2$, cardiac output, and systemic vascular resistance. Consequently, this section will consider the rationale for pulmonary vascular pressure monitoring, when it is inappropriate to use central venous pressure monitoring instead of pulmonary vascular pressure monitoring, the clinical value of inserting pulmonary artery catheters, and, finally, the complications of pulmonary artery catheter insertion.

1. Left Ventricular Preload and Left Ventricular Function

The Frank-Starling myocardial function curve states that as initial ventricular fiber length is increased, which is the ventricular preload, ventricular performance increases (force of fiber contraction increases) (Fig. 7–2). In the intact heart, initial fiber length is the end-diastolic fiber length, which is determined by the left ventricular end-diastolic volume (Fig. 7–3). Left ventricular end-diastolic volume can be measured intraoperatively by esophageal probe echocardiography, but the measurement is not widely available, and it can be technically difficult to obtain quantitatively accurate volumes.

Left Ventricular Function Curve

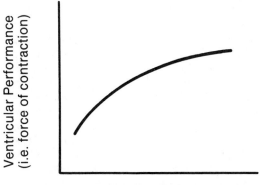

Figure 7–2. The Frank-Starling principle states that ventricular performance (i.e., force of contraction) is directly proportional to the preload (i.e., fiber length, ventricular end diastolic volume [VEDV]).

Indices of Left Ventricular Preload

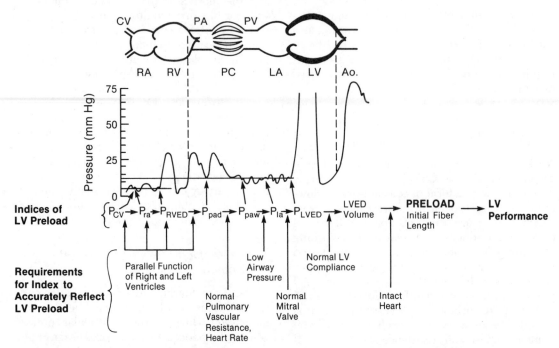

Figure 7–3. The figure dynamically describes the various indices of left ventricular preload. In the top portion of the diagram the various central vascular and cardiac chambers are schematically portrayed in the sequence that blood flows through them. The cardiac valves portray the end diastolic moment; the pulmonary and aortic valves are closed, and the mitral valve is open. In the graph below the cardiac chambers, the characteristic vascular pressure contours in each vascular compartment are depicted directly below each compartment. Below this graph the various indices of left ventricular preload are labelled; they consist mainly of the pressures within the various vascular compartments as well as two non-pressure indices on the right-hand side of the panel (volume and fiber length). At the bottom of the diagram the requirements for each of the indices to reflect accurately left ventricular preload are shown impacting between the index in question and the preceding closer approximation of left ventricular preload.

Consequently, other, more removed, indices of left ventricular preload are used clinically in the vast majority of cases. However, it should be noted that esophageal echocardiography can clearly demonstrate abnormalities of interventricular septal and ventricular wall motion (akinesia and dyskinesia) and valve function. The next few sections describe a series of progressively more removed and less accurate, but usually easier to obtain, indices of left ventricular preload (Fig. 7–3). Any factor that decreases the accuracy of a preceding index of left ventricular preload also decreases the accuracy of all of the succeeding (further removed) indices of left ventricular preload (Fig. 7–3).

The next closest approximation of left ventricular preload to left ventricular end-diastolic volume is left ventricular end-diastolic pressure. As left ventricular end-diastolic volume increases, left ventricular end-diastolic pressure increases (Fig. 7–4); the relationship between

ventricular volume and pressure is called ventricular compliance (compliance = volume/pressure). Thus, when left ventricular compliance is unchanging, left ventricular end-diastolic pressure should be directly proportional to left ventricular end-diastolic volume, fiber length, and ventricular output (Fig. 7–4, middle curve). If left ventricular compliance is decreased (stiffer, less distensible ventricle) so that the position of the left ventricular end-diastolic pressure-volume curve is shifted upward and to the left (Fig. 7–4, upper curve), then any given left ventricular end-diastolic volume will be associated with a higher left ventricular end-diastolic pressure. Conditions that decrease left ventricular compliance are myocardial ischemia, fibrosis, right-to-left interventricular septal shifts (as caused by right ventricular pressure loading [as caused by lung disease, PEEP, volume loading]), pericardial constriction, effusion and tamponade, systemic hyper-

LV Compliance

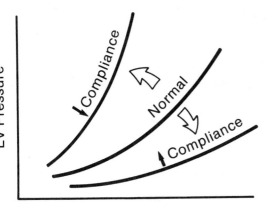

LV Volume

Figure 7–4. Left ventricular (LV) compliance is the slope of the curve relating left ventricular volume to left ventricular pressure. Three curves are shown: normal compliance, decreased compliance, and increased compliance. A ventricle that has decreased compliance is stiff and nondistensible and has a higher pressure than normal for any given volume. A ventricle that has increased compliance is soft and distensible and has a lower pressure than normal for any given volume. LV pressure will not accurately reflect LV volume when LV compliance is changing.

tension, aortic stenosis, and idiopathic hypertrophic subaortic stenosis.[50] If left ventricular compliance is increased (softer, more distensible ventricle) so that the position of the left ventricular end-diastolic pressure-volume curve is shifted downward and to the right (Fig. 7–4, lower curve), then any given left ventricular end-diastolic volume will be associated with a lower left ventricular end-diastolic pressure. Conditions that increase left ventricular compliance are administration of vasodilators such as nitroglycerin and nitroprusside, left-to-right interventricular septal shifts (as caused by right ventricular pressure unloading), congestive cardiomyopathies, and aortic and mitral regurgitation,[50] Thus, when left ventricular compliance changes, changes in left ventricular end-diastolic pressure (and the other, more removed various indices of preload [P_{pad}, P_{paw} and P_{cv}]) may not reflect left ventricular end-diastolic volume and may be difficult to interpret. For example, Figure 7–5 shows the effects of interventricular septal shifts on left ventricular compliance. With right-to-left shifts and decreased left ventricular compliance (Fig. 7–5, lower panel), decreased end-diastolic volumes are associated with increased end-diastolic pressures, and with left-to-right shifts and increased left

ventricular compliance (Fig. 7–5, middle panel), increased end-diastolic volumes are associated with normal or mildly decreased end-diastolic pressures.

Aside from the issue of left ventricular compliance, left ventricular end-diastolic pressure would frequently be a good index of left ventricular preload. However, there is not a good, safe (no puncture of ventricular wall) and easy (avoid retrograde technique) way of measuring left ventricular end-diastolic pressure. Consequently, other, more removed, but easier to obtain, indices of ventricular preload must be used clinically.

2. Various Indices of Left Ventricular End-Diastolic Pressure

A schematic representation of the central circulation is shown in Figure 7–3.[51] Above are the various vascular compartments; below are characteristic pressure contours recorded at each site. At the end of diastole, the pulmonic and aortic valves are closed, and the mitral valve is open. The entire vascular bed between the closed pulmonic and aortic valves behaves like a common fluid-filled pressure chamber. At the end of diastole, pressure should fall to the same level in all segments of the common pressure chamber, provided there is a sufficiently low resistance to blood flow and that there is a sufficient amount of time (slow enough heart rate) for the diastolic pressure run-off. End-diastolic pressure in the left ventricle determines the pressure level to which there is a pulmonary artery diastolic pressure run-off.

Therefore, at the end of diastole and under normal conditions, pressure at all points within the continuous chamber (namely, pressure in the left ventricle (LV), left atrium (LA), pulmonary veins (PV), pulmonary capillaries (PC), and pulmonary artery (PA) is the same. Thus, the pulmonary artery diastolic pressure (P_{pad}) should normally equal pulmonary artery wedge (P_{paw}) and left atrial (P_{la}) pressure, which should equal left ventricular end-diastolic pressure (P_{LVED}). As a corollary, in the absence of end-diastolic pressure gradients, there is no end-diastolic pulmonary blood flow.

a. LEFT ATRIAL PRESSURE

Mitral and aortic valve disease will create a left atrial pressure–to–left ventricular end-diastolic pressure gradient. Mitral stenosis causes left atrial pressure to be higher than left ven-

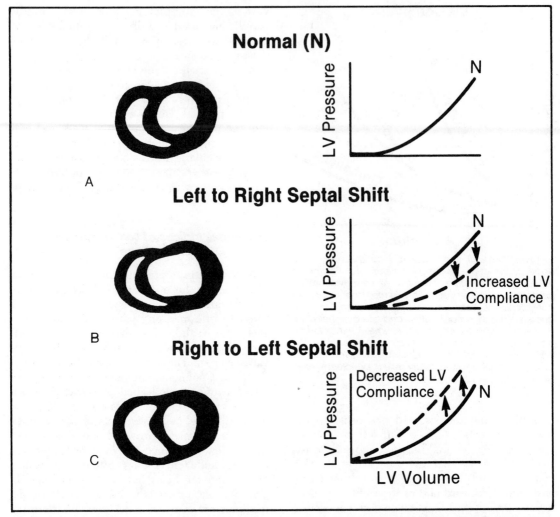

Figure 7–5. The effect of interventricular septal shifting (as might be caused by right ventricular volume and pressure loading and unloading) on left ventricular compliance. A, The interventricular septum in a normal position and accompanied by a normal (N) ventricular compliance curve. B, A left to right interventricular septal shift and an increase in left ventricular compliance (increased volumes with decreased pressures). C, A right to left interventricular septal shift and a decrease in left ventricular compliance (decreased volumes with increased pressure). (Data taken from reference 50.)

tricular end-diastolic pressure, and aortic regurgitation causes left atrial pressure to be lower than left ventricular end-diastolic pressure. These cardiac valve diseases affect the pulmonary artery wedge pressure in the same way as they do left atrial pressure.

b. PULMONARY ARTERY WEDGE PRESSURE

Inflation of the flotation balloon on a pulmonary artery catheter until pulmonary artery blood flow is completely obstructed creates a static column of fluid distal to the catheter tip, which extends across the pulmonary artery and capillaries over to the pulmonary veins (Fig.

7–6). The static column of fluid serves as an extension of the pulmonary artery catheter tip, and allows the catheter tip to "see" pressure on the left side of the pulmonary circulation. The pressure measured by the distal tip of the catheter beyond the obstructing balloon is called the "wedge" pressure (P_{paw}) and is precisely defined as the pressure in the pulmonary venous circulation where flow first begins beyond the static column of fluid. With the exception of the rare condition of pulmonary venous thrombosis, there are virtually no pressure gradients from the pulmonary venous circulation to the left atrium, and, therefore, the wedge pressure essentially measures left atrial pressure. Since the P_{paw} is essentially a direct measurement of pulmonary venous and left atrial pressures, P_{paw} equals left atrial pressure even in patients with very high pulmonary arterial vascular resistance (i.e., the point of resistance is completely proximal to the point of P_{paw} measurement).[52]

Pulmonary arterial wedge pressure (P_{paw}) is considered an accurate reflection of left atrial pressure (P_{la}) provided there is a continuous column of fluid between the wedged pulmonary arterial catheter tip and the left atrium (zone 3, a region within the lung where pulmonary arterial pressure [P_a] exceeds pulmonary venous pressure [P_v], which in turn exceeds alveolar pressure [P_A], $P_a > P_v > P_A$) (Fig. 7–6; see also Fig. 3–1). Positive end-expiratory pressure (PEEP) can result in intermittent collapse (zone 2, $P_a > P_A > P_v$) and perhaps continuous collapse (zone 1, $P_A > P_a > P_v$) of this column

of fluid, depending upon the magnitude of PEEP, the vertical hydrostatic gradient between the wedged pulmonary arterial catheter tip and the left atrium, the transmission of PEEP to the pulmonary vasculature as a function of pulmonary parenchymal compliance, and the pressure changes occurring in the pleural space during the ventilatory cycle. If the fluid column between the pulmonary artery catheter tip and left atrium is collapsed by alveolar pressure (Figs. 7–6 and 7–7), the catheter tip can only sense the interrupting alveolar pressure and reflect PEEP rather than the downstream P_{la}. A study conducted with dogs with normal lungs and normal P_{la} during controlled positive-pressure ventilation demonstrated that a progressive increase in PEEP $\geq$ 5 mm Hg produced a progressive positive discrepancy between P_{paw} and P_{la} (i.e., $P_{paw} > P_{la}$) when the pulmonary arterial catheter was wedged above

Pulmonary Artery Wedge Pressure Measurement

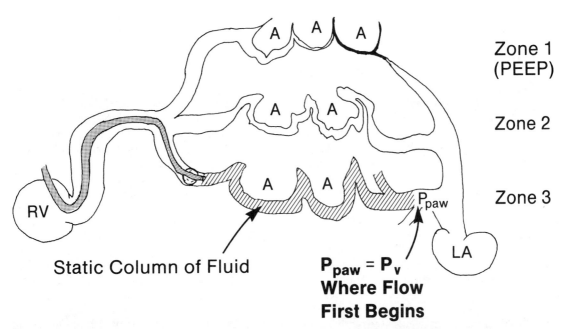

Figure 7–6. The mechanism by which pulmonary artery wedge pressure (P_{paw}) records left atrial pressure. When the balloon on the pulmonary artery catheter is inflated, a static column of fluid is created distal to the catheter tip, which serves as an extension of the catheter over to the venous side of the pulmonary circulation. This system (fluid-filled catheter plus static column of blood) will record the pressure that is present in the pulmonary circulation where flow first begins (beyond the static column of blood). Consequently, the pulmonary artery wedge pressure (P_{paw}) is a pulmonary venous pressure (P_v). Since there is virtually no pressure gradient between the pulmonary veins and the left atrium, the P_{paw} is, for all intents and purposes, equal to left atrial pressure. Since the pulmonary veins are continuously collapsed in zone 1 and intermittently collapsed in zone 2, the P_{paw} may not accurately reflect left atrial pressure in these regions of the lung.

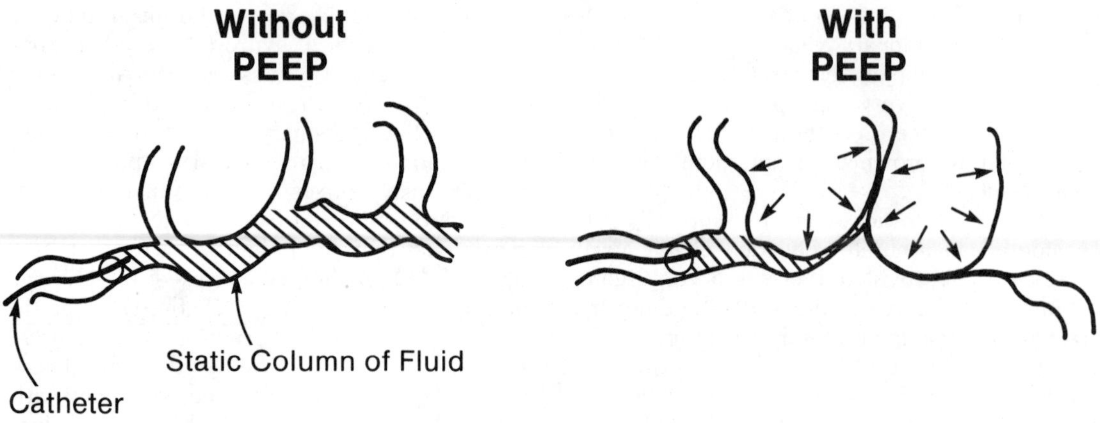

Without PEEP

With PEEP

Static Column of Fluid

Catheter

Factors Causing Preservation of $P_{paw} = P_{la}$ During PEEP

1. Location of catheter in dependent lung (Zone 3)
2. Maintenance of some spontaneous ventilation (venous return)
3. Non-compliant lung (decreased transmission of PEEP)

Figure 7–7. In the clinical situation, zone 1 conditions are created by the application of positive end-expiratory pressure (PEEP). PEEP may collapse the pulmonary capillaries, interrupting the static column of fluid normally created by inflation of the pulmonary artery catheter balloon. Consequently, the pulmonary artery wedge pressure (P_{paw}) will sense alveolar pressure (PEEP) rather than a downstream of vascular pressure (left atrial pressure [P_{la}]). Several commonly present clinical conditions tend to preserve the P_{paw} as a reflection of P_{la} even when PEEP is being used; these consist of dependent lung catheterization, presence of spontaneous ventilation, and noncompliance of the lung.

the left atrium.[53] When the pulmonary artery catheter was wedged below the left atrium it was not possible to create a $P_{paw} - P_{la}$ gradient with even high levels of PEEP.

In summary, high levels of PEEP can cause P_{paw} to be falsely high (i.e., cause the pulmonary artery catheter to "see" the PEEP and not P_{la}) compared with true P_{la} when the pulmonary artery catheter locates in a nondependent position. However, and fortunately, there are three factors that are usually present in critically ill patients that greatly minimize the potential for PEEP-induced $P_{paw} - P_{la}$ gradients. First, most pulmonary artery catheters are located in the dependent regions of the lung (i.e., zone 3).[54, 55] Second, most critically ill patients have somewhat noncompliant lungs that do not readily transmit alveolar pressure.[56, 57] Third, many critically ill patients are ventilated with an intermittent mandatory/spontaneous ventilation pattern that facilitates maintenance of venous return and normal pulmonary venous pressure. Consequently, the P_{paw} is probably an accurate reflection of P_{la} during the application of low to moderate levels of PEEP in critically ill patients.

C. PULMONARY ARTERY DIASTOLIC PRESSURE

Normally, pulmonary artery diastolic pressure equals left ventricular end-diastolic pressure. In Figure 7–8, pulmonary arterial (heavy line) and left ventricular (thin line) blood pressures are superimposed upon one another during three conditions: (1) normal circumstance (A), (2) in the presence of left ventricular failure (B), and (3) in the presence of increased pulmonary vascular resistance (C).[51] In the first two instances both diastolic blood pressures fall to the same level at the end of diastole (single arrow). The pulmonary hypertension shown in Fig. 7–8B is a passive consequence of the increased left ventricular end-diastolic pressure. The vessel walls remain thin and distensible under these conditions and do not impose an appreciable increase in resistance to blood flow. In contrast, the panel on the right illustrates that when pulmonary hypertension stems from abnormal structure or function of the pulmonary vessels, pressure in the pulmonary artery will exceed the left ventricular pressure at the end of diastole, as indicated by the two arrows. Disease has rendered the pulmonary

Normal   **Pulmonary Hypertension**

LV Failure   Increased Pulmonary
Vascular Resistance

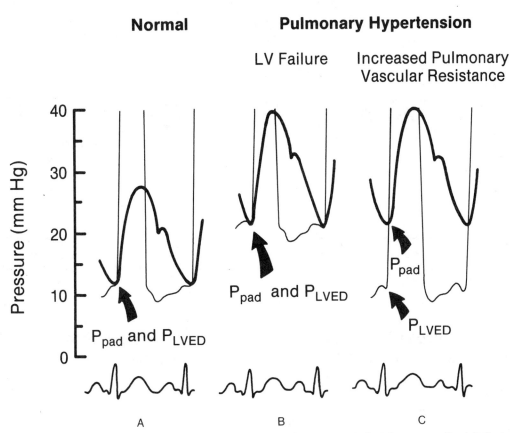

Figure 7–8. A, *Pulmonary diastolic pressure (P_{pad}) equals left ventricular end diastolic pressure (P_{LVED}). B, During left ventricular failure, P_{pad} is passively and mechanically elevated to the same level as P_{LVED}. C, In the presence of increased pulmonary vascular resistance, P_{pad} is elevated above P_{LVED}. (Modified with permission from Enson Y: Pulmonary heart disease: Relation of pulmonary hypertension to abnormal lung structure and function. Bull NY Acad Med 53:551–566, 1977.)*

vessels sufficiently obstructed so that resistance to blood flow is greatly increased. The vertical distance between the two arrows, which represents the end-diastolic pressure gradient between the pulmonary artery and the left ventricle, is proportional to the increase in pulmonary vascular resistance. In summary, when pulmonary vascular resistance is normal, pressure in the pulmonary artery during diastole can run off to and decrease to left ventricular end-diastolic pressure (Fig. 7–9, upper panel); whereas when pulmonary vascular resistance is increased, pressure in the pulmonary artery during diastole cannot run off to and decrease to left ventricular end-diastolic pressure (Fig. 7–9, lower panel).

Increased resistance to flow can be caused by both passive mechanical and active vasoconstrictor mechanisms. The passive mechanical mechanisms consist of capillary and venous compression by interstitial fluid and/or blood and/or fibrosis, endothelial cell edema, capillary

compression by PEEP, arterial obstruction by thrombosis and/or microembolism, and medial hypertrophy. The active vasoconstriction mediators can be alveolar hypoxia, systemically released vasoconstrictor amines and peptides, decreased mixed venous oxygen tension, and acidosis (Fig. 7–10).[58] These changes result in an increase in pulmonary vascular resistance, which is "a universal feature of acute respiratory failure."[59] Tachycardia (heart rate greater than 120/min) can also independently cause an end-diastolic pressure gradient (as much as 10 mm Hg) between the pulmonary artery and left ventricle because of insufficient diastolic run-off time.[60] Thus, in patients with acute respiratory failure who have the above pathologic changes and often an associated tachycardia, it is likely that pulmonary artery diastolic pressure will be higher than left ventricular end-diastolic pressure.

A pulmonary artery catheter should be floated to the most proximal position from which

Pulmonary Artery Diastolic Pressure Monitoring

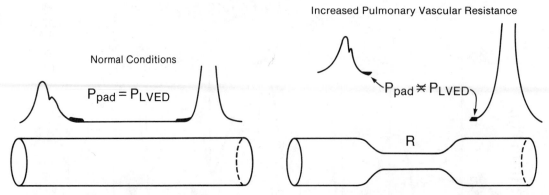

Figure 7–9. *During normal conditions, pressure in the pulmonary artery during diastole (P_{pad}) can decrease to left ventricular end diastolic pressure (P_{LVED}). When pulmonary vascular resistance (R) is increased, P_{pad} cannot run off to or decrease to the P_{LVED} level.*

Causes of Increased Pulmonary Vascular Resistance in Acute and Chronic Lung Disease

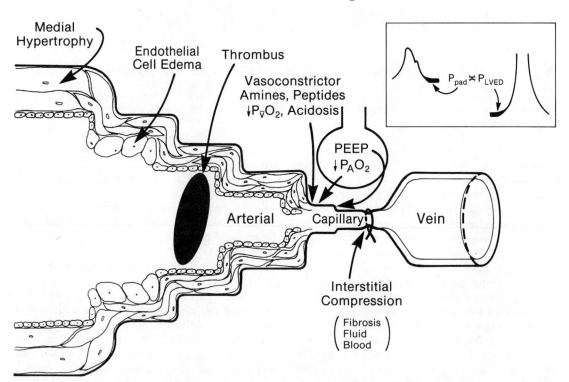

Figure 7–10. *The causes of increased pulmonary vascular resistance during acute and chronic respiratory failure are multiple. In an anatomical progression from the arterial to the venous side of the pulmonary circulation, the causes of increased pulmonary vascular resistance consist of medial hypertrophy, endothelial cell edema, pulmonary thromboembolism, arteriolar constriction by vasoactive amines, peptides, decreased mixed venous oxygen tension ($\downarrow P_{\bar{v}}O_2$), acidosis, and alveolar hypoxia ($\downarrow P_AO_2$). Positive end-expiratory pressure (PEEP) can compress the pulmonary capillaries. Increased interstitial hydrostatic pressure due to transudated fluid and blood, which can later fibrose, can compress the venous side of the pulmonary capillaries. All these causes of increased pulmonary vascular resistance will create a pulmonary artery diastolic (P_{pad}) to left ventricular end diastolic pressure (P_{LVED}) gradient (see inset).*

both a wedge pressure and phasic pulmonary artery pressure can be obtained by simple sequential inflation and deflation of the flotation balloon. If the catheter floats out too far in the peripheral lung parenchyma, it may permanently wedge and greatly increase the risk of pulmonary infarction. If the catheter is floated to a too proximal position in the main pulmonary artery, the catheter tip may intermittently whip or dip into and out of the right ventricle. Under these circumstances, the "diastolic" pressure may be intermittently too low because several of the recorded beats will have actually been right ventricular (diastolic pressure in the right ventricle is close to zero).

3. Various Indices of Right Ventricular End-Diastolic Pressure

If the right and left ventricle have parallel function, then right ventricular end-diastolic pressure should follow left ventricular end-diastolic pressure. The difference in absolute value between the two end-diastolic pressures would be caused only by the difference in compliance between the two ventricles; the right ventricle, being more compliant than the left ventricle, has a lower end-diastolic pressure (see Normal Heart as follows). With this reservation in mind, various indices of right ventricular end-diastolic pressure can be used to assess preload clinically.

a. RIGHT ATRIAL PRESSURE

Tricuspid and pulmonic valve disease will create a right atrial–to–right ventricular end-diastolic pressure gradient. Tricuspid stenosis causes right atrial pressure to be higher than right ventricular end-diastolic pressure, and pulmonic regurgitation causes right atrial pressure to be lower than right ventricular end-diastolic pressure.

b. CENTRAL VENOUS PRESSURE

In order to clearly answer the question of whether or when central venous, as opposed to pulmonary vascular, pressure monitoring can be used (P_{cv} versus P_{pad} and P_{paw} to assess preload, it is necessary to consider the answer separately for a normal heart versus an abnormal heart.

(1) **Normal Heart.** The left ventricle is a thickly muscled (walled) cavity and therefore is relatively noncompliant (Fig. 7–11, right-hand panel). When fluid is systemically infused (pre-

load increased), the increase in left ventricular end-diastolic volume causes a large increase in left ventricular end-diastolic pressure (as measured by P_{pad} or P_{paw}). The right ventricle is a thinly muscled (walled) cavity and therefore is relatively compliant (Fig. 7–11, left-hand panel). The infusion of fluids systemically causes the increase in right ventricular end-diastolic volume to be accompanied by only a relatively small increase in right ventricular end-diastolic pressure (as measured by central venous pressure [P_{CV}]. Thus, when intravascular volume is acutely increased, the P_{CV} increases only a small amount compared with a relatively large increase in the wedge pressure.[61] Indeed, when preload is manipulated in normal patients (fluid infusion or diuresis[62] or by position changes[63]) and simultaneous measurements of the P_{CV} and P_{paw} are made, the initial and final absolute P_{paw} is always approximately 100 per cent greater than P_{CV} (Figs. 7–11 and 7–12). In other words, initial and final P_{paw} is twice as great as the initial and final P_{CV}, and the change in P_{paw} is always approximately twice the change in the P_{CV} (Figs. 7–11 and 7–12). Thus, in a normal heart, there is an orderly and predictable relationship between the filling pressures of the right and left hearts, and the P_{CV} can be used to follow left heart function.

However, in view of the fact that the regression line relating P_{CV} (x-axis) to P_{pad} and P_{paw} (y-axis) in relatively normal patients has an average slope of 2 (which means P_{paw} changes twice as much as the P_{CV}) (Fig. 7–12),[61-63] the P_{paw} may be easier, and perhaps more reliable, to use than the P_{CV} to follow intravascular volume status. In other words, it may be easier to distinguish physiologically meaningful changes above and beyond the usual background noise and variation in the P_{paw} compared with the P_{CV}. In addition, it is not known how other changes (e.g., afterload and changes in myocardial contractility) in normal patients will affect simultaneously measured P_{CV} and P_{pad} and P_{paw}.[64] In summary, because the right and left hearts have an orderly and predictable functional relationship to one another in the normal heart, the P_{CV} may be used as a substitute for pulmonary vascular pressure monitoring in normal patients, but the changes in P_{CV} will be less marked than those that might be observed in P_{paw}.

(2) **Abnormal Heart.** In an abnormal heart, left and right heart ventricular function curves (filling pressure versus output) may be markedly different from one another. For example, it is

P_{CV} versus P_{pad} and P_{paw}

Preload Changes, Normal Heart

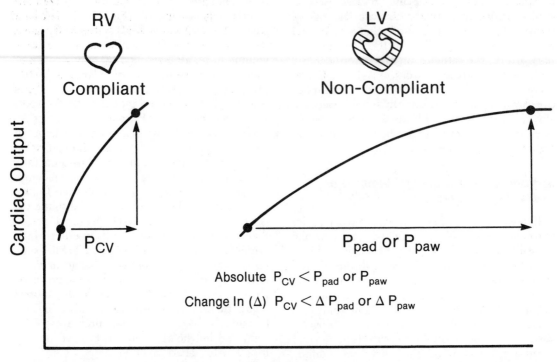

Figure 7–11. *The relationship between central venous pressure (P_{CV}) and pulmonary artery wedge pressure (P_{paw}) and pulmonary artery diastolic pressure (P_{pad}) is normally based on the differences in compliance between the right ventricle (RV) and the left ventricle (LV). The right ventricle is relatively compliant because it is thinly muscled, and the left ventricle is relatively noncompliant because it is thickly muscled. Thus, when preload is changed in a normal heart (such as with fluid infusion), the central venous pressure (as a reflection of right ventricular end diastolic pressure) increases only a small amount for a given increase in cardiac output, whereas the pulmonary artery wedge pressure and pulmonary artery diastolic pressure (as reflections of left ventricular end diastolic pressure) increase a large amount for the same increase in cardiac output. Thus, due to the differences in compliance between the two ventricles, the absolute central venous pressure is always less than the pulmonary artery wedge and pulmonary artery diastolic pressure, and the change in the central venous pressure is always less than the change in pulmonary artery wedge and pulmonary artery diastolic pressure.*

possible to have a failing right ventricle and a normal left ventricle, resulting in a high P_{CV} and a low P_{paw}, whereas with an ischemic left ventricle and a normal right ventricle (which is not an uncommon combination), P_{paw} will be high while P_{CV} may be low (Fig. 7–13). Consequently, the discrepancy between the P_{CV} and the P_{pad} and P_{paw} increases a great deal when intravascular volume is augmented in patients with heart disease,[63, 64] and it is usually misleading to use the P_{CV} as a meaningful guide to the filling pressures of the left side of the heart. Thus, candidates for pulmonary vascular pressure monitoring include all patients who have

any significant myocardial compromise who are undergoing significant perioperative period stress.

4. Clinical Value of the Pulmonary Artery Catheter (Fig. 7–14)

From the foregoing discussion, it is clear that measurements of P_{pad} and P_{paw} are clinically useful; however, the pulmonary artery catheter is valuable in a number of other ways. Left ventricular ischemia causes the left ventricle to become less compliant (stiffer), which may re-

P_{CV} versus P_{paw}

Preload Changes, Normal Heart

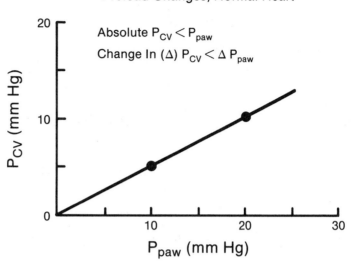

Figure 7–12. Summary of data from references 62 and 63 in which simultaneous measurements of central venous pressure (P_{cv}) and pulmonary artery wedge pressure (P_{paw}) were made during preload changes in patients with normal hearts. The absolute level of the pulmonary artery wedge pressure was always twice that of the central venous pressure, and the change in pulmonary artery wedge pressure was always twice the change in central venous pressure.

P_{CV} versus P_{pad} and P_{paw}

Abnormal Heart

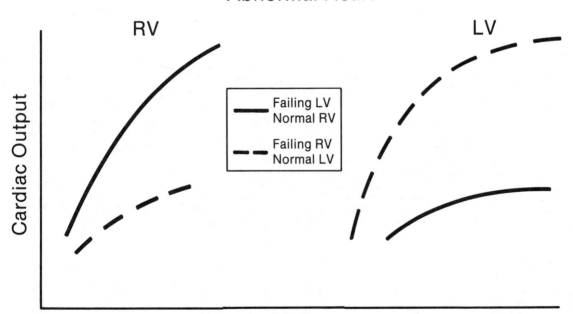

Figure 7–13. Patients with abnormal hearts may have either a normal right ventricular (RV) and an abnormal left ventricular (LV) function curve (most common) (solid line) or an abnormal RV function curve and a normal LV function curve (less common) (dashed line).

Clinical Value of Pulmonary Artery Catheter

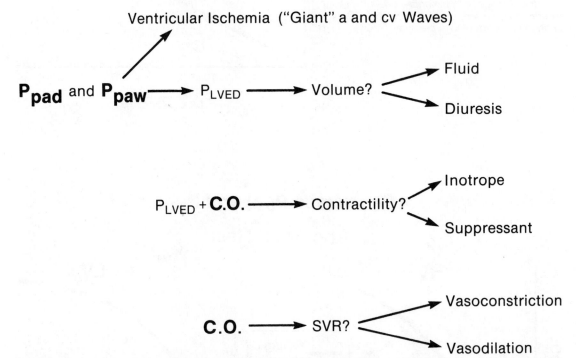

Figure 7-14. The clinical value of the pulmonary artery catheter is great. Measurement of pulmonary artery diastolic (P_{pad}) and pulmonary artery wedge (P_{paw}) pressures can be early indicators of left ventricular ischemia (increase in mean pressure and the appearance of "giant" a and cv waves). These two pressures allow estimation of left ventricular end diastolic pressure (P_{LVED}), which allows for assessment of intravascular volume, and based on this assessment decisions regarding preload changes (position, fluid infusion, or diuresis) can be made objectively. Measurement of the cardiac output (C.O.) along with P_{paw} allows for estimation of myocardiac contractility and for an objective decision to be made as to whether inotropic or suppressant drugs should be used. Measurement of cardiac output along with systemic pressure allows for determination of systemic vascular resistance (SVR) and for an objective decision to be made as to whether vasodilator or vasoconstrictor drugs should be used.

sult in increased pulmonary vascular pressures (P_{pad} and P_{paw}). In addition, and just as important, left ventricular ischemia may also cause a change in the morphology of the a, c, and v waves on the P_{paw} trace (Fig. 7–15). The a wave is caused by atrial contraction, and atrial contraction into a stiff ventricle may cause the appearance of "giant" a waves on the P_{paw} trace (Fig. 7–16). The c wave is caused by bulging of the mitral valve into the left atrium during isovolemic ventricular contraction. If ventricular ischemia also causes the papillary muscles supporting the mitral valve to dysfunction, so that mitral regurgitation occurs, "giant" cv waves will appear on the P_{paw} trace (Fig. 7–16).[65]

Much more commonly, knowledge of P_{pad} and P_{paw} allows for assessment of intravascular volume (preload). Knowledge of pulmonary vascular pressure along with cardiac output (which can be determined easily, rapidly, and repetitively with a thermodilution pulmonary artery catheter) allows for assessment of myocardial contractility. Knowledge of cardiac output along with systemic and pulmonary vascular pressures allows for calculation of systemic and pulmonary vascular resistances, respectively. Knowledge of cardiac output along with heart rate allows for calculation of stroke volume. Measurement of $P_{\bar{v}}O_2$ (pulmonary artery blood) allows for

calculation of $\dot{Q}_s/\dot{Q}_t$, and $P_{\bar{v}}O_2$ alone can be used as an indirect gross measure of cardiac output and oxygen consumption.

Figure 7–17 illustrates the great hemodynamic insight that pulmonary artery catheter monitoring can provide. The upper panel of the figure shows examples of typical and uncomplicated hemodynamic data for two common pathologic conditions (hypovolemia versus cardiac failure due to myocardial infarction). In both hemodynamic syndromes, or constellations, systemic pressure (P_{sa}), central venous pressure (P_{CV}), heart rate (HR), cardiac output (CO) and systemic vascular resistance (SVR) are identical, or at least quite similar, and the differential diagnosis between the two conditions is not possible without measurement of pulmonary vascular pressure. With simple hypovolemia the heart is normal, and the CVP and P_{paw} correlate, whereas with myocardial infarction the heart is abnormal and the CVP and P_{paw} do not correlate. Consequently, the pulmonary vascular pressures are shaded in and are the key differentiating factors. Note that the correct diagnosis dictates therapy strategies that are quite different.

Similarly, the lower panel of Figure 7–17 shows that measurement of P_{sa}, CVP, and heart rate may not be dramatically different during

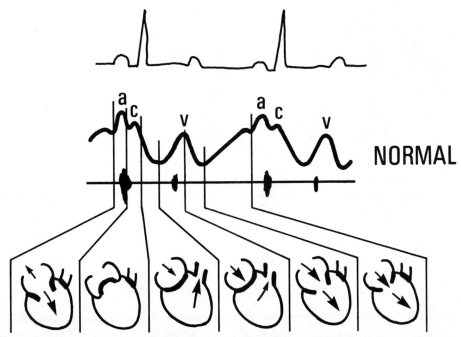

Figure 7–15. The cardiac cycle and the genesis of a, c, and v waves. The a wave is caused by atrial contraction. The c wave is caused by the bulging of the atrioventricular valve into the atrium during isovolemic ventricular contraction. The v wave is caused by venous filling.

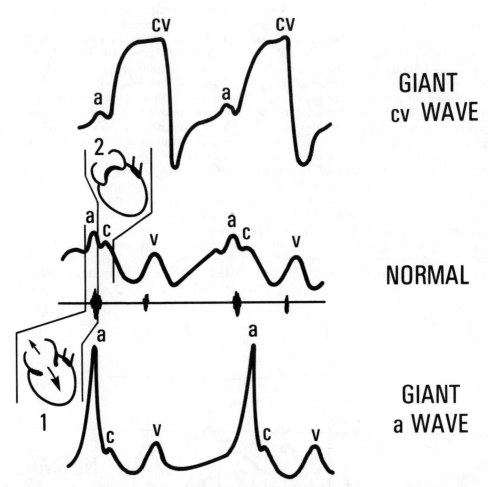

Figure 7-16. Giant a waves are caused by atrial contraction into a noncompliant stiff ventricle (as may be caused by ventricular ischemia). Giant cv waves are really giant c waves and are due to atrioventricular valve regurgitation when the supporting papillary muscles dysfunction (as may be caused by ventricular ischemia).

DECISION ANALYSIS – HEMODYNAMIC DATA

P_{sa}	P_{CV}	HR	CO	SVR	P_{paw}	DIAGNOSIS	THERAPY
↓	↓	↑	↓	↑	↓	HYPOVOL-EMIA	GIVE VOLUME
↓	↓ or N	↑	↓	↑	↑	CARDIAC FAILURE (MI)	1. ↑ CONTRACTILITY 2. ? VOLUME 3. ? VASODILATE

DECISION ANALYSIS – HEMODYNAMIC DATA

P_{sa}	P_{CV}	HR	CO	SVR	P_{paw}	DIAGNOSIS	THERAPY
N or ↓	N or ↓	↑	↑	↓↓	N	SEPSIS	VASOCONTRICTION
N or ↑	N or ↑	↑	↓	↑↑	↑	CARDIAC FAILURE (↑ afterload)	VASODILATION

Figure 7–17. Data from a pulmonary artery catheter can be the differentiating factor among clinical syndromes that otherwise might appear hemodynamically similar. The shaded boxes provide the key hemodynamic data for diagnostic analysis and therapeutic decision making. See text for fuller explanation and definition of abbreviations.

sepsis and cardiac failure (due to very increased systemic afterload). However, measurement of cardiac output and systemic vascular resistance clearly differentiates between the two conditions and would result in very different treatment strategies.

5. Special Pulmonary Vascular Monitoring Considerations Related to Thoracotomy in the Lateral Decubitus Position

Pulmonary arterial catheters usually (greater than 90 per cent) float to and locate in the right lung.[54] Consequently, during a right thoracotomy (left lateral decubitus position), the pulmonary artery catheter will be in the nondependent lung and, therefore, either in a collapsed lung if one-lung ventilation is employed or possibly in a zone 1 or 2 region of the lung if large tidal volume two-lung ventilation is employed. Conversely, when a left tho-

racotomy is performed (patient in the right lateral decubitus position), the pulmonary artery catheter will be in the dependent lung and will probably be in a zone 3 region. Thus, it is theoretically possible that the pulmonary artery catheter might function differently or yield different pulmonary vascular pressure and cardiac output data during right versus left thoracotomies and during two-lung versus one-lung ventilation.

Indeed, with the pulmonary artery catheter tip located in the right lung, the cardiac output is lower during right thoracotomy with one-lung ventilation (right lung collapsed) than during left thoracotomy with one-lung ventilation (left lung collapsed) in patients who were otherwise similar (Fig. 7–18A).[66] Consequently, it is possible that when the pulmonary artery catheter is located in the collapsed lung, where blood flow patterns may be distorted or the function of the thermistor interfered with (not free in the lumen of the vessel), the measured

Conditions During Thoracotomy in Lateral Decubitus Position When Pulmonary Artery Catheter Data May be Inaccurate

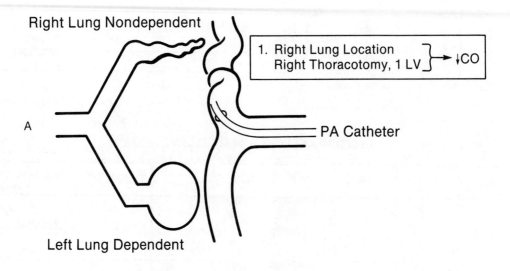

Right Lung Nondependent

1. Right Lung Location
   Right Thoracotomy, 1 LV $\rightarrow$ $\downarrow$CO

A

PA Catheter

Left Lung Dependent

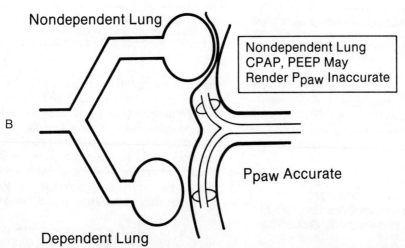

Nondependent Lung

Nondependent Lung
CPAP, PEEP May
Render P$_{paw}$ Inaccurate

B

P$_{paw}$ Accurate

Dependent Lung

Figure 7–18. Conditions during thoracotomy in the lateral decubitus position when pulmonary artery catheter data may be inaccurate. A, During right thoracotomy with a pulmonary artery (PA) catheter located in the collapsed right lung (one-lung ventilation [1LV]), the cardiac output (C.O.) may be lower than when the right lung is ventilated. The thermistor in the collapsed lung may be exposed to abnormal flow patterns or vascular wall interference. B, When the pulmonary artery catheter is in the nondependent lung and the nondependent lung is exposed to CPAP or PEEP, the pulmonary artery wedge pressure (P$_{paw}$) may be inaccurate. Nondependent lung CPAP or PEEP may cause zone 1 conditions in the nondependent lung. The P$_{paw}$ is probably always reasonably accurate when the pulmonary artery catheter is in the dependent lung, even if the dependent lung is exposed to PEEP.

output is indeed lower. This hypothesis is supported by the concurrent finding that continuously measured mixed venous oxygen saturation is also decreased during right thoracotomies compared with left thoracotomies when the pulmonary artery catheter is located in the collapsed nondependent lung. The decrease in mixed venous oxygen saturation may have been caused by stagnant blood flow and, therefore, not truly representative of whole patient mixed venous oxygen saturation.[66] When the nondependent lung is ventilated with varying levels of PEEP (in contrast to nondependent lung collapse), there is no difference in the cardiac output measured simultaneously from thermistors located in the nondependent and dependent lungs.[67] This finding implies that when the pulmonary artery catheter tip is in the nondependent lung and the nondependent lung is ventilated, blood flow to the nondependent lung is undistorted and/or there is no interference with the function of the thermistor.

When the pulmonary artery catheter is in the nondependent lung and the nondependent lung is ventilated with large tidal volume, PEEP, or CPAP, the wedge pressure may not reflect left atrial pressure (Fig. 7–18B).[56] When the pulmonary artery catheter is in the dependent lung and presumably in the zone 3 region, wedge pressure should accurately reflect left atrial pressure even when PEEP is applied to the dependent lung.[56]

In summary, the lateral decubitus position is important with regard to pulmonary artery catheter monitoring in three situations. First, when the nondependent lung is collapsed and the catheter is in the nondependent lung, the measured cardiac output and $P_{\bar{v}}O_2$ may be decreased compared with more normal conditions or the "real" value. Second, when the nondependent lung is ventilated with positive end-expiratory pressure and the catheter is in the nondependent lung, P_{paw} may not equal P_{la}. Third, when the catheter is in the dependent lung, P_{paw} will be a faithful index of P_{la} even if PEEP is used.

6. Risks and Complications of Pulmonary Vascular Pressure Monitoring

Pulmonary vascular pressure monitoring is an invasive and sophisticated procedure and consequently involves numerous potential physical risks and requires intelligent and informed interpretation of the results. The physical risks must be known in order to make an objective risk/benefit ratio decision to insert a pulmonary artery catheter. Failure to understand the rationale for each index of P_{LVED} (P_{la}, P_{paw}, P_{pa}, P_{CV}, as previously discussed, may cause the unwary and unknowing therapist to employ the wrong pressures to arrive at ill-advised, if not contraindicated, therapeutic decisions. The physical risks are related to complications of gaining and maintaining central venous access and actually passing and floating the pulmonary artery catheter into the pulmonary circulation. This section will briefly discuss the physical risks.

a. COMPLICATIONS OF GAINING AND MAINTAINING CENTRAL VENOUS ACCESS (Table 7–4)

The most obvious and often dramatic complication of utilizing pulmonary vascular pressure monitoring has to do with the fact that it is necessary to gain controlled access to the central venous circulation. Frequently, the internal jugular, external jugular, and subclavian veins are used for this purpose. Since the needle that finds and identifies these neck/central veins can inadvertently strike nearby vital organs, it is important to understand these potential complications. First, and probably most common, the carotid and subclavian arteries lie next to and parallel to the corresponding internal jugular and subclavian veins, and the incidence of arterial puncture is approximately 2.0 per cent.[68] The potential for vascular injury is greatly minimized if the finder needle is of a small bore (approximately 22 gauge). Nerves can be damaged at multiple sites, but brachial plexus, stellate ganglion, and phrenic nerve injuries, in particular, have been reported. This

Table 7–4. Complications of Gaining and Maintaining Central Venous Access

1. Carotid and subclavian artery puncture
2. Brachial plexus nerve injury
3. CSF tap
4. Hemo-, pneumo-, and chylothorax
5. Mediastinal and pericardial tamponade
6. Air embolism
7. Thrombophlebitis
8. Fracture and cut catheter in half
9. Electrical hazard
10. Horner's syndrome
11. Phrenic nerve palsy
12. Recurrent laryngeal nerve palsy

author has observed the withdrawal of cerebrospinal fluid on aspiration of an internal jugular vein finder needle. The pleural cavity can be invaded by the probing needle, causing either hemo-, pneumo-, or chylothorax. The pericardium and vessels in the mediastinum can be invaded by the probing needle, causing cardiac tamponade. If the syringe used for venous blood aspiration is disengaged from the finder needle during a spontaneous inspiration, it is possible for environmental air to be sucked into the central venous circulation and result in air embolism.[69] Thrombophlebitis of the veins in question is always possible, and indwelling vascular catheters and sheath introducers can always serve as a source of infection and sepsis.[70-76] Pulmonary artery catheters have been fractured in half[77] and have been cut in two at the time of surgery.[78] Finally, the pulmonary artery catheter provides a direct route for electrical current into the cavities of the heart, and therefore cardiac fibrillation is an ever present hazard. In comparison to neck veins, peripheral extremity veins (cephalic and brachial [antecubital] or femoral veins) are associated with many fewer cannulation complications, but it is much more difficult and complicated to actually pass and to float a catheter into the pulmonary circulation from an extremity vein.[77]

b. COMPLICATIONS OF ACTUALLY PASSING AND FLOATING THE PULMONARY ARTERY CATHETER (Table 7–5)

Rupture of an inflated pulmonary artery catheter balloon has been reported, but no serious embolic sequela have been noted.[76] Arrhythmias are not uncommon during passage of the catheter through the right heart (approximately 15 per cent of pulmonary artery catheter passages cause premature ventricular contractions),

Table 7–5. Complications of Actually Passing and Floating the Pulmonary Artery Catheter

1. Rupture of balloon
2. Arrhythmias (atrial, ventricular)
3. Knotting of catheters (on themselves, with other catheters, around papillary muscles)
4. Permanent wedge (infarction)
5. Perforation of pulmonary vessels (hemorrhage, hemoptysis)
6. Damage to tricuspid and pulmonary valves
7. Hepatic vein rupture

although persistent atrial arrhythmias,[79] complete heart block,[80] and ventricular fibrillation have occurred.[81] Catheters have knotted on themselves,[82, 83] with other indwelling catheters,[84] and around papillary muscles.[85, 86] Passage of pulmonary artery catheters has caused damage to the tricuspid[87] and pulmonary valves.[88] Catheters have permanently wedged in distal pulmonary vessels with subsequent pulmonary infarction in the distribution of the vessel containing the catheter.[89, 90] Pulmonary artery catheters have also perforated pulmonary vessels,[91] causing massive pulmonary hemorrhage[92, 93] and hemoptysis[94] and have perforated the right ventricle, causing pericardial tamponade.[68]

These complications of central venous access and catheter flotation are admittedly rare events, and therefore most of the references[68-94] to these complications are case reports (which involve one patient) rather than a series of patients. Nevertheless, for an intelligent judgment to be made about whether a pulmonary artery catheter should be used in a given patient it is necessary to enter this information into the risk-benefit equation or balance.

7. Lung Water Measurements

The preceding pulmonary artery catheter measurements greatly increase the understanding of how the respiratory and cardiovascular systems work together. Very recently and using a combination of these techniques and methodology, extravascular lung water measurements have become available for clinical use (American Edwards Laboratories 9310 Computer). Extravascular lung water is measured using a thermal change–green dye concentration change double-indicator dilution technique. The two indicators are injected simultaneously into the central venous circulation and are detected by a thermistor-tipped arterial catheter. One indicator, indocyanine green dye, binds to serum albumin and remains intravascular as it passes through the lung. The other indicator, a cold bolus of dextrose solution, diffuses throughout the extravascular space at the same time. Time-related dilution curves are determined and analyzed by the computer. Cardiac output and mean transient time are automatically calculated for each indicator. The product of cardiac output and mean transit time for a given indicator yields the volume distribution for that indicator. The difference between the volume distribution of the two indicators represents the volume of extravascular water in the lungs. The correlation between the double-indicator dilution technique and gravimetrics, the accepted standard, has been good (r = 0.96),[95–98] and it has been possible to perform multiple determinations rapidly and reproducibly. However, it is important to note that the correlation between extravascular lung water measurements and other observable parameters of respiratory function and the effect of various therapeutic modalities has not yet been established.

REFERENCES

1. Benumof JL: Monitoring respiratory function during anesthesia. In Saidman LJ, Smith NT (eds): Monitoring in Anesthesia. Boston, Butterworth Publishers, Inc., 1984, chapter 3, pp 33–77.
2. Cooper JB, Newbower RS, Kitz RJ: An analysis of major errors. Anesthesiology 60:34–42, 1984.
3. Paulus DA, Basta JW, Klie H, Radson EA: Preanesthetic checklist. Anesth Analg 64:264, 1985.
4. Debban DG, Bedford RF: Overdistension of the rebreathing bag: A hazardous test for circle system integrity. Anesthesiology 42:365–366, 1975.
5. Ward CS: The prevention of accidents associated with anesthetic apparatus. Br J Anaesth 40:692–701, 1968.
6. Westenskow DR, Jordan WS, Jordan R, Gillmore ST: Evaluation of oxygen monitors for use during anesthesia. Anesth Analg 60:53–56, 1981.
7. Meyer RM: A case for monitoring oxygen in the expiratory limb of the circle. Anesthesiology 61:347, 1984.
8. Saklad M, Paliotta J, Weyerhauser A: On line monitoring of ventilatory parameters. Clin Anesth 9:335–362, 1973.
9. Egbert LD, Biano D: The educated hand of the anesthesiologist. Anesth Analg 46:195–200, 1967.
10. Kelman GR, Nunn JF: Clinical recognition of hypoxaemia under fluorescent lamps. Lancet 1:1400, 1966.
11. Landsgaard C, Van Slyke DD: Cyanosis. Baltimore, Williams & Wilkins Co, 1923.
12. France CJ, Eger EI, Bendixen HH: The use of peripheral venous blood for pH and carbon dioxide tension determinations during general anesthesia. Anesthesiology 40:311–314, 1974.
13. Harrison EM, Galloon S: Venous blood as an alternative to arterial blood for the measurement of carbon dioxide tensions. Br J Anaesth 37:13–28, 1965.
14. Kassim D, Kenny S: The accuracy of capillary sampling for acid base estimations. Br J Anaesth 37:840–844, 1965.
15. Knudsen EJ, Hansen P: Carbon dioxide tension in nonarterialized capillary and arterial blood during anesthesia. Acta Anaesth Scand 6:29, 1962.
16. Levesque PR: Significance of P_{CO_2} within low pressure endotracheal tube cuffs. Anesth Analg 55:595–596, 1976.
17. Stanley TH: Nitrous oxide and pressures and volumes of high and low pressure endotracheal-tube cuffs in intubated patients. Anesthesiology 42:637–640, 1975.
18. Walts LF, Levin N, Dillon JB: Assessment of recovery from curare. JAMA 213:1894–1896, 1974.
19. Special Symposium: Trancutaneous O_2 and CO_2 monitoring of the adult and neonate. Crit Care Med 9:689–760, 1981.
20. Huch R, Huch A, Lubbers DW: Trancutaneous P_{O_2}. New York, Thieme-Stratton, Inc, 1981.
21. Finer NN: Newer trends in continuous monitoring of critically ill infants and children. Ped Clin North Am 27:553–566, 1980.
22. Tremper KK, Konchigeri HN, Cullen BF, Kapur PA, Thangathurai D, Percival C: Transcutaneous monitoring of oxygen tension in one-lung anesthesia. J Thorac Cardiovasc Surg 88:22–25, 1984.
23. Salmentera M, Heinomen J: Transcutaneous oxygen measurement during one-lung anesthesia. Acta Anesth Scand 28:241–244, 1984.
24. Chubra-Smith NM, Grant RP, Jenkins LC: Transcutaneous oxygen monitoring during endobronchial thoracic anesthesia. Anesth Analg 64:200, 1985.
25. Gothgen I, Degn H, Jacobsen E, Rassmussen JP: Transcutaneous oxygen measurements during thoracic anesthesia. Acta Anesth Scand 24:491–494, 1980.
26. Brodsky JB, Shulman MS, Swan M, Mark JB: Pulse oximetry during one-lung ventilation. Anesthesiology 63:212–213, 1985.
27. Thys DM, Cohen E, Eisenkraft JB, Kaplan JA: The pulse oximeter, a non-invasive monitor of oxygenation during one-lung anesthesia. Anesth Analg 64:292, 1985.
28. Yelderman M, New W Jr: Evaluation of pulse oximetry. Anesthesiology 59:349–352, 1983.
29. Krauss AN, Waldman S, Frayer WW, et al: Noninvasive estimation of arterial oxygenation in newborn infants. J Pediatr 93:275–278, 1978.
30. Saunders NA, Powles ACP, Rebuck AS: Ear oximetry: Accuracy and practicability in the assessment of arterial oxygenation. Am Rev Respir Dis 113:745–749, 1976.
31. Versmold HT, Linderkamp O, Stuffer KH, et al: In vivo response time of transcutaneous P_{O_2} electrodes. A comparison of four devices in newborn infants. Acta Anesth Scand 68 (Suppl):40–48, 1978.
32. McLellan PA, Goldstein RS, Ramcharan V, Rebuck AS: Transcutaneous carbon dioxide monitoring. Am Rev Resp Dis 124:199–201, 1981.
33. Hansen TN, Tooley WH: Skin surface carbon dioxide tension in sick infants. Pediatrics 64:942–945, 1979.
34. Hutchinson CDS, Rocca G, Honeybourne D: Estimation of arterial oxygen tension in adult subjects using a transcutaneous electrode. Thorax 36:473–477, 1981.
35. Rafferty TD, Marrero O, Nardi D, Schacter EN, Mentelos R, Hastings A, Roselli D: Relationship between transcutaneous and arterial carbon dioxide tension in adult patients anesthetized with nitrous oxide fentanyl and nitrous oxide-enflurane. Anesth Analg 60:504–507, 1981.
36. Tremper KK, Waxman K, Shoemaker WC: Use of transcutaneous oxygen sensors to titrate PEEP. Ann Surg 193:206–209, 1981.
37. Takki S, Aromaa U, Kauste A: The validity and usefulness of the end-tidal P_{CO_2} during anesthesia. Ann Clin Res 4:278–284, 1972.
38. Sykes JK: A mixing device for expired gas. Anaesth 23:446, 1968.
39. Levesque PR, Rosenberg H: Rapid bedside estimation of wasted ventilation (V_D/V_T). Anesthesiology 42:98–100, 1975.
40. Hilberman M, Kamm B, Lasny B, Dietrich HP, Martz K, Osborn JJ: An analysis of potential physiological predictors of respiratory adequacy following cardiac surgery. J Thorac Cardiovasc Surg 71:711–720, 1976.
41. Harrison RA, Davison R, Shapiro BA, Myers SN: Reassessment of the assumed A-V oxygen content dif-

ference in the shunt calculation. Anesth Analg 54:198–202, 1975.

42. Dongre SS, McAslan TC, Shin B: Selection of the source of mixed venous blood samples in severely traumatized patients. Anesth Analg 56:527–532, 1977.

43. Prakash O, Jonson B, Meij S, Bos E, Hugenholtz PG, Nanta J, Hekman W: Criteria for early extubation after intracardiac surgery in adults. Anesth Analg 56: 703–708, 1977.

44. Neumark J, Bardeen A, Sulzer E, Kampine JP: Miniature intravascular PCO_2 sensors in neurosurgery. J Neurosurg 43:172–176, 1975.

45. Downs JB: A technique for direct measurement of intrapleural pressure. Crit Care Med 4:207–210, 1976.

46. Suter PM, Schlobohm RM: Determination of functional residual capacity during mechanical ventilation. Anesthesiology 41:605–607, 1974.

47. Laws AK: Effects of induction of anesthesia and muscle paralysis on functional residual capacity of the lungs. Can Anaesth Soc J 15:325–331, 1968.

48. Colgan SD, Whang TB: A method for measuring the functional residual capacity and dynamic lung compliance during oxygen and halothane inhalation. Anesthesiology 28:559–563, 1967.

49. Jonmarker C, Jansson L, Jonson B, Larsson A, Werner O: Measurement of functional residual capacity by sulfahexafluride washout. Anesthesiology 63:89–95, 1985.

50. Carlile PV: Pitfalls in the interpretation of hemodynamic data. Progress in Crit Care Med 2:69–86, 1985.

51. Enson Y: Pulmonary heart disease: Relation of pulmonary hypertension to abnormal lung structure and function. Bull NY Acad Med 53:551–566, 1977.

52. Levin RI, Glassman E: Left atrial-pulmonary artery wedge pressure relation: Effect of elevated pulmonary vascular resistance. Am J Cardiol 55:856–857, 1985.

53. Roy R, Powers SR, Feutsel PJ, et al: Pulmonary wedge catheterization during positive end-expiratory pressure ventilation in the dog. Anesthesiology 46:385–390, 1970.

54. Benumof JL: Where do pulmonary artery catheters go: Intrathoracic distribution. Anesthesiology 46:336–338, 1977.

55. Kronberg GM, Quan SF, Schlobohm RM, et al: Anatomical location of pulmonary artery catheters in supine patients. Anesthesiology 51:467–469, 1979.

56. Berryhill RE, Benumof JL: PEEP-induced discrepancy between pulmonary arterial wedge pressure and left atrial pressure: The influence of controlled vs. spontaneous ventilation and compliant vs. noncompliant lungs. Anesthesiology 46:383–386, 1979.

57. Hasan FM, Weiss WB, Braman SS, Hoppin FG Jr.: Influence of lung injury on pulmonary wedge–left atrial pressure correlation during positive end-expiratory pressure ventilation. Am Rev Resp Dis 131:246–250, 1985.

58. Petty TL: Adult respiratory distress syndrome. Semin Resp Med 3:219–224, 1982.

59. Zapol WM, Snider MT: Pulmonary hypertension in severe acute respiratory failure. N Engl J Med 296:476–480, 1977.

60. Enson Y, Wood JA, Mantaras NB, et al: The influence of heart rate on pulmonary arterial–left ventricular pressure relationships at end-diastole. Circ 56:533–539, 1977.

61. Field J, Shiroff RA, Zelis RF, Babb JD: Limitations in the use of the pulmonary capillary wedge pressure. Editorial. Chest 70:451–453, 1976.

62. Samii K, Conseiller C, Viars P: Central venous pressure

and pulmonary wedge pressure: A comparative study in anesthetized surgical patients. Arch Surg 111: 1122–1125, 1976.

63. Mangano DT: Monitoring pulmonary arterial pressure in coronary artery disease. Anesthesiology 53:364–370, 1980.

64. Lowenstein E, Teplick R: To (PA) catheterize or not to (PA) catheterize—that is the question. Editorial. Anesthesiology 53:361–363, 1980

65. Kaplan, JA, Wells PH: Early diagnosis of myocardial ischemia using the pulmonary arterial catheter. Anesth Analg 60:789–793, 1981.

66. Cohen E: Hemodynamics and oxygenation during one-lung anesthesia: Right vs. left. Anesthesiology 63:(in press).

67. Hasan FM, Malanga A, Corrao WM, Braman FS: Effect of catheter position on thermodilution cardiac output during continuous positive-pressure ventilation. Crit Care Med 12:387–390, 1984.

68. Shah KB, Rao TLK, Laughlin S, El-Etr AA: A review of pulmonary artery catheterization in 6245 patients. Anesthesiology 61:271–275, 1984.

69. Doblar DD, Hinkle JC, Fay ML, Condon BF: Air embolism associated with pulmonary artery catheter introducer kit. Anesthesiology 56:307–309, 1982.

70. Chastre J, Cornud F, Bouchama A, et al: Thrombosis after pulmonary artery catheterization via the internal jugular vein. N Engl J Med 306:278–281, 1982.

71. Benumof JL: Thrombosis after pulmonary artery catheterization via the internal jugular vein. N Engl J Med 306:1486–1487, 1982.

72. Collin J, Collin C, Constable FL, Johnston IDA: Infusion thrombophlebitis and infection with various catheters. Lancet 2:150, 1975.

73. Greene JF, Fitzwater JE, Clemmer TP: Septic endocarditis and indwelling pulmonary artery catheters. JAMA 233:891, 1975.

74. Pace NL, Horton W: Indwelling pulmonary artery catheters. Their relationship to aseptic thrombotic endocardial vegetations. JAMA 233:893, 1975.

75. Opie JC: Contamination of internal jugular lines. Anesthesia 35:1060–1065, 1980.

76. Buckbind N, Ganz W: Hemodynamic monitoring: Invasive techniques. Anesthesiology 45:146, 1976.

77. Parulkar DS, Grundy EM, Bennett EJ: Fracture of a float catheter. Br J Anaesth 50:201–203, 1978.

78. Pease RD, Scanlon TS, Herron AL, Benumof JL: Intraoperative transection of a Swan-Ganz catheter. Anesth Analg 58:519–521, 1979.

79. Geha DG, Davis NJ, Lappas DG: Persistent atrial arrhythmias associated with placement of a Swan-Ganz catheter. Anesthesiology 39:651, 1973.

80. Abernathy WS: Complete heart block caused by the Swan-Ganz catheter. Chest 65:349, 1974.

81. Cairns JA, Holden D: Ventricular fibrillation due to passage of a Swan-Ganz catheter. Am J Cardiol 35:589, 1975.

82. Daum S, Schapira M: Intracardiac knot formation in a Swan-Ganz catheter. Anesth Analg (Cleve.) 52:862, 1973.

83. Lipp H, O'Donoghue K, Resnekov L: Intracardiac knotting of a flow-directed balloon catheter. N Engl J Med 284:220, 1971.

84. Swaroop S: Knotting of two central venous monitoring catheters. Am J Med 53:386, 1972.

85. Meister SG, LFurr Cm, Engel TR, Jones M, Frankl WS: Knotting of a flow-directed catheter about a cardiac structure. Cathet Cardiovasc Diagn 3:171–175, 1971.

86. Schwartz KV, Garcia FG: Entanglement of Swan-Ganz

catheter around an intracardiac structure. JAMA 273:1198, 1977.

87. Smith WR, Glauser FL, Jemison P: Ruptured chordae of the tricuspid valve. The consequence of flow-directed Swan-Ganz catheterization. Chest 70:790–792, 1976.

88. O'Toole JD, Wurtzbacker JJ, Weaver NE, et al: Pulmonary valve injury and insufficiency during pulmonary artery catheterization. N Eng J Med 301:1167–1168, 1979.

89. Foote GA, Schabel SI, Hodges M: Pulmonary complications of the flow directed balloon-tipped catheter. N Engl J Med 290:927, 1974.

90. Colvin MP, Savege TM, Lewis CT: Pulmonary damage from a Swan-Ganz catheter. Br J Anaesth 47:1107, 1975.

91. Chun GMH, Ellestad MH: Perforation of the pulmonary artery by a Swan-Ganz catheter. N Engl J Med 284:1041, 1971.

92. Golden MS, Pinder T, Anderson WT: Fatal pulmonary hemorrhage complicating use of a flow direct balloon-tipped catheter in a patient receiving anticoagulant therapy. Am J Cardiol 32:865, 1973.

93. Pape LA, Haffajee CI, Markis JE: Fatal pulmonary hemorrhage after use of the flow directed balloon-tipped catheter. Ann Int Med 90:344–347, 1979.

94. Lapin ES, Murray JA: Hemoptysis with flow-directed cardiac catheterization (letter) JAMA 220:1246, 1972.

95. Tranbaugh RF, Lewis FR, Christensen JM, et al: Lung water changes after thermal injury. Ann Surg 192:479–490, 1980.

96. Lewis FR, Elings VI: Microprocessor determination of lung water using thermal-green dye double indicator dilution. Surgical Forum 29:182, 1978.

97. Feeley TW, Mihm FH, Futhaner D, Rosenthal MH: Extravascular thermal volume as an estimate of lung water. Presented at the meeting of the American Society of Anesthesiologists, October 1979.

98. Lewis FR, Elings VB, Sturm JA: Bedside measurement of lung water. J Surg Res 27:250–261, 1979.

Choice of Anesthetic Drugs and Techniques

8

I. INTRODUCTION

The choice of anesthetic drug and technique in the vast majority of thoracic surgery cases is based on the preoperative cardiopulmonary evaluation. Some drugs and techniques may favor the overall perioperative function of one organ at the expense of another. For example, the halogenated drugs may prevent or minimize bronchospasm but at the same time may decrease myocardial contractility, whereas the narcotics may preserve myocardial contractility but may not prevent bronchospasm in patients with reactive airways. Since different patients will have varying degrees of dysfunction of different organs and anesthetic drugs differentially affect the various organs, the most appropriate anesthetic will depend upon the patient.

This chapter first briefly considers the usual and major pulmonary and cardiac problems that patients undergoing thoracic surgery may have (with both lungs ventilated) as well as the most important effect anesthetic drugs might have on these problems. Next, the specific effect of anesthetic drug and technique on gas exchange for the special one-lung ventilation situation (in particular, on hypoxic pulmonary vasoconstriction) will be covered. Finally, the chapter rec-

ommends anesthetic drugs and techniques that should simultaneously minimize the pulmonary and cardiac problems but yet incorporate enough flexibility to emphasize the function of one organ over another, should that be considered necessary. As with most of the other chapters in this book, respiratory considerations are emphasized more than cardiac considerations.

II. THE MOST COMMON AND IMPORTANT CARDIOPULMONARY CONSIDERATIONS FOR PATIENTS UNDERGOING THORACIC SURGERY

A. Pulmonary Considerations (Two-Lung Ventilation)

1. Reactive Airways

The mechanisms by which increases in airway resistance may be stimulated have been summarized[1] and include mechanical and chemical mucosal stimulation (causing various neural reflexes that are mediated by medullary centers, local arcs, and the autonomic nervous system), anaphylactoid bronchoconstriction, histamine-induced bronchoconstriction, alpha-adrenergic predominance, vagal (cholinergic) predominance, and exercise-induced broncho-constriction. In this discussion, the term "re-active airways" applies to patients who come to surgery with pre-existing bronchospasm or will likely react to the mechanical stimulation of endotracheal tube insertion and/or tracheobron-chial tree manipulation with bronchospasm.

Patients undergoing thoracic surgery are likely to have an increased incidence of reactive airways for two reasons. First, the vast majority of patients have a long and significant smoking history and therefore have varying degrees of chronic obstructive pulmonary disease, excess secretions, and increased reversible airway re-sistance (bronchoconstriction). The presence of the increased airway resistance can often be readily demonstrated by improvement in expi-ratory airflow rates following the preoperative administration of bronchodilating drugs. In-deed, there is a strong dose-response relation between the amount of secretions, cough, bron-choconstriction, severity of chronic obstructive pulmonary disease, and the risk of mortality from chronic obstructive pulmonary disease and the number of cigarettes smoked per day, the number of years of smoking, and the depth of smoke inhalation.[2] Second, thoracic surgery often demands direct manipulation of the tra-cheobronchial tree. Although much of the direct surgical contact is external (on the adventitia), the manipulations (clamping, compression be-tween the fingers) usually cause mucosal stim-ulation, as does endotracheal intubation, and can therefore cause bronchospasm. In fact, even normal healthy patients undergoing this type of surgical stimulation of the lung parenchyma and airways can develop bronchospasm,[3] especially if too lightly anesthetized.

a. EFFECT OF ANESTHETIC DRUGS ON AIRWAY REACTIVITY (Table 8–1)

The following discussion of the pharmacology of anesthetic drugs is limited to those aspects that suggest their use or avoidance in patients with reactive airways. Some of the drugs used in anesthetic practice (especially the halogen-ated drugs) decrease the reactivity of airways. However, there must be some initial smooth muscle constriction in order for a bronchodilat-ing anesthetic to have any effect on broncho-motor tone. Thus, measurements of airway re-sistances in normal men have generally failed to show a bronchodilatory effect of halothane.[4]

Table 8–1. Effect of Anesthetic Drugs on Airway Reactivity

Anesthetic Drug				
Class	Drug	Bronchodilation	Bronchoconstriction	Comment
Inhalation	Isoflurane	+ +	0	Drug of choice
	Halothane	+ +	0	See text
	Enflurane	+ +	0	See text
	N_2O	0	0	→ Light anesthesia
Narcotics	Fentanyl	0	0	Drug of Choice
	Meperidine	0	+	Releases histamine
	Morphine	0	+ +	Releases histamine
Induction	Ketamine	+	0	Drug of choice for asthmatic
	Pentothal	0	+ ?	Light anesthesia?
Relaxants	Vecuronium	0	0	Drug of choice
	Pancuronium	0	0	Drug of choice
	Succinylcholine	0	0	Drug of choice
	Atracurium	0	+ ?	Releases histamine, high doses
	Metocurine	0	+	Releases histamine, high-moderate doses
	d-tubocurarine	0	+ +	Releases histamine, normal doses
Adjuncts	Lidocaine	+	0	Useful pre- and intraoperatively
	Neostigmine	0	+ + +	Must use atropine concomitantly
	Atropine	+	0	See text

+, + +, + + + = mild, moderate, severe effect, respectively.

Similarly, in patients with normal bronchomotor tone on cardiopulmonary bypass, the administration of halothane both by the airway and systemically (via the pump circuit) does not alter the resistive work of breathing (as it does in patients with increased bronchomotor tone; see the following).[5]

However, when bronchoconstriction is provoked in patients by either hypocapnia[6] or inhalation of ultrasonic aerosols,[7] halothane and enflurane reliably decrease bronchomotor tone. The mechanism of bronchodilation by the halogenated drugs most probably takes place by direct action on the airway musculature and/or local reflex arcs rather than via centrally controlled reflex pathways. This contention is best supported by the fact that systemic (intravenous) administration of halothane via cardiopulmonary by-pass pump does not decrease hypocapnia-induced increased airway resistance, whereas inhaled halothane (during cardiopulmonary by-pass) does.[5,8] Since halothane has a direct relaxant effect on bronchial smooth muscle, it is not surprising that in animals it can block acetylcholine-, histamine-, alpha-adrenergic-, and antigen-induced increases in bronchial muscle tension.[9] Isoflurane is probably just as efficacious as halothane or enflurane in decreasing elevated bronchomotor tone.[9]

Since the halogenated drugs are the most potent bronchodilating anesthetic drugs used today, they must be considered the anesthetic drug of choice for patients with reactive airways. If the halogenated drug is used as a primary induction agent for a patient with reactive airways, then halothane might be considered the induction drug of choice, since it is less pungent than isoflurane. However, isoflurane is a better choice for the maintenance of anesthesia for three reasons. First, isoflurane has a high arrhythmogenic threshhold, which has increased importance in patients with reactive airways because they may more likely receive aminophylline and beta$_2$-agonists and may more likely become acidotic (all of which may cause arrhythmias). Second, isoflurane is not metabolized as much as halothane (it has less or no hepatic toxicity). Third, isoflurane provides much more cardiovascular stability and potency than enflurane. Consequently, isoflurane should be regarded as the halogenated drug of choice for maintenance anesthesia in patients with reactive airways.

Fentanyl does not have any effect on bronchomotor tone, which is consistent with the fact that, in humans, fentanyl does not change plasma histamine concentrations.[10] On the other hand, morphine is known to release histamine and to increase central vagal tone. In dogs, bronchoconstriction due to morphine has been shown to be reduced by either administration of an antihistamine intravenously or by bilateral vagotomy.[11] Similarly, meperidine has been shown in dogs to have a bronchoconstricting effect similar to that of morphine.[11] Consequently, in patients with reactive airways for whom a narcotic supplement to nitrous oxide (which has no effect on bronchomotor tone) or halogenated drug anesthesia is desired, or to use a narcotic alone in high doses, fentanyl is the preferred choice. However, it should be remembered that a N_2O narcotic-relaxant anesthetic, as ordinarily administered with low to moderate doses of narcotic, produces a light anesthesia and will not prevent bronchospasm in patients with reactive airways.

Ketamine and thiopental are intravenous anesthetic drugs that are mainly associated with the induction of anesthesia. For the patient with reactive airways ketamine is believed to be more advantageous than most other anesthetic drugs used for induction. In dogs, ketamine protects against antigen-induced bronchospasm, while thiopental does not; the protective effect can be blocked by propanalol, suggesting that the mechanism of action of ketamine is, perhaps, due to beta-adrenergic stimulation.[12] Thus, ketamine has been used very successfully in patients with a history of asthma,[13] whereas thiopental has clinically been associated with more bronchospasm than any other anesthetic drug (perhaps due to light levels of anesthesia that leave airway reflexes relatively intact).[14] Consequently, ketamine (1 to 2 mg/kg) may be the drug of choice for induction of anesthesia in patients with bronchospastic disease requiring a rapid induction of anesthesia.

With the exception of d-tubocurarine, all of the muscle relaxants may be used in patients with reactive airways. D-tubocurarine releases histamine and increases airway resistance in humans.[15] Metocurine can also release histamine in ordinary clinical doses but not nearly as much as d-tubocurarine. Atracurium may release histamine but only in very high doses. Succinylcholine is structurally related to acetylcholine and could theoretically release histamine, but clinically it is unassociated with bronchospasm, even in asthmatics. Pancuronium and vecuronium do not release histamine.

Lidocaine, given immediately prior to intubation (1 to 2 mg/kg IV), is a useful drug in the prevention of reflex bronchoconstriction provoked by instrumentation of the airway. Similarly, lidocaine by infusion (1 to 3 mg/kg/hr) may be useful in diminishing the reactivity of airways throughout surgery in patients with limited cardiac reserve who would not hemodynamically tolerate the usual doses of the usual anesthetics. Intravenous administration of lidocaine has also been successfully used to treat bronchospasm during anesthesia.[16] Lidocaine, inhaled in an ultrasonic aerosol, has been shown to produce mild bronchodilation in healthy subjects, whereas normal saline induced mild bronchoconstriction.[17] In a similar study, lidocaine administered by aerosol both prevented and reversed increases in airway resistance provoked by ultrasonically nebulized water.[18] The lidocaine was thought to be acting directly on bronchial smooth muscle. Thus, it appears that administration of lidocaine both via the airway or intravenously has a role in preventing and protecting against the development of bronchospasm in patients with reactive airways.

Neostigmine, physostigmine, and pyridostigmine are cholinesterase-blocking drugs that can be expected to produce an increase in airway resistance by increasing cholinergic activity. In clinical practice, of course, atropine is used to block this effect when anticholinesterases are administered to reverse the effects of neuromuscular blocking drugs.

Atropine, the classic cholinergic blocker, not only reverses effects of anticholinesterase drugs but can also directly dilate the airways. A decrease in airway resistance was found following intravenous administration of atropine (0.84 mg/70 kg) to patients anesthetized with 75 per cent nitrous oxide and oxygen.[19] In addition to its potential effect on airway resistance, atropine has been shown to increase respiratory dead space in both dogs and humans, presumably by dilating larger bronchi.[20]

Table 8–1 summarizes the effect of inhalation and intravenous anesthetic drugs on bronchomotor tone and, in view of the preceding discussion, ranks the various drugs of each class in terms of their efficacy for the patient with reactive airways. Ketamine appears to be the induction drug of choice, with thiopental a close second. Intravenous lidocaine is probably a useful adjunct in the peri-induction period. Isoflurane appears to be the halogenated drug of choice for maintenance anesthesia. Fentanyl is the narcotic of choice. Relaxation can be facilitated by succinylcholine, but if a rapid intubation is not necessary, vecuronium or pan-

curonium may be the relaxants of choice, with atracurium a reasonably close second choice. Nitrous oxide is a benign drug for the patient with reactive airways (if anesthesia caused by other drugs is adequate), but in view of the fact that a large number of patients undergoing thoracic surgery will have one-lung ventilation and therefore require a high F_IO_2, use of nitrous oxide is limited in these patients.

2. Gas Exchange Impairment

Chapter 4 describes in great detail the pathophysiology of two-lung ventilation in the open-chest paralyzed patient in the lateral decubitus position. In summary, the nondependent lung may be well ventilated owing to an increase in compliance but may be poorly perfused owing to gravitational effects. The dependent lung may be poorly ventilated owing to a decrease in compliance but may be well perfused. Consequently, there may be mismatching of ventilation and perfusion in the open chest, paralyzed patient in the lateral decubitus position. The low ventilation-perfusion ratio in the dependent lung can be improved with selective dependent lung positive end-expiratory pressure (PEEP) while the nondependent lung is ventilated with zero end-expiratory pressure (ZEEP). The differential lung ventilation combination of dependent lung PEEP and nondependent lung ZEEP provides better arterial oxygenation compared with ventilation of both the nondependent and dependent lungs with ZEEP.

Chapter 4 also describes in great detail the pathophysiology of one-lung ventilation in the lateral decubitus position. The one-lung ventilation condition creates a large obligatory right-to-left shunt that is not present during the two-lung ventilation condition. This right-to-left shunt during one-lung ventilation, however, is minimized by the presence of hypoxic pulmonary vasoconstriction in the nondependent nonventilated lung. Section III of this chapter will consider in great detail the effects of anesthetic drugs on hypoxic pulmonary vasoconstriction in the nonventilated nondependent lung.

B. Cardiac Considerations

1. Coronary Artery Disease

Patients undergoing thoracic surgery, especially those beyond their fourth decade, should be approached with an increased index of suspicion that coronary artery disease may be present. Ten major cohort studies, accounting for over 20 million person years of observation in several countries, supports the statement in the 1983 Surgeon General's report that "cigarette smoking should be considered the most important of the known modifiable risk factors for coronary heart disease in the United States."[21] These studies showed that men 40 to 59 years of age who were smoking a pack or more per day at the time of initial examination had a risk for a first major coronary event that was 2.5 times as great as that of nonsmokers, with a strong dose-response relation.[22] Studies both in the United States and abroad have demonstrated consistently that women whose smoking patterns are similar to those in men have a similar increased risk of death from coronary heart disease and for common morbidity from the disease, such as angina pectoris, compared with nonsmokers.[21,23] The risk of death from coronary heart disease among both male and female smokers is increased by early initiation of smoking, long total exposure to smoking, and deep smoke inhalation.

Although smoking, hypertension, and hypercholesterolemia confer approximately the same average increase in the risk of coronary heart disease in populations, smoking in the presence of other risk factors for coronary heart disease appears to create a synergistic effect on mortality from the disease.[21] The lifestyle of many smokers also includes caffeine and nicotine addiction and obsessive-compulsive type A behavior and results in an increased incidence of systemic hypertension; the combination of smoking and systemic hypertension increases the risk of coronary artery disease. Pipe and cigar smokers have a risk of experiencing a major coronary event and subsequent morbidity from chronic heart disease that is intermediate between that for nonsmokers and cigarette smokers.[21]

Smoking cessation results in a decreased risk of mortality from coronary heart disease, and the degree of risk reduction is determined by the length of time after cessation, the amount smoked, and the duration of smoking before cessation. Although the risk of coronary heart disease attributable to smoking declines by approximately 50 per cent 1 year after cessation, it approaches that of a person who has never smoked only after a decade or more.[21]

The anesthetic management and choice of anesthesia for patients with coronary artery disease is based on the factors that determine myocardial oxygen supply and demand (Table 8–2). Myocardial oxygen demand is increased by tachycardia (the most oxygen-expensive factor), increased myocardial wall tension, and increased contractile state of the heart (as caused by degree of sympathetic nervous system activity). Diastolic myocardial wall tension is determined by preload (left ventricular end-diastolic pressure, the second most oxygen-expensive factor), and systolic myocardial wall tension is determined by afterload (systemic systolic blood pressure and vascular resistance). Myocardial oxygen supply is determined by the product of coronary artery blood flow and the oxygen content of coronary artery blood. Coronary artery blood flow is increased by an increased diastolic filling time (slow heart rate, most important oxygen-supply factor), and the coronary artery perfusion pressure. The coronary perfusion pressure is equal to coronary artery diastolic pressure (there is no perfusion during systole) minus the preload (which is ventricular end-diastolic pressure or the outlet or back pressure, and is the second most important oxygen-supply factor). The oxygen content of arterial blood is a function of the amount of hemoglobin (most important), position of the oxygen-hemoglobin dissociation curve (P_{50}), and the ventilation-perfusion relationships within the lung (which determines P_aO_2). Thus, common precipitating factors for myocardial ischemia are tachycardia (increases oxygen demand and decreases oxygen supply), increased preload (increases oxygen demand and decreases oxygen supply), hypertension (increases systolic wall tension more than increasing oxygen supply from the increase in perfusion pressure), and hypotension (decreases oxygen supply more than oxygen consumption). It follows that anesthetic management should minimize

Table 8–2. Determinants of Myocardial Oxygen Supply and Demand

Myocardial Oxygen Demand	Myocardial Oxygen Supply
Heart rate*	Coronary artery blood flow
	Heart rate–diastolic filling time*
Wall tension	
Preload (VEDP)— diastole*	Perfusion pressure (diastolic pressure– preload)
Afterload–systole	
Contractile state	CaO_2 (Hb, P_{50}, $\dot{V}/\dot{Q}$)

* = most important factors; VEDP = ventricular end-diastolic pressure.

myocardial oxygen demand by continuing pre-operative beta blockers until the time of surgery, minimize preinduction anxiety, keep heart rate low, maintain adequate levels of anesthesia, and use myocardial depressant drugs when indicated. Anesthetic management should also maximize myocardial oxygen supply by keeping diastolic blood pressure normal or increased, keep heart rate low, assure adequate arterial oxygenation, and use venous and arterial vasodilators to reduce preload and afterload, respectively, and to relieve coronary artery spasm.

a. EFFECT OF ANESTHETIC DRUGS ON CARDIOVASCULAR FUNCTION (Table 8–3)

This discussion is not intended as a review of the general pharmacology of anesthetic drugs; rather, it discusses those features of anesthetic drugs that suggest their use or avoidance in patients with coronary artery disease. Depending on the drug and the amount used, anesthetic technique may alter all of the determinants of myocardial oxygen supply and demand.

The narcotics, especially fentanyl, have minimal primary hemodynamic effects if adequate doses are used (or are supplemented by other drugs). High doses of fentanyl (greater than 60 μg/kg) provide remarkable hemodynamic stability for coronary artery bypass surgery and, in this group of patients, low to moderate doses of fentanyl (15 μg/kg) will also provide stable anesthesia for induction and intubation, provided the fentanyl is administered rapidly (within 12 sec).[24] The decrease in heart rate with fentanyl is a desirable characteristic in patients with coronary artery disease. Meperidine has a negative inotropic effect and positive chronotropic effect.

The halogenated drugs have a number of unfavorable cardiovascular effects. A major cardiovascular disadvantage of the halogenated drugs is a 20 to 40 per cent decrease in systemic blood pressure. Since cardiac output is decreased 20 to 40 per cent by halothane and enflurane, and not at all by isoflurane, and in the context of a 20 to 40 per cent decrease in systemic blood pressure caused by all drugs, systemic vascular resistance is only minimally affected by halothane and enflurane but is decreased by isoflurane. Since filling pressures are increased by halothane and enflurane, and not at all by isoflurane, and in the context of a decrease in cardiac output caused by halothane and enflurane, but not by isoflurane, cardiac

Table 8–3. Effect of Anesthetic Drugs on Cardiovascular Function

Anesthetic Drug		Blood Pressure	Systemic Vascular Resistance	Cardiac Output	Cardiac Contractility	Central Venous Pressure	Heart Rate	Sensitization of the Heart to Epinephrine
Class	Drugs							
Inhalation 1.0 to 1.5 MAC	Isoflurance	↓↓	↓↓	0	0	0	↑	0?
	Halothane	↓↓	0	↓↓	↓	↑	0↓	↑↑↑
	Enflurane	↓↓	↓	↓↓	↓↓	↑	↑↑	±↑
	N₂O	↑	↑	↓	↓	0	±	0
Narcotics	Fentanyl	0	0	0	0	±	↓	0
	Meperidine	↓	↓	↓	↓	↓	±↓	0
	Morphine	↓	↓	↓	0	↓	±↓	0
Induction	Ketamine	↑	↑	↑	↑*	0	↑	0
	Pentothal	↓	±	↓	↓	↓	↑	0
Relaxants	Vecuronium	0	0	0	0	0	0	0
	Pancuronium	↑	±	↑	↑	0	↑	0
	Succinylcholine	0	0	0	0	0	± ↑→↓	?
	Atracurium	0	0	0	0	0	0	0
	Metocurine	±↓	0	0	0	0	0	0
	d-tubocurarine	↓	↓	0	0	↓	↑	0
Adjuncts	Lidocaine	±↑	±↓	0	0	0	0	↓↓
	Diazepam	0	0	±↓	±↓	0	0	0

0 = no change; ↓ and ↓↓ = 10 to 20 per cent and 20 to 40 per cent decrease; ↑, ↑↑, ↑↑↑ = progressively greater increases; ± = small changes that depend on circumstances and reflex activity; * = ketamine has a direct myocardial depressant action that becomes evident when its sympathetic stimulating effects are blocked or when the sympathetic nerves are maximally stimulated, as in severe hypotension.

contractility is decreased by halothane and enflurane and not at all by isoflurane. Halothane greatly sensitizes the myocardium to catecholamines, and arrhythmias may be prominent in patients with irritable ventricular foci (which may be due to ischemia caused by coronary artery disease). Enflurane causes a 20 to 40 per cent and isoflurane a 10 to 20 per cent increase in heart rate, which may be very and moderately disadvantageous, respectively, to the patient with coronary artery disease. Isoflurane may act as a nonspecific coronary vasodilator, which can theoretically result in a "coronary steal"; that is, vasodilation and an increase in blood flow in normal areas can occur at the expense of blood flow to ischemic areas that have a fixed vascular resistance.[25]

The neuromuscular blocking drugs have hemodynamic effects, but they are not generally of large magnitude. Pancuronium has the most undesirable effects for the patient with coronary artery disease because it can stimulate the sympathetic nervous system, causing tachycardia and increased blood pressure and cardiac output. *D*-tubocurarine also has undesirable effects for the patient with coronary artery disease because of the development of hypotension and tachycardia. Succinylcholine may mimic acetylcholine at nicotinic and muscurinic receptors; consequently, a dose-related tachycardia followed by bradycardia may be seen, owing to sequential stimulation of these receptors, respectively. The other relaxants have only minimal effects on cardiovascular function.

Ketamine can cause a significant stimulation of the sympathetic nervous system that results in an increase in contractility, tachycardia, and hypertension, whereas thiopental can cause significant depression of myocardial contractility and hypotension. Consequently, both of these intravenous anesthetic induction drugs have major disadvantages in patients with coronary artery disease. However, the sympathomimetic effect of ketamine may be used to good advantage in hypovolemic patients.

III. CHOICE OF ANESTHESIA AND ARTERIAL OXYGENATION DURING ONE-LUNG VENTILATION

A. Effect of Anesthetics on Hypoxic Pulmonary Vasoconstriction (HPV)

As discussed in chapters 3 and 4, an undesirable property of general anesthesia is inhibition of HPV in the nonventilated nondependent lung by the anesthetic drug. All of the inhalation and many of the injectable anesthetics have been studied with regard to their effect on HPV. Halothane has been the most extensively studied agent (Table 8–4).[26–43] The experimental preparations utilized may be divided into four basic categories, which are (1) in vitro, (2) in vivo–not intact (pumped perfused lungs, no systemic circulation or neural function), (3) in vivo–intact (normally perfused lungs, normal systemic circulation), and (4) humans (volunteers or patients). It appears, according to this break down of experimental preparation, that inhibition of HPV by halothane is a universal finding in the in vitro and in vivo–not intact preparations. However, in the more normal or physiologic in vivo–intact and human studies, halothane has caused no or only a very slight decrease in HPV response. Thus, it appears that a fundamental property of halothane is its inhibition of HPV in experimental preparations, which can be controlled for other physiologic influences (e.g., pulmonary vascular pressure, cardiac output, mixed venous oxygen tension, CO_2 level, and temperature) that can have an effect on the HPV response. In the more biologically complex in vivo models other factors seem to be involved that greatly diminish the inhibitory effect of halothane on HPV. Important methodologic differences between the in vitro and in vivo–not intact preparations and the in vivo–intact and human models that could account for the observed differences in halothane effect on HPV are presence (or absence) of perfusion pulsations, perfusion fluid composition, size of perfusion circuit;[39] baroreceptor influences, absence of bronchial blood flow (which abolishes all central and autonomic nervous activity in the lung),[44] chemical influences (i.e., pH, Po_2), humoral influences (i.e., histamine and prostaglandin release from body tissues), lymph flow influences, and, very importantly, unaccounted for or uncontrolled changes in physiologic variables, such as cardiac output, mixed venous oxygen tension and pulmonary vascular pressures, which might have directionally opposite effects on HPV, and the use of different species.[45–47]

Ether has been the next most studied drug, and it appears that the quantitative effect of ether on HPV is also dependent on the type of experimental preparation used. Thus, the in vitro and in vivo–not intact models show much more inhibition of HPV by anesthetic drug (ether) than the in vivo–intact and human

Table 8–4. *Effect of Halothane on Hypoxic Pulmonary Vasoconstriction (HPV) in Various Experimental Preparations*

Anesthetic Drug	Experimental Preparation	Species	Regional (R) vs. Whole (W) Lung Hypoxia	Dose (Converted to MAC)	Effect on HPV/Magnitude of Change*	Reference
Halothane	Vessel strips	Rabbit	W	1.2 to 2.4	↓/Dr–to ?	27
	Heart-lung	Rat	W	1.3 to 2.1	↓/Dr–to 100%	28
	Heart-lung	Rat	W	1 to 3	↓/Dr–to 100%	29
In vitro:	Heart-lung	Rat	W	2	100%	30
	Heart-lung	Rat	W	0 to 2	↓/Dr–to 90%	31
	Heart-lung	Rat	W	2 to 4	↓/Dr–to 90%	26
	Lung	Cat	W	0.5 to 2.5	↓/Dr–to 95%	32
In vivo:	Not intact,	Cat	W	0.5	↓/50%	33
	pump perfused	Cat	W	1 to 3	↓/Dr–to 60%	34
		Dog	W	1.5	↑/Moderate	35
		Dog	W	0.5 to 1	Slight HPV/Slight ↓	36
		Dog	R	to 1.7	↓ Slight	37
In vivo:	Intact,	Dog	R	1	↓ Slight	38
	normally perfused	Dog	R	0.5 to 1.5	0	39
		Dog	R	1 to 3	Slight ↑ or 0	40
		Dog	R	0 to 2	↓ Slight	41
		Goat	W	1	↓/90%	42
	Human	Human	R	0.5 to 2.0	↓/20 to 30% ?	43

*↓ = decrease; ↑ = increase; ↓/Dr–to % = HPV was progressively decreased to the maximum shown in column 6 over the concentration range shown in column 5.

models (Table 8–5).[26,28,29,32,34,48,49] Although the number of studies involving halogenated drugs other than halothane, namely isoflurane,[31,40,41,50–54] enflurane,[26,31,55,56] methoxyflurane,[27–29,57,58] fluroxene,[40,41] and trichloroethylene,[32] have been too small to permit recognition of an experimental preparation result pattern, most of these anesthetics have demonstrated inhibition of HPV (at least in the in vitro models) (Table 8–5). Nitrous oxide seems to cause a small, somewhat consistant inhibition of HPV (Table 8–5).[29,36,40,41,59,60] All injectable anesthetics studied to date have no effect on HPV (Table 8–5).[28,29,37,40,56,61–63]

To summarize previous animal studies, it appears that a fundamental property of inhalational anesthetics is to decrease HPV. However, in intact animal preparations some biologic or physiologic property seems to remove or greatly lessen the inhibitory effect of anesthetic drugs on HPV. It may be that the cause(s) of the difference in effect of anesthetic drugs on regional HPV from preparation to preparation, anesthetic to anesthetic, and species to species (see the following) are closely related to the mechanism of HPV, which is still unknown.

B. Effect of Anesthetics on Arterial Oxygenation During One-Lung Ventilation

An often-made extrapolation of the much more numerous in vitro and in vivo–not intact HPV studies is that anesthetic drugs might impair arterial oxygenation during one-lung anesthesia by inhibiting HPV in the nonventilated lung. One of the previously mentioned studies on the effect of isoflurane on regional canine HPV was especially well controlled and showed that when all nonanesthetic drug variables that might change regional HPV are kept constant, isoflurane inhibits single-lung HPV in a dose-dependent manner.[52] Additionally, the study is valuable because the authors offer the reader an easily comprehensible quantitative summary of the relationship between dose of isoflurane administered and degree of inhibition of the single-lung canine HPV response. If the summary can be extrapolated or applied to the clinical one-lung ventilation situation (at least as an approximation), insights can be gained into what might be expected with regard to arterial oxygenation when such patients are

Table 8–5. *Effect of Ether, Isoflurane, Enflurane, Methoxyflurane, Fluroxene, Trichlorethylene, Nitrous Oxide, and Injectable Anesthetics on Hypoxic Pulmonary Vasoconstriction (HPV)*

Anesthetic Drug	Experimental Preparation		Species	Regional (R) vs. Whole (W) Lung Hypoxia	Dose (Converted to MAC)	Effect on HPV/ Magnitude of Change*	Reference
Ether	In vitro:	Heart-lung	Rat	W	0.5 to 1.0	↓/Dr–to 100%	28
		Heart-lung	Rat	W	1 to 2	↓/Dr–to 100%	29
		Heart-lung	Rat	W	4 to 6	↓ 60 + 70%	26
		Lung	Cat	W	0.5 to 5.0	↓ 90 to 95%	32
		Lung	Cat	W	1	↓ 85%	48
	In vivo:	Not intact, pump perfused	Cat	W	2.5 to 5.0	↓/Dr–to 95%	34
	In vivo:	Intact, normally perfused	Dog	R	1.5 to 3.0	↓/55%	49
	Human		Human	R	1 to 2	↓/33%	42
Isoflurane	In vitro:	Heart-lung	Rat	W	0.2	↓/Dr–to 90%	31
	In vivo:	Not intact, pump perfused	Dog	R	0 to 2	0	51
	In vivo:	Intact, normally perfused	Dog	R	1 to 3	↓/Dr–to 60%	40
			Dog	R	1 to 2	↓/Dr–to 50%	41
			Dog	R	1 to 2	0	50
			Dog	R	0 to 2.4	↓/Dr–to 50%	52
			Dog	R	1.3	0	53
	Human		Human	R	1.0 to 1.5	0	54
Enflurane	In vitro:	Heart-lung	Rat	W	0 to 2	↓/Dr–to 90%	31
		Heart-lung	Rat	W	1 to 3	↓/60%	26
		Heart-lung	Rat	W	1 to 3	↓/Dr–to 100%	55
Methoxy-flurane	In vitro:	Vessel strips	Rabbit	W	1 to 5	VARIABLE	27
		Heart-lung	Rat	W	0.3 to 0.5	↓/Dr–to 100%	28
		Heart-lung	Rat	W	0.3 to 1.3	↓/Dr–to 50%	29
		Lung	Cat	W	1 to 10	↓/Dr–to 100%	57
	In vivo:	Intact, normally perfused	Dog	R	3	0	58
Fluroxene	In vivo:	Intact, normally perfused	Dog	R	1 to 3	↓/Dr–to 80%	40
			Dog	R	1 to 2	↓/Dr–to 55%	41
Trichlorethylene	In vitro:	Lung	Cat	W	0.5–2.5	↓/Dr–to 90%	32
N₂O	In vitro:	Heart-lung	Rat	W	1.4	0	29
	In vivo:	Not intact, pump perfused	Cat	W	0.1 to 0.3	↓/Dr–to 50%	59
	In vivo:	Intact, normally perfused	Dog	W	0.3	↑/Moderate	36
			Dog	R	0.6	↓/30%	40
			Dog	R	0.3	↓/10%	41
			Dog	R	0.5	↓/40%	60
Injectable Anesthetics†	In vitro:	Heart-lung	Rat	W	↑	0	28
		Heart-lung	Rat	W		0	29
		Heart lung	Rat	W		0	61
	In vivo:	Not intact, pump perfused	Cat	W	†	0	62
			Dog	R		0	62
	In vivo:	Intact, normally perfused	Dog	R		0	37
			Dog	R	↓	0	40
	Humans		Humans	R		0	63

*↓ = decrease; ↑ = increase; Dr–to % = HPV was progressively decreased to the maximum shown in colum 6 over the concentration range shown in column 5.

†Drugs used in these experiments were fentanyl, meperidine, morphine, thiopental, pentobarbital, hexobarbital, doperidol, diazepam, chlorpromazine, ketamine, pentazocine, lidocaine, buprenorphine. For doses and blood levels, see the references in the far right column.

anesthetized with isoflurane. In order to put these insights into sharp clinical focus, it is necessary to first understand what should happen to blood flow, shunt flow, and arterial oxygenation, as a function of a normal amount of HPV, when two-lung ventilation is changed to one-lung ventilation in the lateral decubitus position. Once the stable one-lung ventilation condition has been described, it is then possible, using the data from the previously mentioned study to see how isoflurane administration would affect the one-lung ventilation blood flow distribution, shunt flow, and arterial oxygen tension.

1. Two-Lung Ventilation: Blood Flow Distribution

Gravity causes a vertical gradient in the distribution of pulmonary blood flow in the lateral decubitus position for the same reason that it does in the upright position. Consequently, blood flow to the dependent lung is significantly greater than blood flow to the nondependent lung. When the right lung is nondependent, it should receive approximately 45 per cent of total blood flow as opposed to the 55 per cent that it received in the upright and supine positions. When the left lung is nondependent, it should receive approximately 35 per cent of total blood flow as opposed to the 45 per cent

that it received in the upright and supine positions (closed-chest data with normal pulmonary artery pressure) (Fig. 8–1).[64,65] If these blood flow distributions are combined (both the right and left lungs being nondependent an equal number of times), average two-lung ventilation blood flow distribution in the lateral decubitus position would consist of 40 per cent of total blood flow perfusing the nondependent lung and 60 per cent of total blood flow perfusing the dependent lung (Fig. 8–1, right-hand panel and Figs. 8–3 and 8–4, left-hand panels).

It is possible that nondependent lung blood flow may increase slightly when the nondependent hemithorax is open for two reasons.[66] First, if the compliance of the nondependent lung increases so much that nondependent lung alveolar pressure decreases significantly, nondependent lung blood flow may increase relative to dependent lung blood flow. Second, if the nondependent lung falls away from the open chest wall, the vertical distance between the heart and the nondependent lung may decrease, which in the face of a constant pulmonary artery pressure might result in an increased perfusion of the nondependent lung. Consequently, the 40/60 per cent nondependent/dependent lung blood flow ratio during closed chest two-lung ventilation may be a slight underestimation of the ratio during open chest two-lung ventilation.

Blood Flow Distribution: Two Lung Ventilation

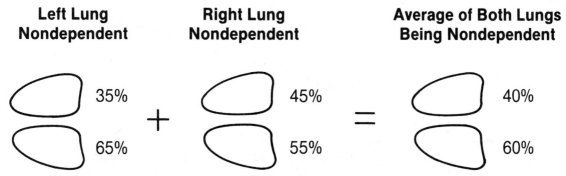

Figure 8–1. This schematic diagram shows that when the left lung is the nondependent lung, the distribution of blood flow between the nondependent and dependent lungs is 35/65 per cent. When the right lung is the nondependent lung the blood flow distribution between the nondependent and dependent lungs is 45/55 per cent. When the left and right lungs are nondependent an equal number of times, then the average one-lung ventilation blood flow distribution would consist of a nondependent and dependent lung blood flow ratio of 40/60 per cent.

2. One-Lung Ventilation: Blood Flow Distribution, Shunt Flow, and Arterial Oxygen Tension

When the nondependent lung is nonventilated (made atelectatic), HPV in the nondependent lung will increase nondependent lung pulmonary vascular resistance and decrease nondependent lung blood flow. In the absence of any confounding or inhibiting factors to the HPV response, a single-lung HPV response should decrease the blood flow to that lung by 50 per cent (Figs. 8–2, 8–3, and 8–4).[67] Consequently, the nondependent lung should be able to reduce its blood flow from 40 to 20 per cent of total blood flow, and the nondependent/dependent lung blood flow ratio during one-lung ventilation should be 20/80 per cent (Fig. 8–4, middle panel).

All the blood flow to the nonventilated nondependent lung is shunt flow, and therefore one-lung ventilation creates an obligatory right-to-left transpulmonary shunt flow that was not present during two-lung ventilation. If no shunt existed during two-lung ventilation conditions (ignoring the normal 1 to 3 per cent shunt flow due to the bronchial, pleural, and thebesian circulations), we would expect the ideal total shunt flow during one-lung ventilation to be a minimal 20 per cent of total blood flow. With a normal hemodynamic and metabolic state the arterial oxygen tension should be approximately 280 mm Hg (Fig. 8–5).[68]

Table 4–1 shows a quantitative example of a model of blood flow to each lung during two-lung and one-lung ventilation, with an increasing initial two-lung ventilation shunt through both lungs. As the initial nondependent lung shunt flow increases (i.e., during two-lung ventilation), the amount of nondependent lung blood flow able to participate in nondependent lung HPV and the amount of nondependent lung HPV blood flow diversion decrease, and the one-lung ventilation shunt increases. As the initial dependent lung shunt flow increases (i.e., during two-lung ventilation), the amount of one-lung ventilation shunt also increases irrespective of nondependent lung HPV.

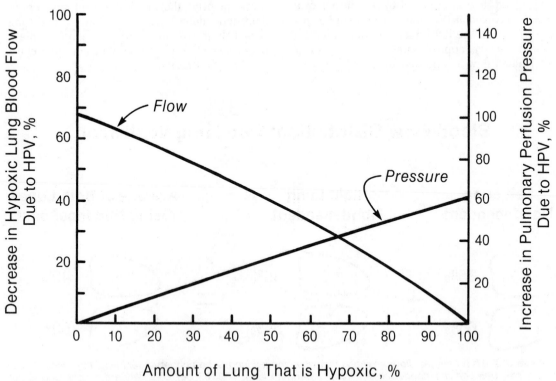

Figure 8–2. On the x-axis is the amount of lung that is hypoxic. On the left hand y-axis is the expected amount of blood flow reduction to the hypoxic lung due to HPV. On the right hand y-axis is the amount of perfusion pressure increase expected due to HPV. When 40 per cent of the lung is hypoxic, the blood flow reduction to the hypoxic lung should be very near 50 per cent. (Redrawn with permission from Marshall BE, Marshall C: Continuity of response to hypoxic pulmonary vasoconstriction. J Appl Physiol 49:189–196, 1980.)

Conversion of Two-Lung to One-Lung Ventilation: Blood Flow Distributions

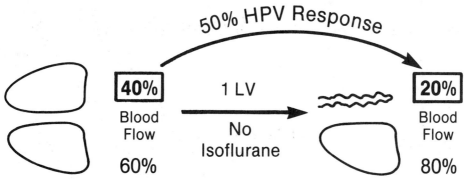

Figure 8–3. *This schematic diagram shows that the two-lung ventilation nondependent/dependent lung blood flow ratio is 40/60 per cent (left-hand side). When two-lung ventilation is converted to one-lung ventilation (as indicated by atelectasis of the nondependent lung), the HPV response decreases the blood flow to the nondependent lung by 50 per cent so that the nondependent/dependent lung blood flow ratio is now 20/80 per cent (right-hand side).*

Effect of 1 MAC Isoflurane Anesthesia on Shunt During One Lung Ventilation (1LV) of Normal Lungs

$$\boxed{\% \downarrow \text{HPV}} = 22.8\,(\% \text{ Alveolar Isoflurane}) - 5.3 = 22.8\,(1.15) - 5.3 = \boxed{21\%}$$

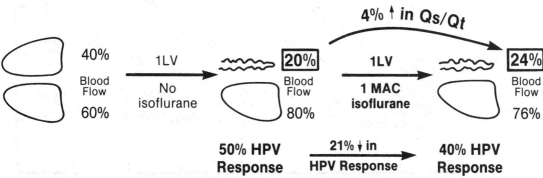

Figure 8–4. *This schematic diagram shows that the two-lung ventilation nondependent/dependent lung blood flow ratio is 40/60 per cent (left-hand side). When two-lung ventilation is converted to one-lung ventilation (as indicated by atelectasis of the nondependent lung), the HPV response decreases the blood flow to the nondependent lung by 50 per cent, so that the nondependent/dependent lung blood flow ratio is now 20/80 per cent (middle). According to the data of Domino et al,[52] administration of 1 MAC isoflurane anesthesia should cause a 21 per cent decrease in the HPV response, which would decrease the 50 per cent blood flow reduction to a 40 per cent blood flow reduction HPV response. Consequently, the nondependent/dependent lung blood flow ratio would now become 24/76 per cent, representing a 4 per cent increase in the total shunt across the lungs (right-hand side). (Reproduced with permission from Benumof JL: Isoflurane anesthesia and arterial oxygenation during one-lung ventilation. Anesthesiology 64:419–422, 1986.)*

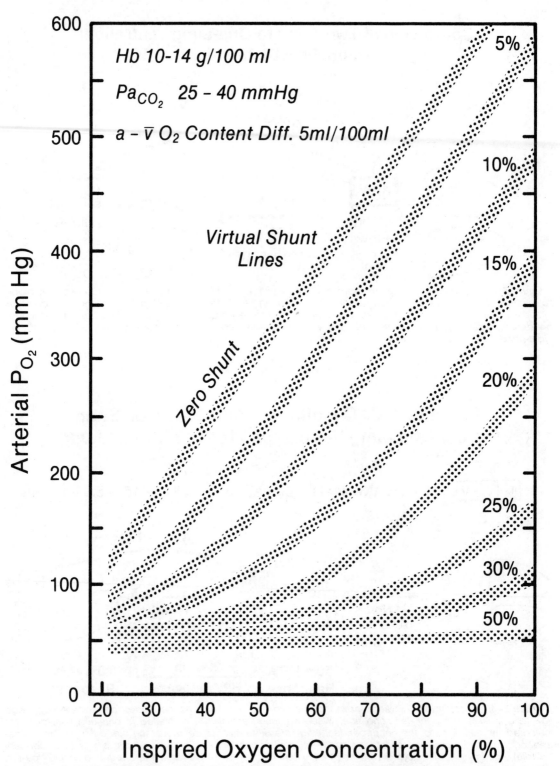

Figure 8–5. On the x-axis is the inspired oxygen concentration. On the left hand y-axis is the expected arterial PO_2 for a family of intrapulmonary shunts. The tick intervals on the right-hand y-axis are the same as those for the left-hand y-axis. As shunt increases, the family of isoshunt lines becomes flatter and closer together, and for a given F_IO_2 an increase in shunt has a decreasing effect on decreasing arterial PO_2. The model assumes relatively normal hemoglobin, P_aCO_2, and a-v̄ O_2 content difference (upper left-hand corner). (Redrawn with permission from Lawler PGP, Nunn JF: A reassessment of the validity of the isoshunt graph. Br J Anaesth 56:1325–1335, 1984.)

3. Effect of Isoflurane on the One-Lung Ventilation Blood Flow Distribution, Shunt Flow, and Arterial Oxygen Tension

Domino et al found: per cent inhibition of regional HPV response equals 22.8 (per cent alveolar isoflurane) minus 5.3.[52] As previously described, under normal conditions collapse of the nondependent lung in the lateral decubitus position causes a nondependent lung HPV response to decrease nondependent lung blood flow by 50 per cent; that is, from 40 to 20 per cent of total flow (Figs. 8–2, 8–3, and 8–4). Using these values as a model of the normal two-lung to one-lung ventilation conversion process, we can construct a table (Table 8–6) that sequentially relates per cent alveolar isoflurane to per cent inhibition of the nondependent lung HPV response, to the resultant nondependent lung HPV response (expressed as a per cent decrease in nondependent lung blood flow), to the resultant increase in atelectatic nondependent lung blood flow (which is the shunt during one-lung ventilation), to an absolute increase in shunt, to a decrease in arterial oxygenation during one-lung ventilation (from 280 mm Hg [F_IO_2 = 1.0] to some lower value).

Table 8–6 and the right-hand panel of Figure 8–4 show that 1 MAC isoflurane anesthesia would inhibit the nondependent lung HPV response by approximately 21 per cent, which would decrease the nondependent lung HPV response from a 50 to 40 per cent nondependent lung blood flow reduction, which would increase nondependent lung blood flow from 20 to 24 per cent of total blood flow, causing shunt to increase by 4 per cent of the cardiac output and P_aO_2 to decrease a moderate amount to 205 mm Hg (F_IO_2 = 1.0) (Fig. 8–5). Table 8–6

shows that one-half MAC isoflurane anesthesia would cause a very small increase in the total one-lung ventilation shunt and a small decrease in P_aO_2, whereas 2 MAC isoflurane anesthesia would cause a moderate increase in the total one-lung ventilation shunt and a large decrease in P_aO_2. Since isoflurane causes undesirable hemodynamic effects at high doses (greater than 1 MAC), and moderate doses of fentanyl (20 μg/kg) have a relative absence of hemodynamic effect, isoflurane anesthesia is usually administered in a 1 MAC or less concentration and is often supplemented with moderate doses of narcotics (or vice versa) (see Recommended Anesthesia Induction and Maintenance Drugs and Techniques).

There are a number of important nonanesthetic drug factors that might make the administration of isoflurane anesthesia have less of an effect on shunting and arterial oxygenation during one-lung ventilation than the preceding analysis would suggest. First, and most important, the absolute level of shunt is almost always higher in surgical patients than the minimal 20 per cent used in the preceding analysis of one-lung ventilation (see Table 4–1). The effect of a given increase in shunt on P_aO_2 depends on the absolute level of the initial shunt and the inspired oxygen concentration (Fig. 8–5).[68] With an F_IO_2 of 1.0, an increase in shunt from 20 to 24 per cent of the cardiac output decreases the P_aO_2 a moderate amount. However, if the two-lung and one-lung ventilation shunt is increased, perhaps owing to pre-existing or anesthesia-induced lung disease, the same isoflurane-induced increase in shunt will cause much less of a decrease in P_aO_2 (the larger iso-shunt lines of Fig. 8–5 are much flatter and closer together). For example, if the one-lung ventilation shunt without isoflurane is 30 per cent

Table 8–6. The Effect of Isoflurane Anesthesia on P_aO_2 During One-Lung Ventilation

MAC	Alveolar Isoflurane (Per Cent)	Inhibition of Nondependent Lung HPV Response (Per Cent)	Resultant Nondependent Lung HPV Response (Per Cent ↓ in Nondependent Lung Blood Flow)	Resultant Nondependent Lung Blood Flow (Per Cent of Cardiac Output)	Increase in Shunt Due to Inhibition of Nondependent Lung HPV (Per Cent of Cardiac Output)	P_aO_2 (F_IO_2 = 1.0) (mm Hg)
0	0	0	50	20	0	280
0.5	0.58	8	46	22	2	250
1.0	1.15	21	40	24	4	205
1.5	1.69	33	33	27	7	140
2.0	2.30	47	26	29	9	110

HPV = hypoxic pulmonary vasoconstriction; MAC = minimum alveolar concentration.

and 34 per cent with isoflurane, the decrease in P_aO_2 will be very small and perhaps not detectable, given the usual accuracy of clinical methodology.

In fact, in clinical one-lung ventilation studies involving intravenously anesthetized patients with this level of shunting, administration of 1 MAC isoflurane (and halothane) anesthesia during stable one-lung ventilation conditions causes no detectable decrease in P_aO_2.[69,70] In one of these clinical studies,[69] stable one-lung ventilation conditions in the lateral decubitus position were established in patients who were anesthetized with only intravenous drugs. While stable one-lung ventilation was maintained, inhalational anesthetics were administered (halothane and isoflurane end-tidal concentrations were greater than 1 MAC for at least 15 minutes) and then discontinued (halothane and isoflurane end-tidal concentrations decreased to near zero). In the other study[70] steady state one-lung ventilation conditions in the lateral decubitus position were established in patients who were anesthetized with only inhalational drugs (halothane and isoflurane end-tidal concentrations were constantly greater than 1 MAC for more than 40 min). While one-lung ventilation was continued, inhalational anesthesia was then discontinued, and intravenous anesthesia was administered (halothane and isoflurane end-tidal concentrations decreased to near zero). There was no significant difference in P_aO_2 during inhalation anesthesia with either halothane or isoflurane compared with intravenous anesthesia during one-lung ventilation in either of the two experimental sequences. In addition, there were no significant changes in physiologic variables, such as cardiac output, pulmonary vascular pressure, and mixed venous oxygen tension, that might secondarily alter nondependent lung HPV. Thus, irrespective of whether inhalational anesthesia is administered before or after intravenous anesthesia during one-lung ventilation, inhalation anesthesia does not further impair arterial oxygenation. These findings are consistent with the interpretation that 1 MAC halothane and isoflurane do not inhibit HPV in patients with a moderate level of shunting enough to cause a significant decrease in P_aO_2 during one-lung ventilation in the lateral decubitus position.

Further considering the implications of Figure 8–5, some anesthesiologists use an F_1O_2 less than 1.0 during one-lung ventilation (which I do not recommend). As can be seen from Figure 8–4, the family of iso-shunt lines is much closer together at $F_1O_2 = 0.5$ than at $F_1O_2 = 1.0$, and the decrease in P_aO_2 with a given increase in shunt is much less (but the absolute level of P_aO_2 is uncomfortably low).

Second, as pointed out by Domino et al,[52] the secondary effects of anesthesia with isoflurane may counteract the direct HPV-inhibitory effect of the drug. Thus, a decrease in cardiac output, mixed venous oxygen tension, and pulmonary artery pressure, all of which may accompany isoflurane anesthesia, would intensify nondependent lung HPV at the same time isoflurane was decreasing it. Third, the presence of chronic irreversible disease in the vessels of the nondependent lung may render these vessels incapable of an HPV response.[71,72] Fourth, the presence of disease in the dependent lung (either pre-existing or anesthesia-induced), which increases dependent lung vascular resistance, will make the dependent lung less able to accept redistributed blood flow and thereby decrease the nondependent lung HPV response.[67,73–75] The smaller the HPV response, the less of an effect isoflurane anesthesia can have on the HPV response. Fifth, surgical interference with blood flow to the nondependent lung will also decrease the effect that isoflurane anesthesia can have on the one-lung ventilation shunt. Sixth, species differences[45–47] and differences in the study and clinical one-lung ventilation methodology (nitrogen ventilation versus atelectasis, administration of isoflurane to the hypoxic lung versus the normoxic or hyperoxic lung, and large versus small alveolar–to–mixed venous isoflurane tension gradients, respectively) may alter the precise relationship between per cent inhibition of single-lung HPV and the alveolar concentration of isoflurane.

In summary, as demonstrated by Domino et al, isoflurane anesthesia has a direct inhibiting effect on regional hypoxic pulmonary vasoconstriction in dogs.[52] In the simple case, where physiologic variables (cardiac output, mixed venous oxygen tension, pulmonary vascular pressures, and carbon dioxide tension) are normal and the amount of lung disease is minimal, the effect of isoflurane on shunting during one-lung ventilation is reasonably predictable and moderately small. In the complex case, where physiologic variables are abnormal and/or the amount of lung disease is extensive, the effect of isoflurane on shunting during one-lung ventilation is much less predictable but almost certainly still small. Nevertheless, it should be remembered that it is the compromised patient who will be most intolerant of any further anesthesia-induced inhibition of HPV. For this kind of patient, the effect of isoflurane anesthesia on shunting must be carefully considered, arterial oxygenation must be closely monitored, and therapeutic measures to decrease shunting, such as nondependent lung CPAP and return to two-lung ventilation, should be quickly instituted, if necessary.

IV. RECOMMENDED ANESTHESIA INDUCTION AND MAINTENANCE DRUGS AND TECHNIQUES

A. Summary of Advantages of Anesthetic Drugs

1. Inhalational Anesthetics

General anesthesia with controlled ventilation is the safest method of anesthetizing patients for the vast majority of elective thoracic procedures. While a variety of general anesthesia techniques can be used, the volatile halogenated anesthetic drugs are good choices for several reasons. First, the halogenated drugs have a salutary effect on airway irritability. The mechanism of this action is controversial, but, as previously discussed, there is evidence that these drugs can block specific forms of bronchoconstriction[9,76] as well as have a nonspecific bronchodilating effect that is related to the depth of anesthesia.[5] Obtundation of airway reflexes in patients who have reactive airways (i.e., smokers) and who may have their airways directly manipulated by the surgeon is a highly desirable property of the general anesthesia produced by these drugs. Second, the use of volatile halogenated drugs allows for delivery of a high inspired oxygen concentration without loss of anesthesia. Although a nitrous oxide-oxygen-narcotic–relaxant anesthesia technique can be used, nitrous oxide necessitates a significant decrease in the inspired oxygen concentration and increases the chance of developing hypoxemia (especially if one-lung ventilation is employed).[77] Unless very high doses of narcotics are used, airway reflexes and reactivity may remain at a high level. Third, since the volatile halogenated drugs can be rapidly eliminated, concern over postoperative hypoventilation in extubated patients may be diminished. Doses of intravenous anesthetics, such as the narcotics, ketamine, and the barbiturates, which render the patient areflexic to surgical stimulation, may cause the patient to require a period of postoperative ventilation. Fourth, in the usual clinical doses (near 1 MAC), the halogenated anesthetic drugs provide a reasonable degree of cardiovascular stability. This may be of particular importance in patients with coronary artery disease and systemic hypertension. Fifth, the halogenated drugs do not appear to decrease P_aO_2 any more than intravenous anesthetics during one-lung ventilation (see the following).[69,70]

2. Intravenous Anesthetics

The narcotics, especially fentanyl, have a number of desirable properties that could be used to advantage for patients undergoing thoracic surgery. First, fentanyl has no adverse hemodynamic effects and, therefore, is a useful drug to use in patients who have significant coronary artery disease. Second, if significant blood levels exist at the end of surgery, the narcotics can allow an intubated patient to have a smooth transition from surgery into the postoperative period. Third, the narcotics, if used in moderate dosage, greatly diminish the amount of volatile halogenated drug anesthesia required to achieve surgical levels of anesthesia. Fourth, high doses of narcotics or moderate doses in conjunction with halogenated drugs allow for the use of a high inspired oxygen concentration without loss of anesthesia. Fifth, the narcotics are thought not to diminish regional hypoxic pulmonary vasoconstriction and, therefore, should permit optimal oxygenation during one-lung ventilation.

Ketamine, in combination with nitrous oxide and a muscle relaxant, has also been used for anesthesia in thoracic surgery.[78] While we do not ordinarily employ ketamine for elective thoracic procedures, the drug is very useful for the induction of general anesthesia in critically ill patients undergoing emergency thoracic surgery for several reasons. First, ketamine has sympathomimetic properties[79] that are highly desirable because many emergency thoracic procedures are associated with hypovolemia (gunshot and stab wounds of the chest, blunt trauma, and massive hemoptysis). However, it should be remembered that ketamine will depress cardiovascular function (systemic blood pressure, contractility) if the degree of hypovolemia is severe and the patients are sympathetically exhausted. Second, ketamine has a rapid onset of action and can be used safely, along with cricoid pressure, to induce anesthesia in patients with full stomachs. Third, ketamine may reduce bronchospasm in asthmatic patients;[13] the clinical extrapolation of this effect to thoracic surgical patients is uncertain at this time. Fourth, ketamine does not impair arterial oxygenation during one-lung ventilation (perhaps owing to lack of effect on hypoxic pulmonary vasoconstriction).[63]

B. Recommended Anesthetic Drugs and Technique

It should be obvious from the foregoing discussions that there are advantages and disadvantages to both the inhalation and intravenous anesthetic drugs. The following recommended anesthetic technique takes advantage of the desirable properties and minimizes the undesirable properties of these drugs. Thus, the halogenated drugs are used for their effect on bronchomotor tone, to administer 100 per cent oxygen, and to allow for early extubation while not decreasing hemodynamic function and arterial oxygenation, whereas fentanyl is used to ensure hemodynamic stability while not jeopardizing early extubation if desired. If it is thought that the patient will not be extubated early or if greater hemodynamic stability is desired, anesthesia consisting of more fentanyl and less halogenated drug can be used.

1. The Induction of Anesthesia (Fig. 8–6)

The patient is preoxygenated by spontaneously breathing 100 per cent oxygen through a black rubber anesthesia mask that is connected to an anesthesia circle system. Fentanyl is administered intravenously until the respiratory rate is approximately 8 to 10 breaths/min. This usually corresponds to a dose of 10 to 15 μg/kg and is usually administered over 3 min. When the respiratory rate is relatively slow and deep, and response to commands are becoming sluggish, a small dose of pentathol (2 to 3 mg/kg) or ketamine (1 to 2 mg/kg) (if the patient is thought to have an especially reactive airway or to be minimally to moderately hypovolemic) is administered, which renders the patient unconscious and usually apneic. The airway is then established, and ventilation is controlled with intermittent positive-pressure oxygen via the black rubber mask. While the patient is being ventilated with positive pressure, concentrations of 2.5 to 0.5 per cent isoflurane are administered. The higher isoflurane concentration is used initially for a short period of time (overpressure, 1 to 2 min), and as the patient

demonstrates signs of deepening anesthesia, the inspired isoflurane concentration is decreased. In view of the fact that general anesthetics significantly decrease the ventilatory response to CO_2 (to a much greater degree in patients with mechanical ventilatory impairment compared with normal patients), patients are not allowed to breathe spontaneously until the end of the procedure; alarming degrees of hypercapnia have been observed in similar circumstances when spontaneous ventilation was allowed.[80]

Early during the period of positive-pressure ventilation with isoflurane, paralysis is induced with either pancuronium 0.02 mg/kg and metocurine 0.08 mg/kg, or vecuronium 0.1 mg/kg, or atracurium 0.5 mg/kg. The development of full paralysis is monitored with a neuromuscular blockade monitor. During the period of deepening isoflurane anesthesia and paralysis, blood pressure is supported with an infusion of approximately 10 ml/kg crystalloid. If more cardiovascular support is required, the first drugs used (while fluid is being infused) are ephedrine 0.05 to 0.1 mg/kg, atropine 0.02 mg/kg, and calcium 5 mg/kg. When the patient has been judged to be adequately (surgical stage) anesthetized (as judged by changes in blood pressure, heart rate, and eye signs [the eyes should be central, conjugate, fixed, staring, without tears, and with nondilated pupils]) and paralyzed in the above manner, lidocaine 1 mg/kg is administered intravenously, laryngoscopy is performed, the tracheobronchial tree sprayed with a laryngotracheobronchial spray system, and the trachea intubated with a double-lumen tube (see chapter 9). The intravenous and intratracheal lidocaine should diminish both the airway and cardiovascular response to endotracheal intubation.[81] The patient is then ventilated with maintenance doses of isoflurane and administered maintenance doses of narcotics and relaxants. Use of maintenance paralysis decreases isoflurane requirements, possibly allowing for a more rapid emergence from anesthesia.[82]

2. The Maintenance of Anesthesia

Anesthesia is maintained with both isoflurane (concentration approximately 0.5 to 1.0 MAC) and narcotics. Isoflurane is primarily used if the patient is thought to stand a reasonable chance of being extubated within the first couple hours postoperatively. Narcotics (fentanyl) are primarily used if the patient is thought not to have a reasonable chance of being extubated in the

Anesthetic Technique for Typical
One Lung Ventilation Thoracic Surgery Cases

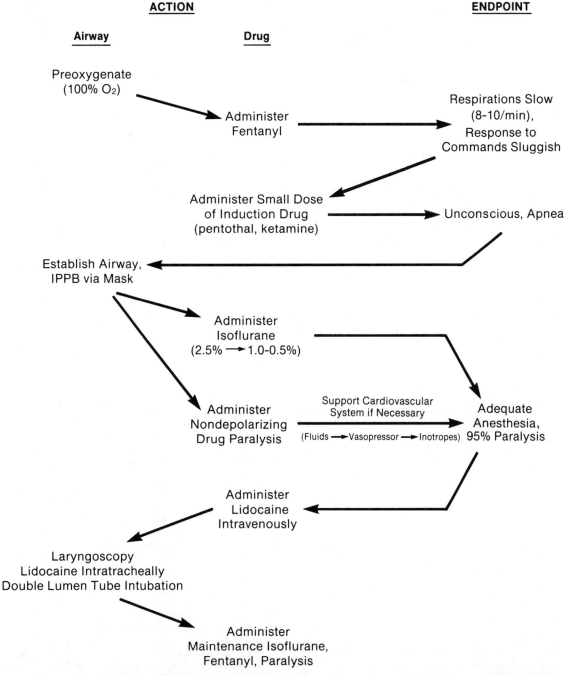

Figure 8–6. *This action-endpoint flow diagram describes the anesthetic technique used for a typical one-lung ventilation thoracic surgery case. The actions are divided into those that are primarily concerned with airway management versus those that involve administration of a drug. All drug administrations are associated with an endpoint. See text for full explanation.*

immediate postoperative period and will require a significant period of postoperative ventilation. Relaxants (primarily pancuronium) are administered in small doses to keep the level of neuromuscular blockade, as judged by a neuromuscular blockade monitor, near the 90 per cent paralysis level.

If the patient is thought to have a reasonable chance of being extubated in the first postoperative hour, the patient is turned supine, the double-lumen tube changed to a single-lumen tube, paralysis reversed, and spontaneous ventilation is allowed to recur. Fentanyl is administered in extremely small increments (0.3 µg/kg) while the patient is breathing spontaneously. The goal of the fentanyl administration is to have the patient breathing relatively slowly (approximately 10 to 12 breaths/min) and deeply when surgery is completed. The presence of a moderate narcotic base allows the patient to be returned to the recovery room for a short period of mechanical ventilatory support (if needed) and weaned and extubated in a relatively smooth manner.

REFERENCES

1. Aviado DM: Regulation of bronchomotor tone during anesthesia. Anesthesiology 42:68, 1975.
2. Fielding JE: Smoking: Health effects and control. N Engl J Med 313:491–498, 1985.
3. Bennett DJ, Torda TA, Horton DA, et al: Severe bronchospasm complicating thoracotomy. Arch Surg 101:555, 1970.
4. Brakensiek AL, Bergman JA: The effect of halothane and atropine on total respiratory resistance in anesthetized man. Anesthesiology 53:341, 1970.
5. Patterson RW, Sullivan SF, Malm JR, et al: The effects of halothane on human airway mechanics. Anesthesiology 29:900, 1968.
6. McAslan C, Mima M, Norden I, et al: Effect of halothane and methoxyflurane on pulmonary resistance to gas flow during lung bypass. Scand J Thorac Cardiovasc Surg 5:193, 1971.
7. Waltemath CL, Bergman NA: Effect of ketamine and halothane on increased respiratory resistance provoked by ultrasonic aerosols. Anesthesiology 41:473, 1974.
8. Meloche R, Norlander O, Norden I, Herzog P: Effects of carbon dioxide and halothane on compliance in pulmonary resistance during cardiopulmonary bypass. Scand J Thorac Cardiovasc Surg 3:69, 1969.
9. Hirshman CA, Edelstein G, Peetz S, Wayne R, Downes H: Mechanism of action of inhalational anesthesia on airways. Anesthesiology 56:107, 1982.
10. Moss J, Rosow CE, Savarese JJ, et al: Role of histamine in the hypotensive action of d-tubocurarine in humans. Anesthesiology 55:19–25, 1981.
11. Shemano I, Wendel H: Effects of meperidine hydrochloride and morphine sulfate on the lung capacity of intact dogs. J Pharmacol Exp Ther 149:379–384, 1965.
12. Hirshman CA, Downes H, Farbood A, et al: Ketamine block of bronchospasm in experimental canine asthma. Br J Anaesth 51:713–718, 1979.
13. Corssen G, Gutierrez J, Reeves JG, et al: Ketamine in the anesthetic management of asthmatic patients. Anesth Analg 51:588–596, 1972.
14. Clarke RSJ, Dundee JW, Garrett RT, McArdle GK, Sutton JA: Adverse reactions to intravenous anesthesia. Br J Anaesth 47:575, 1975.
15. Crago RR, Bryan AC, Laws AIC, Winestock AE: Respiratory flow resistance after curare and pancuronium measured by forced oscillations. Canad Anaesth Soc J 19:607–614, 1972.
16. Brandus V, Joffe S, Benoit CV, Wolff WI: Bronchial spasm during general anesthesia. Canad Anaesth Soc J 17:269–274, 1970.
17. Gal TJ: Airway responses in normal subjects following topical anesthesia with ultrasonic aerosols with 4 per cent lidocaine. Anesth Analg 59:123–129, 1980.
18. Loehning RW, Waltemath CL, Bergman NA: Lidocaine and increased respiratory resistance produced by ultrasonic aerosols. Anesthesiology 44:306–310, 1976.
19. Don HF, Robson JG: The mechanics of the respiratory system during anesthesia: The effects of atropine and carbon dioxide. Anesthesiology 26:168–178, 1965.
20. Severinghaus JW, Stupfel M: Respiratory dead space increase following atropine in man and atropine, vagal or ganglionic blockade and hypothermia in dogs. J Appl Physiol 8:81–87, 1955.
21. Department of Health and Human Services: The health consequences of smoking: Cardiovascular disease. A report of the Surgeon General. Rockville, Maryland, 1983.
22. The Pooling Project Research Group: Relationship of blood pressure, serum cholesterol, smoking habit, relative weight, and ECG abnormalities to incidence of major coronary events: Final report of the Pooling Project. J Chronic Dis 31:201–306, 1978.
23. Department of Health and Human Services: A report of the Surgeon General: The health consequences of smoking for women. Rockville, Maryland, 1980.
24. Bazaral MG, Wagner R, Abi-Nader E, Estafanous FG: Comparison of the effects of 15 and 60 µg/kg fentanyl used for induction of anesthesia in patients with coronary disease. Anesth Analg 64:312–318, 1985.
25. Reiz S, Balfors E, Sorensen MB, Ariola S Jr, Freidman A, Truedsson H: Isoflurane—A powerful coronary vasodilator in patients with coronary artery disease. Anesthesiology 59:91, 1983.
26. Bjertnaes LJ, Mundal R, Hauge A, Nicolaysen A: Vascular resistance in atelectatic lungs: Effect of inhalation anesthetics. Acta Anaesth Scand 24:109–118, 1980.
27. Gorsky B, Schneider AJL: Interaction of anesthetics and hypoxia on pulmonary vessels. Abstracts of Scientific Papers, 1972 Annual ASA meeting, p 179.
28. Bredesen J, Bjertnaes L, Hauge A: Effects of anesthetics on the pulmonary vasoconstrictor response to acute alveolar hypoxia. Microvasc Res 10:236, 1975.
29. Bjertnaes LJ: Hypoxia-induced vasconstriction in isolated perfused lungs exposed to injectable or inhalation anesthetics. Acta Anaesth Scand 21:133–147, 1977.
30. Bjertnaes LJ, Hauge A, Torgrinsen T: The pulmonary vasoconstrictor response to hypoxia. The hypoxia-sensitive site studied with a volatile inhibitor. Acta Physiol Scand 109:447–462, 1980.
31. Marshall C, Lindgren L, Marshall BE: The effect of inhalation anesthetics on HPV. Anesthesiology 59: A527, 1983.

32. Sykes MK, Davies DM, Chakrabarti MK, Loh L: The effects of halothane, trichlorethylene and ether on the hypoxic pressor response and pulmonary vascular resistance in the isolated, perfused lung. Br J Anaesth 45:655–663, 1973.

33. Gibbs JM, Sykes MK, Tait AR: Effects of halothane and hydrogen ion concentration on the alteration of pulmonary vascular resistance induced by graded alveolar hypoxia in the isolated perfused cat lung. Anaesth Intens Care 2:231–239, 1974.

34. Loh L, Sykes MK, Chakrabarti MK: The effects of halothane and ether on the pulmonary circulation in the isolated perfused cat lung. Br. J Anaesth 49:309–314, 1977.

35. Babjak AF, Forrest JB: Effects of halothane on the pulmonary vascular response to hypoxia in dogs. Canad Anaesth Soc J 26:6–14, 1979.

36. Buckley MJ, McLaughlen JS, Fort L III, Saigusa M, Morrow DH: Effects of anesthetic agents on pulmonary vascular resistance during hypoxia. Surg Forum 15:183–184, 1964.

37. Lumb TD, Silvay G, Weinreich AI, Shiang W: A comparison of the effects of continuous ketamine infusion and halothane on oxygenation during one lung anesthesia in dogs. Canad Anaesth Soc J 26:394–401, 1979.

38. Hall SM, Chapleau M, Cairo J, Levitsky MG: The effect of high frequency ventilation on halothane ablation of hypoxic pulmonary vasoconstriction. Fed Proc 42:595, 1983.

39. Sykes MK, Gibbs JM, Loh L, Marin JBL, Obdrzalek J, Arnot RN: Preservation of the pulmonary vasoconstrictor response to alveolar hypoxia during the administration of halothane to dogs. Br J Anaesth 50:1185–1196, 1978.

40. Benumof JL, Wahrenbrock EA: Local effects of anesthetics on regional hypoxic pulmonary vasoconstriction. Anesthesiology 43:525–532, 1975.

41. Mathers J, Benumof JL, Wahrenbrock EA: General anesthetics and regional hypoxic pulmonary vasoconstriction. Anesthesiology 46:111–114, 1977.

42. Pavlin EG, Reed RL, Winn RK: Pulmonary vascular pressure-flow curves in intact goats demonstrate hypoxic pulmonary vasoconstriction is abolished by halothane. Anesthesiology 63:A532, 1985.

43. Bjertnaes LJ: Hypoxia-induced pulmonary vasoconstriction in man: Inhibition due to diethyl ether and halothane anesthesia. Acta Anaesth Scan 22:570–588, 1978.

44. Allison PR, Daly I de B, Waaler BA: Bronchial circulation and pulmonary vasomotor nerve responses in isolated perfused lungs. J Physiol 157:462, 1961.

45. Grover RF, Vogel JHK, Averill KH, Blount SG: Pulmonary hypertension. Individual and species variability relative to vascular reactivity. Am Heart J 66:1–3, 1963.

46. Tucker A, McMurtry IF, Alexander AF, Reeves JT, Grover RF: Lung mast cell density and distribution in chronically hypoxic animals. J Appl Physiol 42:174–178, 1977.

47. Tucker A, McMurtry IF, Reeves JT, Alexander AF, Will DH, Grover RF: Lung vascular smooth muscle as a determinant of pulmonary hypertension at high altitude. Am J Physiol 228:762–767, 1975.

48. Hurtig JB, Tait AR, Sykes ML: Reduction of hypoxic pulmonary vasoconstriction by diethyl ether in the isolated perfused cat lung: The effect of acidosis and alkalosis. Canad Anaesth Soc J 24:433–444, 1977.

49. Sykes MK, Hurtig JB, Tait AR, Chakrabarti MK: Reduction of hypoxic pulmonary vasoconstriction during diethyl ether anesthesia in the dog. Br J Anaesth 49:293–299, 1977.

50. Saidman LJ, Troudsale FR: Isoflurane does not inhibit hypoxic pulmonary vasoconstriction. Anesthesiology 57:A472, 1982.

51. Gardaz JP, Morel PH, Py P, Gemperle M: Isoflurane and regional pulmonary vascular resistance during lobar ventilation hypoxia and collapse in dogs. Anesthesiology 63:A531, 1985.

52. Domino KB, Borowec L, Alexander CM, Williams JJ, Chen L, Marshall C, Marshall BE: Influence of isoflurane on hypoxic pulmonary vasoconstriction in dogs. Anesthesiology 64:423–429, 1986.

53. Chuda RM, Yao FS, Harvey RC: Cardiopulmonary function during one-lung anesthesia with alfentanil or isoflurane in the dog. Anesthesiology 63:A562, 1985.

54. Jolin-Carlsson A, Bindslev L, Hedenstierna G: Hypoxia-induced pulmonary vasoconstriction in the human lung. The effect of isoflurane anesthesia. Karolinsk Hospital ISBN 91–7900–016–9 Repro Print Stockholm, 1986 pages IV:I–IV:10.

55. Bjertnaes LJ, Mundal R: The pulmonary vasoconstrictor response to hypoxia during enflurane anesthesia. Acta Anaesth Scand 24:252–256, 1980.

56. Rees DI, Gaines GY: One-lung anesthesia—a comparison of pulmonary gas exchange during anesthesia with ketamine or enflurane. Anesth Analg 63:521–525, 1984.

57. Sykes MK, Davies DM, Loh L, Jastrzebski J, Chakrabarti MK: The effect of methoxyflurane on pulmonary vascular resistance and hypoxic pulmonary vasoconstriction in the isolated perfused cat lung. Br J Anaesth 48:191–194, 1976.

58. Marin JLB, Carruthers B, Chakrabarti MK, Sykes MK: Preservation of the hypoxic pulmonary vasoconstrictor mechanism during methoxyflurane anesthesia in the dog. Br J Anaesth 51:99–105, 1979.

59. Hurtig JB, Tait AR, Loh L, Sykes MK: Reduction of hypoxic pulmonary vasoconstriction by nitrous oxide administration in the isolated perfused cat lung. Canad Anaesth Soc J 24:540–549, 1977.

60. Sykes MK, Hurtig JB, Tait AR, Chakrabarti MK: Reduction of hypoxic pulmonary constriction in the dog during administration of nitrous oxide. Br J Anaesth 49:301–307, 1977.

61. Bjertnaes L, Hauge A, Kriz M: Hypoxia induced pulmonary vasoconstriction: Effects of fentanyl following different routes of administration. Acta Anaesth Scand 24:53–57, 1980.

62. Gibbs JM, Johnson H: Lack of effect of morphine and buprenorphine on hypoxic pulmonary vasoconstriction in the isolated perfused cat lung and the perfused lobe of the dog lung. Br J Anaesth 50:1197–1201, 1978.

63. Weinreich AI, Silvay G, Lumb PD: Continuous ketamine infusion for one-lung anesthesia. Canad Anaesth Soc J 27:485–490, 1980.

64. Wulff KE, Aulin I: The regional lung function in the lateral decubitus position during anesthesia and operation. Acta Anesth Scand 16:195–205, 1972.

65. Rehder K, Wenthe FM, Sessler AD: Function of each lung during mechanical ventilation with ZEEP and with PEEP in man anesthetized with theopental-meperidine. Anesthesiology 39:597–606, 1973.

66. Werner O, Malmkvist G, Beckman A, Stahle S, Nordstrom L: Gas exchange and haemodynamics during thoracotomy. Br J Anaesth 56:1343–1349, 1984.

67. Marshall BE, Marshall C: Continuity of response to hypoxic pulmonary vasoconstriction. J Appl Physiol 59:189–196, 1980.
68. Lawler PGP, Nunn JF: A reassessment of the validity of the iso-shunt graph. Br J Anaesth 56:1325–1335, 1984.
69. Rogers SN, Benumof JL: Halothane and isoflurane do not decrease P_aO_2 during one-lung ventilation in intravenously anesthetized patients. Anesth Analg 64:946–954, 1985.
70. Augustine SD, Benumof JL: Halothane and isoflurane do not impair arterial oxygenation during one-lung ventilation in patients undergoing thoracotomy. Abst Anesth 61:A484, 1984.
71. Casthely PA, Lear F, Cottrell JE, Lear E. Intrapulmonary shunting during induced hypotension. Anesth Analg 61:231–235, 1982.
72. Zapol WM, Snider MT: Pulmonary hypertension in severe acute respiratory failure. N Engl J Med 296:476–480, 1972.
73. Scanlon TS, Benumof JL, Wahrenbrock EA, Nelson WL: Hypoxic pulmonary vasoconstriction and the ratio of hypoxic lung to perfused normoxic lung. Anesthesiology 49:177–181, 1978.
74. Marshall BE, Marshall C, Benumof JL, Saidman LJ: Hypoxic pulmonary vasoconstriction in dogs: Effects of lung segment size and alveolar oxygen tensions. J Appl Physiol 51:1543–1551, 1981.
75. Zasslow MA, Benumof JL, Trousdale FR: Hypoxic pulmonary vasoconstriction and the size of hypoxic compartment. J Appl Physiol 53:626–630, 1982.
76. Coon RL, Kampine JP: Hypocapnic bronchoconstriction and inhalation anesthetics. Anesthesiology 43:635–641, 1975.
77. Boutrous AR, Weisel MR: Arterial blood oxygenation during thoracotomy using 70 per cent nitrous oxide in oxygen. Anesthesiology 28:705–710, 1968.
78. Vaughan RW, Stephen CR: Abdominal and thoracic surgery in adults with ketamine, nitrous oxide, and d-tubocurarine. Anesth Analg 53:271, 1974.
79. Tweed WA, Minuck M, Mywin D: Circulation responses to ketamine anesthesia. Anesthesiology 77:613, 1972.
80. Pietak S, Weenig CS, Hickey RF, et al: Anesthetic effects on ventilation in patients with chronic obstructive pulmonary disease. Anesthesiology 72:160, 1975.
81. Denlinger JK, Ellison N, Ominsky AJ: Effects of intratracheal lidocaine on circulatory responses to tracheal intubation. Anesthesiology 41:409, 1974.
82. Forbes AR, Cohen NH, Eger EI: Pancuronium reduces halothane requirement in man. Anesth Analg 58:497, 1979.

Separation of the Two Lungs (Double-Lumen Tube Intubation)

I. INTRODUCTION

The complete functional separation of the two lungs is often the most important anesthetic consideration for patients undergoing thoracic surgery. The procedure can occasionally be life-saving, and very frequently it greatly facilitates the conduct of surgery. Newly introduced disposable plastic double-lumen tubes, which are relatively nontraumatic and easy to insert, and the advent of fiberoptic bronchoscopy, which makes location of a double-lumen tube under direct vision possible and therefore a precise, repeatable, low-risk maneuver, have greatly increased the efficacy and use of double-lumen tubes. This chapter sequentially discusses the indications for separation of the two lungs, conventional techniques of double-lumen tube insertion and determination of position, use of the fiberoptic bronchoscope to insert a double-lumen tube, and determination of precise double-lumen tube position by fiberoptic bronchoscopy. The chapter ends with a brief consideration of other methods, such as bronchial blockers and endobronchial intubation, to separate the two lungs.

II. INDICATIONS FOR SEPARATION OF THE TWO LUNGS

There are several absolute and relative indications for separation of the two lungs during thoracic operations or procedures (Table 9–1).

A. Absolute Indications

Separation of the two lungs for any of the absolute indications discussed here should be considered a life-saving maneuver because failure to separate the two lungs under any of these conditions could result in a life-threatening complication or situation. There are three absolute indications for separating the two lungs (Table 9–1 and Fig. 9-1). First, separation of one lung from the other is absolutely necessary in order to prevent spillage of pus or blood from an infected (abscessed) lung or bleeding lung, respectively, to a noninvolved lung. Acute contamination of a lung with either blood or pus from the other lung usually results in severe massive (bilateral) atelectasis, pneumonia, and sepsis. Second, there are a number of unilateral

Table 9-1. Indications for Separation of the Two Lungs (Double-Lumen Tube Intubation) and/or One-Lung Ventilation

Absolute
1. Isolation of one lung from the other to avoid spillage or contamination
   A. Infection
   B. Massive hemorrhage
2. Control of the distribution of ventilation
   A. Bronchopleural fistula
   B. Bronchopleural cutaneous fistula
   C. Surgical opening of a major conducting airway
   D. Giant unilateral lung cyst or bulla
   E. Tracheobronchial tree disruption
3. Unilateral bronchopulmonary lavage
   A. Pulmonary alveolar proteinosis

Relative
1. Surgical exposure—high priority
   A. Thoracic aortic aneurysm
   B. Pneumonectomy
   C. Upper lobectomy
2. Surgical exposure—low priority
   A. Middle and lower lobectomies and subsegmental resections
   B. Esophageal resection
   C. Thoracoscopy
   D. Procedures on the thoracic spine
3. Postcardiopulmonary bypass status after removal of totally occluding chronic unilateral pulmonary emboli

lung problems that can prevent adequate ventilation of the other noninvolved side. A large bronchopleural or bronchopleural cutaneous fistula or a surgically opened conducting airway has such a low resistance to gas flow that a tidal inspiration delivered by positive pressure will exit via the low resistance pathway, and it will become impossible to ventilate the other, more normal, lung adequately. A giant unilateral bulla or cyst may rupture if exposed to positive-pressure ventilation and result in a tension pneumothorax or pneumomediastinum. Finally, positive-pressure ventilation of a lung with a tracheobronchial tree disruption can result in dissection of gas into the pulmonary interstitial space or mediastinum, resulting in a tension pneumomediastinum. Third, separation of the two lungs is absolutely necessary in order to perform unilateral bronchopulmonary lavage in patients with pulmonary alveolar proteinosis (and rarely, asthma and cystic fibrosis).

B. Relative Indications

There are a large number of relative indications for separation of the two lungs, and they are all for the purpose of facilitating surgical exposure by collapsing the lung in the operative hemithorax. These relative indications can be divided into high priority and low priority categories (Table 9–1 and Fig. 9–2). Of the relative indications, repair of a thoracic aortic aneurysm is usually the highest priority because it requires exposure of the thoracic aorta as it runs the entire length of the left hemithorax. A pneumonectomy, especially if performed through a median sternotomy,[1] is greatly aided by the wide exposure of the lung hilum that is afforded by collapse of the operative lung. Similarly, an upper lobectomy, which is technically the most difficult lobectomy, and many mediastinal exposures, may be made much easier by eliminating ventilation to the lung on the side of the procedure. The surgical items in the low priority category do not routinely require collapse of the lung on the operative side but still significantly aid surgical exposure and eliminate the need for the surgeon to handle (retract, compress, pack away) the operative lung. Severe intraoperative retraction of the lung on the operated side can traumatize the operative lung and impair gas exchange both intra-[2, 3] and postoperatively.[4, 5] The lower priority items consist of middle and lower lobectomies, less extensive pulmonary resections, thoracic spinal procedures that are approached anteriorly through the chest, and esophageal surgery. However, even relatively small operations such as wedge and segmental resections benefit by double-lumen tube insertion because of the ability to alternate easily and quickly between lung collapse and inflation, which is sometimes required to better visualize lung morphology and to facilitate identification and separation of important planes and fissures. Examination of the pleural space (thorocoscopy) is considerably aided by collapse of the ipsilateral lung. Finally, the separation of the lungs following removal of totally occluding and predominantly unilateral chronic pulmonary emboli (postcardiopulmonary bypass) can be very helpful because of the possibility of massive transudation of hemorrhagic fluid across the alveolar capillary membrane in the region of the lung supplied by the previously occluded vessel (reperfusion of a previously and chronically nonperfused vascular bed). Should significant and predominantly unilateral post-thromboembolectomy postcardiopulmonary bypass pulmonary edema occur, the patient should be returned to cardiopulmonary bypass, and a double-lumen endotracheal tube should be inserted so that differential lung ventilation may be used (see chapters 11 and 19).

Absolute Indications for
Lung Separation/One Lung Ventilation

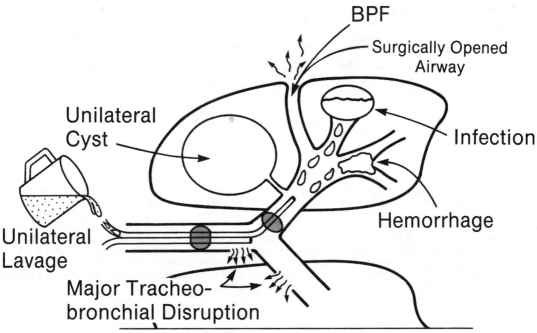

Figure 9–1. This schematic diagram shows the absolute indications for lung separation and/or one-lung ventilation. Hemorrhage and infection in one lung can contaminate and soil the other lung. A low-resistance ventilation pathway, such as a bronchopleural fistula (BPF) or a surgically opened major airway, can make positive pressure ventilation of the other lung impossible. A giant unilateral cyst or bulla can rupture if exposed to positive pressure ventilation and can result in a tension pneumothorax. Unilateral lung lavage requires the instillation of large amounts of saline into one lung while the other lung is being ventilated. Major tracheobronchial disruption can lead to mediastinal and pulmonary interstitial emphysema if exposed to positive pressure.

Relative Indications for Lung Separation/ One Lung Ventilation

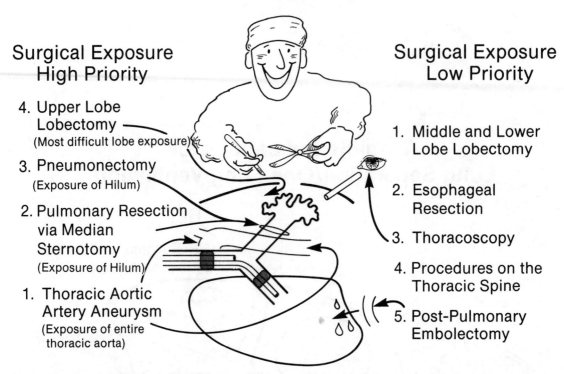

Surgical Exposure High Priority

4. Upper Lobe Lobectomy
(Most difficult lobe exposure)

3. Pneumonectomy
(Exposure of Hilum)

2. Pulmonary Resection via Median Sternotomy
(Exposure of Hilum)

1. Thoracic Aortic Artery Aneurysm
(Exposure of entire thoracic aorta)

Surgical Exposure Low Priority

1. Middle and Lower Lobe Lobectomy

2. Esophageal Resection

3. Thoracoscopy

4. Procedures on the Thoracic Spine

5. Post-Pulmonary Embolectomy

Figure 9–2. This schematic diagram depicts the relative indications for lung separation and/or one-lung ventilation. The indications are all for facilitating surgical exposure and can be divided into high priority and low priority categories. The high priority items for lung collapse are thoracic aortic artery aneurysm repair (requires exposure of the entire thoracic aorta, which is greatly facilitated by collapsing the left lung), pneumonectomy (requires wide exposure of the lung hilum), and upper lobe lobectomy (technically the most difficult lobe to expose). The lower priority items for lung collapse are middle and lower lobe lobectomy and esophageal surgery. Inspection of a hemithorax by thoracoscopy, if performed under general anesthesia, is greatly facilitated by collapse of the ipsilateral lung. Procedures on the thoracic spine that are approached anteriorly via the chest are facilitated by collapse of the lung on the operative side. Lung separation is useful if unilateral pulmonary edema occurs following removal of a chronic, totally occluding, unilateral pulmonary embolus (postcardiopulmonary bypass).

III. DOUBLE-LUMEN TUBE INTUBATION

Double-lumen endotracheal tubes have evolved to become considered as the technique of choice for most cases of lung separation and will be discussed here in great detail. Bronchial blockers and endobronchial tubes are not often used today and are only briefly described at the end of the chapter. There are many reasons double-lumen tubes are favored over bronchial blockers and endobronchial tubes for lung separation. First, double-lumen tubes are relatively easily placed by even inexperienced anesthesiologists, whereas a much higher degree of skill is required to position bronchial blockers and endobronchial tubes correctly. Second, double-lumen tubes allow easy, repeated, and

rapid conversion from two-lung ventilation to one-lung ventilation and vice versa at any time during surgery, whereas bronchial blockers and endobronchial tubes preclude two-lung ventilation. Third, double-lumen tubes allow for suctioning of both lungs, whereas bronchial blockers and endobronchial tubes preclude suctioning of the collapsed lung. Fourth, double-lumen tubes allow CPAP to be applied to the nonventilated lung, whereas with bronchial blockers and endobronchial tubes no ventilatory maneuvers can be used on the lung under operation.

There are two relatively minor disadvantages to double-lumen tubes, and both are related to the fact that the lumens of a double-lumen tube may be narrow. First, suctioning may be more difficult down a narrow lumen, but this is usually not a problem with the new disposable Robertshaw type double-lumen tubes, which have nonadhering suction catheters that slide easily down the lumens of the double-lumen tube. Second, although airway resistance may be increased with a narrow lumen, the increased airway resistance can be easily overcome by positive-pressure ventilation.[6]

A. The Various Double-Lumen Endotracheal Tubes

Double-lumen tubes are essentially two catheters bonded together and each lumen is intended to ventilate one of the two lungs. Double-lumen tubes are made as left- and right-sided tubes. A left-sided tube means that the left lung catheter is placed into the left mainstem bronchus, whereas the right lung catheter ends in the trachea; therefore, for a left-sided tube, the left lung catheter is longer than the right lung catheter (Fig. 9–3). A right-sided tube means that the right lung catheter is placed into the right mainstem bronchus, whereas the left lung catheter ends in the trachea; therefore, for a right-sided tube, the right lung catheter is longer than the left lung catheter (Fig. 9–3). All the double-lumen tubes have a proximal cuff for the trachea and a distal cuff for a mainstem bronchus; the endobronchial cuff causes separation and sealing off of the two lungs from each other, and the tracheal cuff causes separation and sealing off of the lungs from the environment. The part of the right lung catheter of the right-sided double-lumen tube that is in the right mainstem bronchus must be slotted to allow for ventilation of the right upper lobe (Fig. 9–3) because the right mainstem bronchus is too short to accommodate both the right lumen tip and the right endobronchial cuff (see Fig. 9–20). All the double-lumen endotracheal tubes have two curves that lie in planes approximately 90° apart from one another. The two curves are designed to facilitate placement of the distal catheter tip into the appropriate mainstem bronchus.

The double-lumen tubes that have been used for lung separation and one-lung ventilation include the Carlens, White, Bryce-Smith, and Robertshaw. The Robertshaw double-lumen endotracheal tube is by far the most commonly used tube, and the use of the disposable polyvinylchloride Robertshaw tube has completely replaced the red rubber Robertshaw tube (the former is easier to pass, is positioned more quickly, and causes less mucosal damage).[7] Consequently, the modern polyvinylchloride tube will be described in great detail. The other double-lumen tubes (the first three mentioned) are seldom used (although some anesthesiologists still use the Carlens tube), are largely of historical interest, and will only be briefly described here.

The left-sided Carlens tube (Fig. 9–4) was the first double-lumen endotracheal tube utilized for one-lung ventilation.[8] The tube has a carinal hook to aid in its proper placement and to minimize tube movement after placement. Potential problems with carinal hooks include increased difficulty (more rotations) and laryngeal trauma during intubation, amputation of the hook during passage, malpositioning of the

Double-Lumen Tubes

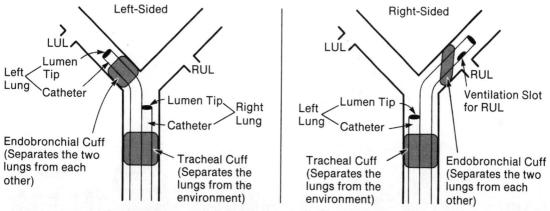

Figure 9–3. This schematic diagram depicts the essential features and parts of right-sided and left-sided double-lumen tubes. (RUL = right upper lobe; LUL = left upper lobe.)

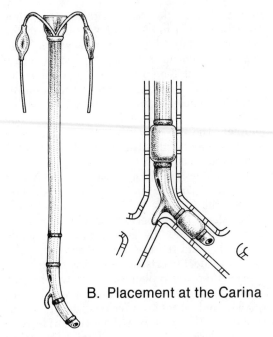

B. Placement at the Carina

A. Carlens Tube

Figure 9–4. A, *Sketch of the red rubber Carlens double-lumen tube.* B, *Close-up of the placement of the red rubber Carlens double-lumen tube at the carina. Note that the left endobronchial lumen and carinal hook straddle the carina.*

tube due to the hook (see Margin of Safety in Positioning Double-Lumen Tubes), and physical interference when performing a pneumonectomy.[9] Therefore, some anesthesiologists prefer to use the tube with the hook cut off. The tube is available in four sizes: 41, 39, 37, and 35 French (which correspond to an internal diameter for each lumen of approximately 6.5, 6.0, 5.5 and 5.0 mm, respectively). The cross-sectional shape of each lumen is oval, and this accounts for the occasional difficulty in passing a suction catheter down the lumen.

The White tube was essentially a modified right-sided Carlens tube and was used for right mainstem bronchus intubation.[10] The right mainstem bronchial cuff is slotted in order to provide for ventilation of the right upper lobe. As with the Carlens tube, suctioning may occasionally prove to be difficult, and the carinal hook can cause a variety of physical problems.

The Bryce-Smith tube (Fig. 9–5) represents another modification of the Carlens tube and was intended to reduce trauma to the larynx and tracheobronchial tree.[11] This tube was originally designed for placement in the left mainstem bronchus, although a right-sided tube was soon developed as well.[12] The cuff for the right mainstem bronchus is slotted in order to allow

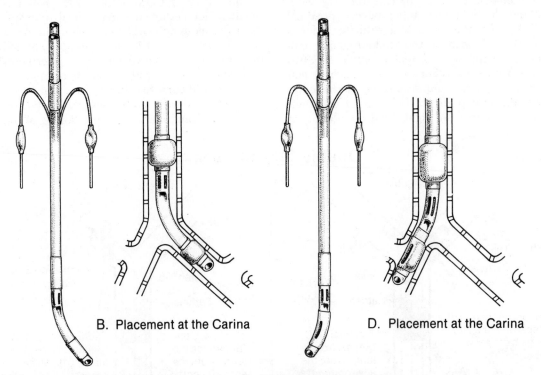

B. Placement at the Carina   D. Placement at the Carina

A. Left Bryce-Smith Tube   C. Right Bryce-Smith Tube

Figure 9–5. A, *Sketch of the left Bryce-Smith double-lumen tube.* B, *Close-up of the placement of the left Bryce-Smith double-lumen tube at the carina.* C, *Sketch of the right Bryce-Smith tube.* D, *Close-up of the placement of the right Bryce-Smith double-lumen tube at the carina.*

for ventilation of the right upper lobe. These tubes do not have a carinal hook, and both lumens (arranged anteriorly and posteriorly) are round, allowing for greater ease in passing a suction catheter. Bryce-Smith double-lumen endotracheal tubes are available in three sizes according to the internal diameter of the lumen: 7, 6.5, and 6 mm.

1. The Robertshaw Double-Lumen Endotracheal Tube

a. THE ORIGINAL RED RUBBER ROBERTSHAW DOUBLE-LUMEN ENDOTRACHEAL TUBE

The original Robertshaw double-lumen tube, introduced in 1962, was made as a reusable red rubber tube (Fig. 9–6).[13] This tube was designed to provide the largest possible lumen in order to decrease airway resistance and to facilitate removal of secretions. The lumens are D-shaped and lie side by side, like those of the Carlens tube, but are larger in size. As with the other double-lumen endotracheal tubes, it has two curves (in planes 90° apart) that facilitate intubation and proper endobronchial placement. Both a right-and left-sided tube is available, and the absence of a carinal hook allows

for easier tracheal intubation and perhaps correct positioning. The right-sided tube has a slotted endobronchial cuff in order to permit ventilation of the right upper lobe. This endobronchial cuff has an additional area of inflation on the nonslotted side above the slot in order to effect a more reliable seal (in contrast to the endobronchial cuffs of the other right-sided tubes that do not have this inflation area). On the slotted side, inflation of the endobronchial cuff is restricted. However, the right endobronchial cuff design forces the right upper lobe slot to lie flat against the right upper lobe orifice, and if the right upper lobe slot is not perfectly aligned with the right upper lobe orifice, the right upper lobe ventilation slot will be blocked (obstructed) by the right mainstem bronchial wall (and vice versa). Nevertheless, because of its many good features, the original Robertshaw double-lumen tube rapidly gained wide popularity.[14]

b. THE MODERN PLASTIC DISPOSABLE ROBERTSHAW DOUBLE-LUMEN ENDOTRACHEAL TUBE

The Robertshaw type tube is now made of a clear nontoxic tissue-implantable plastic (de-

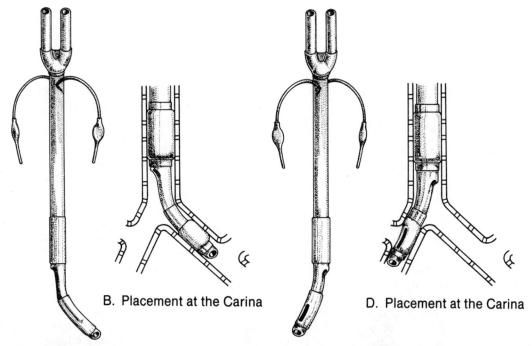

B. Placement at the Carina   D. Placement at the Carina

A. Left Robertshaw Tube   C. Right Robertshaw Tube

Figure 9–6. A, Sketch of the left-sided red rubber Robertshaw double-lumen tube. B, Close-up of the placement of the left-sided red rubber Robertshaw double-lumen tube at the carina. C, Sketch of the right-sided red rubber Robertshaw double-lumen tube. D, Close-up of the placement of the right-sided red rubber Robertshaw double-lumen tube at the carina.

noted by the marking Z-79) and is disposable (Fig. 9–7). The tubes are made in sizes 41, 39, 37, 35 and 28 French (internal diameter of each lumen is approximately 6.5, 6.0, 5.5, 5.0 and 4.5 mm, respectively). These tubes are relatively easy to insert and have appropriate end-of-lumen and cuff arrangements that minimize lobar obstruction. The endobronchial cuff is colored brilliant blue, which is a very important feature for recognition when using a fiberoptic bronchoscope. The ends of both lumens have a black radiopaque line, which is an essential recognition marker when viewing a chest x-ray. The tubes have high volume–low pressure tracheal and endobronchial cuffs. The slanted doughnut-shaped endobronchial cuff on the right-sided double-lumen tube allows the right upper lobe ventilation slot to ride off of (away from) the right upper lobe orifice, which minimizes the chance of right upper lobe obstruction by the tube. The clear tubing is helpful because it permits continuous observation of the tidal movement of respiratory moisture as well as observation of secretions from each lung. The tubes are packaged with malleable stylets and are relatively easy to insert and to position. These tubes have large internal-to-external diameter ratios and therefore allow suctioning to be done relatively easily. They are packaged with their own nonadhering suction catheters. The large internal-to-external diameter ratio also provides a relatively low resistance to ventilation. For these reasons the Robertshaw type tubes are now considered by far the double-lumen endotracheal tube of choice by most anesthesiologists. It is expected that in the near future several companies will be manufacturing this type double-lumen tube.

A left-sided double-lumen endotracheal tube should be used for right thoracotomies requiring collapse of the right lung and ventilation of the left lung (Fig. 9–8). A left- or right-sided tube may be used for left thoracotomies requiring collapse of the left lung and ventilation of the right lung (Fig. 9–8). However, since the right upper lobe ventilation slot of a right-sided tube has to be closely apposed to the right upper lobe orifice in order for unobstructed right upper lobe ventilation to occur, and since there is considerable anatomic variation in the exact position of the right upper lobe orifice and, therefore, length of the right mainstem bronchus (in fact, it is well known that an anomalous right upper lobe can take off from the trachea), use of a right-sided tube for left lung collapse introduces the risk of inadequate

right upper lobe ventilation. For this reason, a left-sided tube is preferable for most cases requiring one-lung ventilation. If clamping of the left mainstem bronchus is necessary, the tube can be withdrawn at that time into the trachea and then used in the same manner as a single-lumen endotracheal tube (ventilate the right lung with both lumens) (Fig. 9–8). Contraindications to use of a left-sided double-lumen tube are carinal and proximal left mainstem bronchial lesions that could be traumatized by the passage of a left-sided tube. These lesions include strictures, endoluminal tumors, tracheobronchial disruptions, and compression of the airway by an external mass. The largest size tube that can comfortably pass the glottis should be used, since a relatively small double-lumen tube may require excessive cuff volume for an endobronchial cuff seal to be obtained (see the discussion of endobronchial cuff problems in section D and Fig. 9–16) and may cause difficulty with suctioning secretions.

In summary, the new plastic disposable Robertshaw type double-lumen tubes are by far the most commonly used double-lumen tubes. Since a right-sided tube incurs the risk of inadequate right upper lobe ventilation, left-sided tubes are used far more commonly than right-sided tubes. Consequently, the rest of this chapter will emphasize the insertion and location of the left-sided Robertshaw type double-lumen tube.

B. The Conventional Double-Lumen Tube Intubation Procedure

Prior to intubation with a double-lumen endotracheal tube, both cuffs and lumen connections are checked. A 3 ml syringe with stopcock should be placed on the end of the bronchial cuff pilot tube, since proper bronchial cuff inflation rarely requires more than 1 to 2 ml of air; a 5 or 10 ml syringe with stopcock should be placed on the tracheal cuff pilot tube. Since the high volume–low pressure cuffs can be easily torn by teeth, the distal tube is coated with a lubricating ointment (preferably containing a local anesthetic) in order to minimize this possibility. If a less than optimal view of the larynx is anticipated, the stylet that comes packaged with the tube is lubricated, inserted into the left lumen, and appropriately curved. The patient is then anesthetized and paralyzed as described in chapter 8. A curved open-phalanged blade (MacIntosh) is usually preferred

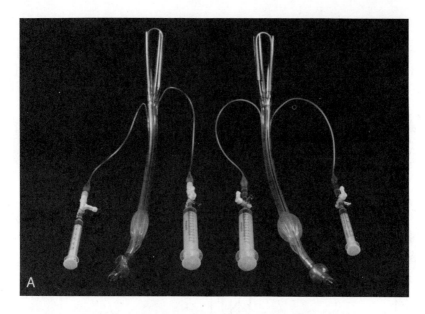

The Advantages of the Modern
Plastic Disposable Robertshaw Double-Lumen
Endobronchial Tubes

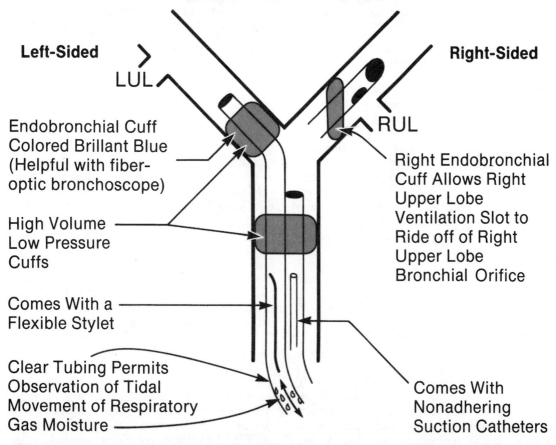

Left-Sided

LUL

Endobronchial Cuff
Colored Brillant Blue
(Helpful with fiber-
optic bronchoscope)

High Volume
Low Pressure
Cuffs

Comes With a
Flexible Stylet

Clear Tubing Permits
Observation of Tidal
Movement of Respiratory
Gas Moisture

Right-Sided

RUL

Right Endobronchial
Cuff Allows Right
Upper Lobe
Ventilation Slot to
Ride off of Right
Upper Lobe
Bronchial Orifice

Comes With
Nonadhering
Suction Catheters

B

Figure 9-7. A, *Photograph of left- and right-sided disposable Robertshaw double-lumen tubes.* B, *Schematic diagram depicts the advantages of left-sided and right-sided modern plastic disposable Robertshaw double-lumen endobronchial tubes. Both lumens of the left-sided double-lumen tube are shown, whereas only the distal endobronchial lumen of the right-sided double-lumen tube is shown.*

Right Lung Surgery and Left-Sided Double Lumen Tube

Left Lung Surgery and Right-Sided Double-Lumen Tube

Left Lung Surgery and Left-Sided Double-Lumen Tube Pulled Back

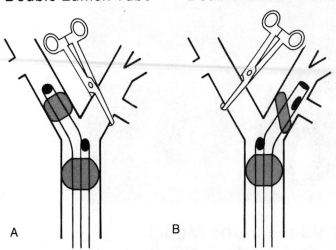
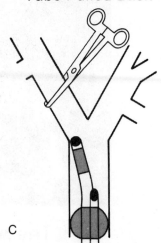

Figure 9–8. Use of left-sided and right-sided double-lumen tubes for left and right lung surgery (as indicated by the clamp). When surgery is going to be performed on the right lung, a left-sided double-lumen tube should be used (A). When surgery is going to be performed on the left lung, a right-sided double-lumen tube can be used (B). However, because of uncertainty as to the alignment of the right upper lobe ventilation slot to the right upper lobe orifice, a left-sided double-lumen tube can also be used for left lung surgery (C). If the left lung surgery requires a clamp to be placed high on the left mainstem bronchus, the left endobronchial cuff should be deflated, the left-sided double-lumen tube pulled back into the trachea, and the right lung ventilated through both of the lumens (use the double-lumen tube as a single-lumen tube).

for laryngoscopy, since it approximates the curvature of the tube and therefore provides the largest possible area through which to pass the tube. However, a straight (Miller) blade may be a better choice in patients with overriding teeth or an excessively anterior larynx.

Double-lumen endotracheal tubes with carinal hooks are first inserted through the vocal cords with the hook facing posteriorly. When the tip of the tube has passed the vocal cords, the tube is rotated 180°, so that the hook passes anteriorly through the glottis. After the tube tip and hook pass the larynx, the tube is rotated 90° so that the tube tip enters the appropriate bronchus.

The Robertshaw double-lumen tube is passed with the distal curvature initially concave anteriorly (Fig. 9–9A). After the tube tip passes the larynx, and while anterior force on the laryngoscope is continued, the stylette (if used) is removed and the tube is carefully rotated 90° (so that the distal curve is now concave toward the appropriate side and the proximal curve is concave anteriorly) to allow endobronchial intubation on the appropriate side (Fig. 9–9B). Continued anterior force by the laryngoscope during tube rotation prevents hypopharyngeal structures from falling in around the tube and

interfering with a free 90° distal tube tip rotation. Failure to obtain close to a 90° rotation of the distal tube tip, while the proximal end does rotate 90°, will cause either a kink or twist in the shaft of the tube and/or prevent the distal end of the lumen from lying free in the mainstem bronchus (i.e., not up against the bronchial wall). After rotation, the tube is advanced until most of it is inserted (the proximal end of the common or two-lumen binding mold should be near or at the level of the teeth in a normal-sized person) and/or moderate resistance to further passage is encountered, indicating that the tube tip has been firmly seated in a mainstem bronchus (Fig. 9–9C). Double-lumen endotracheal tubes may also be passed successfully via tracheostomy, although it should be remembered that the tracheal cuff may be at the tracheal stoma or lie partly outside the trachea in this situation.[15, 16]

Once the tube tip is thought to be in an endobronchial position, the following checklist is carried out to ensure proper functioning of the tube. Inflate the tracheal and endobronchial cuffs until moderate tension is palpated in the external pilot balloons (the endobronchial cuff should not require more than 2 to 3 ml of air), deliver several positive-pressure ventilations and auscultate and observe the chest bilaterally to determine that the trachea, rather than the esophagus, has been intubated and that both lungs are being ventilated (Fig. 9–9C). In addition to seeing the tube go through the vocal cords, correct intubation position is checked by feeling and observing the anesthesia reservoir bag to make sure it has the appropriate compliance and movement, maintaining normal pulse oximetry and end-tidal CO_2 values, and perhaps palpating the tracheal cuff in the neck. If only unilateral breath sounds or chest movement are present, it is likely that both of the lumens of the tube have entered a mainstem bronchus (if both of the lumens enter the left mainstem bronchus, the findings may mimic an esophageal intubation and vice versa). In this situation,

quickly deflate the cuffs, withdraw the tube 1 to 2 cm at a time, inflate the cuffs, and reassess ventilation until bilateral breath sounds are heard. If bilateral breath sounds are not heard, and the tube has been withdrawn a significant amount, the entire procedure must be repeated, beginning with establishing the airway and oxygen ventilation via mask, laryngoscopy, and reinsertion of the double-lumen tube through the vocal cords. If bilateral breath sounds are present, then one side is clamped, and breath sounds and chest movement should disappear on the ipsilateral side and remain on the contralateral side. Next, the clamped side should be unclamped and the breath sounds and chest movement should reappear on that side. During unilateral clamping the breath

Passage of Left-Sided Double-Lumen Tube

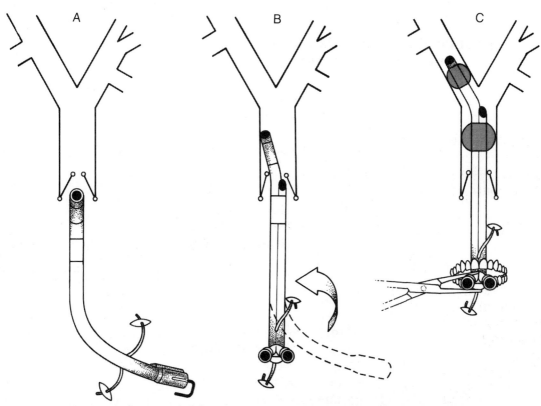

Figure 9–9. This schematic diagram depicts the passage of the left-sided double-lumen tube in a supine patient. A, The tube is held with the distal curvature concave anteriorly and the proximal curve concave to the right and in a plane parallel to the floor. The tube is then inserted through the vocal cords until the left cuff passes the vocal cords. The stylet is then removed. B, The tube is rotated 90° counter-clockwise so that the distal curvature is concave anteriorly and the proximal curvature is concave to the left and in a plane parallel to the floor. C, The tube is inserted until either a moderate resistance to further passage is encountered or the end of the common molding of the two lumens is at the teeth. Both cuffs are then inflated, and both lungs are ventilated. Finally, one side is clamped while the other side is ventilated and vice versa (see text for further explanation).

sounds on the ventilated side should be compared with and calibrated against unilateral chest wall movements and the inspiratory disappearance and expiratory appearance of respiratory gas moisture in the clear tubing of the ventilated side (Fig. 9–10). In addition, the compliance of the lung should be gauged by using hand ventilation. The unilateral clamping and unclamping should then be repeated on the opposite side to assure adequate lung separation and cuff seal.

Recently, a new, single-unit double-lumen tube adaptor has been described that permits each lumen independently to be either open to the mechanical ventilator or the atmosphere or completely blocked (as though it were clamped) by simply turning a dial to the desired setting without the need for airway disconnection and/or external clamping maneuvers (Fig. 9–11).[17] When the dial is turned either to lung ventilation or open to the atmosphere, either lung may receive PEEP, CPAP, fiberoptic

bronchoscopy, and/or suctioning. These features greatly facilitate the testing for lung separation as well as use of all of the other one-lung ventilation/anesthesia maneuvers that are demanded by modern anesthetic practice (see chapter 11).

In summary, when double-lumen endotracheal tube position is correct, the breath sounds are normal and follow the expected unilateral pattern with unilateral clamping, the chest rises and falls in accordance with the breath sounds, the ventilated lung feels reasonably compliant, no leaks are present, and respiratory gas moisture appears and disappears with each tidal ventilation (Fig. 9–10). Conversely, when the double-lumen endotracheal tube is malpositioned, any or all of the following may occur: the breath sounds are poor and correlate poorly with unilateral clamping, the chest movements do not follow the expected pattern, the ventilated lung feels noncompliant, leaks are present, or the respiratory gas moisture in the clear

Correct Position of Double-Lumen Tube and Unilateral Clamping

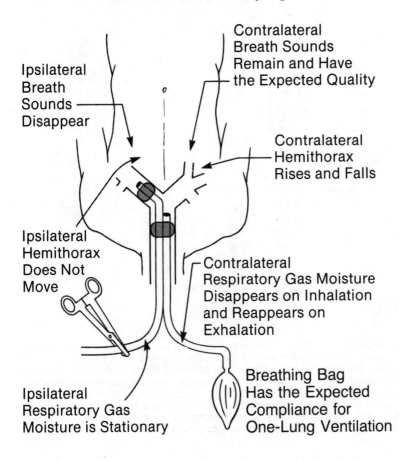

Ipsilateral Breath Sounds Disappear

Contralateral Breath Sounds Remain and Have the Expected Quality

Contralateral Hemithorax Rises and Falls

Ipsilateral Hemithorax Does Not Move

Contralateral Respiratory Gas Moisture Disappears on Inhalation and Reappears on Exhalation

Ipsilateral Respiratory Gas Moisture is Stationary

Breathing Bag Has the Expected Compliance for One-Lung Ventilation

Figure 9–10. This schematic diagram shows the results of unilateral clamping when the double-lumen tube is in the correct position.

Possible Double-Lumen Tube Adaptor Settings

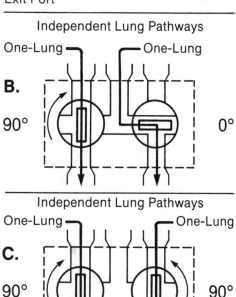

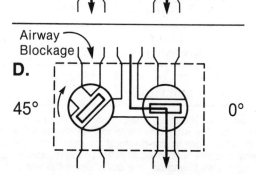

Figure 9–11. Double-lumen tube adapter and possible adapter settings. A, On the anesthesia machine side of the double-lumen tube adapter there are three entry ports, each fitted with a 15 mm male connector. On the patient side of the double-lumen tube adapter there are two exit ports, each fitted with a 15 mm female connector; each exit port connects with one of the lumens of the double-lumen tube. When the two stopcock (circles) handles (rectangles within the circles) are in a horizontal position (0°), the central entry port is connected to both the exit ports; this pathway can be used to ventilate and to administer PEEP to both lungs (heavy dark arrow lines). B, When one of the stopcock handles has been turned 90° into a vertical position so that one of the lateral entry ports connects to the ipsilateral exit port, one lung can be ventilated (with or without PEEP), exposed to CPAP, suctioned, or viewed with a fiberoptic bronchoscope through this pathway while the other lung is managed via the central entry port pathway. C, When both stopcock handles are turned 90° into the vertical position, both lungs may be managed differently and separately via the lateral entry-exit port pathways. D, When one of the stopcocks is turned to a 45° angle there is no entry-exit port pathway; the lung is then locked into whatever volume and gas composition it previously contained.

tubing is relatively stationary. It is very important to realize, however, that even if the double-lumen tube is thought to be properly positioned based on clinical signs, subsequent fiberoptic bronchoscopy will reveal a 48 per cent incidence of malpositioning.[18]

When it is felt that the double-lumen endotracheal tube is malpositioned based on clinical signs, it is theoretically possible to diagnose the malposition of the tube more precisely by a combination of several unilateral clampings, chest auscultation, and left endobronchial cuff inflation-deflation maneuvers (Fig. 9–12). With reference to a left-sided double-lumen endotracheal tube, there are three possible gross malpositions: in too far on the left (both lumens in the left mainstem bronchus), out too far (both lumens in the trachea), and in or down the right mainstem bronchus (at least the left lumen is in the right mainstem bronchus). When the right (tracheal) side is clamped and the tube is in too far on the left side, breath sounds will be heard only on the left side. When the tube is out too far and the right side is clamped, breath sounds will be heard bilaterally. When the tube is in or down the right side and the right mainstem bronchus is clamped, breath sounds will be heard only on the right side. When the left side is clamped and the left endobronchial cuff is inflated, the right lumen is blocked by the left cuff in all three malpositions. Consequently, with the left side clamped and the left cuff inflated, none or very diminished breath sounds will be heard bilaterally in all three malpositions. When the left side is clamped and the left cuff is deflated, so that the right lumen is no longer blocked by the left cuff, breath sounds will be heard only on the left side when the tube is in too far on the left, breath sounds will be heard bilaterally if the tube is out too far, and breath sounds will be heard only on the right side when the tube is

Double-Lumen Tube Malpositions

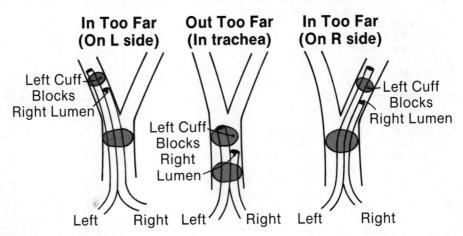

Procedure	Breath Sounds Heard		
Clamp Right Lumen Both Cuffs Inflated	Left	Left and Right	Right
Clamp Left Lumen Both Cuffs Inflated	None or Very ↓↓	None or Very ↓↓	None or Very ↓↓
Clamp Left Lumen Deflate Left Cuff	Left	Left and Right	Right

Figure 9–12. There are three major (involving a whole lung) malpositions of a left-sided double-lumen endotracheal tube. The tube can be in too far on the left (both lumens are in the left mainstem bronchus), out too far (both lumens are in the trachea), or down the right mainstem bronchus (at least the left lumen is in the right mainstem bronchus). In each of these three malpositions the left cuff, when fully inflated, can completely block the right lumen. Inflation and deflation of the left cuff while the left lumen is clamped creates a breath sound differential diagnosis of tube malposition. (See text for full explanation). (L = left; R = right; ↓ = decreased.)

Use of Fiberoptic Bronchoscope to
Insert Left-Sided Double-Lumen Tube

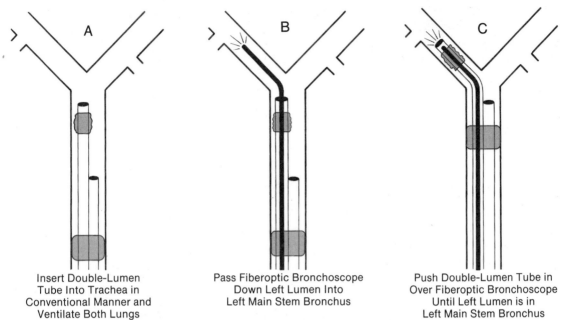

Insert Double-Lumen
Tube Into Trachea in
Conventional Manner and
Ventilate Both Lungs

Pass Fiberoptic Bronchoscope
Down Left Lumen Into
Left Main Stem Bronchus

Push Double-Lumen Tube in
Over Fiberoptic Bronchoscope
Until Left Lumen is in
Left Main Stem Bronchus

Figure 9–13. This schematic diagram portrays use of the fiberoptic bronchoscope to insert a left-sided double-lumen tube. The double-lumen tube can be put into the trachea in a conventional manner, and both lungs can be ventilated by both lumens (A). The fiberoptic bronchoscope may be inserted into the left lumen of the double-lumen tube through a self-sealing diaphragm in the elbow connector to the left lumen; this allows continued positive pressure ventilation of both lungs through the right lumen without creating a leak. After the fiberoptic bronchoscope has been passed into the left mainstem bronchus (B), it is used as a stylet for the aftercoming left lumen (C). The fiberoptic bronchoscope is then withdrawn. Final precise positioning of the double-lumen tube is performed with the fiberoptic bronchoscope in the right lumen (see Fig. 9–14).

in the right side. The left cuff inflation/deflation findings provide the key diagnostic data because they essentially define the position of the right tracheal lumen by blocking and unblocking it with the left cuff.

There are, however, several situations in which unilateral clamping, auscultation, and cuff inflation and deflation maneuvers for determining the integrity of lung separation are either unreliable or impossible. First, and most importantly, when the patient is in the lateral decubitus position, has had a skin preparation, and is draped, access to the chest wall is impossible, and the anesthesiologist cannot listen to the chest. Second, the presence of unilateral or bilateral lung disease, which either preexisted before anesthesia and surgery or was induced by anesthesia, may markedly obscure the crispness of the chest auscultation endpoints. Third, the diagnosis of exactly where the double-lumen endotracheal tube has located may be confused when the tube is just slightly malpositioned. Fourth, the tube may have moved because of some event such as coughing,

turning into the lateral decubitus position, and tracheal manipulation and hilar retraction by the surgeon. Finally, some combination of the above circumstances may culminate in uncertainty as to where the double-lumen tube has located. The solution to any uncertainty as to the exact position of the double-lumen tube is to determine the position by use of fiberoptic bronchoscopy (see Use of Fiberoptic Bronchoscope To Determine Precise Double-Lumen Tube Position).

C. Use of Fiberoptic Bronchoscope To Insert the Bronchial Lumen of a Double-Lumen Tube Into a Mainstem Bronchus

The insertion of the bronchial lumen of a double-lumen tube into the appropriate mainstem bronchus may be aided by the use of a fiberoptic bronchoscope (Fig. 9–13). The double-lumen tube is first placed in the trachea in a conventional manner (laryngoscopy, manual tube insertion) until the tracheal cuff just passes the vocal cords, the tracheal cuff is inflated, and both lungs are ventilated with both lumens (use the double-lumen tube as if it were a single-lumen tube). A pediatric fiberoptic bronchoscope can then be inserted into the bronchial lumen through a self-sealing diaphragm in the elbow connector to the bronchial lumen (which permits continued positive-pressure ventilation through that lumen around the fiberoptic bronchoscope) and passed into the appropriate mainstem bronchus. The tracheal cuff is then deflated and the bronchial lumen is passed over the fiberoptic bronchoscope stylet into the appropriate mainstem bronchus. The fiberoptic bronchoscope is then withdrawn from the bronchial lumen and passed down the tracheal lumen to determine the precise double-lumen tube position (see the following section).

Alternatively, once the double-lumen tube is in the trachea, the fiberoptic bronchoscope can be inserted into the tracheal lumen through a self-sealing diaphragm in the elbow connector to the tracheal lumen (which permits continued positive-pressure ventilation through that lumen around the fiberoptic bronchoscope) and passed just proximal to the tracheal carina. While the carina and the two mainstem bronchial orifices are in view, the double-lumen tube can be advanced and the degree of lateral rotation adjusted so that the left lumen enters the left mainstem bronchus. Final precise positioning (see the following section) can be done with the fiberoptic bronchoscope remaining in the tracheal lumen.

D. Use of Fiberoptic Bronchoscope To Determine Precise Double-Lumen Tube Position

As noted previously, even when a double-lumen tube is thought to be in proper position based on clinical signs, subsequent fiberoptic bronchoscopy will reveal a 48 per cent incidence of malpositioning.[18] Indeed, when the position of the double-lumen tube is checked only by clinical signs, 25 per cent of the time there will be intraoperative problems with either deflating the nondependent lung, ventilating the dependent lung, or completely separating the two lungs.[19] The exact position of a left-sided double-lumen endotracheal tube can be ascertained at any time, in less than a minute, by simply passing a pediatric fiberoptic bronchoscope through the tracheal lumen of the double-lumen tube. It is rarely necessary also to have to pass the fiberoptic bronchoscope down the left endobronchial lumen. With reference to a left-sided double-lumen tube, looking down the right (tracheal) lumen the endoscopist should see a clear straight-ahead view of the tracheal carina, the left lumen going off to the left, and the upper surface of the left endobronchial balloon just below the tracheal carina (Figs. 9–14 and 9–15). (The importance of seeing the upper surface of the left endobronchial cuff below the tracheal carina will be emphasized in the following section.) It is important that the volume of air used to fill the left endobronchial left cuff does not cause the endobronchial cuff to herniate over the tracheal carina or cause the tracheal carina to deviate to the right (Figs. 9–15 and 9–16); both cuff herniation and carinal deviation can be readily appreciated looking down the tracheal lumen. Looking down the left lumen (which is sometimes done when inserting a left-sided double-lumen tube with a fiberoptic bronchoscope [see section C immediately above] and in all cases of bronchopulmonary lavage in which perfect tube position and tight cuff seal are extremely critical) the endoscopist should see a very slight narrowing of the left lumen (due to endobronchial cuff pressure) as well as the bronchial carina distal to the end of the tube (Fig. 9–15). The endoscopist should not see excessive left

Use of Fiberoptic Bronchoscope Down the Right Lumen to Determine Precise Left-Sided Double-Lumen Tube Position

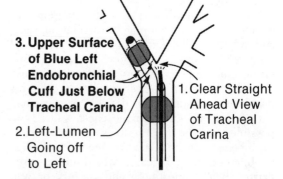

3. Upper Surface of Blue Left Endobronchial Cuff Just Below Tracheal Carina

2. Left-Lumen Going off to Left

1. Clear Straight Ahead View of Tracheal Carina

Figure 9–14. *This schematic diagram portrays use of the fiberoptic bronchoscope down the right lumen to determine precise left-sided double-lumen tube position. The endoscopist should see a clear straight-ahead view of the tracheal carina, the left lumen going off into the left mainstem bronchus and, most importantly (in bold print), the upper surface of the blue left endobronchial cuff just below the tracheal carina.*

Use of Fiberoptic Bronchoscope to Determine Precise Left-Sided Double-Lumen Tube Position

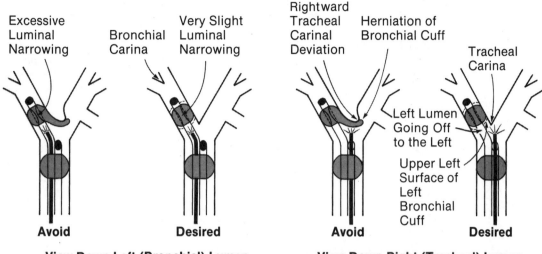

Excessive Luminal Narrowing

Bronchial Carina

Very Slight Luminal Narrowing

Rightward Tracheal Carinal Deviation

Herniation of Bronchial Cuff

Tracheal Carina

Left Lumen Going Off to the Left

Upper Left Surface of Left Bronchial Cuff

Avoid   **Desired**   **Avoid**   **Desired**

View Down Left (Bronchial) Lumen   **View Down Right (Tracheal) Lumen**

Figure 9–15. This schematic diagram depicts the complete fiberoptic bronchoscopy picture of left-sided double-lumen tubes (both the desired view and the view to be avoided from both of the lumens). When the bronchoscope is passed down the right lumen of the left-sided tube, the endoscopist should see a clear straight-ahead view of the tracheal carina and the upper surface of the blue left endobronchial cuff just below the tracheal carina. Excessive pressure in the endobronchial cuff, as manifested by tracheal carinal deviation to the right and herniation of the endobronchial cuff over the carina, should be avoided. When the bronchoscope is passed down the left lumen of the left-sided tube, the endoscopist should see a very slight left luminal narrowing and a clear straight-ahead view of the bronchial carina off in the distance. Excessive left luminal narrowing should be avoided.

Excessive Left Cuff Inflation: Problems

Figure 9–16. Excessive inflation of the left cuff of a left-sided double-lumen tube can cause impaired ventilation of both the right and left lungs. Right lung ventilation may be impaired by left cuff herniation over the tracheal carina (due to excessive left cuff volume) and by tracheal carinal deviation to the right (due to excessive left cuff pressure). Left lung ventilation may be impaired by invagination of the left lumen caused by excessive left cuff pressure.

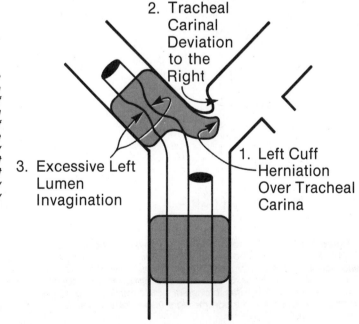

2. Tracheal Carinal Deviation to the Right

1. Left Cuff Herniation Over Tracheal Carina

3. Excessive Left Lumen Invagination

luminal narrowing (due to excessive left cuff pressure) (Fig. 9–16). Thus, aside from gross malposition, important undesirable findings on endoscopy are related to excessive left cuff inflation and pressure and consist of cuff herniation over the tracheal carina, carinal deviation to the right (both of which may block the right mainstem bronchial orifice and impair right lung ventilation), and excessive left lumen constriction (invagination), which may impair left lung ventilation (Fig. 9–16).[20] In addition, when an inappropriately undersized tube is used, the large endobronchial cuff volume required for endobronchial cuff seal tends to force the entire double-lumen tube cephalad, making a functional bronchial seal more difficult.[21]

With reference to a right-sided double-lumen tube, looking down the left (tracheal) lumen the endoscopist should see a clear straight-ahead view of the tracheal carina, with the right lumen going off to the right (Fig. 9–17A). The upper surface of the right endobronchial balloon may not be visible below the tracheal carina. Look-

ing down the right lumen, the endoscopist should see a very slight narrowing of the right lumen as well as the right middle-lower lobe bronchial carina distal to the end of the tube. Most importantly, the endoscopist should locate the right upper lobe ventilation slot and be able to look directly into the right upper lobe orifice through the right upper lobe ventilation slot by simply flexing the tip of the fiberoptic bronchoscope superiorly (Fig. 9–17B). There should be no overriding of the right upper lobe ventilation slot on the bronchial mucosa, and the bronchial mucosa should not be covering any of the right upper lobe ventilation slot. The fact that there is little room for error in aligning the right upper lobe ventilation slot with the right upper lobe orifice will be emphasized in the following section.

The right upper lobe ventilation slot may be easily located by first finding the bronchial lumen radiopaque marker. The radiopaque marker appears as either a white or black line on the inside of the bronchial lumen, which

Use of Fiberoptic Bronchoscope to Determine Precise Right-Sided Double-Lumen Tube Position

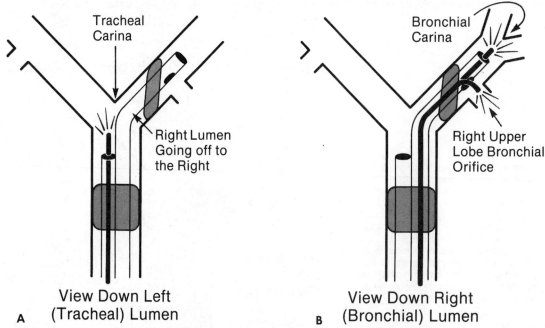

Figure 9–17. This schematic diagram portrays use of a fiberoptic bronchoscope to determine precise right-sided double-lumen tube position. A, When the fiberoptic bronchoscope is passed down the left (tracheal) lumen, the endoscopist should see a clear straight-ahead view of the tracheal carina and the right lumen going off into the right mainstem bronchus. B, When the fiberoptic bronchoscope is passed down the right (bronchial) lumen, the endoscopist should see the bronchial carina off in the distance; when the fiberoptic bronchoscope is flexed cephalad and passed through the right upper lobe ventilation slot, the right upper lobe bronchial orifice should be visualized.

ends at the proximal end of the right upper lobe ventilation slot. If one simply follows the radiopaque line, it will lead the endoscopist to the right upper lobe ventilation slot.

In the author's experience in eight out of ten cases the clinical signs (breath sounds, chest movements, compliance of the lung(s), movement of respiratory gas moisture) indicate that the lungs are apparently clearly and without doubt completely separated when the double-lumen tube is first inserted with the patient in the supine position. However, in view of the finding that 48 per cent of double-lumen tubes are malpositioned to some extent in the supine position, even though clinical signs indicate there is no problem,[18] it is strongly advisable to check the position of the tube with a fiberoptic bronchoscope in the supine position (especially considering that the procedure takes less than a minute). Even if no problem is identified, the procedure still allows the endoscopist to become familiar with the patient's anatomy and facilitates the more important endoscopy performed after turning the patient into the lateral decubitus position. In approximately two out of ten cases there is doubt about tube location in the supine position, and in these patients the fiberoptic bronchoscope is always used to correct the double-lumen tube malposition. The fiberoptic bronchoscope is always used to determine double-lumen tube position after the patient has been turned into the lateral decubitus position. Of course, a determined effort is made to prevent dislodgement of the tube during turning by holding onto the tube at the level of the incisors and by keeping the head absolutely immobile in a neutral or slightly flexed position. Head extension can cause movement of the tube in a cephalad direction, which may result in bronchial decannulation; head flexion can cause movement of the tube in a caudad direction, which may result in an upper lobe obstruction or in both lumens being in a mainstem bronchus (see the next section).[22, 23] Finally, the fiberoptic bronchoscope is used anytime during the procedure when there is a question about double-lumen tube position. This is not an infrequent occurrence and is usually caused by surgical manipulation and traction on either the hilum, carina, or trachea.

1. Margin of Safety in Positioning Double-Lumen Tubes

A correctly positioned double-lumen tube does not cause obstruction of any conducting airway. This section will discuss the length of adult male and female tracheobronchial trees, over which differently sized and manufactured double-lumen tubes can be moved and still be correctly positioned; this length is defined as the margin of safety.[24]

a. LEFT-SIDED DOUBLE-LUMEN TUBES

The outermost acceptable position of a left-sided double-lumen tube occurs when the left endobronchial cuff is just below the tracheal carina. If a left-sided double-lumen tube is pulled out any further, the left endobronchial cuff will obstruct the trachea and the right mainstem bronchus (Fig. 9–18A). The innermost acceptable position occurs when the distal tip of the left lumen is at the left upper lobe bronchus, because further insertion will obstruct the left upper lobe (Fig. 9–18B). The margin of safety in positioning a left-sided double-lumen tube is the difference between these outermost and innermost acceptable positions.

The margin of safety for left-sided double-lumen tubes may be quantitatively analyzed as follows (Fig. 9–19): The length of a left-sided double-lumen tube between the right and left lumen tips is designated as B. The length of a left-sided double-lumen tube between the cephalad (proximal) surface of the left cuff and left lumen tip is designated as A. The length of the left mainstem bronchus is designated as LMS. The margin of safety for a left-sided double-lumen tube is LMS – A.

The LMS for male and female cadavers is 54 ± 7 mm and 50 ± 7 mm, respectively (Fig. 9-20A).[25] The in vivo bronchoscopically determined LMS for males and females is 50 ± 7 mm and 45 ± 7 mm, respectively, with a slight clinically and statistically significant positive correlation with height (Fig. 9–21).[24] Note that in both the cadaver and in vivo studies there is a wide scattering of lengths and a very large standard deviation. Since the cadaver studies contain many more patients than the in vivo bronchoscopy studies, the following analysis will use the cadaver values for length LMS.

Table 9–2 shows the mean value for lengths (mm) A and B and the margin of safety (LMS – A) for various left-sided double-lumen tubes for males and females. The margin of safety for the various left-sided double-lumen tubes ranges from 12 to 29 mm. Figure 9–22A shows an example of a common situation using a 37 French clear plastic left-sided double-lumen tube in an average-sized female. With the left

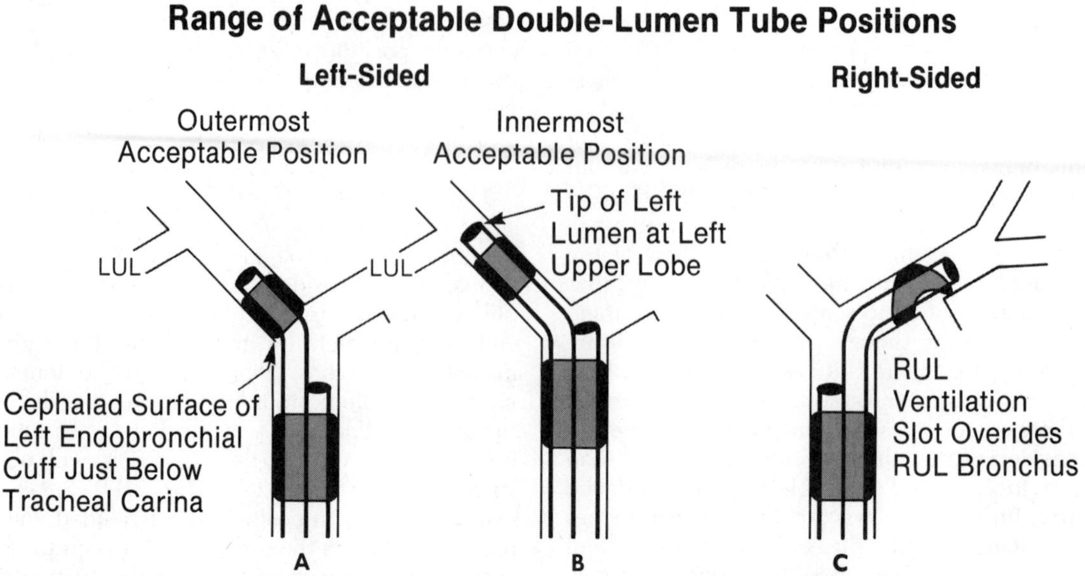

Range of Acceptable Double-Lumen Tube Positions

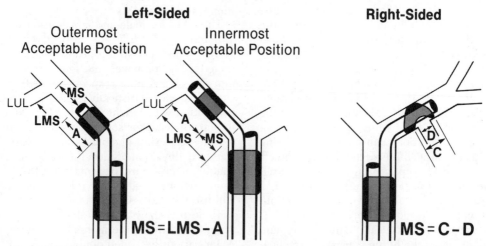

Left-Sided

Right-Sided

Outermost
Acceptable Position

Innermost
Acceptable Position

Tip of Left
Lumen at Left
Upper Lobe

LUL

LUL

Cephalad Surface of
Left Endobronchial
Cuff Just Below
Tracheal Carina

RUL
Ventilation
Slot Overrides
RUL Bronchus

A   B   C

Figure 9–18. This schematic diagram defines the range of acceptable double-lumen tube positions for both left-sided and right-sided tubes. A, The outermost acceptable position for a left-sided tube occurs when the cephalad surface of the left endobronchial cuff is just below the tracheal carina, for any further outward movement would cause the left endobronchial cuff to block the right mainstem bronchial orifice. B, The innermost acceptable position of a left-sided double-lumen tube occurs when the tip of the left lumen is at the left upper lobe (LUL), for if the tube were inserted any further, the left lumen would block the left upper lobe. C, A right-sided double-lumen tube does not have a range of acceptable positions because there is only one position when the right upper lobe (RUL) ventilation slot appropriately overrides the right upper lobe bronchial orifice.

Margin of Safety (MS) in Positioning Double-Lumen Tubes

Left-Sided

Right-Sided

Outermost
Acceptable Position

Innermost
Acceptable Position

LUL

MS

LMS

A

LUL

A

LMS   MS

D

C

MS = LMS – A

MS = C – D

Figure 9–19. This schematic diagram depicts the margin of safety (MS) in positioning both left-sided and right-sided double-lumen tubes. (LUL = left upper lobe; RUL = right upper lobe; A = distance between cephalad surface of left cuff to tip of left lumen; LMS = length of left mainstem bronchus; C = length of right upper lobe ventilation slot; D = diameter of right upper lobe bronchial orifice. For a left-sided double-lumen tube, MS = LMS − A; for a right-sided double-lumen tube MS = C − D.)

Distribution of Mainstream Bronchial Length

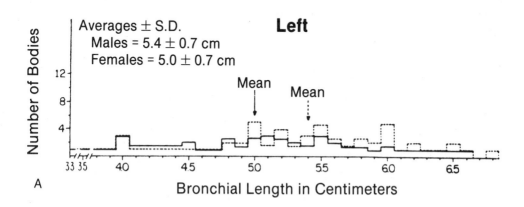

A

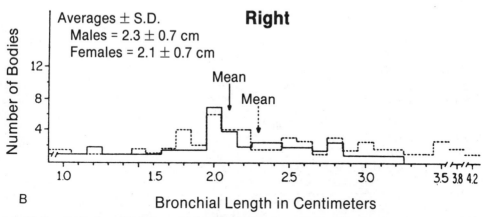

B

Figure 9–20. *The distribution of left* (A) *and right* (B) *mainstem bronchial lengths found in the cadaver study cited in reference 21. The dashed line histogram is for males, and the solid line histogram is for females. Note the extreme variation and large standard deviation around the means for both male and female.*

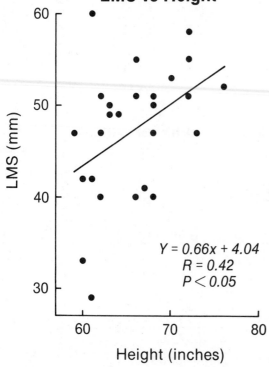

In-Vivo Measurements of LMS vs Height

$$Y = 0.66x + 4.04$$
$$R = 0.42$$
$$P < 0.05$$

Figure 9–21. *In vivo fiberoptic bronchoscopy measured length of the left mainstem bronchus (LMS) plotted as a function of the height of the patients. A weak but statistically significant correlation was found.*

endobronchial cuff placed just below the tracheal carina, and using average values for double-lumen tube and LMS lengths, the margin of safety is 21 mm. However, since the distance between the right and left lumen tips for the clear plastic tube (69 mm) is longer than the length of the left mainstem bronchus (50 mm) in this typical example, it is possible for the

right lumen to be above the tracheal carina while the left lumen tip obstructs the left upper lobe (Fig. 9–22B). Figure 9–23 shows a postoperative chest roentgenogram of a patient who underwent a right upper lobectomy and demonstrates this problem: A left-sided double-lumen tube is in situ, the right lumen tip is above the tracheal carina, and the remaining right lung is well aerated while the left upper lobe is partially collapsed.

In addition to a significant variability in length LMS, there is also a fairly significant variability (up to 20 per cent) among same-sized and manufactured individual left-sided double-lumen tubes in length A and B. Length A and B also change inconsistently with changes in left-sided double-lumen tube size. The explanation for the 20 per cent variation in distances A and B in the clear plastic double-lumen tubes is that the cutting of the proximal lumen and the placement of the endobronchial cuff is done by hand at the end of the manufacturing process.

The variation in double-lumen tube lengths A and B and left mainstem bronchial length (LMS) greatly reinforces the need to determine double-lumen tube location with a fiberoptic bronchoscope. The variation in these lengths

Table 9–2. *The Double-Lumen Tube Lengths A and B (see text) and Margin of Safety (MS; LMS – A) in mm for Male (M) and Female (F) for Various Sized and Manufactured Double-Lumen Tubes*

L-DLT				LMS-A (MS)	
Manufacturer	Fr	A	B	M	F
National Catheter	41	28	70	26	22
Corp.	39	26	70	28	24
n = 6	37	29	69	25	21
	35	25	66	29	25
Carlens	41	32	67	22	18
n = 3	39	32	65	22	18
	37	31	64	23	19
	35	27	60	27	23
Leymed	44	38	90	16	12
n = 6	38	33	82	21	17
	32	27	72	27	23

37 French Left-Sided Double-Lumen Tube and Adult Female Left Main Stem Bronchial Dimensions and Relationships

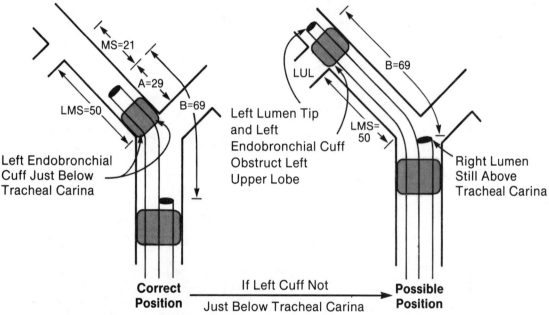

Figure 9–22. This schematic diagram shows the relationship of the lumen tips and cuffs of a correctly and an incorrectly positioned 37 French left-sided double-lumen tube to the tracheobronchial tree of an average-sized adult female. When the left endobronchial cuff is just below the tracheal carina (correct position), the margin of safety (MS) is 21 mm because the length of the left mainstem bronchus (LMS) exceeds the distance between the cephalad surface of the left cuff and the tip of the left lumen (distance A). However, since the distance between the right and left lumens (distance B) exceeds the length of the left mainstem bronchus, it is possible to still have the right lumen above the tracheal carina while the left lumen tip and the left endobronchial cuff obstruct the left upper lobe (LUL). Thus, as a left-sided tube is inserted further (so that the left cuff cannot be visualized below the carina), the first airway likely to be obstructed will be the left upper lobe.

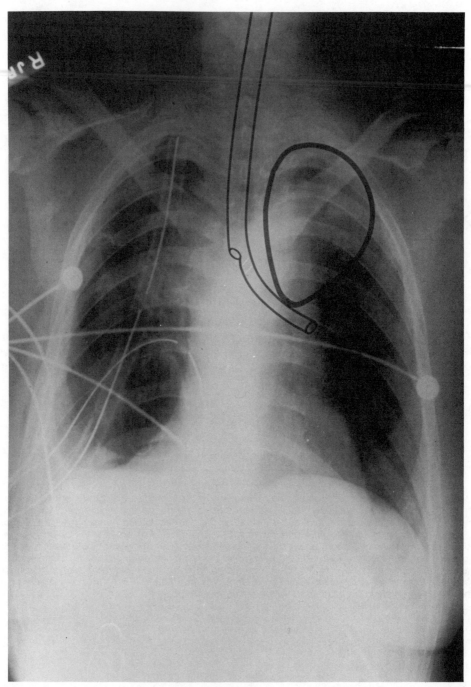

Figure 9–23. This x-ray shows an example of a patient with the problem schematically depicted in Figure 9–22. The right lumen is above the tracheal carina, and the right lung is well ventilated, while the left lumen tip is deeply inserted into the left lung, and the left upper lobe is opacified.

has three more important implications. First, a patient with a small LMS will have a smaller margin of safety. In fact, if a patient with a small LMS (two standard deviations less than the cadaver mean) and a large distance A and B (20 per cent greater than the mean value in Table 9–2) received a 37 French plastic tube, there would be no margin of safety, even if the left endobronchial cuff is positioned just below the tracheal carina (Fig. 9–24); this situation has the smallest margin of safety realistically possible. Second, and conversely, if a patient with a long LMS (two standard deviations greater than the cadaver mean) received a 37 French plastic double-lumen tube with a short distance B (20 per cent less than the mean value in Table 9–2), the right lumen could be in the left mainstem bronchus (right mainstem bronchus obstructed) while the left lumen tip was still above the left upper lobe (Fig. 9–25). However, it must be emphasized that no matter which manufactured tube or sized tube is used and no matter how long or short the left main-

Example of Right Lumen Tip Being in Left Main Stem Bronchus when Left Lumen Tip is Above Left Upper Lobe When Left Main Stem Bronchus (LMS) is Long and Length B is Short

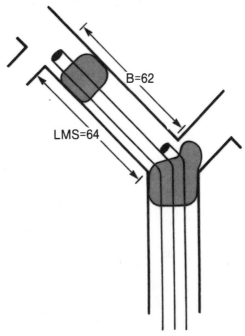

Figure 9–25. This schematic diagram shows that it is possible for the right lumen to be in the left mainstem bronchus when the left lumen tip is still above the left upper lobe if the left mainstem bronchus (LMS) is long and length B is short.

stem bronchus is (within the range of extremes observed in the cadaver studies), when the upper surface of the left endobronchial balloon is just below the tracheal carina, it is not possible for the left lumen tip to obstruct the left upper lobe or the right (tracheal) lumen to be near a mainstem bronchus. Third, in view of the fact that head flexion and extension can move the tip of a left-sided double-lumen tube in or out 27 mm,[23] these considerations show that it is easily possible to cause left upper lobe obstruction with head flexion and bronchial decannulation with head extension (Fig. 9–26).

b. RIGHT-SIDED DOUBLE-LUMEN TUBES

A right-sided double-lumen tube is acceptably positioned if the right upper lobe ventilation slot is aligned with the right upper lobe orifice (Figs. 9–3 and 9–18). The analysis of right-sided double-lumen tube margin of safety is as follows: The length of the right upper lobe venti-

Example of No Margin of Safety (MS) When Left Main Stem Bronchus (LMS) is Short and Length A is Large

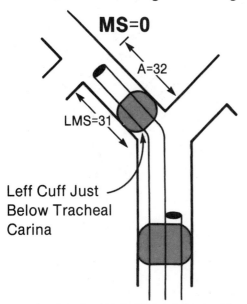

Figure 9–24. This schematic diagram shows that there will be no margin of safety (MS) when a double-lumen tube is used that has a large length A in a patient who has a short left mainstem bronchus (LMS), even though the left endobronchial cuff is positioned just below the tracheal carina. Nevertheless, with the left endobronchial cuff just below the tracheal carina, the left upper lobe is unobstructed.

Left Double Lumen Tube Position and Head Flexion and Extension

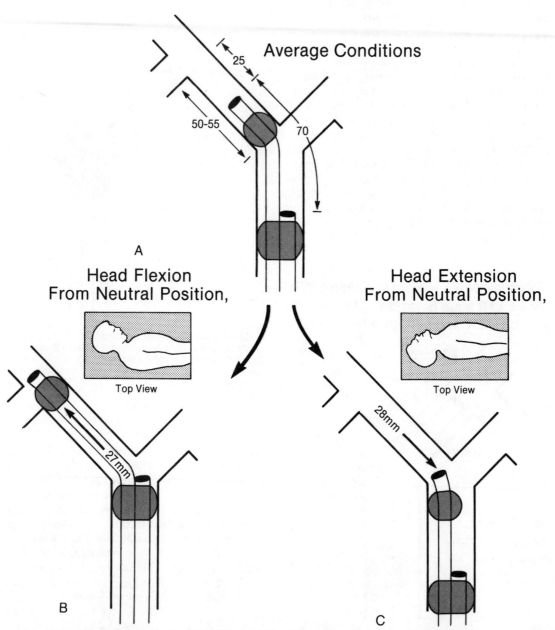

Figure 9–26. *Head flexion moves an endotracheal tube inward, and head extension moves an endotracheal tube outward. A, Correct position of a left-sided double-lumen tube along with average values (in mm) for left mainstem bronchus, right to left lumen tip and left lumen tip to left upper lobe lengths; the latter length is the margin of safety. When the left cuff is just below the tracheal carina, the margin of safety is 25 mm. B, Extreme head flexion can cause left upper lobe obstruction. C, Extreme head extension can cause left mainstem bronchial decannulation.*

lation slot is designated as C, and the diameter of the right upper lobe orifice is designated as distance D. Thus, the margin of safety for a right-sided double-lumen tube is the C – D difference. The mean values for C for medium-sized Leymed and clear plastic disposable right-sided double-lumen tubes are 21 and 11 mm, respectively. The mean value for D for adults is 10 mm (Fig. 9–27).[26] Therefore, the margins of safety (C – D) for the Leymed and clear plastic right-sided double-lumen tubes are only 11 and 1 mm, respectively. However, it should be remembered that the unique slanted dough-nut shape of the right endobronchial cuff of the disposable right-sided double-lumen tube (Mallinkrodt) allows the right upper lobe ventilation slot to ride off of the right upper lobe orifice, thereby increasing (from 1 mm) to an unknown extent the margin of safety in positioning this particular right-sided tube.

This analysis of right-sided double-lumen tube margin of safety has three clinical implications. First, the small margin of safety for right-sided double-lumen tubes, along with the large variation in the length of the right mainstem bronchus indicates that whenever all other considerations are equal, a left-sided double-lumen tube is preferable to a right-sided dou-ble-lumen tube. Second, tolerance of head movement with a right-sided double-lumen tube will be obviously much less than for a left-sided double-lumen tube. Third, if a right-sided double-lumen tube has to be used, the clear plastic disposable ones may be best because of the slanted doughnut shape of the right endo-bronchial cuff (Mallinkrodt), which decreases the likelihood of right upper lobe obstruction (see Fig. 9–7).

In summary, the analyses of margin of safety in positioning left- and right-sided double-lu-men tube indicate that if a question arises concerning double-lumen tube position (using conventional unilateral clamping and ausculta-tion methods), blind attempts to adjust the position of the double-lumen tube have a very good chance of being unsuccessful and/or un-certain. Instead the double-lumen tube position should be checked by fiberoptic bronchoscopy and for a left-sided double-lumen tube the endobronchial cuff should be positioned just below the tracheal carina (and, therefore, left upper lobe obstruction will not be possible). When a double-lumen tube is used for clinical research purposes, a fiberoptic bronchoscope must be used to confirm the proper double-lumen tube position to prevent otherwise un-recognizable upper lobe obstruction and to eliminate this possibility of gathering uninter-pretable and nonrepresentative data.

Tracheobronchial Tree Diameters

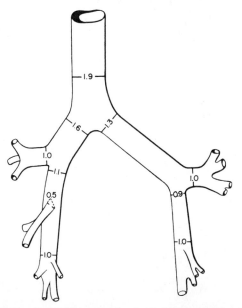

Figure 9–27. Mean tracheobronchial tree diameter (in cm) (taken from reference 22). Note that the diameter of the right upper lobe bronchial orifice is 1 cm.

2. Relationship of Fiberoptic Bronchoscope Size To Double-Lumen Tube Size

The clear plastic disposable right- and left-sided double-lumen endotracheal tubes are manufactured in five sizes: 28, 35, 37, 39, and 41 French. A 5.6 mm outside diameter diag-nostic fiberoptic bronchoscope will not pass down the lumens of any sized double-lumen tube. A 4.9 mm external diameter fiberoptic bronchoscope passes easily through the lumens of the 41 French tube, passes moderately easily with lubrication through the 39 French tube, causes a tight fit that needs a liberal amount of lubrication and a strong pushing force to pass through the 37 French tube, and does not pass through the lumen of the 35 French tube. A silicon-based fluid (such as that made by the American Cystoscope Co.) is the best lubricant for a fiberoptic bronchoscope because it does not dry out or crust and does not interfere with the view even if it coats the tip of the broncho-scope. Fortunately, from the point of view of using a 4.9 mm outside diameter fiberoptic bronchoscope, a 37 French tube or larger can be used in almost all adult females and 39 French tube or larger can be used in almost all adult males. A 3.6 to 4.2 mm outside diameter (pediatric) fiberoptic bronchoscope passes easily through the lumens of all sized double-lumen endotracheal tubes and, because the bronchoscope has an increased amount of space, the maneuverability of the tip of the bronchoscope is greatly increased. Therefore, the 3.6 to 4.2 mm outside diameter bronchoscope is obviously the bronchoscope of choice for double-lumen tubes. Table 9–3 summarizes these fiberoptic bronchoscope–double-lumen tube relationships. Several companies (Olympus, Machida, Pentax) presently manufacture 4.9 and 3.6 to 4.2 mm outside diameter fiberoptic bronchoscopes that are of adequate length and have a suction channel.

E. Use of Chest X-Ray To Determine Double-Lumen Tube Position

The chest roentgenogram can be used to determine double-lumen tube position. The usefulness of a chest roentgenogram may be greater than conventional unilateral auscultation and clamping in some patients, but it is always less precise than fiberoptic bronchoscopy. In order to use the chest roentgenogram, the double-lumen tube must have radiopaque markers at the end of the right and left lumens. The key to discerning double-lumen tube position on the chest roentgenogram is seeing where the marker at the end of the tracheal lumen is in relation to the tracheal carina. The end of the tracheal lumen marker must be above the tracheal carina; however, this does not guarantee correct position because this technique may not reveal a subtle obstruction of an upper lobe (see Fig. 9–23 and Margin of Safety in Positioning Double-Lumen Tubes). If the tracheal carina cannot be seen (which is often the case with a portable anterior-posterior film), then the chest roentgenogram method of determining double-lumen tube position is not usable. Furthermore, the chest roentgenographic method is time consuming (for film transport, film development), costly, and awkward to perform and may dislodge the tube (the cassettes are often difficult to place under the operating room table and may require movement of the patient).

F. Quantitative Determination of Cuff Seal Pressure Hold

The use of fiberoptic bronchoscopy to determine double-lumen tube position does not provide evidence or a guarantee that the two lungs are functionally separated (i.e., against a fluid and/or air pressure gradient). There are times, such as during the performance of unilateral pulmonary lavage, when the anesthesiologist must be absolutely certain that functional separation has been achieved. Complete separation of the two lungs by the left endobronchial cuff can be demonstrated in a left-sided tube by clamping the connecting tube to the right lung proximal to the right suction port and attaching a small tube (i.e., intravenous extension tubing) to the open right suction port (by appropriate adaptors) (Fig. 9–28). The free-end of this tube is submerged in a beaker of water. When the left lung is statically inflated to any pressure considered necessary, and the left endobronchial cuff is not sealed, air will enter the left lung as well as escape out from around the unsealed left cuff, up the right lumen to the

Table 9–3. Relationship of Fiberoptic Bronchoscope Size To Double-Lumen Tube Size

Fiberoptic Bronchoscope Size Outside Diameter (mm)	Double-Lumen Tube Size (French)	Fit of Fiberoptic Bronchoscope Inside Double-Lumen Tube
5.6	All sizes	Does not fit
4.9	41	Easy passage
	39	Moderately easy passage
	37	Tight fit, needs lubricant,* hard push
	35	Does not fit
3.6–4.2	All sizes	Easy passage

*Lubricant recommended is a silicon-based fluid made by the American Cystoscope Company.

Air Bubble Method for Detection of Cuff Seal/Leak

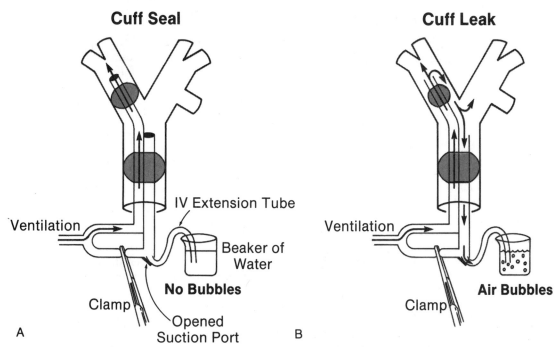

Figure 9–28. *This schematic diagram shows the air bubble detection method for checking adequacy of the seal of the left endobronchial cuff of a left-sided double-lumen tube. When the left lung is selectively ventilated or exposed to any desired distending pressure, and the left cuff is adequately sealed, no air will escape around the left cuff and out the open right suction port and, thus, no bubbles will be observed passing through the beaker of water (A). When the left lung is ventilated or exposed to any desired distending pressure and the left endobronchial cuff is not adequately sealed, air will escape around the left cuff and out the open right suction port, and, thus, air bubbles will be observed passing through the beaker of water (B).*

small connecting tube, and bubble through the beaker of water (Fig. 9–28B). If the left endobronchial cuff is sealed, no bubbles should be observed passing through the beaker of water (Fig. 9–28A). Following demonstration of functional lung separation, the right connecting tube is unclamped, the right suction port is closed, and ventilation to both lungs is resumed. To test for lung separation with the pressure gradient across the endobronchial balloon reversed, the left airway connecting tube is clamped proximal to the left suction port, the left suction port is opened to the beaker of water via the small tube, the right lung is statically inflated to any desired pressure, and the absence or presence of air bubbles in the beaker of water is noted. It should be remembered that even though the left endobronchial cuff may be adequately sealed, it is possible that during these maneuvers compression of the nonventilated lung by the ventilated lung may initially cause some small amount of

bubbling in the beaker, which will cease with repeated inflation of the ventilated lung (no bubbles should be seen following several inflations).[20, 21] The absence of airflow from the nonventilated lung suction port is a very simple but sensitive indicator of functional separation of the two lungs.

G. Complications of Double-Lumen Endotracheal Tubes

In addition to an impediment to arterial oxygenation that is inherent in the use of double-lumen endotracheal tubes for one-lung anesthesia, the tubes themselves are occasionally the cause of other serious complications (Table 9–4). Most of the complications reported in the literature involve the use of the Carlens tube, which reflects, in part, the long history of clinical use of this tube.

In a group of 200 patients in whom the Carlens tube was used, a 1.5 per cent incidence

Table 9–4. Complications of Double-Lumen Tubes

1. Malpositioning
2. Tracheobronchial tree disruption
3. Traumatic laryngitis
4. Suturing of double-lumen tube to intrathoracic structure

of traumatic laryngitis occurred, which was probably due to malposition of the carinal hook at the time of intubation.[9] Incorrect intraoperative positioning of the tube was encountered in at least six patients in this pre–fiberoptic bronchoscopy series and was felt to be responsible for one intraoperative death. Another death that occurred during the use of a Carlens tube during pneumonectomy was caused by the inadvertent suturing of a pulmonary vessel to the tube.[27] The possibility of a suture through the endotracheal tube should be considered whenever excessive resistance to extubation is encountered; the consideration of this complication may warrant re-exploration of the chest. The possibility of this complication occurring during pneumonectomy should be minimized if an opposite-sided double-lumen endotracheal tube is used or if the double-lumen endotracheal tube is withdrawn into the trachea just before the bronchus is clamped.

In a series of approximately 2700 thoracic procedures in which a red rubber Carlens tube was used, five cases of traumatic tracheobronchial rupture were discovered.[28] In three cases the rupture was noted intraoperatively and in the other two it was discovered early in the postoperative period. All patients underwent successful direct repair of the injuries. The authors suggested that factors leading to this injury included the use of inappropriately sized double-lumen tubes, tube malpositioning, and rapid and excessive inflation of tube cuffs (Table 9–5). These reports emphasize that postoperative bronchoscopy should be performed to rule out the diagnosis of tracheobronchial rupture when an unexplained serious pneumothorax or pneumomediastinum persists after thoracotomy.

Bronchial rupture has also occurred with the use of the red rubber Robertshaw double-lumen endotracheal tube. An intraoperative diagnosis of bronchial rupture was made by the detection of mediastinal bubbles and subsequent direct inspection of the left bronchus; intraoperative repair resulted in an uneventful recovery.[29] The authors suggest that this complication can be

avoided by proper selection of tube size, deflation of the endobronchial cuff prior to turning to the lateral decubitus position, and checking the integrity of the previously intubated bronchus at the time of testing the bronchial stump for leaks (Table 9–5). Obviously, great care must be taken when moving the patient from the supine to the lateral decubitus position to prevent tube movement, which cannot only cause tube malposition but also tracheobronchial tree damage (Table 9–5).

Bronchial rupture has also occurred with the use of the red rubber White double-lumen tube.[30] In this case of right mainstem bronchial rupture, nitrous oxide diffusion into the right endobronchial cuff causing excessive right endobronchial cuff volumes was felt to be the cause. The authors, therefore, recommend that the cuffs be inflated with a sample of the inspired mixture of gases rather than room air, or that cuff pressures be monitored, so that variation in cuff pressure can be observed and corrected (Table 9–5). As a simple method of monitoring cuff pressures and dealing with excessive cuff volumes and pressures, the tension in the pilot balloons to the cuffs can be periodically palpated and gas removed from the cuffs if the tension appears to be increasing (same standard of practice as with single-lumen tubes) (Table 9–5). The authors also noted that bronchial rupture is more likely to occur in patients with congenital abnormalities of the bronchus, weakness of the bronchial wall caused by infiltration of tumor, by infection, or by poor quality tissues (sepsis, alcoholism, drug abuse), and distortion of the bronchial tree by enlarged mediastinal lymph glands or by extrabronchial tumors (Table 9–5). In addition, the authors felt that the bevel of the tube or carinal hook can potentially dissect underneath the mucosa. Finally, the authors correctly warn of the dangers of ad-

Table 9–5. Endobronchial Cuff Considerations to Minimize Tracheobronchial Wall Damage (Disruption)

1. Be particularly cautious in patients with bronchial wall abnormalities.
2. Pick an appropriately sized tube.
3. Be certain tube is not malpositioned.*
4. Avoid overinflation of endobronchial cuff.*
5. Deflate endobronchial cuff during turning.
6. Inflate endobronchial cuff slowly.
7. Inflate endobronchial cuff with inspired gases.
8. Do not allow tube to move during turning.*

*Most important considerations.

vancing the stylet beyond the vocal cords and of using force to further advance the tube whenever resistance is encountered.

A common thought in the preceding reports is that excessive air volume and pressure in the bronchial balloon may be a major factor in the genesis of tracheobronchial tree tears following double-lumen tube insertion. Consequently, this complication was the logical inspiration for the development of clear plastic, tissue implantable double-lumen tubes with high volume–low pressure cuffs (as it was the earlier inspiration for single-lumen tubes). Indeed, when the tracheobronchial tree is inspected with a fiberoptic bronchoscope after double-lumen tube insertion, much less mucosal damage is caused by the tissue-implantable, low-pressure, cuffed tubes than with the red rubber, high-pressure, cuffed tubes.[7] However, in spite of these expected findings, tracheobronchial tree disruption has also occurred following the use of the tissue-implantable, low-pressure, cuffed double-lumen tubes,[31, 32] and the precautions listed in Table 9–5 must be considered even with the new modern double-lumen tubes.

H. Relative Contraindications To Use of Double-Lumen Endotracheal Tubes

There are several situations in which lung separation by a double-lumen tube may be relatively contraindicated because insertion of the double-lumen tube is either difficult or dangerous (Table 9–6). These situations include patients who have a full stomach (risk of aspiration), patients who have a lesion (airway stricture,[33] endoluminal tumor) that is present somewhere along the pathway of the double-lumen tube and thus could be traumatized, small patients in whom a 35 French tube is too large to fit comfortably through the larynx and for whom a 28 French tube (which is now manufactured) is considered too small, patients whose upper

Table 9–6. Relative Contraindications to Use of Double-Lumen Tube

1. Presence of lesion along double-lumen tube pathway.
2. Difficult/impossible conventional direct vision intubation.
3. Extremely critically ill patients with single-lumen tube in situ who cannot tolerate even a short period off mechanical ventilation.
4. Full stomach/high risk of aspiration.
5. Some combination of above.

airway anatomy precludes safe insertion of the tube (recessed jaw, prominent teeth, bull neck, anterior larynx), patients extremely critically ill who have a single lumen tube already in place and will not tolerate being taken off mechanical ventilation and PEEP (even for the short period of time of one minute), and patients having some combination of all these problems. Under these circumstances, it is still possible to separate the lungs safely and adequately by using a single-lumen tube and fiberoptic bronchoscopic placement of a bronchial blocker or by fiberoptic bronchoscopic placement of a single-lumen tube in a mainstem bronchus.

IV. BRONCHIAL BLOCKERS (WITH SINGLE-LUMEN ENDOTRACHEAL TUBES)

Lung separation can be effectively achieved with the use of a single-lumen tube and a fiberoptically placed bronchial blocker (Fig. 9–29). This is often necessary in children, since double-lumen endotracheal tubes are too large to be used in these patients. The smallest double-lumen tube available is a 28 French and may be potentially used in patients in the range of 10 to 14 years and weighing 30 to 45 kg. Bronchial blockers that are balloon-tipped luminal catheters have the advantage of allowing suctioning and injection of oxygen down the central lumen. Bronchial blockers have the disadvantage of sometimes requiring rigid bronchoscopy for placement, and, because they have high-pressure spherically inflating balloons, there is a tendency for them to back out of the bronchus into the trachea (see the following).

The bronchial blocker most often used for adults is a Fogarty occlusion (embolectomy) catheter with a 3 ml balloon.[34] The Fogarty catheter comes with a stylet in place so that it is possible to place a curvature at the distal tip. If no endotracheal tube is in place, the operator exposes the larynx and places a single-lumen tube with a high-volume cuff in the trachea. The Fogarty catheter is then placed alongside of the single-lumen tube. A fiberoptic bronchoscope is passed down to the end of the single-lumen tube through a self-sealing diaphragm in the elbow connector (which permits continued positive-pressure ventilation around the fiberoptic bronchoscope), and the Fogarty catheter is visualized below the tip of the single-lumen tube. The proximal end of the bronchial blocker is then twirled in the fingertips until the distal

Lung Separation With Single Lumen Tube, Fiberoptic Bronchoscope and Right Lung Bronchial Blocker

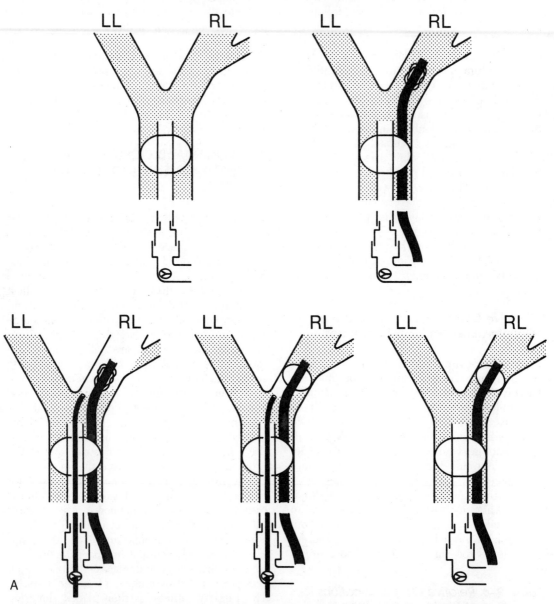

Figure 9–29. This figure shows how to separate the two lungs with a single-lumen tube, fiberoptic bronchoscope, and a left lung (A) and a right lung (B) bronchial blocker. The sequence of events is as follows: A single-lumen tube is inserted, and the patient is ventilated (upper left diagram, A and B). A bronchial blocker is passed alongside of the indwelling endotracheal tube (upper right diagram, A and B). A fiberoptic bronchoscope is passed through a self-sealing diaphragm in the elbow connecter to the endotracheal tube and is used to place the bronchial blocker into the appropriate mainstem bronchus under direct vision (lower left diagram, A and B). The balloon on the bronchial blocker is also inflated under direct vision and is positioned just below the tracheal carina (lower middle diagram, A and B). During the lower panel sequence (insertion and use of fiberoptic bronchoscope) the self-sealing diaphragm allows the patient to continue to be ventilated with positive pressure ventilation (around the fiberoptic bronchoscope but within the lumens of the endotracheal tube). (LL = left lung; RL = right lung.)

Illustration continued on opposite page

Lung Separation With Single Lumen Tube, Fiberoptic Bronchoscope and Left Lung Bronchial Blocker

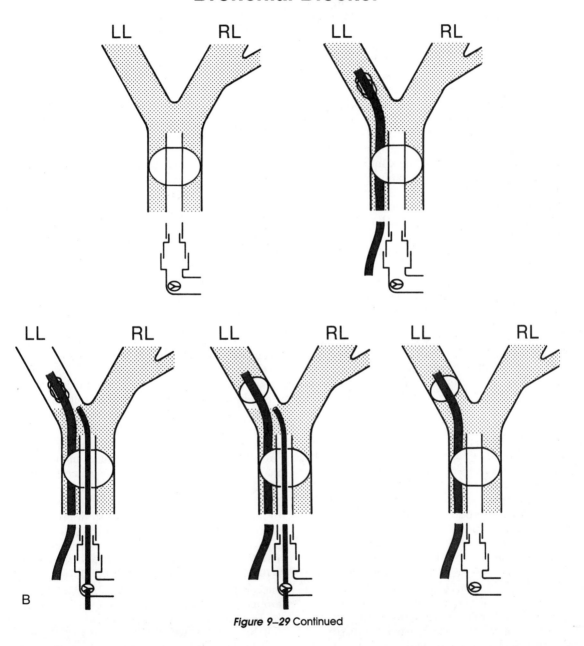

Figure 9–29 Continued

tip locates in the desired mainstem bronchus. The catheter balloon is then inflated under direct visualization, and the fiberoptic bronchoscope is withdrawn through the self-sealing diaphragm.

The bronchial blocker technique has been modified so that the bronchial blocker can be passed along with (at the same time as) the single-lumen endotracheal tube.[35, 36] With this commercial modification (Univent, Fuji Systems Corp., Tokyo, Japan), the bronchial blocker is housed in a small channel bored through the anterior wall of the endotracheal tube, which allows the bronchial blocker to be transmitted to the distal trachea by the endotracheal tube. The bronchial blocker is then visualized by the fiberoptic bronchoscope and is manipulated into the desired mainstem bronchus as previously described (although the original authors inappropriately recommend doing this blindly, i.e., turning the concavity of the single-lumen tube toward the appropriate mainstem bronchus, advancing the bronchial blocker distally, and inflating the balloon without visualization of the location of the balloon). Finally, other balloon-tipped luminal catheters (such as a Magill or Foley type catheter) may be used as bronchial blockers.

For bronchial blockade in very small children (10 kg or less) a Fogarty embolectomy catheter with a balloon capacity of 0.5 ml or a Swan-Ganz catheter (1 ml balloon) should be used.[37] Of course these catheters have to be positioned under direct vision, usually with a rigid bronchoscope. Pediatric patients of intermediate size will require intermediately sized occlusion catheters and a judgment on the mode of placement (i.e., rigid versus fiberoptic bronchoscope) (see chapter 17).

Disadvantages of bronchial blockage compared with double-lumen endotracheal tube lung separation include the inability to suction and/or to ventilate the lung distal to the blocker, increased placement time, and the definite need for a fiberoptic or rigid bronchoscope. In addition, if a mainstem bronchial blocker backs out into the trachea, the seal between the two lungs will be lost, and two catastrophic complications may occur. First, if the bronchial blocker was being used to seal off a fluid (blood or pus) in one lung, then both lungs may become contaminated with the fluid. Second, the trachea will be at least partially obstructed by the blocker, and ventilation will be greatly impaired. Therefore, bronchial blockage requires that the anesthesiologist continuously

and intensively monitor the compliance and breath sounds of the ventilated lung. Because of these potentially catastrophic problems, bronchial blockers are rarely used for elective procedures for adults today.[14]

V. ENDOBRONCHIAL INTUBATION WITH SINGLE-LUMEN TUBES

In adults presenting with hemoptysis, endobronchial intubation with a single-lumen tube is often the easiest, quickest way of effectively separating the two lungs, especially if the left lung is bleeding. If the left lung is bleeding, one can simply take an uncut single-lumen endotracheal tube and advance it inward until moderate resistance is felt (Fig. 9–30A). In the vast majority of patients the single-lumen tube will locate in the right mainstem bronchus, thereby blocking off the bleeding left lung and allowing for selective ventilation of just the right lung. Under these circumstances it is very possible that the right upper lobe bronchus will be blocked off as well, resulting in ventilation of just the right middle and lower lobes. Ventilation of just a soiled right lung or ventilation of just the right middle and lower lobes (even if they are unsoiled) incurs the risk of serious hypoxemia due to the very large transpulmonary shunt that is necessarily created by the single lung endobronchial intubation.

If the right lung is bleeding, a fiberoptic bronchoscope can be passed through a self-sealing diaphragm in the single-lumen tube elbow connector and directed into the left mainstem bronchus. Persistent large soft catheter suctioning of the carinal area through the single-lumen tube prior to use of the fiberoptic bronchoscope and suctioning through the fiberoptic bronchoscope (through the single-lumen tube) may be required in order to visualize the tracheal carina (Fig. 9–30B). The single-lumen tube can then be passed over the fiberoptic bronchoscope into the left mainstem bronchus, thereby sealing off the bleeding right lung and allowing for selective ventilation of the left lung. Passing the fiberoptic bronchoscope through a self-sealing diaphragm allows for the continuance of positive-pressure ventilation and PEEP around the bronchoscope. However, it should be realized that visualization of the carina may not be possible when the bleeding is copious and that the only hope for the patient may lie in rapid thoracotomy and control of bleeding from within the chest. In addition, under these

Single Lumen Tube: Lung Bleeding

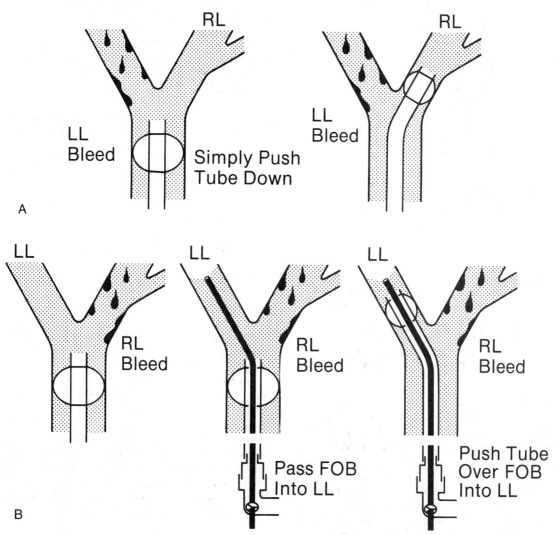

Figure 9–30. *This figure shows how to separate the two lungs with a single-lumen tube in the presence of massive lung bleeding. When the left lung is bleeding (A) an uncut single-lumen tube may simply be inserted its full length, and, in the vast majority of cases, it will enter the right mainstem bronchus, thereby effectively sealing off the right lung from the left lung. However, one can expect that the cuff of the single-lumen tube will obstruct the right upper lobe. When the right lung is bleeding (B), a fiberoptic bronchoscope, which is jacketed on its proximal end with an endotracheal tube, can be passed through a self-sealing diaphragm in the elbow connector to the endotracheal tube (which allows continued positive pressure breathing) and, if a moment's view of the tracheal carina can be obtained, passed into the left mainstem bronchus. Using the fiberoptic bronchoscope as a stylet, the endotracheal tube can be passed over the fiberoptic bronchoscope into the left mainstem bronchus. The fiberoptic bronchoscope is then withdrawn. (LL= left lung; RL = right lung; FOB = fiberoptic bronchoscope.)*

very adverse conditions conventional passage of a double-lumen tube may more rapidly and effectively separate the two lungs than trying to visualize anatomy with a fiberoptic bronchoscope. Alternatively, a right mainstem endobronchial tube, which has tracheal and right endobronchial cuffs and a right upper lobe ventilation slot, can be passed, but the endobronchial tube has limitations that the double-lumen tube does not have (see discussion of this tube and Fig. 9–31 immediately following).

For adults, a variety of reusable endobronchial tubes have been developed for insertion into a mainstem bronchus to provide one-lung

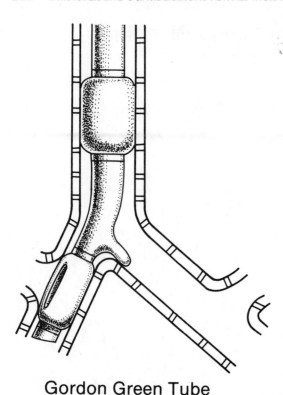

Gordon Green Tube

Figure 9–31. Schematic diagram of the placement of a Gordon Green endobronchial tube at the carina.

anesthesia during thoracic surgery (see Table 1–1). Some of these can be placed blindly, while others require placement via an intubating bronchoscope. These tubes have the advantage of having a large diameter and therefore a low-airway resistance. Major disadvantages include the inability to suction the operative site, difficulty in positioning the bronchial cuff, the possibility of the thin-walled tube kinking in the posterior pharynx, and the very considerable hazard of inadequately ventilating the right upper lobe after right endobronchial intubation. The Gordon-Green tube, having both a tracheal and endobronchial cuff, offers several advantages if a right-sided endobronchial tube is selected (see Fig. 9–31).[38] A carinal hook facilitates blind positioning. Inflation of the bronchial cuff isolates the left lung; when the right endobronchial balloon is not inflated, the entire lung can be ventilated by backflow around the distal balloon. Finally, the endobronchial cuff is slotted in order to provide ventilation to the right upper lobe during one-lung ventilation. In spite of these advances in tube design, endobronchial tubes are generally less satisfactory than double-lumen endotracheal tubes and are used infrequently today.[14]

In children the simplest method for achieving lung separation is to pass a standard single-lumen tube into a mainstem bronchus. Right mainstem bronchial intubation is easily achieved blindly; left mainstem bronchial intubation may require fiberoptic bronchoscopy (see preceding), fluoroscopy, or guidance of the tube by the surgeon from within the chest (see chapter 17 and Figs. 17–7 and 17–8).

In summary, double-lumen endotracheal tubes are the method of choice for separating the lungs in adult patients. If there is any question, the precise location of a double-lumen tube can be determined by fiberoptic bronchoscopy at any time. There are a number of situations in which insertion of a double-lumen tube may be difficult and/or dangerous, and under these circumstances consideration should be given to separating the lungs with a single-lumen tube alone or in combination with a bronchial blocker. However, when using a single-lumen tube in a mainstem bronchus or when using a bronchial blocker, ability to suction the operative site and control oxygen uptake (the blocked lung cannot be ventilated with oxygen at any time) is limited. In addition, the placement of the single-lumen tube into one or the other mainstem bronchi and the proper placement of a bronchial blocker require fiberoptic bronchoscopy. Therefore, no matter which method of separating the lungs is chosen, there is a real need for the immediate availability of a small diameter fiberoptic bronchoscope (for checking the position of the double-lumen tube, placing a single-lumen tube in the left mainstem bronchus, and placing a bronchial blocker) that has a suction port (in order to clear secretions and blood from the airway).

REFERENCES

1. Urschel HC Jr, Razzuk MA: Median sternotomy as a standard approach for pulmonary resection. Ann Thorac Surg 41:130–134, 1986.
2. Anderson HW, Benumof JL: Intrapulmonary shunting during one-lung ventilation and surgical manipulation. Anesthesiology 55:A377, 1981.
3. Thomson DF, Campbell D: Changes in arterial oxygen tension during one-lung anesthesia. Br J Anaesth 45:611–616, 1973.
4. Boysen PG: Pulmonary resection and postoperative pulmonary function. Chest 77:718–719, 1980.
5. Boysen PG, Block AG, Moulder PV. Relationship between preoperative pulmonary function tests and complications after thoracotomy. Surg Gynecol Obstet 152:813–815, 1981.
6. Lack JA: Endobronchial tube resistances. Br J Anaesth 46:461, 1974.

7. Clapham MCC, Vaughan RS: Bronchial intubation. A comparison between polyvinyl chloride and red rubber double lumen tubes. Anaesthesia 40:1111–1114, 1985.
8. Bjork VO, Carlens E: The prevention of spread during pulmonary resection by the use of a double-lumen catheter. J Thorac Surg 20:151, 1950.
9. Newman RW, Finer GE, Downs JE: Routine use of the Carlens double-lumen endobronchial catheter: An experimental and clinical study. J Thorac Cardiovasc Surg 42:327, 1961.
10. White GMJ: A new double-lumen tube. Br J Anaesth 32:232, 1960.
11. Bryce-Smith R: A double-lumen endobronchial tube. Br J Anaesth 31:274, 1959.
12. Bryce-Smith R, Salt R: A right-sided double-lumen endobronchial tube. Br J Anaesth 32:230, 1960.
13. Robertshaw FL: Low resistance double-lumen endotracheal tubes. Br J Anaesth 34:576, 1962.
14. Pappin JC: The current practice of endobronchial intubation. Anaesth 34:57–64, 1979.
15. Simpson PM: Tracheal intubation with a Robertshaw tube via a tracheostomy. Br. J Anaesth 48:373–375, 1976.
16. Seed RF, Wedley JR: Tracheal intubation with a Robertshaw tube via a tracheostomy (letter). Br J Anaesth 49:639, 1977.
17. Anderson HW, Benumof JL, Ozaki GT: New improved double lumen tube adaptor. Anesthesiology 56:54–56, 1982.
18. Smith G, Hirsch N, Ehrenwerth J: Sight and sound: Can double-lumen endotracheal tubes be placed accurately without fiberoptic bronchoscopy? Anesth Analg 65:S1–S170, 1986.
19. Read RC, Friday CD, Eason CN: Prospective study of the Robertshaw endobronchial catheter in thoracic surgery. Ann Thorac Surg 24:156, 1977.
20. Alfery DD, Benumof JL, Spragg RG: Anesthesia for bronchopulmonary lavage. In Kaplan J (ed): Thoracic Anesthesia. New York, Churchill-Livingstone, 1982, pp 403–419.
21. Spragg RG, Benumof JL, Alfery DD: New methods for performance of unilateral lung lavage. Anesthesiology 57:535–538, 1982.
22. Conrady PA, Goodman LR, Cainge R, et al: Alteration of endotracheal tube position: Flexion and extension of the neck. Crit Care Med 4:8, 1976.
23. Saito S, Dohi S, Naito H: Alteration of double-lumen endobronchial tube position by flexion and extension of the neck. Anesthesiology 52:696–697, 1985.
24. Keating JL, Benumof JL: An analysis of margin of safety in positioning double-lumen tube. Anesthesiology 63:A563, 1985.
25. Jesseph JE, Merendino KA: The dimensional interrelationships of the major components of the human tracheobronchial tree. Surg Gynecol Obstet 105:210–214, 1957.
26. Merendino KA, Keriluk LB: Human measurements involved in tracheobronchial resection and reconstruction procedures. Surgery 35:590–597, 1954.
27. Dryden GE: Circulatory collapse after pneumonectomy (an unusual complication from the use of a Carlens catheter): Case report. Anesth Analg 56:451, 1977.
28. Guernelli N, Bragaglia RB, Briccoli A, et al: Tracheobronchial ruptures due to cuffed Carlens tubes. Ann Thorac Surg 28:66, 1979.
29. Heiser M, Steinberg JJ, MacVaugh H, et al: Bronchial rupture, a complication of use of the Robertshaw double-lumen tube. Anesthesiology 51:88, 1979.
30. Foster JNG, Lau OJ, Alimo EB: Ruptured bronchus following endobronchial intubation. Br J Anaesth 55:687–688, 1983.
31. Wagner DL, Gammage GW, Wong ML: Tracheal rupture following the insertion of a disposable double-lumen endotracheal tube. Anesthesiology 63:698–700, 1985.
32. Burton NA, Fall SM, Lyons T, Graeber GM: Rupture of the left main-stem bronchus with a polyvinylchloride double-lumen tube. Chest 83:928–929, 1983.
33. Cohen JA, Denisco RA, Richard TS, et al: Hazardous placement of a Robertshaw-type endobronchial tube. Anesth Analg 65:100–101, 1986.
34. Ginsberg RJ: New technique for one lung anesthesia using an endobronchial blocker. J Thorac Cardiovasc Surg 82:542–546, 1981.
35. Inoue H, Shohtsu A, Ogawa J, et al: New device for one lung anesthesia: Endotracheal tube with moveable blocker. J Thorac Cardiovasc Surg 83:940–941, 1982.
36. Kamaya H, Krishna PR: New endotracheal tube (Univent tube) for selective blockade of one lung. Anesthesiology 63:342–343, 1985.
37. Veil R: Selective bronchial blocking in a small child. Br J Anaesth 41:453–454, 1969.
38. Green R, Gordon W: Right lung anesthesia. Anesthesia for left lung surgery using a new right endobronchial tube. Anaesthesia 12:86, 1957.

Routine Surgical Considerations That Have Anesthetic Implications

10

I. INTRODUCTION

There are a number of common surgical considerations that have important routine management implications for the anesthesiologist (Table 10–1). First, the anesthesiologist should be aware of the planned patient position and how to position the patient correctly. Knowledge of the position of the patient may influence or determine the timing of such anesthetic procedures as epidural catheter placement, location of intravenous and monitoring lines, and whether anesthesia is induced on the transporting gurney or on the operating room table. In addition, the anesthesiologist is responsible, at least in part, for positioning the patient and avoiding complications related to patient position. Second, the anesthesiologist should be familiar with the various thoracic incisions. The time of making the incision is important to the anesthesiologist, for this is when he must closely observe the patient and operating field (watch for signs of inadequate anesthesia, the color of the shed blood, and the opening of the pleura [which entails stopping breathing and initiating one-lung ventilation]). The anesthesiologist must also closely observe the closure of the pleura (sigh patient to reverse atelectasis, expel air and fluid from the pleural space) and the skin incision so that the administration or discontinuance of drugs (reversal of paralysis, discontinuance of inhalational drugs, administration of intravenous narcotics) can be made with maximum precision. Third, the anesthesiologist

should have some idea of the sequence of events that occur during the surgical procedure so that autonomic reflexes, arrhythmias, blood loss, and changes in gas exchange may be more readily anticipated and responded to. Consequently, this chapter will consider, in sequence, positioning of the patient, the various thoracic incisions, and briefly the common major thoracic operations.

II. POSITIONING THE PATIENT

Following the induction of anesthesia and double-lumen tube insertion, the patient is ready to be positioned for the surgical procedure. Although it is not the primary responsibility of the anesthesiologist to position the patient, in practice this duty falls at least in part on the anesthesiologist. In addition, the anesthesiologist is liable for complications caused by patient position and, therefore, the anesthesiologist should actively contribute to preventing these complications. Consequently, this section is written with these duties in mind and describes the correct positioning of the patient for the various thoracic incisions (see next section).

A. Posterior Lateral Thoracotomy

A standard posterior lateral thoracotomy is the incision of choice for the majority of intra-

Table 10–1. Surgical Events that Require the Anesthesiologist's Attention

1. Positioning
2. Skin incision
   a. Color of shed blood
   b. Signs of inadequate anesthesia
3. Pleural incision
   a. Freedom of movement of lung beneath pleura
   b. Cessation of breathing
   c. Initiation of one-lung ventilation
4. Pulmonary resection
   a. Prevent any patient movement while vessels are being secured
   b. Note whether pulmonary veins are taken before pulmonary arteries (causes entrapment of much more blood within specimen)
   c. Test integrity of bronchial stump with sigh
5. Pleural closure
   a. Sigh to reverse atelectasis
   b. Sigh to expel air and fluid from pleural space while last stitch is being placed
6. Skin closure
   a. Time administration or discontinuance of anesthetic drugs

thoracic operations and requires that the patient be placed in the lateral decubitus position (Fig. 10–1). A folded gauze pad or towel is placed under the axilla to prevent compression of the axillary structures against the rib cage. The hands and arms are first outstretched in the position of an athlete performing the hammer throw, and then both forearms are bent cephalad and supported on pads placed below the lower elbow and between the two elbows. This brings the vertebral border of the scapula forward, thus permitting the incision to be extended superiorly as high as necessary. The thigh closest to the table is flexed slightly and the knee bent; the thigh and leg in the superior position are kept straight. This pose maintains the hips and trunk in a vertical plane. A pillow is placed between the thighs, knees, and legs to avoid pressure on the dependent extremity by the sheer weight of the nondependent extremity. Some surgeons prefer a small pillow

Lateral Decubitus Position for Posterior Lateral Thoracotomy

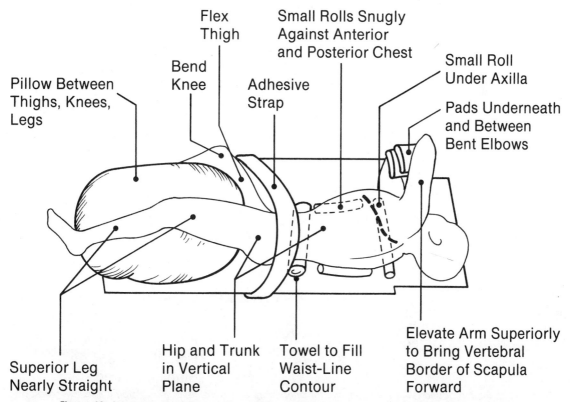

Figure 10–1. Lateral decubitus position for the performance of a posterior lateral thoracotomy.

roll or foam-rubber pad to fill the contour of the waistline above the operating table and perhaps to extend the uppermost intercostal spaces. Small blanket rolls are placed anteriorly and posteriorly, snugly tied to each other, and pulled against the chest wall front and back. A 3- or 4-inch strap of adhesive tape is placed across the hip and attached to the table to steady the patient in position. Such fixation places no pressure on the skin of the patient and permits tilting of the table as required (Fig. 10–1).

B. Anterior Thoracotomy

With the patient in the supine position the hemithorax to be operated upon is elevated 30° on a folded blanket, sponge-rubber pad, or the newer pad filled with plastic beads (see Fig. 10–2). The patient's ipsilateral arm may be elevated and carefully fixed to a cross brace, without causing pressure on the neurovascular structures of the arm or excessive stretch on the brachial plexus. In other instances, the ipsilateral elbow can be bent slightly, and the hand can be placed palm down under the hip, to hold the arm away from the lateral chest wall, again avoiding pressure upon, or angulation of, blood vessels and nerves.

C. Posterior Thoracotomy

The standard posterior thoracotomy, made with the patient in a prone position, is not used often today. The patient lies prone on the table and a foam-rubber or blanket pad is placed under the side opposite that to be operated upon, elevating it slightly (about 10°) (see Fig. 10–5A). Supports may be placed underneath the upper chest and pelvis to allow free diaphragmatic movement. The arm is moved cephalad so that the scapula is drawn away from the site of surgery. Many years ago, Overholt and Langer (1949) had a table especially designed for this position to permit the surgeon to sit while performing the operation. For a number of reasons, not the least of which are pressure injuries to skin, brachial plexus, and axillary vessels, this position is not presently used.

D. Median Sternotomy

The patient is supine with arms by the sides (see Fig. 10–6A). A towel roll is placed underneath and across the shoulders, and the head is slightly extended on the neck and placed in a sponge doughnut for stability. The shoulder roll

Supine Position for Anterior Thoracotomy

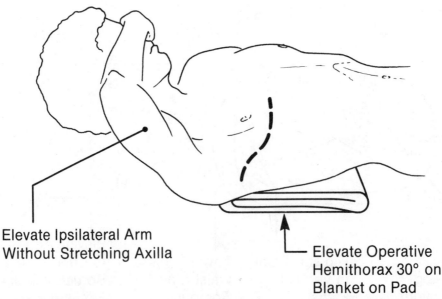

Elevate Ipsilateral Arm
Without Stretching Axilla

Elevate Operative
Hemithorax 30° on
Blanket on Pad

Figure 10–2. Supine position with elevated arm for performance of an anterior thoracotomy. The elevated arm can be stabilized on an ether screen.

and head extension provide access to the superternal notch, where the incision is begun.

E. The Minithoracotomies

There are numerous surgical diagnostic procedures that require small incisions. The scalene node biopsy is made with the patient in the supine position with the head turned slightly to the opposite side of the incision. Mediastinoscopy is performed in the supine position with the patient's head in moderate extension (incision is made over the supersternal notch). Medianstenotomy is made in the supine position (incision is over the second costal cartilage). Other diagnostic procedures such as pleural biopsy, thoracentesis, needle biopsy of the pleura, and thoracoscopy are most often done under local anesthesia. If these procedures are performed under general anesthesia, they are done in the lateral decubitus position, with the affected side up to facilitate the examination. For an open lung biopsy, the incision may be made anywhere in the thorax, as determined preoperatively by the roentgenographic distribution of the disease process. In most patients with diffuse lung disease, an anterior incision provides excellent exposure with minimal postoperative discomfort; thus, the patient is most often in the supine position, and a short submammary skin incision is utilized. The "minithoracotomy" utilizes a small transaxillary approach. The procedure is performed with the patient in the lateral decubitus position, with the arm being extended upward over the patient's head.

III. THORACIC INCISIONS[1]

The anesthesiologist must pay close attention to the operating field during the initial and final phases of thoracotomy (Table 10–1). The attention at the initial incision is directed to the color of the shed blood, signs of sympathetic nervous system stimulation, and the opening of the pleura (observe how freely the lung moves below the pleura, stop ventilating the patient to avoid having the surgeon incise the lungs beneath the pleura, and time the initiation of one-lung ventilation). Attention to the closure of the incision is important in order to expand the lungs fully under direct observation just prior to closure (reverse atelectasis) and as the last stitch closing the pleura is tied (expel all possible air and fluid from the pleural space) and to time the administration or discontinuance of the various anesthetic drugs, depending on whether a smooth transition to postoperative mechanical ventilation in the recovery room or intensive care unit is desired as opposed to extubation in the immediate postoperative period. The usual incisions providing access to the thorax are posterior lateral, anterior, and posterior thoracotomy and median sternotomy.

A. Posterior Lateral Thoracotomy

A standard posterior lateral thoracotomy is the incision of choice for the majority of intrathoracic operations. This incision provides good access to all areas of the lung, lung hilum, and most of the mediastinum.

With the patient in the lateral decubitus position (see Positioning the Patient), the skin incision is begun at the anterior axillary line at the level at which the surgeon wishes to enter the chest, usually the fifth intercostal space, and runs posteriorly several finger breadths below the angle of the scapula, then turns superiorly to run midway between the vertebral border of the scapula and the spinous processes of the vertebrae (Fig. 10–3A). Dissection is then made to expose the rib cage by dividing the serratus anterior, latissimus dorsi, trapezius, and, perhaps, the rhomboid muscles (Fig. 10–3B). Entry into the pleural space can then be gained by either resecting a rib or utilizing an intercostal space. If the rib is to be resected, the periosteum is incised and then elevated from the bone. The rib is divided with a rib shears at the costotransverse junction posteriorly and at the anterior axillary line. It is necessary to ligate and to divide the intercostal bundles if the rib is to be divided, to obviate tearing these vessels when the ribs are subsequently spread. If the intercostal incision is used, it is extended down to the pleura, while injury to the intercostal vessels and nerve is avoided. Entry into the pleural space is gained by making an incision through the bed of the resected rib or through the exposed pleura in the intercostal space. In either instance, positive pressure should be removed from the airway system to permit the lung to collapse away (inward) from the thoracic wall. If adhesions are present between the visceral and parietal pleura (i.e., the lung does not move "freely" in the pleural space), these must be divided, and if vascular, they must be ligated.

Posterior Lateral Thoracotomy

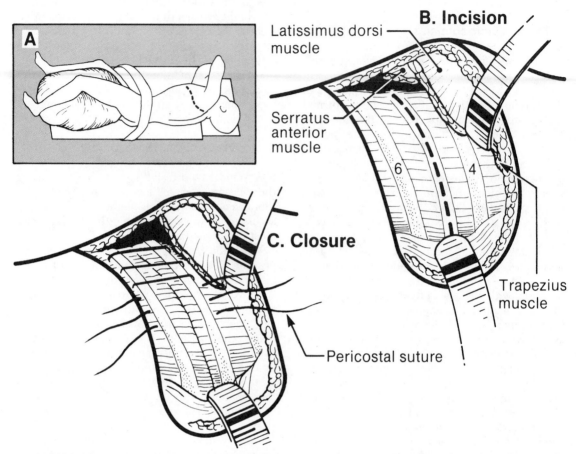

A

B. Incision

Latissimus dorsi muscle

Serratus anterior muscle

6 4

C. Closure

Trapezius muscle

Pericostal suture

Figure 10–3. Posterior lateral thoracotomy. A, Outline of incision proceeding anteriorly to posteriorly following the course of the fifth or the sixth rib and then around the angle of the scapula to head superiorly between the scapula and vertebral column. B, The extracostal muscles have been divided or retracted, and the incision through the periosteum of the fifth rib is shown. C, Closure of the thoracotomy wound, with pericostal sutures in place.

Closure of the posterior lateral thoracotomy is made by first placing several sutures pericostally above and below the ribs adjacent to the intercostal incision (Fig. 10–3C). The intercostal nerve, artery, and vein can be dissected free from the costal groove or protected by inclusion of a thick layer of the intercostal muscle. There may be less pain in the postoperative period if the intercostal nerve is excluded from the pericostal suture. No attempt is made to approximate the parietal pleura as a separate layer, and the parietal pleura is included in the suture of the intercostal muscles. These muscles are approximated with either continuous or interrupted sutures. All layers of the divided extracostal muscles should be reapproximated anatomically.

B. Anterior Thoracotomy

A standard anterior thoracotomy provides speed of entry into the chest and minimal disturbance of respiratory and circulatory functions, and closure is relatively easy. It provides adequate exposure to the anterior mediastinum, to the anterior portions of the upper lobes, and to areas necessary for some cardiac procedures. Lower lobe segments are difficult to expose through this incision, especially on the left, where the heart would have to be retracted, leading to decreased cardiac output and arrhythmias.

The incision extends from the lateral edge of the sternum in a curvilinear manner to the midaxillary line (Fig. 10–4A). In men, the incision parallels the intercostal space to be entered, and in women, it is made along the inframammary fold. The pectoralis major and minor are then divided and retracted (Fig. 10–4B). The intercostal muscles are divided down to the parietal pleura, so that the surgeon can determine whether a "free" pleural space is present by observing lung motion with respiration. If this space is present, the pleura can be incised safely and the lung permitted to retract from the chest wall. Frequently, when performing an anterior thoracotomy, it is unnecessary to resect or to divide a rib to gain adequate exposure, although one or two costal cartilages may be divided for greater access to the pleural space.

The incision through the pleura and intercostal muscles is carried posteriorly toward the axilla, and the fibers of the serratus are split back to the long thoracic nerve, which is pre-

served. The latissimus dorsi muscle is usually not divided but can be retracted posteriorly, if necessary, to obtain greater exposure.

Closure of the anterior thoracotomy is essentially the same as that described for the posterior lateral incision (Fig. 10–4C). The pectoralis major and minor muscles must be anatomically reattached.

C. Posterior Thoracotomy

The standard posterior thoracotomy made with the patient in a prone position is not often used today. The advantages claimed for this incision in the past included better ventilation of the lung not under operation and reduced possibility of aspiration of infective secretions into the unoperated side. However, the risk of injury to the skin, brachial plexus, and axillary

Anterior Thoracotomy

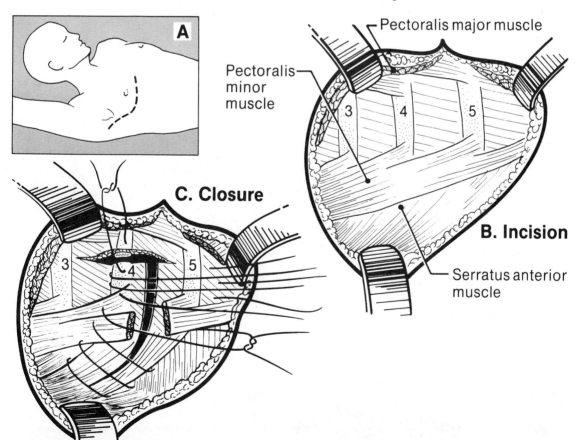

Figure 10–4. Anterior thoracotomy. A, *Outline of skin incision.* B, *Pectoralis major muscle separated and retracted to expose the anterior chest wall.* C, *Placement of sutures pericostally above and below the adjacent ribs to close the intercostal incision as well as to approximate the divided costal cartilage.*

vessels is high. In addition, without use of a double-lumen tube, the prevention of aspiration is not certain. The patient is difficult to position, and exposure is poor for anteriorly located lesions and is especially poor for exposure of the anterior hilar and mediastinal structures.

The skin incision for the posterior thoracotomy extends from the level of the spine of the scapula superiorly, along the midline between the spinous processes of the vertebrae and the vertebral border of the scapula, and swings laterally around the angle of the scapula to about the midaxillary line or slightly posterior to that point (Fig. 10–5A). The muscles are incised as previously described for a standard posterior lateral thoracotomy (Fig. 10–5B). The closure of the incision is similar to that used in the posterior lateral approach (Fig. 10–5C).

D. Median Sternotomy

Longitudinal median sternotomy is the procedure of choice for exposure of the anterior mediastinum, great vessels, and the heart. By and large, other incisions, such as transverse sternotomy with bilateral thoracotomy and partial sternotomy with partial resection of the clavicle or disarticulation at the sternal clavicular joint, have been abandoned. Recently, median sternotomy has gained popularity as an approach to the excision of bilateral pulmonary processes such as excision of bilateral multiple metastatic pulmonary nodules and bilateral pulmonary bullous disease.[2,3] Since the median sternotomy approach has been thought to be associated with less postoperative pain and respiratory dysfunction, it has even been recom-

Prone Posterior Position Thoracotomy

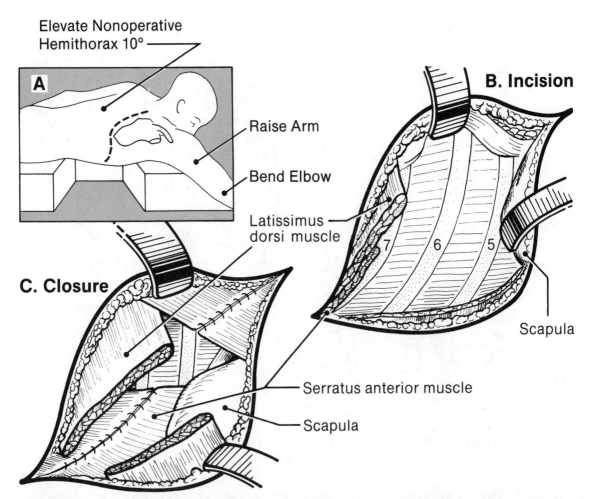

Elevate Nonoperative Hemithorax 10°

A

Raise Arm

Bend Elbow

Latissimus dorsi muscle

B. Incision

7   6   5

Scapula

C. Closure

Serratus anterior muscle

Scapula

Figure 10–5. Posterior thoracotomy. A, Outline of skin incision. B, Latissimus dorsi and serratus anterior muscles are divided, and the scapula and upper margins of the muscles are retracted cephalad. C, Reapproximation of muscles by sutures.

Median Sternotomy Supine Position

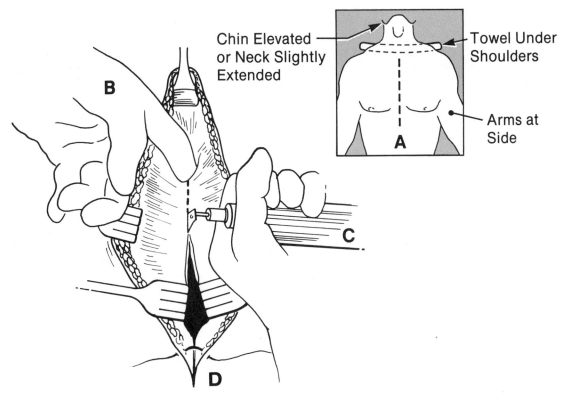

Figure 10–6. Median sternotomy. A, Incision from just below the supersternal notch to below the top of the xiphoid. B, Blunt dissection of the posterior aspect of the sternum at the supersternal notch. C, Division of the sternum from below upward with the use of an oscillating saw. D, Closure of the divided sternum with wire sutures.

mended for routine pulmonary resections.[4] Although pulmonary resections may be accomplished by this route, the anatomic disadvantages are similar to those of the standard anterior thoracotomy noted previously and usually require one-lung ventilation (collapse of the operative lung).

The skin incision is made from just below the top edge of the manubrium at the supersternal notch to about 2 to 3 inches below the xiphoid process (Fig. 10–6A). The incision is not carried higher, since if a tracheostomy is necessary, it may be performed without making the tracheostomy incision part of the sternotomy wound. When the tracheostomy incision is part of the sternotomy wound, comtamination of the wound from the trachea can readily occur. By retracting the skin, the supersternal notch is exposed without difficulty. The supersternal notch and subxiphoid area are developed with blunt dissection (Fig. 10–6B). The xiphoid process is split in the midline, and a power oscillating saw is used to divide the sternum (Fig. 10–6C). After the sternum is divided com-

pletely, the retrosternal space is cleared progressively of the loosely adherent pleura, which is identified easily by asking the anesthesiologist to inflate the lungs, so as to fill the pleural space.

For optimum healing, the sternum must be closed meticulously to ensure as nearly an immobile unit as possible. If the pleura has been opened, the chest must be drained, bilaterally if necessary. The sternum is reapproximated with six or eight heavy wires passed through each side of it. The soft tissues are then reapproximated with interrupted sutures. Firm adhesive strapping may be applied externally for additional support.

E. Minithoracotomy

Techniques of minithoracotomy include limited-anterior thoracotomy, transaxillary thoracotomy, and superclavicular thoracotomy. Such incisions are used for excision of limited disease processes in the apex of the lung, excision of the first rib, and biopsy of limited or diffuse disease in the pulmonary parenchyma, which is otherwise not amenable to diagnosis. Each of these approaches offers an alternative approach to a more extensive major thoracotomy. Each is well tolerated postoperatively, and minimum debility is noted after its use.

F. Drainage of the Pleural Space

After thoracotomy, the pleural space should be drained, especially when there has been resection of lung tissue or a portion of the chest wall. For tube placement in a posterioinferior location, a skin incision 2-cm long is made just anterior to the posterior axillary line in about the eighth intercostal space. A heavy duty 8-inch hemostat or forceps is inserted into the skin incision at an angle and is pushed through the intercostal muscles so that the forceps enters the pleural space cephalad to the skin incision. The forceps then pulls the distal end of the chest drain out of the chest cavity; this prevents contamination of the proximal end of the drain (the indwelling end) by contact with the skin. By palpating the level of the dome of the diaphragm, the proximal end of the tube is positioned so that the proximal tip of the tube is at the dome and the side opening of the tube is in the sulcus. For anterior tube placement the tube is inserted just lateral to the border of the pectoralis major muscle. A skin incision is made at the level of the third intercostal space, and with cephalad direction, the tube usually enters the chest through the second intercostal space. The tip of the catheter is fixed to the anterior parietal pleura by a slip knot to keep the tip from becoming angulated medially and lying adjacent to the great vessels of the mediastinum, where, by constant motion, penetration of the wall of the vessel could conceivably occur. If such movement of the tip of the tube is noted on postoperative roentgenograms of the chest, the tube should be withdrawn promptly. The loosely tied slip knot suture permits easy removal of the tube. A firm stitch is used to anchor any chest drain to the skin, and a separate loose mattress suture is placed around the drain so that this can be cut and tied to seal the wound when the drain is withdrawn postoperatively. See chapter 13 for a complete discussion of the design and function of a modern chest tube drainage system and potential chest tube drainage system complications.

IV. THE COMMON MAJOR ELECTIVE THORACIC OPERATIONS

In a typical modern thoracic surgery service, pulmonary resections are the most frequent major cases done, with esophageal and thoracic aortic surgery making up most of the remainder. Operations such as thoracoplasty, drainage of empyema, thoracoscopy, and phrenic nerve crush/evulsion are infrequently performed or abandoned today. Consequently, this section will describe pulmonary resections (pneumonectomy, lobectomy, segmentectomy) in moderate detail, and the conduct of surgery for esophageal and thoracic aortic operations in brief detail.

A. Pulmonary Resections[5]

1. Pneumonectomy

Following one of the standard thoracic incisions (see preceding section), entrance is made into the pleural space. The pleura is then incised as it reflects upon the hilus anteriorly, superiorly, and posteriorly. On the right, the azygos vein may be isolated and divided to give greater access to the hilus superiorly. Generally, the pulmonary artery is the first structure to be isolated and divided (rather than the pulmonary vein, which would lead to increased blood loss [retained within the specimen]). After control of the pulmonary artery, the superior and then the inferior pulmonary veins are dissected, isolated, and divided, and the cut ends are secured. All the remaining tissue reflections are divided, and the mainstem bronchus is freed up to its junction with the trachea. A bronchial clamp is placed just distal to this junction and the bronchus divided proximal to the clamp. The bronchial stump is then closed with a stapling device, and the anesthesiologist may be asked to test the integrity of the bronchial closure with a sustained positive pressure breath (the surgeon may also immerse the bronchial stump in saline to see if gas bubbles through the saline). Not infrequently, one or two bronchial arteries will need to be ligated after the bronchus has been divided. It is important that bleeding from the bronchial vessels be controlled, since these vessels may cause significant postoperative blood loss. After closure of its proximal end, the bronchial stump is covered with adjacent tissue, such as a pleural flap, the azygos vein, a pedicle graft of pericardial fat, or adjacent pericardium. This is done to provide the stump with a viable tissue cover to help prevent the possible development of a leak from the stump, which normally heals by secondary intention.

Tracheal-sleeve pneumonectomy has been used to excise high line carcinomas of either mainstem bronchus. Resection of the tracheal carina with the ipsilateral lung is carried out and the contralateral bronchus is then anastamosed to the distal end of the trachea. When extensive pleural disease coexists with parenchymal disease that requires a pneumonectomy, a pleuropneumonectomy may be performed. Essentially, a plane of cleavage is developed between the endothoracic fascia and the parietal pleura, and the pleura and lung are freed as one from the chest wall, diaphragm, and mediastinal structures down to the hilus. From this stage on, the vessels and bronchus are managed as in a standard pneumonectomy.

2. Lobectomy

After the pleural space is entered (see Thoracic Incisions), the pleura is incised as it reflects upon the hilar structures. The oblique (major) fissure is then opened to expose the interlobar portion of the pulmonary artery. The arterial branches of the lobe to be resected are then divided, double ligated, transfixed, and divided. After control of the arteries, the veins draining the lobe are identified and managed in a similar fashion. The lobar bronchus is then isolated and clamped distally to the proposed line of division. After division of the bronchus, the proximal end of the stump is closed with a stapling device. Coverage of the stump with adjacent tissue is practiced by most thoracic surgeons, although the remaining lung tissue generally will cover the stump effectively when the remaining lung is re-expanded. Removal of the lobe is then completed by division of any remaining connections to the other lobe or lobes. The integrity of the bronchial suture line is tested by pouring saline into the pleural cavity to cover the stump while sustained positive pressure of 30 to 40 cm H_2O is maintained by manual compression of the rebreathing bag. Some gas usually escapes during this maneuver, but it is generally from the raw, now separated, surface of the remaining lung and not from the bronchial stump.

A radical lobectomy may be utilized in certain instances for treatment of carcinoma of the lung. In this procedure the lymphatic nodes in the mediastinum are removed en bloc with the lobe. This is most easily and satisfactorily performed on the right upper lobe, although it may be done almost as well on the left upper lobe. Both right and left lower radical lobectomies are more difficult to perform, and it is doubtful whether an adequate radical lymphatic dissection is truly possible in these anatomic locations. A lobectomy may also include a sleeve resection of a portion of the mainstem bronchus. This is indicated for the preservation of lung tissue either when the pathologic lesion to be removed is benign or when the patient has insufficient pulmonary reserve to tolerate a pneumonectomy. The initial steps of the operative procedure are carried out as in a standard lobectomy. The arterial and venous branches to the lobe are isolated, ligated, and divided. Next, the lobar bronchus and adjacent mainstem bronchus are dissected free from the remaining vascular structures. A clamp is placed proximally on the mainstem bronchus, and the bronchus is then divided just distal to the clamp. The mainstem bronchus is divided a second time distal to the lobar orifice, and this segment of the bronchus is removed along with the resected lobe. The cut ends of the bronchus are then tailored, as necessary, to fit each other and are reapproximated.

3. Segmentectomy

The initial steps in a segmentectomy (removal of a discrete bronchopulmonary segment) are carried out in the same manner as that in a lobectomy. After exposing the hilar structures and opening the major fissure, the pulmonary artery is identified, and the arterial branch of the segment or segments to be removed are identified, isolated, secured, and divided. After control of the arterial supply, the segmental veins and the bronchus are divided, although at times the order of these procedures may be reversed. Before dividing the bronchus, differential deflation and inflation of the segment to be removed should be done by clamping and unclamping to help delineate the intersegmental planes. It is to be remembered that filling of the deflated segment may occur from the adjacent segments by means of collateral ventilation. Once the segmental planes are identified, the bronchus is divided and the proximal stump is closed with a stapling device. Additional coverage of the stump is not usually carried out. Separation of the diseased segment is accomplished by blunt dissection. Vascular and small airway connections between the adjacent segments must be clamped, divided, and ligated.

4. Wedge and Limited Resections

Wedge resection consists of excision of a diseased portion of the lung (usually small) irrespective of bronchopulmonary segmentology. Entry is made into the pleural space, and the area of lung to be resected is identified. Stapling devices are applied so that the specimen will consist of a margin of surrounding normal lung parenchyma as well as the lesion. The specimen is removed by cutting along the staples. These procedures are usually short.

In a limited or local resection (small discrete tumors that can be enucleated), the visceral pleura is incised over the mass, and the mass is removed by blunt and sharp dissection, with the raw surface, blood vessels, and minor bronchial structures being individually clamped and ligated or stapled. The visceral pleura is reapproximated with suture. These procedures are usually also short.

B. Surgery of the Thoracic Esophagus[6] and Aorta[7]

Resectional surgery of the midthoracic esophagus is technically very complicated (immediate mortality is high—approximately 20 per cent) and usually involves an additional proximal cervical incision (to approach the upper third of the esophagus) and a distal abdominal incision (to approach the lower third of the esophagus). The midthoracic esophagus can be approached through either a left-sided or right-sided thoracotomy (since the midthoracic portion of the esophagus, except for its most distal part, is primarily on the right side of the mediastinum). Advantages of a left thoracotomy include the ability to split open the left diaphragm, mobilize the stomach, and bring it up into the chest without having to change the patient's position. A right thoracotomy has the advantage of allowing the surgeon to perform a bypass between the esophagus and the fundus of the stomach with complete relief from dysphagia in the presence of an unresectable lesion. Also, if the azygos vein is infiltrated by tumor, it is safer to dissect it from the right side. The disadvantages of a right thoracotomy are that the position of the patient must be changed after the abdominal part of the operation (performed first) is completed. In addition, after an extensive procedure in the abdomen and an opening of the chest, the lesion may be found to be nonresectable. Esophageal surgery involves a number of other controversies; they include questions of delayed versus immediate reconstruction and the use of colon or stomach to restore continuity.

Similarly, repair of thoracic aortic aneurysms requires a high degree of technical sophistication and also usually involves proximal and distal perfusion connections and considerations (see chapter 16 for an extensive discussion). Since the aortic arch lies over the esophagus on the left, a left fifth intercostal space thoracotomy is usually used for thoracic aortic surgery. The mediastinal pleura is usually opened over its entire length to allow for mobilization of the entire thoracic aorta. Significant controversy exists about the best method for bypassing the thoracic aorta (see chapter 16). Further description of the ensuing steps of proximal and distal control of the esophagus and aorta are beyond the scope of this chapter.

REFERENCES

1. Lees WM: Thoracic incisions. In Shields TW (ed): General Thoracic Surgery. 2nd ed. Philadelphia, Lea and Febiger, 1983, pp 305–314.
2. Takita H, Merrin C, Didolkar MS, Douglass HO, Edgerton F: The surgical management of multiple lung metastasis. Ann Thorac Surg 24:359–364, 1977.
3. Cooper JD, Nelam JM, Pearson FG: Extended indications for median sternotomy in patients requiring pulmonary resection. Ann Thorac Surg 26:413–418, 1978.
4. Urschel HC Jr.: In discussion of paper by Cooper JD, Nelam JM and Pearson FG (ref. 3): Extended indications for median sternotomy in patients requiring pulmonary resection. Ann Thorac Surg 26:419, 1978.
5. Shields TW: Pulmonary resections. In Shields TW (ed): General Thoracic Surgery. 2nd ed. Philadelphia, Lea and Febiger, 1983, pp 315–330.
6. Shield TW, Postlethwait RW: Resection of the esophagus. In Shields TW (ed): General Thoracic Surgery. 2nd ed. Philadelphia, Lea and Febiger, 1983, pp 354–362.
7. Ruhland DM, Benumof JL: Anesthesia for emergency thoracic surgery. In Donegan J (ed): Anesthesia for Emergency Surgery. New York, Churchill-Livingstone, 1987 (in press).

Conventional and Differential Lung Management of One-Lung Ventilation

11

I. INTRODUCTION

Both the patient's lungs are ventilated with intermittent positive-pressure ventilation during the induction of anesthesia, before and after insertion of the double-lumen endotracheal tube, during positioning of the patient (in the lateral decubitus position in the vast majority of cases), and during the chest wall incision. However, once the pleura has been incised, it is usually useful and helpful to the surgeon to collapse the lung that is being operated on (the nondependent lung) to facilitate surgical exposure. Before describing the various one-lung ventilation management techniques, it is important to review briefly the one-lung ventilation situation to understand how the various one-lung management techniques might influence the distribution of blood flow between the two lungs during one-lung ventilation. Conventional ventilatory management of the one-lung ventilation situation is described first—conventional management of one-lung ventilation provides satisfactory gas exchange in the majority of cases. In a few situations conventional management of one-lung ventilation does not prevent severe hypoxemia, and in these few cases the addition of differential lung ventilation to conventional mechanical ventilation almost always resolves the problem. Accordingly, the chapter ends with a combined conventional and differential lung management plan for providing adequate arterial oxygenation during one-lung ventilation.

II. THE ONE-LUNG VENTILATION SITUATION

Anesthesia for thoracic surgery is most commonly performed with the patient in the lateral decubitus position, with the nondependent hemithorax comprising the operative field. When one-lung ventilation is employed, the nondependent lung is the nonventilated and collapsed (atelectatic) lung, and the dependent lung is the ventilated lung. In this section (which essentially summarizes part of chapter 4) it is important to remember that with a constant cardiac output, whatever increases blood flow to one lung usually decreases blood flow to the other, and vice versa.

A. The Nondependent Nonventilated Lung

The nondependent nonventilated lung has a ventilation-perfusion ratio of zero. Consequently, one-lung ventilation creates an obligatory right-to-left transpulmonary shunt through the nonventilated nondependent lung that is not present during two-lung ventilation (Fig. 4–7). Thus, one-lung ventilation results in a much larger alveolar-to-arterial oxygen tension difference and lower arterial oxygen tension (P_aO_2) than does two-lung ventilation.[1] Fortunately, blood flow to the nondependent nonventilated lung is usually reduced by both passive mechanical and active vasoconstriction mechanisms that are usually operant and, thereby, prevent the shunt from increasing and the P_aO_2 from decreasing as much as might be expected on a two-lung ventilation blood flow distribution basis (Fig. 11–1). The passive mechanical factors that decrease blood flow to the nondependent lung consist of the force of gravity, surgical interference with blood flow (retraction and compression of vessels, tying off of vessels), and a low dependent lung airway pressure. The active vasoconstrictor mechanism decreasing blood flow to the nondependent lung is nondependent lung hypoxic pulmonary vasoconstriction (Fig. 11–1).

B. The Dependent Ventilated Lung

Unfortunately, the dependent lung may have a reduced lung volume and may be poorly ventilated for several reasons (Fig. 11–1) (see chapters 3 and 4). First, in the lateral decubitus position the ventilated dependent lung usually has a reduced lung volume owing to the combined factors of induction of general anesthesia and circumferential (and, perhaps, severe) compression by the weight of the mediastinum from above, by the abdominal contents pressing against the diaphragm from the caudad side, and by suboptimal positioning effects (rolls,

packs, shoulder supports) pushing in from the operating room table. Reduced lung volume usually results in low ventilation-perfusion and atelectatic regions (see Fig. 3–24). Second, absorption atelectasis can also occur in regions of the dependent lung that have low ventilation-perfusion ratios when they are exposed to high inspired oxygen concentration.[2,3] Third, difficulty in secretion removal may also cause the development of poorly ventilated and atelectatic areas in the dependent lung. Finally, maintaining the lateral decubitus position for prolonged periods of time may cause fluid to transudate into the dependent lung (which may be vertically below the left atrium) and cause further decreased lung volume and increased airway closure in the dependent lung.[4] A decrease in lung volume and an increase in airway closure in the dependent lung additively creates areas that have low ventilation-perfusion ratios or atelectasis.[2] The development of low ventilation-perfusion and atelectatic areas in the dependent lung can elicit dependent lung hypoxic pulmonary vasoconstriction, resulting in increased dependent lung pulmonary vascular resistance that will divert blood flow to the nondependent lung, thereby increasing the shunt across the lungs.

In view of these factors, which can affect the amount of nondependent-lung blood flow, the

One Lung Ventilation: Determinants of Blood Flow Distribution

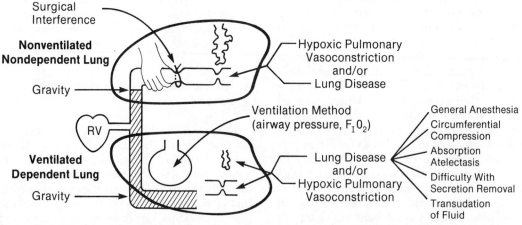

Figure 11–1. This schematic diagram shows the major determinants of blood flow distribution during one-lung ventilation. Blood flow to the nonventilated nondependent lung is reduced by the force of gravity, surgical interference (compression, tying off of vessels), hypoxic pulmonary vasoconstriction, and/or lung disease (vascular obliteration, thrombosis). Blood flow to the ventilated dependent lung is increased by gravity; however, dependent lung blood flow and vascular resistance may be altered in either direction depending on the method of ventilation (amount of airway pressure, F_IO_2, and the amount of dependent lung disease and/or hypoxic pulmonary vasoconstriction). Factors that may increase the amount of dependent lung disease intraoperatively are listed on the extreme right of the figure (see also chapter 3).

Method of Ventilation of the Dependent Lung During One-Lung Ventilation Can Determine Amount of Nondependent Lung Blood Flow

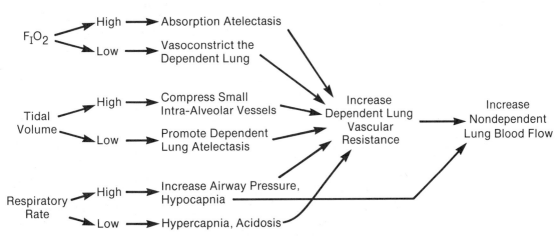

Figure 11–2. The method of ventilation of the dependent lung during one-lung ventilation can be a major determinant of the amount of nondependent lung blood flow.

method used to ventilate the dependent lung is especially important for several reasons (Fig. 11–2). First, if the dependent-lung method of ventilation involves an excessive amount of airway pressure, due to either use of high PEEP levels or very large tidal volumes, then dependent-lung vascular resistance may be increased, which would increase nondependent-lung blood flow. The deleterious effects of increased nondependent-lung blood flow (shunt) may outweigh the beneficial effects of the opening of atelectatic and low ventilation-perfusion areas in the dependent lung. Second, if the dependent lung is hyperventilated (which may require an excessive amount of airway pressure), the resultant hypocapnia may inhibit hypoxic pulmonary vasoconstriction (see chapter 4). Third, if the dependent lung is ventilated with too small of a tidal volume, dependent lung atelectasis may develop. Fourth, a high inspired oxygen concentration to the dependent lung may vasodilate the dependent lung, enhancing nondependent lung hypoxic pulmonary vasoconstriction.[5,6] On the other hand, a high inspired oxygen concentration to the low ventilation-perfusion–dependent lung may promote dependent lung absorption atelectasis.[3,7]

III. CONVENTIONAL MANAGEMENT OF ONE-LUNG VENTILATION

The proper initial conventional management of one-lung ventilation is logically based on the preceding determinants of blood flow distribution during one-lung ventilation. In view of the fact that one-lung ventilation incurs a high risk of causing systemic hypoxemia, it is extremely important that dependent lung ventilation, as it affects these determinants, be optimally managed. This section considers the usual management of one-lung ventilation in terms of the most appropriate inspired oxygen concentration, tidal volume, respiratory rate, and dependent lung PEEP level that should be used (Table 11–1).

A. Inspired Oxygen Concentration

Although the theoretical possibilities of absorption atelectasis and oxygen toxicity exist, the benefits of ventilating the dependent lung with 100 per cent oxygen far exceed the risks (Fig. 11–3). A high F_IO_2 in the single ventilated lung may critically increase the P_aO_2 from arrhythmogenic and life-threatening levels to safer levels. In addition, a high F_IO_2 in the dependent lung will cause vasodilation, thereby increasing the dependent lung capability of accepting blood flow redistribution due to nondependent-lung HPV.[6–8] Direct chemical 100 per cent oxygen toxicity will not occur during the time frame of the operative period,[9] and absorption atelectasis in the dependent lung[3] is unlikely to occur in view of the remaining one-lung ventilation management characteristics (moderately large tidal volumes with intermit-

Table 11–1. *Initial Conventional Ventilatory Management of One-Lung Anesthesia*

1. Maintain two-lung ventilation as long as possible.
2. Begin one-lung ventilation with tidal volume of 10 ml/kg.
3. Adjust the respiratory rate so that $P_aCO_2 = 40$ mm Hg.
4. Use $F_IO_2 = 1.0$.
5. Utilize frequent or continuous arterial PO_2 and PCO_2 monitoring.

tent positive-pressure, low-level PEEP) listed as follows. Although not previously studied during one-lung ventilation, use of a dependent lung F_IO_2 of 0.8 to 0.9 may be ideal in view of the fact that an F_IN_2 of 0.1 to 0.2 greatly reduces the possibility of absorption atelectasis (by allowing some nitrogen to splint open the low $\dot{V}/\dot{Q}$ regions),[3] whereas a reduction in F_IO_2 of 0.1 to 0.2 (from 1.0) will probably cause only a small decrease in P_aO_2 (observe the flatness of the high isoshunt lines in Fig. 3–30).

B. Tidal Volume

The dependent lung should be ventilated with a tidal volume of 10 ml/kg. Use of a tidal volume much less than 10 ml/kg might promote dependent-lung atelectasis. Use of a tidal volume much greater than 10 ml/kg might excessively increase dependent lung airway pressure and vascular resistance[10] and thereby increase nondependent lung blood flow (decrease nondependent-lung HPV).[11–13]

A dependent-lung tidal volume of 10 ml/kg represents a volume that is in the middle of a range of tidal volumes (8 to 15 ml/kg) that have been found to not greatly affect arterial oxygenation during one-lung ventilation. The dependent lung tidal volume was systematically changed from 8 to 15 ml/kg during one-lung ventilation, and blood gases and transpulmonary shunt were measured at the following times: sample 1, lateral decubitus position with the chest closed and two-lung tidal volume of 15 mg/kg; sample 2, chest open with the same two-

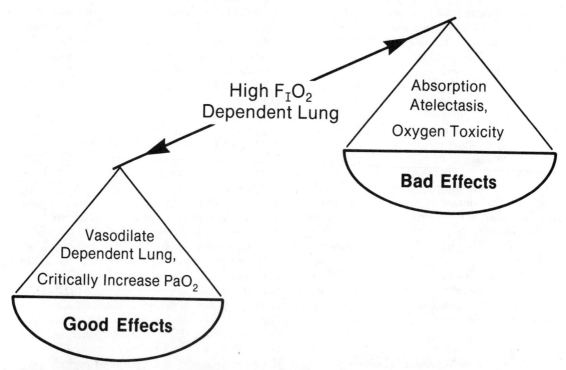

The Good Effects of a High F_IO_2 to Ventilate Dependent Lung Outweigh the Bad Effects

Figure 11–3. The good effects of a high F_IO_2 to the ventilated dependent lung outweigh the bad effects. The good effects consist of vasodilation in the dependent lung, which increases dependent lung blood flow (and decreases nondependent lung blood flow) and may critically increase the PaO_2. The bad effects are theoretical and consist of dependent lung absorption atelectasis and oxygen toxicity.

lung ventilation; sample 3, 10 minutes after collapse of the nondependent lung and with dependent lung tidal volume of 15 ml/kg; sample 4, 10 minutes after tidal volume to the dependent lung was reduced from 15 to 8 ml/kg; sample 5, 10 minutes after dependent lung tidal volume was increased from 8 to 15 mg/kg; sample 6, 10 minutes after occlusion of the pulmonary artery to the upper lung.[14] This study reported a consistent decrease in P_aO_2 and increase in shunt during one-lung anesthesia (sample 3 compared with sample 2). Changes in P_aO_2 with alterations in the tidal volume (sample 4 compared with samples 3 and 5) in individual patients were variable and unpredictable in both degree and direction (although the mean value for the group did not change). Thus, it appears that changing the tidal volume from 15 to 8 ml/kg during one-lung ventilation has an unpredictable but usually not a great impact on arterial oxygenation.

C. Respiratory Rate

The respiratory rate should be set so that the P_aCO_2 remains at 40 mm Hg. Since a dependent lung tidal volume of 10 ml/kg represents a 20 per cent decrease from the usual two-lung tidal volume of 12 ml/kg, the respiratory rate usually needs to be increased by 20 per cent in order to maintain carbon dioxide hemostasis. The trade-off between decreased tidal volume and increased respiratory rate is usually a constant minute ventilation; although ventilation and perfusion are considerably mismatched during one-lung ventilation, an unchanged minute ventilation during one-lung ventilation (compared with two-lung ventilation) can continue to eliminate a normal amount of carbon dioxide because of the high diffusibility of carbon dioxide.[10,15-17] In fact, Figure 11-4 shows that lowering the minute ventilation by approximately one half (tidal volume reduced from 15 to 8 ml/kg while respiratory rate is constant) has little effect on P_aCO_2 (see chapter 4 for explanation). Hypocapnia should be avoided because use of the airway pressure in the dependent lung necessary to produce systemic hypocapnia may excessively increase dependent lung vascular resistance. Furthermore, hypocapnia may directly inhibit HPV in the nondependent lung.[18,19]

D. Dependent Lung PEEP

No, or just a very low level of, dependent lung PEEP (less than 5 cm H_2O) should be used initially because of concern of unnecessarily increasing dependent lung vascular resistance (see Selective Dependent-Lung PEEP).

In summary, at the commencement of one-lung ventilation, 100 per cent oxygen (although it may be argued on theoretical grounds that 80 to 90 per cent oxygen decreases the risk of absorption atelectasis and only minimally, or not at all, increases the risk of hypoxemia), a tidal volume of 10 ml/kg, and a 20 per cent increase in respiratory rate are used as initial ventilation settings (Table 11-1). Ventilation and arterial oxygenation are monitored by use of frequent arterial blood gases, end-tidal carbon dioxide concentration, and pulse oximetry or transcutaneous tensions. If there is a problem with either ventilation or arterial oxygenation, then one or more of the differential lung management techniques is used.

IV. DIFFERENTIAL LUNG MANAGEMENT OF ONE-LUNG VENTILATION

A. Selective Dependent Lung PEEP

Since the ventilated dependent lung often has a decreased lung volume during one-lung ventilation (Figs. 4-6 and 11-1), it is not surprising that several attempts have been made to improve oxygenation by treating the ventilated lung with PEEP.[11-13,20-23] The most accepted mechanism by which PEEP is thought to be of benefit is that PEEP causes an increase in lung volume at end-expiration (by definition, the functional residual capacity, or FRC) (Fig. 3-25). The increase in FRC contributes to the prevention of airway and alveolar closure at end-expiration and to the recruitment of airways and alveoli during inspiration. The increases in lung volume and airway and alveolar openings result in increases in lung compliance, ventilation, and the ventilation-perfusion ratio of the single ventilated lung (Fig. 11-5).[24,25] Consequently, it may be expected that the application of PEEP to the compressed dependent lung would improve dependent lung volume and ventilation-perfusion relationships.

An accepted risk of PEEP is that the PEEP-induced increase in lung volume can cause compression of the small intra-alveolar vessels. If the PEEP-induced intra-alveolar vessel compression is geographically widespread, then total pulmonary vascular resistance increases and cardiac output decreases. If the intra-alveolar vessel compression is limited to the ventilated lung, then the pulmonary vascular resis-

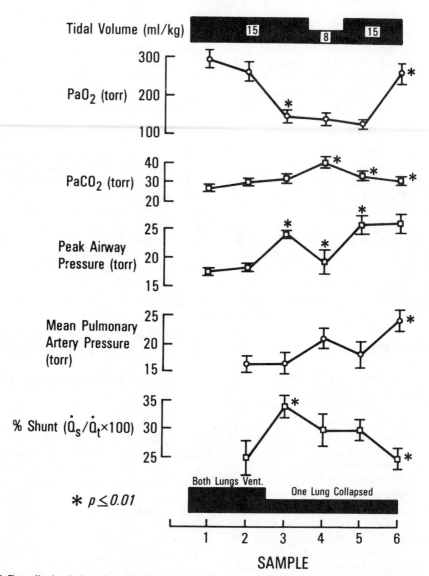

Figure 11–4. The effects of changing tidal volume on arterial blood gas values, peak airway pressure, pulmonary artery pressure, and shunt during one-lung ventilation. PaO2 and percentage shunt are not significantly affected by changing the tidal volume from 15 to 8 ml/kg or vice versa (From Flacke JW, Thompson DS, Reed RC: Influence of tidal volume and pulmonary artery occlusion on arterial oxygenation during endobronchial anesthesia. South Med J 69:619, 1976. Redrawn and reprinted by permission from the Southern Medical Journal.)

tance of the lung just being ventilated and receiving PEEP will increase, which will cause diversion of blood flow away from the ventilated lung to the nonventilated lung (Fig. 11–5), and the shunt will increase, and P_aO_2 will decrease. With regional lung PEEP, pulmonary vascular resistance for the whole lung does not greatly increase, and the cardiac output does not decrease.[11,13] The fact that increases in both PEEP and tidal volume in the dependent ventilated lung have an additive effect in decreasing P_aO_2 during one-lung ventilation greatly supports the

one-ventilated lung volume versus vascular resistance hypothesis.[11] Consistent with these observations is the fact that the application of 10 cm H_2O PEEP to the dependent lung during one-lung ventilation decreases P_aO_2 in some patients but has had no significant systemic hemodynamic effect in any patient.[26,27]

In summary, the effect of dependent lung PEEP on arterial oxygenation is a trade-off between the positive effect of increasing dependent lung FRC and ventilation-perfusion ratio and the negative effect of increasing de-

One Lung Ventilation: Dependent Lung PEEP

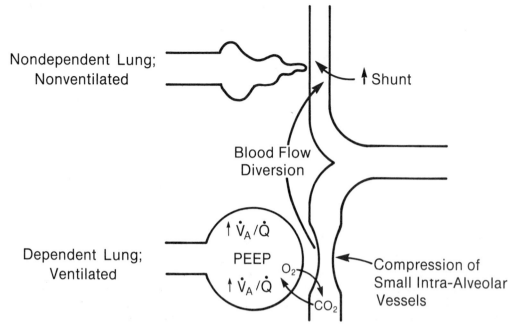

Figure 11–5. Selective positive end-expiratory pressure (PEEP) to the ventilated-dependent lung can increase dependent lung ventilation-perfusion ratios ($\uparrow \dot{V}_A/\dot{Q}$). However, dependent lung PEEP can also cause compression of the small intra-alveolar vessels in the dependent lung, causing blood flow diversion to the nonventilated nondependent lung, thereby increasing the shunt through the nonventilated nondependent lung. Therefore, the overall arterial oxygenation effect of dependent lung PEEP will be a trade-off between the good effect of an increase in dependent lung $\dot{V}_A/\dot{Q}$ and the bad effect of increased nonventilated lung blood flow.

pendent lung vascular resistance and shunting blood flow to the nonventilated lung. Thus, the various one-lung ventilation PEEP studies have contained patients who have had an increase,[12,20,28] no change,[12,21,22,28] or a decrease[12,20,23,28] in oxygenation. It may be expected that in patients with a very diseased dependent lung (low lung volume and low ventilation-perfusion ratio), the positive effect of selective dependent lung PEEP (increased lung volume and increased ventilation-perfusion ratio) might outweigh the negative effects of selective dependent lung PEEP (shunting of blood flow to the nonventilated, nondependent lung), whereas in patients with a normal dependent lung the negative effects of dependent lung PEEP would outweigh the benefits. Indeed, in one study in which 10 cm H_2O PEEP was selectively applied to the dependent lung, P_aO_2 increased in those patients with P_aO_2 less than 80 mm Hg ($F_IO_2 = 0.5$), whereas P_aO_2 decreased or remained constant in patients with P_aO_2 higher than 80 mm Hg ($F_IO_2 = 0.5$).[28] Presumably, in the patients with P_aO_2 lower than 80 mm Hg ($F_IO_2 = 0.5$) the dependent

lung had a low functional residual capacity (low ventilation-perfusion ratio and atelectatic regions) and, therefore, the positive effect of increased dependent-lung volume predominated over the negative effect of shunting blood flow to the nonventilated lung. Conversely, the patients with the higher P_aO_2 presumably had a dependent lung with an adequate functional residual capacity and ventilation-perfusion ratio, and the negative effect of shunting blood flow to the nonventilated lung predominated over the positive effect of increased dependent lung volume. Although in none of these studies was a dose (ventilated lung PEEP)-response (P_aO_2, $\dot{Q}_s/\dot{Q}_t$ value) relationship described, it seems reasonable to postulate on the basis of these results that the therapeutic margin of using PEEP to just the ventilated lung to increase P_aO_2 during one-lung ventilation is quite narrow. PEEP to just the dependent ventilated lung may be delivered by the same anesthesia machine apparatus that is ordinarily used to deliver PEEP to the whole lung. Other studies have shown that high tidal volumes,[29] variations in the inspiratory-to-expiratory ratio,[21] and intermittent manual hyperventilation of the lower lung are not beneficial in increasing P_aO_2 during one-lung ventilation.[21]

B. Selective Nondependent Lung CPAP

Positive pressure can be selectively and statically applied to just the nonventilated nondependent lung. Since under these conditions the nonventilated lung is only slightly but constantly distended by oxygen, an appropriate term for this ventilatory arrangement is nonventilated-lung continuous positive airway pressure (CPAP). Recently, two reports, one in humans[23] and one in dogs,[30] have shown that the application of CPAP (without tidal ventilation) to only or just the nonventilated lung significantly increased oxygenation. The latter study was performed with the dogs in the lateral decubitus position and showed that low levels of CPAP (5 to 10 cm H_2O) to the nonventilated nondependent lung greatly increased P_aO_2 and decreased shunt, while blood flow to the nonventilated lung remained unchanged; presum-

ably, this level of CPAP does not compress the small intra-alveolar vessels in the nondependent lung. Thus, it is not at all surprising to find that the institution of 10 cm H_2O nondependent lung CPAP in patients has had no significant hemodynamic effect.[26,27] In summary, low levels of CPAP simply maintain the patency of nondependent lung airways, allowing some oxygen distention of the gas-exchanging alveolar space in the nondependent lung (Fig. 11–6) without significantly affecting the pulmonary vasculature. In all clinical studies[23,26,27,31] the application of 5 to 10 cm H_2O CPAP has not interfered with the performance of surgery and may, in fact, facilitate intralobar dissection; this is not surprising in view of the fact that the initial compliance of a collapsed lung is only 10 ml/cm H_2O, and 5 to 10 cm H_2O CPAP should only create a slightly distended lung that occupies a volume of 50 to 100 ml, which is hardly or not at all noticed by the surgeon.

On the other hand, in the canine study,[30] 15 cm H_2O of nondependent lung CPAP caused changes in P_aO_2 and shunt similar to those of 5 to 10 cm H_2O nondependent lung CPAP, while

One Lung Ventilation: Nondependent Lung CPAP

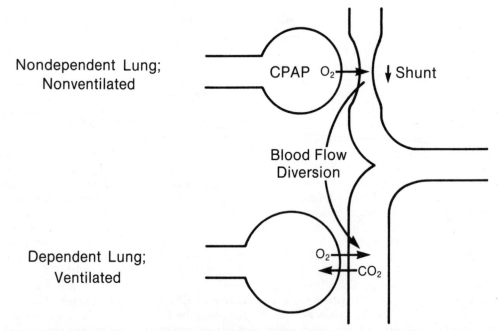

Figure 11–6. Selective continuous positive airway pressure (CPAP) to the nonventilated nondependent lung (static distension without tidal movement) allows this lung to participate in oxygen uptake and markedly decreases the shunt through the nonventilated nondependent lung. Even if the nonventilated nondependent lung CPAP causes blood flow diversion to the ventilated dependent lung, the diverted flow still can participate in oxygen uptake and CO_2 elimination in the ventilated dependent lung. Usually 5 to 10 cm H_2O of nondependent lung CPAP is all that is clinically needed, and this amount of CPAP does not cause any significant surgical interference.

blood flow to the nonventilated nondependent lung decreased significantly. Therefore, high levels of nonventilated lung CPAP act by permitting oxygen uptake in the nonventilated lung as well as by causing blood flow diversion to the ventilated lung, where both oxygen and carbon dioxide exchange can take place (Fig. 11–6). Since low levels of nonventilated lung CPAP are as efficacious as high levels of nonventilated lung CPAP and have less surgical interference and hemodynamic implications, it is logical to first use low levels of nonventilated CPAP.

In all patients in all clinical studies to date, 5 to 10 cm H_2O of nondependent lung CPAP has significantly increased P_aO_2 during one-lung ventilation.[23,26,27,31,33–35] It should be concluded that the single most efficacious maneuver to increase P_aO_2 during one-lung ventilation is to apply 5 to 10 cm H_2O CPAP to the nondependent lung. In my experience, low levels of nonventilated CPAP have corrected severe hypoxemia ($P_aO_2 < 50$ mm Hg) greater than 90 per cent of the time, provided the double-lumen tube was correctly positioned. However, the nondependent lung CPAP must be applied during the deflation phase of a large tidal volume so that the deflating lung can lock into a CPAP level with uniform expansion and avoid the need to overcome critical opening pressures.

In both the human[23] and dog[30] studies, oxygen insufflation at zero airway pressure did not significantly improve P_aO_2 and shunt, and this result was probably due to the inability of zero transbronchial airway pressure to maintain airway patency and overcome critical opening pressures. Although one study in patients has concluded that insufflation of O_2 at zero airway pressure does increase P_aO_2, the study is difficult to interpret, since the patients did not serve as their own control.[32]

Several selective nondependent lung CPAP systems that are easy to assemble have been recently described.[22,33–35] All these nondependent lung CPAP systems have three features in common (Fig. 11–7). First, there must be a source of oxygen to flow into the nonventilated

Nondependent Lung CPAP Systems Has Three Essential Components

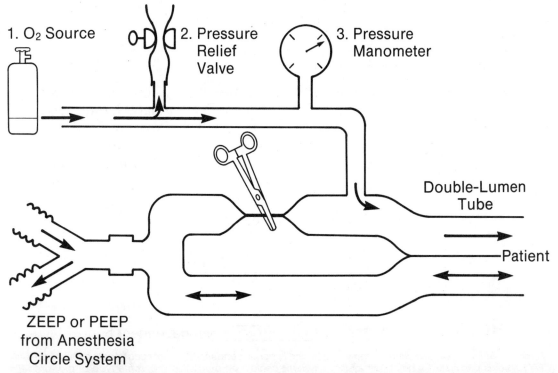

Figure 11–7. The three essential components of a nondependent lung continuous positive airway pressure (CPAP) system consist of (1) an oxygen source, (2) a pressure relief valve, and (3) a pressure manometer to measure the CPAP. The CPAP is created by the free flow of oxygen into the lung versus the restricted outflow of oxygen from the lung by the pressure relief valve. (ZEEP = zero end-expiratory pressure.)

lung. Second, there must be some sort of re-strictive mechanism (hand-screw valve, pop-off valve, weight-loaded valve) to prevent the egress of oxygen out of the nonventilated lung so that the nonventilated lung may become distended. Thus, a free-flowing pressurized source of oxygen flows into a lung, but the escape of the oxygen is restricted; the unre-stricted flow in and the restricted flow out creates a constant distending pressure. Third, the distending pressure must be measured by a manometer. In practice it is simplest to keep the restrictive mechanism constant and adjust the distending pressure with a relatively fine sensitivity by changing the oxygen flow rate. If the nondependent lung CPAP system has a reservoir bag included, the nondependent lung may also be ventilated with intermittent posi-tive-pressure whenever desired.

The exact arrangement of the oxygen source, the restrictive mechanism, and the manometer is not important. For example, Figure 11–8A

shows that these three essential nondependent lung CPAP components may be arranged, pro-ceeding distally to proximally (toward the dou-ble-lumen tube), as anesthesia reservoir bag, restrictive mechanism, pressure manometer, and oxygen source,[33] whereas Figure 11–8B shows a similar type of nondependent lung CPAP system but with the place of the anes-thesia reservoir bag and restrictive mechanism reversed (unpublished personal experience). The presence of an anesthesia reservoir bag in the nondependent lung CPAP system allows for the capability of delivering an independent tidal breath or sigh to the nondependent lung. Fig-ure 11–9 shows two nondependent lung CPAP systems that do not include an anesthesia res-ervoir bag. In the first non–reservoir bag CPAP system (Fig. 11–9A) the arrangement of the necessary three components is oxygen source, pressure manometer, and the restrictive mech-anism,[34] whereas in the second non–reservoir bag CPAP system (Fig. 11–9B) the restrictive

Nondependent Lung CPAP Systems With Reservoir Bags

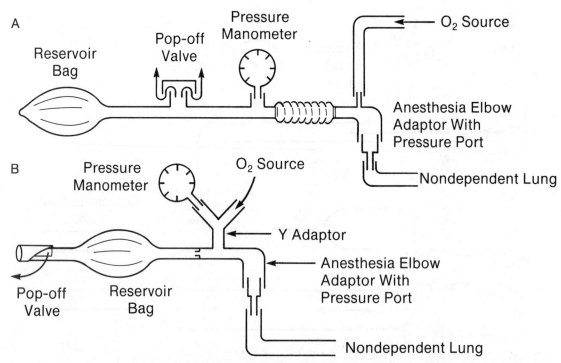

Figure 11–8. This schematic diagram shows two (A and B) nondependent lung continuous positive airway pressure (CPAP) systems with reservoir bags. Both of these systems contain an oxygen source, some type of pressure relief valve, and a pressure manometer to measure the CPAP. The presence of a reservoir bag allows for intermittent positive pressure breathing and sighing, if desired. (A is from reference 22, and B is the system used by the author.)

Nondependent Lung CPAP Systems Without Reservoir Bags

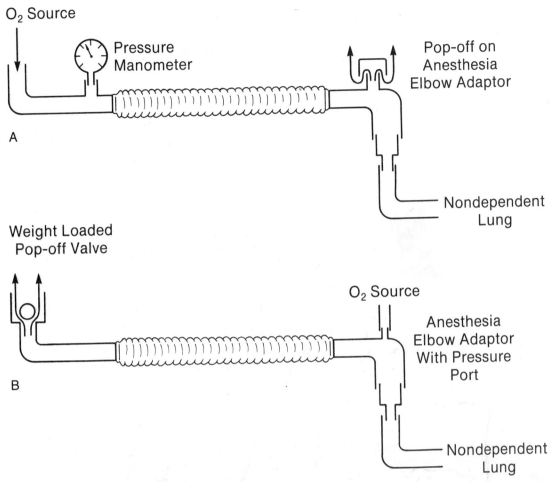

Figure 11–9. *This schematic diagram shows two (A and B) nondependent lung continuous positive airway pressure (CPAP) systems without reservoir bags. Both contain an oxygen source and a pressure relief valve, but the upper panel has a pressure manometer to measure the CPAP, whereas the lower panel does not. (A is from reference 34, and B is from reference 35.)*

mechanism is most distal and the oxygen source most proximal.[35] In most of these systems using these readily available restrictive valves, an oxygen flow rate of 5 to 10 L/min creates a nondependent lung CPAP of 5 to 10 cm H_2O.

The inflow of the fresh gas into a statically distended airway/alveolar air space will wash out some carbon dioxide from the lung. To date, it is not known how much carbon dioxide is removed by causing nondependent lung CPAP with 5 to 10 L/min of oxygen. Obviously, the higher the oxygen flow rate, the greater the washout of carbon dioxide, and as the oxygen flow increases, an approach to continuous high-flow apneic ventilation (see chapter 12), in

which adequate gas exchange can be maintained without any tidal exchange, will be made.

C. Differential Lung PEEP, CPAP

In theory, and from the preceding considerations, it appears that the ideal way to improve oxygenation during one-lung ventilation is to apply differential lung CPAP/PEEP (Fig. 11–10) (see section D for the step-by-step approach). In this situation, the ventilated (dependent) lung is given PEEP in the usual conventional manner in an effort to improve ventilated lung volume and ventilation-perfu-

One Lung Ventilation: Differential Lung CPAP/ PEEP

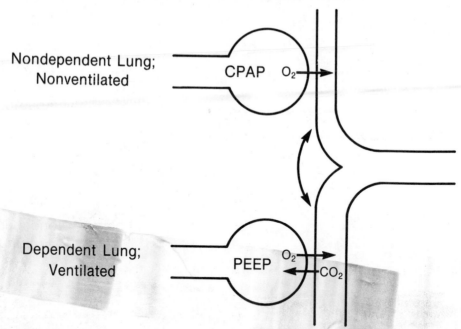

Figure 11–10. *Differential lung continuous positive airway pressure (CPAP)/positive end-expiratory pressure (PEEP) during one-lung ventilation allows for all the lung to participate in oxygen uptake and markedly reduces the shunt during one-lung ventilation. The situation depicted here is a combination of the situations shown in Figures 11–5 and 11–6 (see the legends of those figures for further explanation). With differential lung CPAP/PEEP, the distribution of blood flow is not critically important because all the lung can participate in oxygen uptake.*

sion relationships. Simultaneously, the nonventilated (nondependent) lung receives CPAP in an attempt to improve oxygenation of the blood perfusing this lung. Therefore, with differential lung PEEP or PEEP/CPAP, it does not matter where the blood flow goes nearly as much as during simple one-lung ventilation, since wherever it goes (to either ventilated or nonventilated lung) it has at least some chance to participate in gas exchange with alveoli that are expanded with oxygen. In indirect support of this contention, arterial oxygenation has been increased significantly in patients during thoracotomy in the lateral decubitus position (utilizing two-lung ventilation) when PEEP has been added to the ventilated dependent lung, while the nondependent lung was also able to participate in gas exchange by virtue of being ventilated at zero end-expiratory pressure (ZEEP).[25] In direct support of this contention, in patients undergoing thoracotomy and one-lung ventilation, arterial oxygenation was unchanged by the application of 10 cm H_2O dependent lung PEEP alone (consistent with an equal positive/negative effect trade-off), was sig-

nificantly improved by 10 cm H_2O nondependent lung CPAP alone, and was further and even more significantly increased by use of 10 cm H_2O nondependent lung CPAP and 10 cm H_2O dependent lung PEEP together (differential lung ventilation).[26,27] The use of 10 cm H_2O nondependent lung CPAP together with 10 cm H_2O dependent lung PEEP in patients caused only small, clinically hemodynamic effects.[26,27]

There are now multiple reports of significant increases in oxygenation obtained with the application of differential lung ventilation and positive end-expiratory pressure (either PEEP/PEEP, PEEP/CPAP, or CPAP/CPAP) through double-lumen endotracheal tubes to patients in the intensive care unit with acute respiratory failure due to predominantly unilateral lung disease.[36–49] In all cases conventional two-lung therapy (mechanical ventilation, PEEP, CPAP) was administered via a standard single-lumen tube and either failed to improve or actually decreased oxygenation. In most cases the amount of positive end-expiratory pressure initially administered to each lung was inversely proportional to the compliance of each lung;

ideally, this positive end-expiratory pressure arrangement should result in equal FRC in each lung. In some cases, the amount of positive end-expiratory pressure that each lung received was later readjusted and titrated in an effort to find a differential lung positive end-expiratory pressure combination that resulted in the lowest right-to-left transpulmonary shunt. It has not been necessary to ventilate the two lungs synchronously, and good success has been obtained with asynchronous independent lung ventilation.[48,49] Apparently, the mediastinum does not move enough when the lungs expand at different times to cause significant hemodynamic effects. In addition, the compliance of each lung may be increased by asynchronous independent lung ventilation, since each lung does not have to compete with the other lung for space within the thorax. Special equipment has been developed to facilitate the application of differential lung positive end-expiratory pressure and tidal ventilation.[23,39,45,50] The use of a double-lumen tube adapter that permits selection of, access to, and blockage of each lung independently[50] is particularly helpful in administering differential lung ventilation.

D. Selective Nondependent Lung High-Frequency Ventilation

The studies of selective nondependent lung CPAP indicate that delivery of any amount of oxygen to the nondependent lung alveolar space will cause some oxygen uptake from the nondependent lung and decrease the nondependent lung right-to-left shunt. Consequently, it is not surprising that selective high-frequency ventilation of the nondependent lung (see chapter 12 for extensive discussion of this ventilation modality), while the dependent lung is ventilated with conventional intermittent positive-pressure breathing, increases P_aO_2 compared with simple collapse of the nondependent lung and conventional mechanical ventilation of the dependent lung (Fig. 11–11).[51] However, since the same increase in arterial oxygenation may be obtained by selective nondependent lung CPAP with much simpler equipment compared with high-frequency ventilation apparatus, it is more logical to use selective nondependent lung CPAP than high-frequency ventilation to improve arterial oxygenation during "one-lung ventilation."

Nondependent Lung High Frequency Ventilation

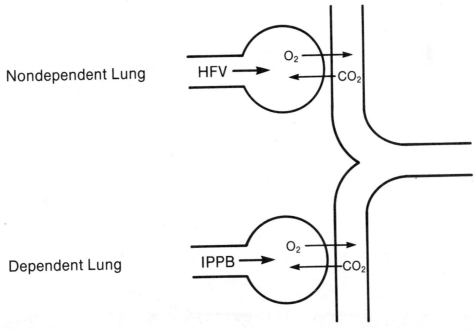

Figure 11–11. *The nondependent lung can be ventilated with high frequency ventilation (HFV) in order to improve arterial oxygenation during ventilation of the dependent lung with intermittent positive pressure breathing (IPPB).*

However, there are two relative indications for the combination of nondependent lung high-frequency ventilation and dependent lung intermittent positive-pressure breathing (see chapter 12).[42] First, if the nondependent lung has a major bronchopleural fistula, high-frequency ventilation may be indicated because it may minimize airway leak. Second, if prolonged surgery has to be performed on a major nondependent lung conducting airway, high-frequency ventilation may be indicated because it may permit a much smaller catheter to pass through the operating field. This ventilatory modality is extensively discussed in chapter 12.

V. RECOMMENDED COMBINED CONVENTIONAL AND DIFFERENTIAL LUNG MANAGEMENT OF ONE-LUNG VENTILATION

Figure 11–12 summarizes the recommended plan for obtaining satisfactory arterial oxygenation during one-lung anesthesia. Two-lung ventilation is maintained for as long as possible (usually until the pleura is opened). When one-lung ventilation is commenced, a tidal volume of 10 ml/kg is used, and the respiratory rate is adjusted so that $P_aCO_2 = 40$ mm Hg. A high inspired oxygen concentration ($F_IO_2 = 0.8$ to 1.0) should be used, and arterial blood gases should be monitored frequently.

If severe hypoxemia is present following this initial conventional approach, then two major causes of hypoxemia, namely malposition of the double-lumen tube and poor hemodynamic status, must be ruled out. If the double-lumen tube is correctly positioned and the hemodynamic status is satisfactory, then simple tidal volume and respiratory rate adjustments should be made.[14] For example, if the tidal ventilation is thought to be too high, it should be decreased, and if the tidal ventilation is thought to be too low, it should be increased. If these simple maneuvers do not quickly resolve the problem, the studies of selective nondependent lung CPAP[23,26,27,30,31,33-35] and differential lung PEEP[36-49] suggest that the next treatment should be to apply 5 to 10 cm H_2O of CPAP to the nondependent lung (Fig. 11–13). Nondependent lung CPAP should be applied during the deflation phase of a large tidal volume breath in order to overcome critical opening pressures in the atelectatic lung. If oxygenation

Overall One Lung Ventilation Plan

1. Maintain Two Lung Ventilation Until Pleura is Opened

2. Dependent Lung
$F_IO_2 = 1.0$
$TV = 8-10$ ml/kg
$RR = $ So That $P_aCO_2 = 40$ mm Hg
$PEEP = 0-5$ mm Hg

3. If Severe Hypoxemia Occurs
(a) Check Position of Double-Lumen Tube With Fiberoptic Bronchoscopy
(b) Check Hemodynamic Status
(c) Nondependent Lung CPAP
(d) Dependent Lung PEEP
(e) Two Lung Ventilation
(f) Clamp Pulmonary Artery ASAP (For Pneumonectomy)

Figure 11–12. The figure shows an overall one-lung ventilation plan. (TV = tidal volume; RR = respiratory rate; PEEP = positive end-expiratory pressure; CPAP = continuous positive airway pressure; ASAP = as soon as possible.)

Nondependent Lung CPAP and Dependent Lung PEEP Search

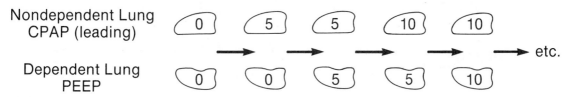

Nondependent Lung
CPAP (leading)

    0   5   5   10   10

→   →   →   →   → etc.

Dependent Lung
PEEP

    0   0   5   5   10

Figure 11–13. A search for optimal nondependent lung continuous positive airway pressure (CPAP) and dependent lung positive end-expiratory pressure (PEEP) is performed by leading with nondependent lung CPAP and following with dependent lung PEEP. Leading with nondependent lung CPAP removes the deleterious arterial oxygenation blood flow diversion effects of dependent lung PEEP.

does not improve with nondependent lung CPAP (which it does in the large majority of cases), 5 to 10 cm H_2O of PEEP to the ventilated dependent lung should then be applied. If dependent lung PEEP does not improve oxygenation, nondependent lung CPAP should be increased to 10 to 15 cm H_2O while the

dependent lung is maintained at 5 to 10 cm H_2O of CPAP. If arterial oxygenation is still not satisfactory, then the nondependent lung CPAP level should be matched with an equal amount of dependent lung PEEP. In this way, a differential lung CPAP/PEEP search for the maximum compliance and a minimum right-to-left

Ligation of Nondependent Lung Pulmonary Artery During One-Lung Ventilation Restores a Matching of Ventilation to Perfusion

**One-Lung Ventilation
With PA Ligation**

**Two-Lung
Ventilation**

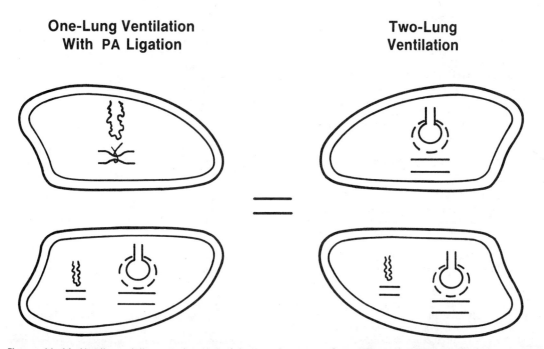

Figure 11–14. Ligation of the nondependent lung pulmonary artery during one-lung ventilation restores a matching of ventilation-perfusion ratios; the nondependent lung is now neither ventilated nor perfused. Consequently, arterial oxygenation during one-lung ventilation with pulmonary artery (PA) ligation is nearly the same as during two-lung ventilation.

transpulmonary shunt is done in an attempt to find the optimal end-expiratory pressure for each lung and the patient as a whole.

If severe hypoxemia is still present following the application of differential lung CPAP/PEEP (which would be extremely rare), it should be remembered that the nondependent lung may be intermittently ventilated with positive pressure with oxygen. Finally, most of the ventilation-perfusion imbalance is eliminated during a pneumonectomy by tightening a ligature around the nonventilated lung pulmonary artery as early as possible, which directly eliminates all shunt flow through the nonventilated lung (Fig. 11–12). Indeed, clamping the pulmonary artery to a collapsed lung functionally resects the entire lung, and the P_aO_2 is restored back to a level not significantly different from a two-lung ventilation or postpneumonectomy one-lung ventilation value (Fig. 11–14).

REFERENCES

1. Tarhan S, Lundborg RO: Carlens endobronchial catheter versus regular endotracheal tube during thoracic surgery: A comparison of blood gas tensions and pulmonary shunting. Can Anaesth Soc J 18:594–599, 1971.
2. Benumof JL: Respiratory physiology and respiratory function during anesthesia. In Miller R (ed): Anesthesia. 2nd ed. New York, Churchill-Livingstone, 1986, chapter 40, pp 1371–1462.
3. Dantzker DR, Wagner PD, West JB: Instability of lung units with low V̇/Q̇ ratios during O_2 breathing. J Appl Physiol 38:886–895, 1975.
4. Ray JF III, Yost L, Moallem S, Sanodos GM, Villamena P, Paredes RM, Clauss RH: Immobility, hypoxemia and pulmonary arteriovenous shunting. Arch Surg 109:537–541, 1974.
5. Benumof JL, Pirlo AF, Trousdale FR: Inhibition of hypoxic pulmonary vasoconstriction by decreased P_vO_2: A new indirect mechanism. J Appl Physiol 51:871–874, 1981.
6. Johansen I, Benumof JL: Flow distribution in abnormal lung as a function of F_iO_2 (abstr). Anesthesiology 51:369, 1979.
7. Lumb TD, Silvay G, Weinreich AI, Shiang W: A comparison of the effects of continuous ketamine infusion and halothane on oxygenation during one-lung anesthesia in dogs. Canad Anaesth Soc J 26:394–401, 1979.
8. Scanlon TS, Benumof JL, Wahrenbrock EA, Nelson WL: Hypoxic pulmonary vasoconstriction and the ratio of hypoxic lung to perfused normoxic lung. Anesthesiology 49:177–181, 1978.
9. Winter PM, Smith G: The toxicity of oxygen. Anesthesiology 37:210–241, 1972.
10. Kerr JH: Physiological aspects of one lung (endobronchial) anesthesia. Int Anesth Clin 10:61–78, 1972.
11. Benumof JL, Rogers SN, Moyce PR, Berryhill RE, Wahrenbrock EA, Saidman LJ: Hypoxic pulmonary vasoconstriction and whole-lung PEEP in the dog. Anesthesiology 51:503–507, 1979.
12. Katz JA, Laverne RG, Fairley HB, Thomas AN: Pulmonary oxygen exchange during endobronchial anesthesia: Effects of tidal volume and PEEP. Anesthesiology 56:164–171, 1982.
13. Finley TN, Hill TR, Bonica JJ: Effect of intrapleural pressure on pulmonary shunt to atelectatic dog lung. Am J Physiol 205:1187–1192, 1963.
14. Flacke JW, Thompson DS, Read RC: Influence of tidal volume and pulmonary artery occlusion on arterial oxygenation during endobronchial anesthesia. South Med J 69:619–626, 1976.
15. Bachand RR, Audet J, Meloche R, et al: Physiological changes associated with unilateral pulmonary ventilation during operations on one lung. Can Anaesth Soc J 22:659–664, 1975.
16. Kerr J, Smith AC, Prys-Roberts C, et al: Observations during endobronchial anaesthesia. I. Ventilation and carbon dioxide clearance. Br J Anaesth 45:159–267, 1973.
17. Hatch D: Ventilation and arterial oxygenation during thoracic surgery. Thorax 21:310–314, 1966.
18. Benumof JL, Wahrenbrock EA: Blunted hypoxic pulmonary vasoconstriction by increased lung vascular pressures. J Appl Physiol 38:846–850, 1975.
19. Benumof JL, Mathers JM, Wahrenbrock EA: Cyclic hypoxic pulmonary vasoconstriction induced by concomitant carbon dioxide changes. J Appl Physiol 41:466–469, 1976.
20. Tarhan S, Lundborg RO: Effects of increased expiratory pressure on blood gas tensions and pulmonary shunting during thoracotomy with use of the Carlens catheter. Can Anaesth Soc J 17:4–11, 1970.
21. Khanam T, Branthwaite MA: Arterial oxygenation during one-lung anesthesia (2). Anaesthesia 23:280–290, 1973.
22. Aalto-Setala M, Heinonen J, Salorinne Y: Cardiorespiratory function during thoracic anesthesia: Comparison of two-lung ventilation and one-lung ventilation with and without PEEP. Acta Anaesthesiol Scand 19:287–295, 1975.
23. Capan LM, Turndorf H, Chandrakant P, Ramanathan S, Acinapura A, Shalon J: Optimization of arterial oxygenation during one-lung anesthesia. Anesth Analg 59:847–851, 1980.
24. Rehder K, Wenthe FM, Sessler AD: Function of each lung during mechanical ventilation with ZEEP and PEEP in man anesthetized with thiopental-meperidine. Anesthesiology 39:597–606, 1973.
25. Brown RD, Kafer RED, Roberson VO, Wilcox BR, Murray GF: Improved oxygenation during thoracotomy with selective PEEP to the dependent lung. Anesth Analg 56:26–31, 1977.
26. Eisenkraft JB, Thys DM, Cohen E, Kaplan JA: Hemodynamic effects of CPAP and PEEP during one-lung anesthesia with isoflurane. Anesthesiology 61:A520, 1984.
27. Cohen E, Thys DM, Eisenkraft JB, Kirschner PA, Kaplan JA: Effect of CPAP and PEEP during one-lung anesthesia: Left versus right thoracotomies. Anesthesiology 63:A564, 1985.
28. Cohen E, Thys DM, Eisenkraft JB, Kaplan JA: PEEP during one-lung anesthesia improves oxygenation in patients with low arterial P_aO_2. Anesth Analg 64:201, 1985.
29. Khanom T, Branthwaite MA: Arterial oxygenation during one-lung anesthesia (1): A study in man. Anaesthesia 28:132–138, 1973.
30. Alfery DD, Benumof JL, Trousdale FR: Improving oxygenation during one-lung ventilation: The effects of

PEEP and blood flow restriction to the nonventilated lung. Anesthesiology 55:381–385, 1981.

31. Merridew CG, Jones RDM: Nondependent lung CPAP (5 cm H₂O) with oxygen during ketamine, halothane, or isoflurane anesthesia and one-lung ventilation. Anesthesiology 63:A567, 1985.

32. Rees DI, Wansbrough SR: One-lung anesthesia: Per cent shunt and arterial oxygen tension during continuous insufflation of oxygen to the nonventilated lung. Anesth Analg 61:507–512, 1982.

33. Thiagarajah S, Job C, Rao A: A device for applying CPAP to the nonventilated upper lung during one lung ventilation. I. Anesthesiology 60:253–254, 1984.

34. Hannenberg AA, Satwicz PR, Pienes RS Jr, O'Brien JC: A device for applying CPAP to the nonventilated upper lung during one lung ventilation. II. Anesthesiology 60:254–255, 1984.

35. Brown DL, Davis RS: A simple device for oxygen insufflation with continuous positive airway pressure during one-lung ventilation. Anesthesiology 61:481–482, 1984.

36. Carlon GC, Kahn R, Howland WS, Baron R, Ramaker J: Acute life-threatening ventilation-perfusion inequality: An indication for independent lung ventilation. Crit Care Med 6:380–383, 1978.

37. Venus B, Pratap KS, Op'Tholt T: Treatment of unilateral pulmonary insufficiency by selective administration of continuous positive airway pressure through a double-lumen tube. Anesthesiology 52:74–77, 1980.

38. Powner DJ, Eross B, Grenvik A: Differential lung ventilation with PEEP in the treatment of unilateral lung ventilation. Crit Care Med 5:170–172, 1977.

39. Gallagher TJ, Banner MJ, Smith RA: A simplified method of independent lung ventilation. Crit Care Med 8:396–398, 1980.

40. Glass DD, Tonnesen AD, Gabel JC, Arens JF: Therapy of unilateral pulmonary insufficiency with a double-lumen endotracheal tube. Crit Care Med 4:323–326, 1976.

41. Trew F, Warren BR, Potter WA: Differential lung ventilation in man. Crit Care Med 4:112, 1976.

42. Benjaminsson E, Klain N: Intraoperative dual-mode independent lung ventilation of a patient with bronchopleural fistula. Anesth Analg (Cleve) 60:118–119, 1981.

43. Rafferty TD, Palma J, Motoyama EK, Schachter N, Ciarcia F: Management of a bronchopleural fistula with differential lung ventilation and positive end-expiratory pressure. Respir Care 25:654–657, 1980.

44. Rivara D, Bourgaim L, Rieuf P, Harf A, Lemaire F: Differential ventilation in unilateral lung disease: Effects of respiratory mechanics and gas exchange. Intensive Care Med 5:189–191, 1979.

45. Ray C, Carlon GC, Miodownik S, Glodiner PL: A method of synchronizing two MA-1 ventilators for independent lung ventilation. Crit Care Med 6:99, 1978.

46. Parish JM, Gracey DR, Southorn PA, Pairolero PA, Wheeler JT: Differential mechanical ventilation in respiratory failure due to severe unilateral lung disease. Mayo Clin Proc 59:822, 1984.

47. Murray JF: Treatment of acute total atelectasis: Use of a double-lumen tube. Anaesthesia 40:158–162, 1985.

48. Stow PJ, Grant I: Asynchronous independent lung ventilation: Its use in the treatment of acute unilateral lung disease. Anaesthesia 40:163–166, 1985.

49. Hillman KM, Barber JD: Asynchronous independent lung ventilation (AILV). Crit Care Med 8:390–395, 1980.

50. Andersen HW, Benumof JL, Ozaki GT: New improved double-lumen tube adaptor. Anesthesiology 56:54–56, 1982.

51. Wilks D, Schumann T, Riley R, Klain M, Freeman J: Selective high-frequency jet ventilation of the operative lung improves oxygenation during thoracic surgery. Anesthesiology 63:A568, 1985.

High-Frequency and High-Flow Apneic Ventilation During Thoracic Surgery

12

I. INTRODUCTION

Conventional positive-pressure breathing can interfere with the performance of thoracic surgery in four ways (Fig. 12–1A). First, conventional positive-pressure breathing requires large endotracheal tubes (either single- or double-lumen tubes) that can greatly interfere with the performance of surgery on major conducting airways. Second, the expansion and movement of the nondependent lung by intermittent positive-pressure breathing may greatly interfere with access to the surgical field. Third, movement of the dependent lung due to intermittent positive-pressure breathing will cause the mediastinum, and therefore the floor of the surgical field, to move up and down, which may hamper the performance of surgery. Fourth, the airway pressure in the ventilated dependent lung, if too high, can compress the small intra-alveolar vessels in the dependent lung, increase dependent lung pulmonary vascular resistance, and shunt blood flow to the nonventilated nondependent lung.

In theory, high-frequency and high-flow apneic ventilation do not have these disadvantages

(Fig. 12–1B). Both these forms of ventilation require only small bore catheters (tidal volumes are very small and/or flow rates are very high) and thereby can potentially facilitate the performance of surgery on major conducting airways. Second, the tidal movements with high-frequency and high-flow apneic ventilation are very small or nonexistent, respectively, thereby minimizing movements of both the nondependent and dependent lungs. In addition, both of these forms of ventilation utilize low airway pressures so that it is possible to obtain adequate gas exchange whenever airway resistance is extremely low (as it might be in surgery on a major conducting airway or with a large bronchopleural fistula) without a large air leak. Finally, the lower airway pressure associated with both these forms of ventilation[1] and release of vasodilator prostaglandins with high-frequency ventilation[2] can, in theory, lower dependent lung vascular resistance and improve diversion of blood flow away from an atelectatic nondependent lung. This chapter reviews clinical experience with high-frequency and high-flow apneic ventilation during intrathoracic surgery. The use of high-frequency ventilation for extra-

---

Figure 12–1. (See illustration on opposite page.) A, *Ways in which conventional intermittent positive pressure breathing (IPPB) can potentially interfere with the performance of thoracic surgery. The large endotracheal tubes (either single- or double-lumen) required by conventional IPPB may interfere with the anastomosis of the airway. The relatively large IPPB tidal movements of the nondependent lung may decrease surgical exposure (with inspiration) and cause a large amount of operative field movement. The relatively large IPPB tidal movements of the dependent lung may cause a large amount of mediastinal movement and, therefore, operative field movement. B, The proposed ways high-frequency (HFV) and high-flow apneic ventilation can potentially facilitate the performance of thoracic surgery. The small catheter associated with the use of high-frequency ventilation facilitates the anastomosis of the airway. In addition, HFV of the nondependent lung increases surgical exposure and minimizes movement of the operative field. HFV of the dependent lung decreases mediastinal and operative field movement. The low airway pressures associated with HFV may decrease the air leak out of a bronchopleural fistula.*

Conventional IPPB Can Potentially Interfere with the Performance of Thoracic Surgery

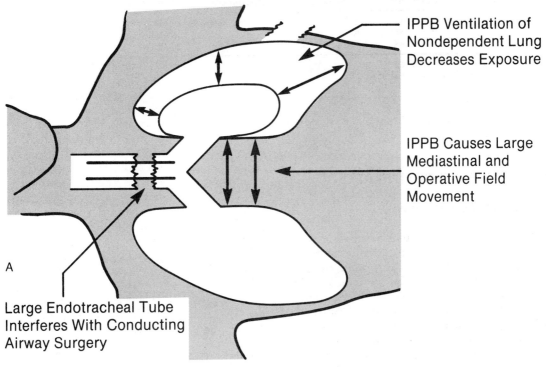

IPPB Ventilation of Nondependent Lung Decreases Exposure

IPPB Causes Large Mediastinal and Operative Field Movement

Large Endotracheal Tube Interferes With Conducting Airway Surgery

Proposed Benefits of High Frequency and High Flow Apneic Ventilation to Facilitate the Performance of Thoracic Surgery

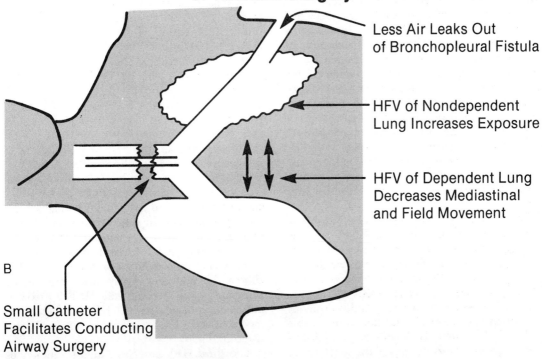

Less Air Leaks Out of Bronchopleural Fistula

HFV of Nondependent Lung Increases Exposure

HFV of Dependent Lung Decreases Mediastinal and Field Movement

Small Catheter Facilitates Conducting Airway Surgery

Figure 12–1 See legend on opposite page

Table 12–1. Characteristics of the Three Types of High-Frequency Ventilation

Type of HFV	Rate/Min	Type of Ventilator	Gas Entrainment	Process	
				Inspiration	Exhalation
HFPPV	60 to 100	Volume	No	Active*	Passive†
HFJV	100 to 400	Jet pulsation	Yes	Active	Passive
HFOV	400 to 2400	Piston pump	Yes	Active	Active

*Active—caused by the ventilator.
†Passive—caused by elastic recoil of lung.

thoracic procedures (i.e., bronchoscopy) is considered in chapter 14.

II. HIGH-FREQUENCY VENTILATION

A. General Considerations

Conventional intermittent positive-pressure ventilation (IPPV) delivers relatively large tidal volumes (10 to 15 ml/kg) at respiratory rates usually less than 30 breaths per minute. With IPPV the basic mechanism of gas transport is by mass movement to the smaller airways and then more distally by mass movement and molecular diffusion.[3] In contrast to IPPV, high-frequency ventilation (HFV) delivers very small tidal volumes (< 2 ml/kg) at rates between 60 and 2400 breaths per minute. Under these circumstances, the proportion of the tidal volume ventilating the deadspace increases so that normal alveolar ventilation can be maintained only by the use of high respiratory rates and minute volumes. With HFV, gas transport by mass movement is still important[4] but may be combined with varying degrees of other mechanisms of gas transport such as enhanced molecular diffusion,[5] high-velocity gas flow,[6] coaxial gas flow (bidirectional flow with gases in the center of the airway moving distally [O_2] and gases on the edge of the airway moving proximally [CO_2],[7] asynchronous regional filling and emptying of alveoli ("pendelluft" movement, resulting in smaller gas volumes effectively reaching more respiratory units),[8] and gas trapping.[9]

High-frequency ventilation is an umbrella term encompassing different delivery systems and respiratory rate ranges. Current methods used to provide high-frequency ventilation are quite diverse, but by using the criteria of ventilation rate and type of gas delivery mechanism, it is possible to separate high-frequency ventilation into three general categories (Table 12–1).[4, 10] The first HFV category, high-frequency positive-pressure ventilation (HFPPV),

employs a volume-controlled ventilator with a low internal compressible volume, which delivers small tidal volumes at rates of 60 to 100 breaths per minute (1 to 1.7 Hz). The negligible internal compliance of the ventilator guarantees that the preset tidal volume (usually approximately equal to the anatomic dead space volume [2 ml/kg]) is the tidal volume that is actually delivered to the patient. The low-compression delivery system enhances gas exchange in the conducting airways by causing a high instaneous gas flow.[6] There is no gas entrainment so that the delivered tidal volume is all fresh gas and the F_IO_2 is the same as the F_IO_2 of the compressed gas. If a standard endotracheal tube is used for HFPPV, PEEP may be added to maximize P_aO_2.[8, 11]

The second HFV category, high-frequency jet ventilation (HFJV), employs pulsation of a small jet of fresh gas introduced from a high pressure source (50 to 60 psi) into the airway via a small catheter (which can be passed alone or through an endotracheal tube) or via an extra lumen in an endotracheal tube at rates usually between 100 and 400 breaths per minute (1.7 to 6.7 Hz). The small catheter tip must be located near the carina (HFJV through catheters located either more distally or proximally do not result in normal CO_2 removal). The jetted fresh gas leaves the narrow injection cannulae at a very high velocity. As it exits from the injection cannulae, the high velocity of the jet flow entrains gas from the endotracheal tube's fresh gas flow or from an injection cannulae sideport gas reservoir (Bernoulli effect).[12] The amount of entrained gas is uncertain and therefore quantification of tidal volume and F_IO_2 is difficult. The jetted and entrained gases (20 to 40 L/min) impact into the much larger volume of relatively immobile gas in the endotracheal tube and conducting airways and cause the gas to move forward.[10, 12] As with HFPPV, oxygenation is enhanced with HFJV when small amounts of PEEP are added (via the endotracheal tube).

The third HFV category, high-frequency oscillation ventilation (HFOV), employs a piston pump or loudspeaker that oscillates gas in the airway back and fourth in a sinusoidal fashion at rates of 400 to 2400 breaths per minute (6.7 to 40 Hz). A fresh gas flow-by (which is entrained) is located between the oscillator and the patient.[13] Delivered tidal volume is very small (50 to 80 ml), and alveolar gas exchange is obtained by enhanced molecular diffusion and coaxial flow.[4, 10, 13]

One other type of HFV system, the flow interrupter, has features of the HFPPV, HFJV, and HFOV categories. Breaths are generated by using a mechanical valve to interrupt very frequently a continuous flow of gas into a low-compression delivery system. Thus, small tidal volumes (HFPPV) with high flow rates (HFJV) at very rapid rates (HFOV) are produced. The interrupters are capable of producing the entire range of HFV respiratory rates, but rates of 100 to 600 per minute have been found to be most effective.[3]

In the last decade, all three types of HFV have been shown to be capable of providing adequate alveolar ventilation and oxygenation in both normal animals and humans and in those with pulmonary disease. In anesthetized animals and in human infants and adults with normal lungs undergoing surgical procedures, arterial blood gases demonstrate adequate alveolar ventilation with high-frequency ventilation.[11, 14–18] Studies performed in animals and humans in acute respiratory failure have also shown that HFV can provide adequate gas exchange.[19–21] In some reports of ventilation during acute respiratory failure, HFV was even more effective than IPPV.[21, 22]

B. Use in Major Conducting Airway Surgery

The most important thoracic surgery advantage of HFV is that the small rapid tidal volumes may be delivered through small airway tubes; thus if a major conducting airway (trachea, carinal area, mainstem bronchus) has to be divided, the transit of a small airway tube through the surgical field causes much less interference with surgery than the pasage of a large standard or double-lumen endotracheal tube. The small airway catheters present the surgeon with an unobstructed, accessible circumference of trachea and bronchus, so that the ends of a divided airway can be properly aligned for the construction of an unstressed and airtight anastomosis. Both HFPPV and

HFJV have been successfully used with small airway catheters for three different types of airway surgery (Fig. 12–2).[23–28]

The first type of airway surgery that has been aided by HFV is carinal resection (in whole or in part) (Fig. 12–2C). During sleeve pneumonectomy (which includes part of carina) a small airway catheter passing through the operative field into the mainstem bronchus of the dependent lung ventilated the dependent lung with either HFJV or, more recently and effectively, with HFPPV.[26] In the author's hands,[26] HFV also minimized bronchial and mediastinal movements, and with HFPPV the continuous outflow of gases through the open bronchus minimized soiling of the ventilated lung with blood from the lung under operation, whereas HFJV created a suction effect (entrainment) that drew blood and debris into the open carinal area down into the bronchous of the lung being ventilated.[26] Additionally, when a left sleeve pneumonectomy was being performed the small catheter inside the right mainstem bronchus eliminated the problem of the right upper lobe collapse associated with the use of right endobronchial tubes. The HFPPV technique described above for sleeve pneumonectomy has also been successfully used for carinal resections with pericardial patch and very low (distal) tracheal resections.[26] In contradistinction to the these findings with HFPPV, HFOV delivered through a standard single-lumen tube has been found to cause changes in the diameter of large airways and to produce a large "mediastinal bounce" with each oscillation that "made surgery on the major airways and around the hilum and mediastinal structures almost impossible."[29]

At the present time, continued investigation in the use of HFV to facilitate carinal surgery still seems warranted, since older previous techniques for providing ventilation for major conducting airway surgery leave a great deal to be desired. Previous techniques used with sleeve pneumonectomy after incision of the airway have included use of a conventional double-lumen endotracheal tube, advancing a single-lumen endotracheal tube through the end of the opened trachea into the appropriate mainstem broncus, or using a separate sterile endobronchial tube through the operative field with a second sterile anesthesia circuit (see chapter 15). Since repeated endobronchial intubation and extubation are necessary during construction of the posterior portion of the anastomosis, the technique is cumbersome and requires alternating periods of apnea and ventilation, which may result in poor gas exchange.[30–33]

Three Types of Airway Surgery Aided by Small HFV Catheter

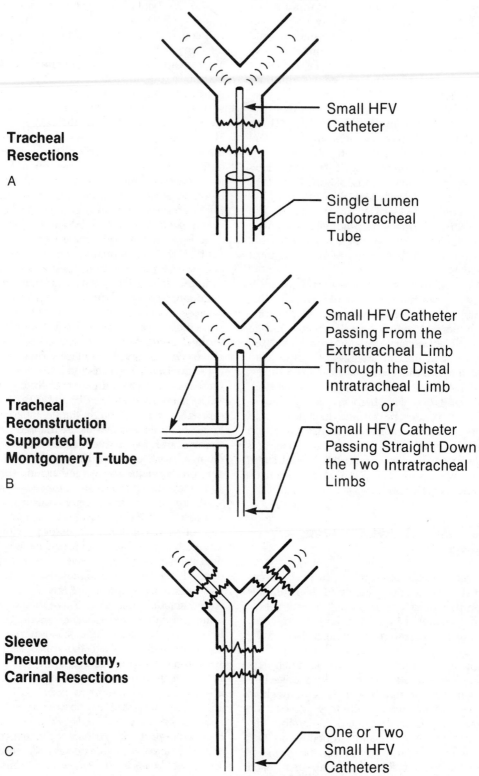

Tracheal Resections

A

Small HFV Catheter

Single Lumen Endotracheal Tube

Tracheal Reconstruction Supported by Montgomery T-tube

B

Small HFV Catheter Passing From the Extratracheal Limb Through the Distal Intratracheal Limb

or

Small HFV Catheter Passing Straight Down the Two Intratracheal Limbs

Sleeve Pneumonectomy, Carinal Resections

C

One or Two Small HFV Catheters

Figure 12–2 See legend on opposite page

The second type of airway surgery aided by HFV is tracheal reconstruction supported by tracheal Montgomery T-tube (Fig. 12–2B). The Montgomery T-tube has two intratracheal limbs (the proximal limb faces the glottis, and the distal limb faces the tracheal carina) and one extratracheal limb, which exits from the tracheal and neck incision to the environment. In one approach, the HFPPV catheter passes straight down through the two intratracheal limbs and gas outflow was via the extratracheal limb.[27] Alternatively, the HFPPV catheter can be introduced through the extratracheal limb and gently flexed downward to direct the catheter to lie above the carina.

Previously, it was difficult to establish an adequate airway for the administration of conventional IPPV with conventional cuffed tracheostomy tubes using the tracheal Montgomery T-tubes.[34, 35] The use of the extratracheal limb as an airway for the delivery of large tidal volume IPPV was associated with a large gas leak through the open proximal intratracheal limb. In order to establish adequate ventilation with conventional IPPV, the superior part of the proximal intratracheal limb had to be occluded by a Fogarty embolectomy catheter (introduced through the extratracheal limb) and by a tight pharyngeal pack (introduced through the oral cavity); this prevented escape of the tidal volume through the open glottis. IPPV has also been administered to a pediatric patient through the proximal intratracheal limb of the tracheal T-tube; the proximal intratracheal limb was intubated with a Cole tube and then the extratracheal limb was occluded to allow for the use of IPPV.[36] These previous conventional IPPV maneuvers and techniques are cumbersome, difficult to apply, and can be dangerous. Blockage of the various T-tube limbs can, for example, occur suddenly and totally obstruct the airway and prevent alveolar ventilation. In addition, use of these IPPV techniques can impair surgical access and complicate the surgery.

The third type of airway aided by HFV is resection of a tracheal stenosis (Fig. 12–2A). In one report a small HFPPV insufflating catheter was inserted through a single-lumen endotracheal tube, which lay above the tracheal stenosis, until the distal end of the HFPPV catheter was beyond the tracheal stenosis.[28] Thus, tracheal resection and end-to-end anastomosis could be accomplished easily around the small catheter. This method has the obvious drawback that the relation between the tracheal stenosis and insufflation catheter must permit a sufficiently large passage for exhalation; the passage must be guaranteed at every moment of the surgical procedure.[28]

C. Use in Bronchopleural Fistula

The second proposed advantage HFV has for thoracic surgery is that the lower inspiratory pressures and tidal volumes may result in a smaller gas leak through pathologic low resistance pathways such as bronchopleural fistulae and tracheobronchial disruptions (Fig. 12–3A). Consequently, air leaks (loss of tidal volume) and mediastinal and interstitial emphysema may be minimized with this form of ventilatory treatment, and HFJV has been successfully used in the treatment of major bronchopleural fistula[37–42] and tracheobronchial disruptions.[23, 43, 44] In most cases of bronchopleural fistula, P_aCO_2 was unacceptably high despite a high minute ventilation on volume-controlled IPPV, whereas HFJV restored normocarbia. However, it appears that the reduction in air leak flow through the fistula is directly related to reduced airway pressure with HFV compared with conventional mechanical ventilation; when peak and mean tracheal pressures are decreased by HFV, fistula leak is decreased, and when peak and mean tracheal pressures are increased by HFV, fistula flow increases.[40–42] Thus, in a series of seven consecutive patients with an average bronchopleural fistual leak of greater than 5 L/min, HFJV (125 to 150/min) caused only two patients to have clinically important

Figure 12–2. The three types of airway surgery aided by small high-frequency ventilation (HFV) catheters are tracheal resections, tracheal reconstructions that require support by a Montgomery T-tube, and carinal procedures (sleeve pneumonectomy, carinal resections). With tracheal resections (A), a simple HFV catheter can be passed beyond the point of airway interruption, but above the tracheal carina, and used to ventilate both lungs with HFV. With tracheal reconstructions supported by a Montgomery T-tube (B), the small HFV catheter can be passed from either the extraluminal limb or from the proximal intraluminal tracheal limb to the distal intraluminal tracheal limb and can be used to ventilate both lungs with HFV. With carinal procedures (C), one or two HFV catheters can be passed into one or both of the mainstem bronchi and can be used to ventilate one or both of the lungs with HFV.

Use of HFV to Treat Bronchopleural Fistula

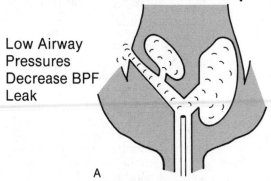

Low Airway
Pressures
Decrease BPF
Leak

A

Alternative Methods to Treat Bronchopleural Fistula

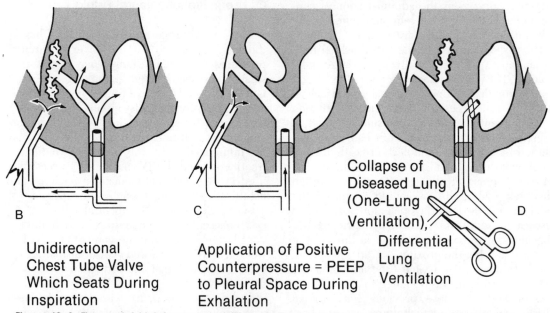

B

Unidirectional
Chest Tube Valve
Which Seats During
Inspiration

C

Application of Positive
Counterpressure = PEEP
to Pleural Space During
Exhalation

D

Collapse of
Diseased Lung
(One-Lung
Ventilation),
Differential
Lung
Ventilation

Figure 12–3. The use of high-frequency ventilation (HFV) to treat bronchopleural fistula (A) is based on the supposition that HFV results in lower airway pressures, and the lower airway pressures decrease the bronchopleural fistula (BPF) air leak. The alternative methods of treating bronchopleural fistula consist of placing unidirectional valves (which seat during inspiration) in the chest tube (helps lock in inspiratory tidal volume) (B), application of positive counterpressure to the pleural space during exhalation (helps lock in positive end-expiratory pressure) (C), and collapse of the diseased lung (one-lung ventilation) for a period of time (D). However, chest tube valves often do not work, owing to the presence of blood or pus, positive counterpressure to the pleural space may have major negative hemodynamic implications, and collapse of the diseased lung for an extended period of time is technically difficult from the point of view of maintaining proper double-lumen tube position and predisposes the collapsed lung to infection.

decreases in airway pressure and air leak fistula flow, and none had significant improvement in gas exchange.[40] The authors recommend measurement of tracheal pressures to predict what is happening to air leak fistula flow.[40] In one case of bronchopleurocutaneous fistula,[37] intraoperative differential lung ventilation, consisting of conventional IPPV for the normal dependent lung and HFJV for the diseased

nondependent lung, was used. HFV has been used prophylactically to prevent the development of a bronchopleural fistula in a patient who had a very friable bronchial stump due to mucormycosis (an opportunistic pulmonary parenchymal infection that occurs in immunocompromised hosts and diabetics and is associated with a high incidence of postoperative bronchopleural fistula).[45] HFPPV and HFOV have been successfully used in dogs with bilateral upper lobe bronchopleural fistulas,[46] but these two types of HFV have not been used in humans with a bronchopleural fistula. In cases of tracheobronchial disruptions, mediastinal and interstitial emphysema was felt to be minimized by the use of HFV.[23, 43, 44]

The previous methods of trying to make conventional IPPV more effective in the presence of pathologic low resistance airway pathways (in addition to using a very large tidal volume) all have major drawbacks (Fig. 12–3B to D). Insertion of unidirectional valves in chest tubes, which seat during inspiration, frequently malfunction due to interference by blood and pus within the chest tube.[47] Application of positive counterpressure to the pleural space during inspiration causes hemodynamic interference.[47] Collapse of the diseased lung with the aid of a double-lumen tube for a prolonged period of time requires very careful monitoring, is technically difficult for the intensive care unit personnel not trained in anesthesia, and predisposes the collapsed lung to infection.[48] Thus, it is likely that investigations in the use of high-frequency ventilation to treat patients with pathologic low resistance airway pathways will continue.

D. Use in Minimizing Movement of the Operative Field

The third proposed advantage for HFV in thoracic surgery is to minimize the tidal movement of the operative field; theoretically, the lower peak inspiratory pressures and tidal volumes of HFV should result in much smaller inflation and deflation movements of the lung. Therefore, HFV of the nondependent lung might provide a relatively "quiet" operative lung field and HFV of the dependent lung could contribute to the "quiet" operative lung field by providing a minimally moving mediastinum (Fig. 12–1). In four reports[49–52] HFPPV was used to ventilate both the nondependent and the dependent lung during thoracic surgery. With the chest open, the nondependent lung had minimal ventilation-synchronous movements and limited lung expansion but still had good aeration and no atelectasis. However, hyperinflation of the lungs occurred in some patients with chronic obstructive pulonary disease, presumably owing to air trapping, and resulted in poor operating conditions.[52] In patients who did not experience hyperinflation, operating conditions for peripheral lung procedures was adequate. Arterial blood gases, analyzed frequently in most reports, showed adequate oxygenation and carbon dioxide removal during HFV despite some brief periods of significant nondependent lung compression by the surgeons. In one report, HFJV was successfully used at 3 Hz to ventilate both lungs, but carbon dioxide retention became a problem at 6 and 12 Hz.[53] During HFPPV the airways could be suctioned without interrupting ventilation. At the conclusion of surgery the nondependent lung fully re-expanded as readily as with conventional techniques. Finally, in one report the dependent lung was selectively ventilated with an HFV flow interrupter (while the operated lung was completely collapsed).[54] Compared with selective dependent lung IPPV, selective dependent lung HFV significantly improved arterial oxygenation, presumably because of lower dependent lung pulmonary vascular resistance (due to either lower dependent lung airway pressures[1] or release of dependent lung vasodilator prostaglandins[2]) and enhanced operating conditions (owing to minimal mediastinal movements). In addition, deflation of the dependent lung endobronchial tube cuff further improved arterial oxygenation owing to overflow of gases from the dependent lung to the nondependent lung, which resulted in recruitment of part of the collapsed lung in gas exchange.

Unfortunately, in none of these reports was the use of HFV compared with conventional one-lung ventilation, with or without nondependent lung CPAP, in terms of operating conditions and efficiency of gas exchange. Since operating conditions and gas exchange are usually excellent with one-lung ventilation and nondependent lung CPAP, it is unlikely that comparative studies will show much improvement with HFV. In addition, the use of HFV to minimize mediastinal and hilar movements must remain controversial in view of the most recent report describing a mediastinal "bounce" with each oscillation, which made surgery around these structures nearly impossible.[52]

In summary, the favorable aspects about HFV for thoracic surgery are adequate pulmonary gas exchange (and, perhaps, increased diversion of blood flow away from the atelectatic lung during ventilation of just the dependent lung),[1] good conditions for peripheral lung surgery, possibly good conditions for major airway conducting surgery, possibly improved gas exchange in cases of bronchopleural fistula, and possibly decreased mediastinal and pulmonary interstitial emphysema in cases of tracheobronchial disruption. As previously mentioned, the first two of these favorable aspects, in the context of the availability of one-lung ventilation, seem superfluous and unnecessary. The unfavorable aspects of high-frequency ventilation for thoracic surgery are possibly unsatisfactory surgical conditions for mediastinal and major airway surgery, hyperinflation in patients with chronic obstructive pulmonary disease, difficulty in monitoring heart and breath sounds with an esophageal stethoscope, inability to judge the adequacy of ventilation from the motion of the chest wall or lungs, use of high flows of anesthetic gases, and difficulty in assessing lung volume. Hence, at the present time, the exact role of HFV in thoracic surgery is uncertain. I am certain, however, that the use of HFV as a routine procedure in thoracic surgery cannot be recommended at the present time.

III. LOW- AND HIGH-FLOW APNEIC VENTILATION

A. Low-Flow Apneic Ventilation

The need for an absolutely quiet surgical field for short periods of time often arises during a thoracotomy in which a standard endotracheal tube and two-lung ventilation is employed. This can be accomplished relatively safely using the principle of apneic mass-movement oxygenation. If ventilation is stopped during the administration of 100 per cent oxygen and the airway is left connected to a fresh gas supply, oxygen will be drawn into the lung by mass-movement to replace the oxygen that crossed the alveolar-capillary membrane (Fig. 12–4A). There is usually no difficulty in maintaining an adequate arterial P_aO_2 (especially if 5 to 10 cm H_2O CPAP is used) during at least 20 minutes of apneic mass-movement oxygenation.

If the flow of oxygen into the lungs is relatively low (less than 0.2 L/kg/min) almost all of the carbon dioxide produced is retained, and the arterial carbon dioxide tension (P_aCO_2) rises approximately 6 mm Hg in the first minute owing to the washin of venous blood into the arterial compartment (venous blood has a carbon dioxide tension 6 mm Hg higher than that of arterial blood) and then 3 to 4 mm Hg each minute thereafter[55, 56] owing to normal CO_2 production (Fig. 12–4A). Based on these considerations, if a patient had a normal CO_2 production, was hyperventilated to a P_aCO_2 of

30 mm Hg, and was then made apneic and oxygen was insufflated into the lungs with a low flow, the P_aCO_2 after 10 minutes of apnea would be 63 to 72 mm Hg. Indeed, one report describes a series of eight patients in whom apneic mass-movement oxygenation was employed for a period of 18 to 55 minutes after normal ventilation.[55] Although the lowest arterial saturation that resulted was 98 per cent, the arterial P_aCO_2 in the five patients in whom it was measured ranged from 103 to 250 mm Hg, and the pH ranged from 6.72 to 6.97. Although severe degrees of hypercapnia and respiratory acidosis may be well tolerated in some healthy patients, it would appear that the safe period of low flow apneic oxygenation during thoracotomy would lie well under 10 minutes.

B. Interrupted High-Flow Apneic Ventilation

If the fresh gas flow into the lungs is very high, it is possible to wash out the carbon dioxide from the alveolar space (Fig. 12–4B). The higher the flow rate, the greater the effective minute ventilation and carbon dioxide removal. At the same time, if the fresh gas were oxygen, whatever oxygen was taken up by the pulmonary perfusion would be replaced, and arterial oxygenation would not be a problem. These high flow apneic ventilation concepts have been tested clinically in humans and experimentally in animals.

1. Low-Frequency Interrupted High Flow

Interrupted high-flow apneic ventilation is essentially equivalent to very short inspiratory time positive-pressure breathing that results from short bursts of extremely high flows of gas through a small ventilating catheter positioned in a mainstem bronchus (Fig. 12–5).[57] The high-pressure (50 psi) gas source is oxygen (available from portable tanks or central supply wall outlets) and is capable of delivering a flow of 100 L/min. Since the flows are so great, the short bursts of oxygen do not cause entrainment of room air. Depending on airway resistance and lung compliance, the inflation is adjusted (to as low as 30 to 40 L/min) through a reducing valve, so that the airway pressure is 25 to 40 cm H_2O. By means of an on/off release button, inflation rates are maintained at 10 to 15 respirations/min, and the adequacy of ventilation is estimated by direct observation of thoracic cage

Low Flow (<0.2 L/kg/min) Apneic Ventilation

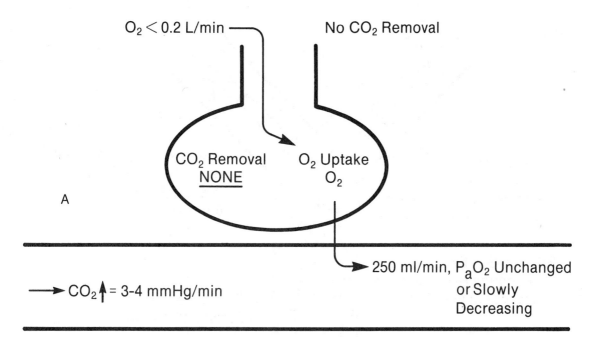

High Flow (1 L/kg/min) Apneic Ventilation

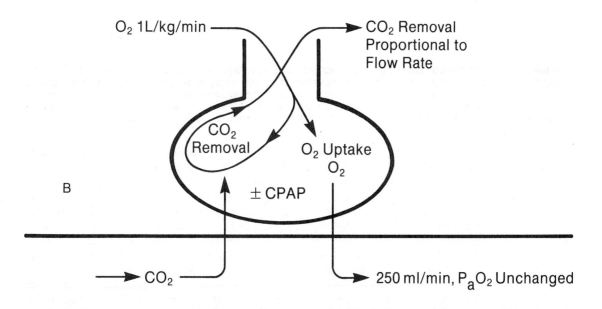

Figure 12–4. Low flow (< 0.2 L/kg/min) apneic ventilation (A) *can provide adequate arterial oxygenation for a period of time but does not remove any carbon dioxide so that hypercapnia is a necessary consequence of this method of ventilation. On the other hand, high flow (1 L/kg/min) apneic ventilation* (B) *maintains arterial oxygenation while at the same time it is able to remove carbon dioxide at a rate that is proportional to the oxygen flow rate. High flow apneic ventilation may be facilitated by use of constant positive airway pressure (CPAP).*

Low Frequency Interrupted High Flow Ventilation

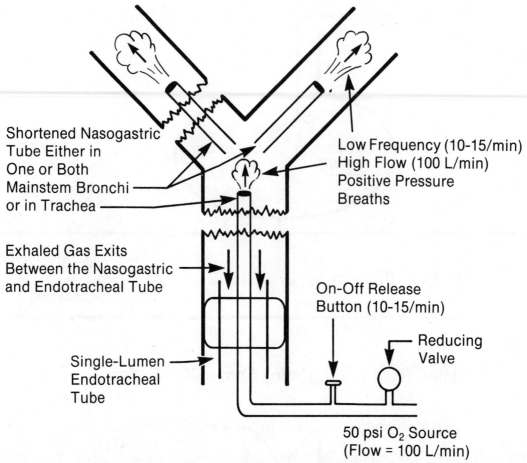

Figure 12–5. *Interruption and release of a very high fresh gas flow (100 L/min) at a low frequency (10 breaths/min) is essentially equivalent to intermittent positive pressure breathing with a very short inspiratory time. A small catheter (nasogastric tube) can be passed through an indwelling single-lumen tube in the trachea and beyond any airway interruption into one or both of the mainstem bronchi and used to ventilate one or both of the lungs. The escape of gas on exhalation is around the small catheter but inside the indwelling single-lumen tube.*

expansion, mediastinal excursion, and arterial blood gas monitoring.

A shortened nasogastric tube, which has been passed down through the lumen of a single-lumen tube into a mainstem bronchus (and, perhaps, through a divided major conducting airway as well), has been used as the ventilation catheter.[57] The appropriate length of the nasogastric tube is 75 to 40 cm, and the nasogastric tube is sized according to the patient's weight. Usually, a steel wire has to be threaded through the lumen of the nasogastric tube to provide some rigidity.

a. USE IN MAJOR CONDUCTING AIRWAY SURGERY

The value of the interrupted high-flow apneic ventilation technique was tested in 18 patients undergoing tracheobronchial reconstruction.[57] The average duration of catheter ventilation was 35 minutes. Seven patients had a tracheal resection (six cervical, one thoracic), nine had a sleeve pneumonectomy, and two additional patients had a carinal resection. The period of catheter ventilation usually began after the airways were divided. The catheter was advanced through either a single-lumen or double-lumen endotracheal tube into the distal airway, and the entire anastomosis was done around the small nasogastric inflation catheter. Throughout the period of interrupted high-flow apneic ventilation, the patients were kept fully paralyzed and anesthesia maintained by intravenous narcotics. At completion of the anastomosis, the catheter was withdrawn, and ventilation was resumed through the existing conventional endotracheal tube. For patients undergoing carinal resection the ventilation was provided by both lungs by using a separate nasogastric catheter for each bronchus. Both catheters were introduced through the endotracheal tube, so that the need for intubation across the operating field was avoided. Pulmonary interstitial and mediastinal emphysema developed during the period of high-flow ventilation in one patient. Although the authors had no clear explanation for this complication, it was possible that the pressure was too high in the airway or that the catheter made a tear in the bronchial mucosa.

The inflation nasogastric catheter technique appears to have specific advantages in regard to simplicity of the equipment and anesthetic technique. At all times, the anesthesiologist has complete control of the airway while oxygenation is maintained by intermittent inflation of the lungs through a small semirigid endotracheal catheter (2 to 6 mm in diameter). The high flow of oxygen does not entrain air, and the inspired fraction of oxygen is predictable. Ventilation rates are maintained at 10 to 15 respirations/min and the inflation pressure (15 to 40 cm H_2O) is regulated by the direct observation of thoracic cage expansion and mediastinal excursion and by arterial blood gas values. The measurment of high arterial oxygen tension in most patients indicates that a lesser concentration of inspired oxygen could be used safely.

Surgical exposure to the trachea is improved by the interrupted high-flow ventilation because there is no intrusion of anesthetic apparatus into the operating field, no endotracheal manipulations need to be done, and reconstruction can be done without interruption around the small inflating nasogastric catheter. This study shows that the high-flow inflation catheter technique fulfills the requirements for safe surgical and anesthetic management during tracheobronchial operations. It appears to be most useful during operations on the intrathoracic trachea and should be considered a valuable alternative to more conventional methods.

2. Continuous High-Flow Apneic Ventilation

Adequate gas exchange has been accomplished in dogs without tidal exchange of gases (apnea) if the airspace is exposed to a very high continuous flow rate of oxygen; carbon dioxide is washed out and oxygen is washed in (Fig. 12–4B).[58-61] Again, as with low frequency interruption of high flows, continuous high-flow apneic ventilation requires that the small catheters

(2.5 mm ID) need to be positioned in a mainstem bronchus (2.5 to 3.0 cm below the carina) and the flow must approximate 1.0 to 1.2 L/kg/min.[58, 59, 61] Continuous flow rates less than 0.7 L/kg/min have been shown to cause carbon dioxide retention.[58, 61] Catheter position is secured by inflating a conventional endotracheal tube cuff (which holds the small catheter between the cuff and the tracheal mucosa). Oxygenation is improved if 4 cm H_2O CPAP is used to the lung that is being oxygenated.[59] Without CPAP the airway pressure due to high gas flow does not exceed 2 mm Hg. The fresh gas is heated and humidified. Under these conditions arterial oxygenation and carbon dioxide removal is well maintained, and the method works well with the chest open as well as closed.[59]

Continuous high-flow apneic ventilation has been partially successful in humans.[62] In five female patients undergoing pelvic procedures, curved endobronchial catheters (2.5 mm OD) were placed 2 cm below the carina with a fiberoptic bronchoscope and secured in place by inflation of an endotracheal tube cuff. Catheter position was verified a second time with the fiberoptic bronchoscope. Continuous high flow apneic ventilation was then started with humidified oxygen at total flows between 0.6 and 0.7 L/kg/min for 30 minutes. Average control P_aO_2 was 321 mm Hg and 30 minute P_aO_2 was 299 mm Hg, whereas control P_aCO_2 was 37 mm Hg and 30 minute P_aCO_2 was 55 mm Hg. The rate of rise of P_aCO_2 was 0.6 mm Hg/min, which compares favorably with the 3.8 mm Hg/min rise in anesthetized humans exposed to continuous low-flow apneic ventilation.[55, 56] Obviously, the technique will have to be improved (higher flow rates, better catheter position) before it can find a useful application in thoracic surgery.

REFERENCES

1. Hall SM, Strawn WB, Levitsky MG: Effect of high-frequency oscillation on blood flow to an atelectatic lung in closed-chested dogs. Crit Care Med 12:447–451, 1984.
2. Wetzel RC, Gordon JB, Gregory TJ, et al: High-frequency ventilation attenuation of hypoxic pulmonary vasoconstriction. Am Rev Resp Dis 132:99–103, 1985.
3. Gillespie DJ: High-frequency ventilation: A new concept in mechanical ventilation. Mayo Clin Proc 58:187–196, 1983.
4. O'Rourke PP, Crone RK: High-frequency ventilation: A new approach to respiratory support. JAMA 250:2845–2847, 1983.
5. Fredberg JJ: Augmented diffusion in the airways can support pulmonary gas exchange. J Appl Physiol 49:232–238, 1980.

6. Eriksson I: The role of conducting airways in gas exchange during high-frequency ventilation—a clinical and theoretical analysis. Anesth Analg 61:483–489, 1982.

7. Haselton FR, Scherer PW: Bronchial bifurcations and respiratory mass transport. Science 208:69–71, 1980.

8. Slutsky AS, Bronw R, Lehr J, et al: High-frequency ventilation: A promising new approach to mechanical ventilation. Med Instrum 15:229–233, 1981.

9. Kolton M, Cattran CB, Kent G, et al: Oxygenation during high-frequency ventilation compared with conventional mechanical ventilation in two models of lung injury. Anesth Analg 61:323–332, 1982.

10. Sjostrand UH, Smith RB: Overview of high-frequency ventilation. Int Anesthes Clin 21:1–10, 1983.

11. Sjostrand U: High-frequency positive-pressure ventilation (HFPPV): A review. Crit Care Med 8:345–364, 1980.

12. Carlon GC, Howland, WS, Ray C, et al: High-frequency jet ventilation: A prospective randomized evaluation. Chest 84:551–559, 1983.

13. Bohn DJ, Marchak BE, Thompson WK, et al: Ventilation by high-frequency oscillation. J Appl Physiol 48:710–716, 1980.

14. Lunkenheimer PP, Rafflenbeul W, Keller H, et al: Application of transtracheal pressure oscillations as a modification of diffusion respiration. Br J Anaesth 44:627, 1972.

15. Klain M, Smith RB: High-frequency percutaneous transtracheal jet ventilation. Crit Care Med 5:280–287, 1977.

16. Butler WJ, Bohn DJ, Bryan AC, et al: Ventilation by high-frequency oscillation in humans. Anesth Analg 59:577–584, 1980.

17. Heijman K, Heijman L, Jonzon A, et al: High-frequency positive pressure ventilation during anesthesia and routine surgery in man. Acta Anaesth Scand 16:176–187, 1972.

18. Heijman L, Nilsson L, Sjostrand U: High-frequency positive-pressure ventilation (HFPPV) in neonates and infants during neuroleptal analgesia and routine plastic surgery, and in postoperative management. Acta Anaesth Scand (Suppl) 64:111–121, 1977.

19. Carlon GC, Klain M, Kalla R, et al: High-frequency positive-pressure ventilation in acute respiratory failure. Crit Care Med 7:128, 1979.

20. Lyrene RK, Wright K, Standaert TA, et al: Rapid oscillation low volume ventilation in oleic acid–induced pulmonary disease. Am Rev Respir Dis 121:294, 1980.

21. Flatau E, Barzilay E, Kaufmann N, et al: Adult respiratory distress syndrome treated with high-frequency positive-pressure ventilation. Israel J Med Sci 17:453–456, 1981.

22. Carlon GC, Ray CJ, Pierri MK, et al: High-frequency jet ventilation for prolonged respiratory support. Anesthesiology 51:S189, 1979.

23. Carlon GC, Ray C Jr, Pierri MK, et al: High-frequency ventilation: Theoretical considerations and clinical observations. Chest 81:350–354, 1982.

24. Carlon GC, Turnbull AD, Alexander JD, et al: High-frequency jet ventilation during tracheal surgery. Crit Care Med 9:163, 1981.

25. El-Baz N, El-Ganzouri A, Gottschalk W, et al: One-lung high frequency positive-pressure ventilation for sleeve pneumonectomy: An alternative technique. Anesth Analg 60:683–686, 1981.

26. El-Baz N, Jensik R, Faber P, et al: One-lung high-frequency ventilation for tracheoplasty and bronchoplasty: A new technique. Ann Thor Surg 34:564–572, 1982.

27. El-Baz N, Holinger L, El-Ganzouri A, et al: High-frequency positive-pressure ventilation for tracheal reconstruction by tracheal T-tube. Anesth Analg 61:796–800, 1982.

28. Eriksson I, Nilsson LG, Nordstrom S, et al: High-frequency positive-pressure ventilation (HFPPV) during transthoracic resection of tracheal stenosis and during preoperative bronchoscopic examination. Acta Anaesth Scand 19:113–119, 1975.

29. Glenski JA, Crawford M, Rehder K: High-frequency, small-volume ventilation during thoracic surgery. Anesthesiology 64:211–214, 1986.

30. Faber LP, Jensik RJ: The planning of tracheal surgery. Surg Clin North Am 50:113–122, 1970.

31. Parrish CM, Jones R: Primary tracheal tumors. Am Surg 26:95–98, 1960.

32. Geffin B, Bland J, Grillo HC: Anesthetic management of tracheal resection and reconstruction. Anesth Analg 48:884–894, 1969.

33. Theman TE, Kerr JH, Nelems JM, et al: Carinal resection. A report of two cases and a description of the anesthetic technique. J Thorac Cardiovasc Surg 71:314–320, 1976.

34. Fredrickson JM: Reinforced T-tube tracheal stent. Arch Otolaryngol 90:120–123, 1969.

35. Montgomery WW: Manual of care of the Montgomery silicone tracheal T-tube. Ann Otol Rhinol Laryngol (Suppl 73) 89:1–8, 1980.

36. Rah KH, Griffith RL III, Jones JR, et al: Anesthetic management of the pediatric patient with a tracheal T-tube. Anesth Analg 60:445–447, 1981.

37. Benjaminsson E, Klain N: Intraoperative dual-mode independent lung ventilation of a patient with bronchopleural fistula. Anesth Analg 60:118–119, 1981.

38. Carlon GC, Ray C, Jr, Klain M, et al: High-frequency positive-pressure ventilation in management of a patient with bronchopleural fistula. Anesthesiology 52:160–162, 1980.

39. Derderian SS, Rajagopal KR, Abbrecht PH, et al: High-frequency positive-pressure jet ventilation in bilateral bronchopleural fistulae. Crit Care Med 10:119–121, 1982.

40. Albelda SM, Hanson-Flaschen JH, Taylor E, Lanken PN, Wollman H: Evaluation of high-frequency jet ventilation in patients with bronchopleural fistulas by quantitation of the airleak. Anesthesiology 63:551–554, 1985.

41. Holzapfel L, Robert D, Lenoir B, Mercatello A, Palmier B, Perrin F, Bertoye A: High-frequency jet ventilation compared with conventional ventilation in patients with acute respiratory failure (abstract). Chest 32:211, 1982.

42. Ritz R, Benson M, Bishop MJ: Measuring gas leakage from bronchopleural fistulas during high-frequency jet ventilation. Crit Care Med 12:836–837, 1984.

43. Carlon GC, Kahn RC, Howland WS, et al: Clinical experience with high-frequency jet ventilation. Crit Care Med 9:1–6, 1981.

44. Turnbull AD, Carlon GC, Howland WS, et al: High-frequency jet ventilation in major airways or pulmonary disruption. Ann Thorac Surg 32:468–474, 1981.

45. Fuhrman T, Reines HD, Kratz J: The use of high-frequency jet ventilation in a patient with pulmonary mucormycosis. Anesthesiol Rev 13:31–32, 1986.

46. Sjostrand UH, Smith B, Hoff BH, et al: Conventional and high-frequency ventilation in dogs with bronchopleural fistula. Crit Care Med 13:191–193, 1985.

47. Downs JB, Chapman RL: Treatment of bronchopleural fistula during continuous positive-pressure ventilation. Chest 69:363–366, 1976.

48. Kirby RR: Ventilatory support and pulmonary baro-trauma. Anesthesiology 50:181–182, 1979.
49. Malina JF, Nordstrom SG, Sjostrand UH, et al: Clinical evaluation of high-frequncy positive-pressure ventilation (HFPPV) in patients scheduled for open-chest surgery. Anesth Analg 60:324–330, 1981.
50. Smith RB, Hoff BH, Rosen L, et al: High-frequency ventilation during pulmonary lobectomy—three cases. Respir Care 26:437–441, 1981.
51. Sjostrand UH, Wattwil LM, Borg UR, et al: Volume-controlled HFPPV as a useful mode of ventilation during open-chest surgery—a report on three cases. Respir Care 27:1380–1385, 1982.
52. Glenski JA, Crawford M, Rehder K: High-frequency small-volume ventilation during thoracic surgery. Anesthesiology 64:211–214, 1986.
53. Seki S, Fukshima Y, Goto K, et al: Facilitation of intrathoracic operations by means of high-frequency ventilation. J Thorac Cardiovasc Surg 86:388–392, 1983.
54. El-Baz N, Kittle CF, Faber LP, et al: High-frequency ventilation with an uncuffed endobronchial tube. J Thorac Cardiovasc Surg 84:823–838, 1982.
55. Frumin MJ, Epstein RM, Cohen G: Apneic oxygenation in man. Anesthesiology 20:789, 1959.
56. Eger EI, Severinghaus JW: The rate of rise of P_aCO_2 in the apneic anesthetized patient. Anesthesiology 22:419, 1961.
57. McClish A, Deslauriers J, Beaulieu M, Desrosieres R, Fugere L, Ginsberg RJ, Hebert C, Heroux M, Martineau A, Piraux M, Proulx Y: High-flow catheter ventilation during major tracheobronchial reconstruction. J Thor Cardiovasc Surg 89:508–512, 1985.
58. Smith RB, Babinski MF, Angell KE: Apneic diffusion oxygenation with high flows of intratracheal oxygen. Resp Care 30:26–29, 1985.
59. Babinski MF, Smith RB, Bunegin L: Continuous flow apneic ventilation during thoracotomy. Anesthesiology 65:399–404, 1986.
60. Bunegin L, Gelineau J, Stone E, et al: The effect of endobronchial catheter position on P_aCO_2 and P_aO_2 during continuous flow apneic ventilation. Crit Care Med 14:370, 1986.
61. Smith RB, Babinski M, Bunegin L, et al: Continuous flow apneic ventilation. Acta Anaesthesiol Scand 28:631–639, 1984.
62. Babinski MF, Sierra OG, Smith RB, et al: Clinical application of continuous flow apneic ventilation. Acta Anaesth Scand 29:750–752, 1985.

Anesthetic Considerations (Other than Management of Ventilation) During and at the End of Thoracic Surgery

13

I. INTRODUCTION

The management of ventilation is the most common major anesthesia problem during thoracic surgery. Chapters 11 and 12 were solely concerned with this problem. One-lung ventilation is absolutely indicated in a number of cases and relatively indicated in most cases. If hypoxemia should occur during conventional management of one-lung ventilation, differential lung management consisting of nonventilated lung CPAP, with or without ventilated lung PEEP, should be instituted. In a few cases involving opening of a major conducting airway, high-frequency and high-flow apneic ventilation may be indicated.

There are a number of other major anesthetic problems that occasionally occur during thoracic surgery. First, since many of these patients are long-term smokers, have reactive airways, and will experience tracheobronchial tree manipulation, there is an increased incidence of bronchospasm. Second, blood and fluid infusion may be problematic. Most thoracic surgery patients do not require replacement of blood loss, and in questionable cases there are survival data (related to recurrence of cancer) to suggest that

blood transfusion should be avoided. There are also data on postpneumonectomy pulmonary edema that suggest that crystalloid infusion should not be overly aggressive. However, some thoracic surgery cases, especially those with extensive local tumor invasion, particularly to the pleura, may involve a great deal of blood loss and require massive transfusion; the blood loss and transfusion requirement may be compounded by the development of hemostatic deficits. Third, some thoracic surgery patients have significant coronary artery disease, and the determinants of myocardial oxygen supply and demand may need to be controlled within narrow limits. Fourth, patients undergoing esophageal surgery have nutritional, regurgitation, and aspiration problems that are unique to esophageal disease. Finally, the transport of a thoracic surgery patient from the operating room to a new location (intensive care unit or recovery room) can be a perilous misadventure. Consequently, the preparation of the patient for transport at the end of a case and the transport of the patient to a new location must be performed with rigorous attention to detail. This chapter discusses the proper anesthetic management of intraoperative bronchospasm, blood loss, hemodynamic changes, common esophageal problems, and transportation of critically ill thoracic surgery patients.

II. MANAGEMENT OF BRONCHOSPASM

The treatment of intraoperative bronchospasm can be divided up into three categories (Fig. 13–1). The first category contains measures that can be done immediately, should be done in the majority of patients, and may correct bronchospasm when it is mild and not very intense. The second category involves administration of major bronchodilating drugs that should be used in patients in whom the first category of therapeutic measures does not work and/or in whom the bronchospasm has a moderate to severe intensity. The third category involves administration of drugs that should be considered as having a minor impact on bronchospasm but might make a difference in patients in whom the first two categories have failed to resolve the bronchospasm completely.

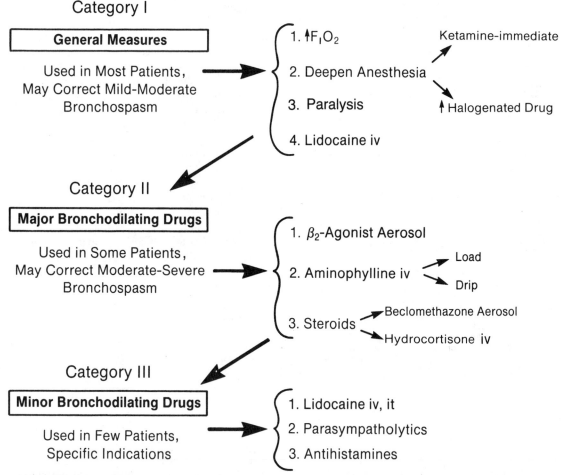

Treatment of Intraoperative Bronchospasm

Category I

General Measures

Used in Most Patients,
May Correct Mild-Moderate
Bronchospasm

1. ↑F_1O_2
2. Deepen Anesthesia → Ketamine-immediate / ↑Halogenated Drug
3. Paralysis
4. Lidocaine iv

Category II

Major Bronchodilating Drugs

Used in Some Patients,
May Correct Moderate-Severe
Bronchospasm

1. β_2-Agonist Aerosol
2. Aminophylline iv → Load / Drip
3. Steroids → Beclomethazone Aerosol / Hydrocortisone iv

Category III

Minor Bronchodilating Drugs

Used in Few Patients,
Specific Indications

1. Lidocaine iv, it
2. Parasympatholytics
3. Antihistamines

Figure 13–1. The treatment of intraoperative bronchospasm can be divided up into three major categories. The first category consists of general measures that are used in most patients and may be expected to correct mild to moderate bronchospasm. Many authors include the use of intravenous lidocaine in this first category. The second category consists of administration of major bronchodilating drugs, which should be used in patients who have moderate to severe bronchospasm. The third category consists of minor bronchodilating drugs that may be helpful in a few patients who have specific indications (such as increased vagal tone, release of histamine). (iv = intravenous; it = intratracheal.)

The first category of therapy involves measures that should be done in most patients and may likely reduce the severity of bronchospasm for the majority of times it occurs during anesthesia (Fig. 13–1, category I). First, the F_IO_2 should be increased as a prophylactic measure against the development of hypoxemia. Second, the level of anesthesia should be deepened. This may be accomplished in two ways. If an immediate effect is desired, sodium pentothal 1 mg/kg or ketamine 0.5 mg/kg IV, can be administered. Alternatively, if halothane or isoflurane are not being used or if they are being used in low doses, the inspired concentration of halogenated drug should be increased. However, deepening anesthesia may not be effective in severe bronchospasm.[1] Third, if paralysis is part of or compatible with the anesthetic plan and the patient is only partially paralyzed and coughing and straining, then he or she should be fully paralyzed, since exaggerated expiratory efforts will worsen small airway obstruction. Finally, serious consideration should also be given to administering intravenous lidocaine 1 mg/kg early to all coughing and/or straining patients (see the following).

The second category of therapy involves the administration of major bronchodilator drugs and should be used in any patient who develops serious bronchospasm (Fig. 13–1, category II). First, the beta-2 agonist drugs are the most potent and rapidly acting bronchodilator drugs.[2] The beta-2 agonist should be delivered by aerosol because of increased bronchial selectivity with decreased side effects (maximal broncho-

dilation can be achieved with barely detectable blood concentrations), whereas intravenous administration results in much higher blood levels and an increased incidence of side effects. The pressurized, metered cannister is convenient and provides accurate dosimetry. The metered aerosol cannisters require a T-piece with 15-mm ends or fittings. The various beta-2 agonists along with their pertinent clinical pharmacology are listed in Table 13–1.

Responses to beta-agonists are mediated by beta-1 receptors, which increase heart rate and cardiac contractility, and beta-2 receptors, which decrease bronchomotor and peripheral vascular tone. Isoproterenol is a very potent bronchodilator, but it is not beta-2 selective and results in tachycardia and arrhythmias. The propensity toward tachycardia and arrhythmias is exaggerated by halothane and minimized by isoflurane. In addition, isoproterenol is not as effective by the tracheal route. The following newer drugs, with substitutions in various parts of the catecholamine structure, differ from isoproterenol in that they have higher beta-2 selectivity, may be administered by the tracheal route, and have a longer action of duration.[2] Albuterol (salbutamol) can be administered as a metered aerosol and, by this route, is as effective a bronchodilator as isoproterenol is intravenously but has minimal cardiovascular effects. Its duration of action is approximately 6 hours. Terbutaline is not available as a metered aerosol, although a water-soluble preparation is available for aerosol use. Metaproterenol and isoetharine are less effective, have less beta-2

Table 13–1. Beta-Agonists and Treatment of Bronchospasm

Beta-Agonist Trade Name	Adrenergic Receptor Activity	Bronchodilator Effectiveness	Onset (Min)	Peak (Min)	Duration (Hours)	Inhaled Via Cannister	Arrhythmia Tachycardia	Side Effects	Comments
Isoproterenol Mistometer Medihaler-Iso	$B_1 + B_2$	+ + +	2 to 5	5	1 to 4	125 μg/puff	+ + + +	Tachyphylaxis ventricular fibrillation, ↓P_aO_2	Very potent
Albuterol Proventil Ventilon	$B_2 > B_1$	+ + +	5 to 10	15	4 to 6	90 μg/puff	+	Muscle tremors	Most effective
Terbutaline Brethine Bricanyl	$B_2 > B_1$	+ +	5 to 15	25	3 to 4	Nebulized, sub q	+ +	Muscle tremors	Not to be used IV or by inhalation
Metaproterenol Alupent Metaprel	$B_2 > B_2$	+	10 to 20	25	3	65 μg/puff	+ +	Muscle tremors	Not used parenterally
Isoetharine Bronkometer	$B_2 > B_1$	+	10 to 25	25	1 to 2	340 μg/puff	+ + +	Tachyphylaxis	Poor choice

selectivity, and are shorter acting than albuterol. They offer no advantage.

Theophylline compounds are beneficial prophylactically in asthmatic patients and therapeutically in bronchospastic patients. Phosphodiesterase inhibition is the major mechanism of action of this drug in contrast to direct beta-2 stimulation; this allows aminophylline to be useful in the patient who is taking beta-blockers or is already using a beta-2 agonist. Side effects include hypotension and/or cardiac arrhythmias, especially during anesthesia with halogenated drugs. The arrhythmias are magnified by halothane and minimized by isoflurane. Should a patient require aminophylline during anesthesia, a loading dose of 5 to 6 mg/kg should be given intravenously and slowly during 15 to 20 min (which is a disadvantage compared with the beta-2 agonists) followed by an infusion of 0.5 to 1.0 mg/kg/hr depending on age (inversely proportional). Theophylline blood levels should be obtained on all patients, and the therapeutic range is 10 to 20 µg/ml.

Corticosteroids may be extremely useful in treating bronchospasm, but it should be realized that the onset of therapeutic action may require 1 to 3 hours,[3] and the mechanism of action in the modulation of airway tone is incompletely understood. Proposed mechanisms include stabilization of membranes, decreased release of chemical mediators, decreased bronchial mucosal edema and inflammatory cells, and potentiation of catecholamine action. The recent advent of an aerosol steroid offers a major advantage in the treatment of asthma. Side effects are greatly minimized but adrenal suppression may still occur. Beclomethasone dipropionate appears to be the best inhaled agent currently available. Hydrocortisone is considered the steroid of choice for parental administration in both the preoperative preparation of patients with reactive airway disease (1 to 2 mg/kg) and the treatment of intraoperative bronchospasm (4 mg/kg).

The third category of therapy involves the administration of compounds that should be expected to have a minor impact on bronchospasm but may, in selected patients, be helpful, especially when administration of the major bronchodilating drugs has not completely resolved the problem (Fig. 13–1, category III). If the increase in airway resistance is thought to be a result of coughing or straining, intravenous lidocaine, 1 mg/kg, should be administered. Additionally, 4 per cent lidocaine may be administered intratracheally (down the tracheal lumen of a double-lumen tube for anesthesia of the carina and one mainstem bronchus, and down the bronchial lumen for anesthesia of the other mainstem bronchus). Both forms of lidocaine administration incur little risk and may be of significant benefit (decrease coughing reflex and bronchospasm and protect against or treat ventricular arrhythmias).

Parasympatholytics (anticholinergics) in large doses are effective at preventing and reversing reflex bronchospasm by blocking the efferent limb of the irritant reflex. In addition, these drugs decrease the volume of secretions. The dose of atropine used in premedication is not large enough to prevent reflex bronchoconstriction but does decrease the volume of secretions. Unfortunately, intravenous administration of large doses of atropine necessary to prevent reflex bronchoconstriction produces undesirable tachycardia. Atropine by inhalation as a 10 mg/ml solution has few side effects and a longer duration than when given by intravenous administration. New aerosol agents, such as ipratropium bromide (SCH 1000 atrovent), appear to be as effective or more so than atropine and have a longer duration of action. Since parasympatholytic drugs have little or no effect on mediator-induced airway constriction, they are far more effective in patients with chronic bronchitis than in those with asthma,[4] perhaps because they decrease the volume of secretions in general and specifically in response to instrumentation of the airway and, therefore, reduce bronchoconstricting reflexes.

Finally, sodium bicarbonate should be administered following blood gas determination if a metabolic acidosis is present (acidosis inhibits the action of catecholamines). Diphenhydramine (a histamine blocker) may be administered to supplement the level of anesthesia. However, administration of an antihistamine should not be expected to have a large effect on the degree of bronchospasm because histamine is usually not the sole mediator involved in producing bronchoconstriction, and the antihistamines do not block reflex airway constriction, which is so important during thoracic surgery. Cromolyn is a mast cell stabilizer and is thought to inhibit release of mediators from the mast cells. The action of the drug is entirely prophylactic, and it is not useful in the treatment of bronchospasm intraoperatively. However, it is a remarkably benign drug in terms of interaction with anesthetics, and patients who are

Assessment of Blood Loss

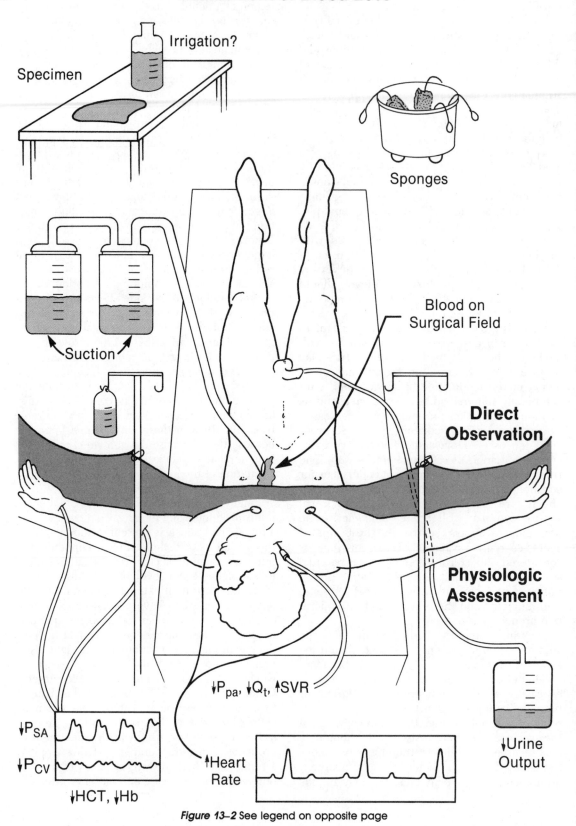

Figure 13–2 See legend on opposite page

receiving this drug should continue to receive it right up to the time of surgery. Mucolytics have no proven value in the treatment of bronchospastic disease. Indeed, they have been shown to provoke reflex bronchoconstriction and are best avoided.

III. MANAGEMENT OF BLOOD LOSS

A. Assessment of Blood Loss

The anesthesiologist should be continuously aware of the amount of blood loss. The assessment of blood loss involves both direct observation and measurement of physiological responses as indirect indicators of blood loss (Fig. 13–2).

1. Direct Observation

Surgical swabs and packs should be observed for the amount of blood staining. Fully stained 4 by 4 gauze sponges and laparotomy pads contain 10 and 50 ml of blood, respectively. If there is a question or concern about the exact amount of blood on the sponges and pads, the sponges and pads should be weighed; each gram greater than the known dry weight represents 1 ml of blood loss. The suction bottles should be frequently observed for blood accumulation. The operative field, the drapes around the operative field, and the floor should also be assessed for blood loss. Furthermore, if uncertainty about the amount of blood loss persists, there should be periodic attempts to look under the drapes and other concealed places for blood loss. With all these forms of direct observation, the anesthesiologist must be aware of how much saline irrigation was used (to wash out pleural cavity, test integrity of bronchial stumps) and how much the irrigation might have contributed to the observed shed volumes. Similar considerations apply to pleural fluid that was present preoperatively and then suctioned intraoperatively. With regard to the aspirated blood in the suction bottles, the hematocrit of the material in the suction bottles can always be meas-

ured and evaluated in light of the blood loss, intravenous fluid infusion, and surgical irrigation and suction history. Usually these data, when processed by the anesthesiologist, circulating nurse, and surgeon, result in a reasonably accurate educated estimate of the blood loss.

Tying off of the pulmonary vessels for lung resection results in blood loss due to entrapment of blood within the specimen. If the pulmonary veins are tied off first, the specimen may be very blood-engorged (due to continued inflow) and with a pneumonectomy the resected lung may contain 500 ml of blood. If the pulmonary arteries are tied off first, then the entrapped blood loss in the specimen is much less. Postoperative drainage adds to this blood loss, and after pneumonectomy the pleural space fills with an unknown but considerable volume of blood and plasma.

2. Physiologic Response to Blood Loss

The patient's physiologic response to fluid and blood loss (Fig. 13–2) is an indirect indicator of how much has been lost and how adequate replacement has been. In the face of continued blood loss and replacement with just crystalloid infusion, serial measurement of the hematocrit and hemoglobin will reveal a progressive decrease. Hemodynamically, blood loss causes a decrease in systemic arterial, central venous, pulmonary arterial systolic, diastolic, and wedge pressures, cardiac output, and urine output. The heart rate and systemic vascular resistance usually increase with blood loss if the depth of anesthesia is not profound. The heart rate may not increase in patients on preoperative beta-blockers.

B. Minimal Blood Loss (<10 Per Cent of Blood Volume): Amount of Crystalloid Fluid Infusion

The amount of crystalloid infused during pulmonary resections, particularly during pneumonectomy, requires special consideration. On

Figure 13–2. The assessment of blood loss involves both direct observation (top half of figure) and physiologic assessment (bottom half of figure). Direct observation of blood loss consists of blood on the surgical field and blood that is contained within suction bottles, on sponges and within the specimen. Assessment of blood loss through direct observation must be modified by the amount of irrigation used. The physiologic assessment consists of quantification of decreases in systemic artery (P_{sa}), central venous (P_{cv}), pulmonary artery (P_{pa}) and pulmonary artery wedge (P_{paw}) pressures and decreases in cardiac output ($\dot{Q}_t$), hematocrit (HCT), hemoglobin (Hb), and urine output; and increases in heart rate and systemic vascular resistance (SVR).

the one hand, as for any major operation, in-sensible fluid, nasogastric and urine fluid, ex-tracellular (third space) wound fluid, and blood losses (less than 10 per cent of blood volume) should be replaced by crystalloid infusion. Fail-ure to do so results in unacceptable hemody-namic depression due to anesthetic drugs and positive-pressure ventilation, inability to toler-ate any further sudden loss of blood, cardiovas-cular lability with changes in anesthetic depth and surgical stimulation, and oliguria.

However, there are both experimental[5] and clinical[6] data suggesting that overinfusion of fluids during pneumonectomy may be particu-larly hazardous with regard to the development of postpneumonectomy pulmonary edema. There are two inter-related reasons why pneu-monectomy may predispose to the formation of pulmonary edema (Table 13–2). First, a de-creased amount of pulmonary vascular bed has to accommodate all of the cardiac output. On the one hand, it has been clearly shown that if the remaining pulmonary vascular bed is nor-mal, then pneumonectomy does not cause an increase in pulmonary extravascular fluid, even if left atrial pressure is deliberately increased to 25 mm Hg.[7] If the remaining pulmonary vascular bed is nondistensible (diseased), the cardiac output is greatly increased (as it may be in the early stress-ridden postoperative period), and/or excessive fluids were infused intraoper-atively, pulmonary hypertension may occur and cause transmembrane transudation of fluid.[5] Second, pneumonectomy results in removal of half of the lymphatics responsible for clearing pulmonary interstitial fluid. The loss of paren-chymal/hilar/mediastinal lymphatic drainage routes, with all other considerations equal, may cause lymphatic clearance thresholds to be more easily exceeded, increasing the risk of pulmonary interstitial fluid accumulation and pulmonary edema.

Postpneumonectomy pulmonary edema has been thought to occur in a few patients.[6] The risk factors for this complication appear to be high(er) perioperative volume of infused fluid

Table 13–2. Theoretical Reasons Why Pneumonectomy May Predispose the Patient Toward the Formation of Pulmonary Interstitial Edema

1. Half the pulmonary vascular bed has to handle all the pulmonary blood flow and volume.
2. Reduced lymphatic channels participate in pulmonary interstitial fluid clearance.

Table 13–3. Treatment of Postpneumonectomy Pulmonary Edema

1. Mechanical ventilation with PEEP.
2. Search for and eliminate septic focus.
3. Examine both right and left ventricles for failure (chapter 7).
4. Treat ventricular failure:
   a. Inotropic drugs
   b. Diuretics
   c. Volume restriction.

and right pneumonectomy, leaving a smaller left lung to cope with the entire cardiac output and, perhaps, higher pulmonary vascular pres-sures. However, as mentioned previously, sim-ple resection of a single lung and minimal to moderate increases in hydrostatic pressure are not likely to be the sole cause of postresection pulmonary edema in patients with relatively normal hearts and remaining lungs,[7] and it may be necessary to have also some factor present that disposes the patient toward edema (pre-existing pulmonary vascular disease, very high cardiac outputs, acute injury to the permeability barrier—sepsis, bronchopneumonia, or trauma) in order for postpneumonectomy pulmonary edema and the adult respiratory distress syn-drome to develop.

In summary, because of the smaller pulmo-nary vascular bed remaining after resection and the interruption of lymphatic drainage, it is reasonable to consider the possibility that pa-tients undergoing pneumonectomy are at greater risk for the development of pulmonary edema from aggressive intravenous fluid admin-istration than other types of surgery patients, especially if the heart and/or the remaining lung is diseased. A reasonable approach would be to start out with infusing 10 ml/kg during the first hour (mainly to make up insensible losses and to minimize cardiovascular depression due to anesthesia) and 5 ml/kg/hr thereafter with ad-justments made according to the estimated blood loss and cardiovascular responses. If pul-monary edema should develop postoperatively, mechanical ventilation with sufficient PEEP to reduce the F_IO_2 to nontoxic levels should be instituted (Table 13–3).[8] Next, a thorough search for a septic focus is warranted; if one is found, it should be promptly removed or drained after appropriate antibiotic therapy has been instituted (Table 13–3).[8] Third, and most vital, one should measure pulmonary vascular pressures and examine both right and left ven-tricles for evidence of failure or overload, which, if present, must be treated with inotropic drugs, diuretics, and volume restriction (Table 13–3).[8] In cases of extreme right ventricular afterloading, it may be appropriate to assess right ventricular performance by either radioisotopic scanning or thermodilution ejection fractions.[9]

C. Moderate Blood Loss (10 to 20 Per Cent Blood Volume): Should Blood Be Infused?

The generally accepted safe lower limit of hemoglobin is 10 g/dl. If a patient started out with a normal hemoglobin level of 14 g/dl, a level of 10 g/dl represents a loss of about 28 per cent of the oxygen-carrying capacity of the blood. Thus, blood losses less than 20 per cent of the blood volume can safely be replaced with nonsanguinous fluids, even with a reasonable margin of error in either the estimation of blood loss or replacement.[10] In addition, in view of the known potentially lethal viral diseases that can be transmitted by blood infusion (hepatitis, autoimmune deficiency syndrome) and the possibility of anaphylactic, hemolytic, and febrile reactions (Table 13–4),[11] it certainly behooves the anesthesiologist to avoid blood transfusion to patients who are initially normal from a cardiovascular point of view when losses are less than 20 per cent of the total blood volume. Concentrations of hemoglobin below 10 g/dl may be accompanied by a progressive increase in the bleeding time,[12] and decreases below 9 g/dl require an increased cardiac output to maintain oxygen transport.[13] However, if the cardiac output does not increase, as may be the situation during anesthesia, and the decrease in hemoglobin concentration is large, then anaerobic metabolism and lactic acidosis may ensue.

Recently, new immunologic and cancer growth data have emerged that reinforce and further support the notion that blood transfusion should be avoided whenever blood loss is less than 20 per cent of the total blood volume and the patient is hemodynamically stable (Table 13–4).[14-19] These studies indicate that perioperative blood transfusion is an important im-

munosuppressant and that immunosuppression may favor growth of cancer.[14] The increased survival of renal allografts following transfusion of whole blood or packed red blood cells indicates that the blood transfusion prior to renal allograft transplant caused immunosuppression. Furthermore, immunosuppressed patients in general are at increased risk for the development of various malignant tumors. For example, it has been found that perioperative blood transfusion is associated with decreased survival of patients undergoing resection for colon and breast cancer due to recurrent or metastatic growths.[15-17]

It now appears, based on two new studies, that intraoperative blood transfusion during non–oat cell lung cancer resection is also associated with decreased survival due to cancer recurrence.[18, 19] In one study,[19] 155 patients undergoing resection for lung carcinoma were analyzed retrospectively, and it was shown that the use of blood transfusion was associated with a significant decrease in survival time in patients undergoing curative resection of lung carcinoma despite multivariate adjustments for age, sex, cell type, right lung versus left lung location, type of operation, and stage of cancer. In the other study,[18] surgical technique–related variables were minimized by limiting the study to one surgeon. Analysis of age, sex, tumor size, histopathology, admission and discharge hematocrit values, estimated operative blood loss, duration of operation, extent of resection, anesthetic agents, and blood transfusion revealed two significant prognostic factors: extent of resection and use or nonuse of transfusions. Transfused patients had lower disease-free rates within 5 years than nontransfused patients. The results of both of these studies indicate that perioperative blood transfusion of patients with lung cancer undergoing resection accelerates the appearance of recurrent or metastatic cancer. The findings are consistent with the hypothesis that blood transfusion, possibly through an immunosuppressive mechanism, is responsible for a poorer prognosis in patients who undergo resection for carcinoma of the lung.

Table 13–4. Reasons Why Blood Should Not Be Transfused When Blood Loss Is Less Than 20 Per Cent of Blood Volume

1. Risk of transmission of viral diseases (hepatitis, AIDS).
2. Reactions (anaphylactic, hemolytic, febrile).
3. Risk of increased cancer recurrence (immunosuppression).

D. Severe Blood Loss (> 20 Per Cent of Blood Volume): Diagnostic and Therapeutic Management Problems

1. Causes of Severe Bleeding

Hemostasis depends upon the interplay of four components: maintenance of vascular integrity, normal number and function of platelets, the coagulation cascade production of fibrin, and the eventual removal of fibrin by fibrinolysis (Fig. 13–3). Derangements in any of these four components may cause excessive bleeding. In surgery, the cause of severe bleeding is almost always loss of vascular integrity, but other (and multiple) abnormalities may contribute to the problem. For example, if bleeding due to loss of vascular integrity has been large and sustained, and massive transfusion with old stored bank blood has been instituted, the infusion of old stored bank blood may, in and of itself, cause a coagulation defect (see Hemostatic Defects Due to Massive Blood Transfusion). In order to institute curative therapy, it is necessary to identify the exact cause of the bleeding. Figure 13–3 shows the systematic work-up and logic that should be employed in the diagnosis and treatment of severe bleeding.

Maintenance of vascular integrity is the primary responsibility of the surgeon (Fig. 13–3). Procedures most likely to incur excessive bleeding due to loss of vascular integrity are resection

The Diagnosis of Cause of Bleeding and the Appropriate Treatment

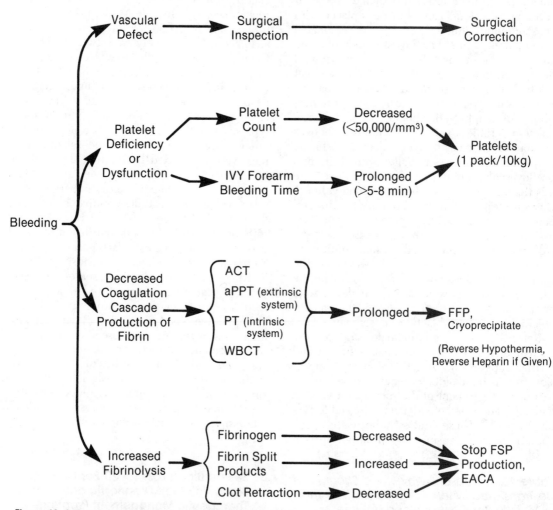

Figure 13–3. There are four major causes of bleeding, which are indicated in the left-hand column. The diagnosis of the cause of bleeding and the results of the various diagnostic tests are indicated in the two middle columns. The appropriate treatment for the cause of bleeding is indicated in the right-hand column. (ACT = activated clotting time; aPTT = activated partial thromboplastin time; PT = prothrombin time; WBCT = whole blood clotting time; FFP = fresh frozen plasma; FSP = fibrin split products; EACA = epsilon aminocaproic acid.)

of tumors with significant local extension (especially to chest wall and mediastinum), resection of tumors that involve bronchial and pulmonary vessels and the pleura, and procedures that require surgical dissection of a thickened inflamed vascular pleura. In order of rapidly decreasing incidence of cause of intraoperative bleeding are the pulmonary arteries and pulmonary, azygous, and subclavian veins.[20] Of course, failed surgical sutures on any large blood vessels will result in rapid massive blood loss. The loss of vascular integrity is diagnosed by inspection, and the treatment is surgical correction. If massive blood loss is anticipated prior to surgery (on a technical basis), preoperative blood donation by the patient (several weeks before surgery) for their own intraoperative use,[21, 22] and/or transfusion of the patient's own shed blood aspirated from the surgical field (autotransfusion),[23] and/or preoperative normovolemic hemodilution (draw off whole blood and simultaneously replace with crystalloid) on the day of surgery[24] may considerably help replacement of lost blood (Table 13–5).

Hemostasis requires an adequate number of normally functioning circulating platelets (Fig. 13–3). Platelets serve as an initial plug for small vascular defects and also as the substrate upon which the enzymatic reaction of the coagulation cascade occurs. They may be deficient in number (dilution, destruction, or sequestration) or deficient in function (drugs, presence of fibrin split products, uremic plasma, von Willebrand's disease) or both. The platelet count measures only platelet number. The bleeding time (Ivy forearm method) evaluates both platelet quantity and function. The test is performed by inflating and maintaining an arm blood pressure cuff at 40 mm Hg and making a 10 mm long, 1 mm deep forearm incision; the blood is lightly blotted with filter paper at 30 second intervals until the clot endpoint is reached (blood no longer appears on the filter paper). The normal forearm bleeding time is 3 to 8 minutes. Since most patients undergoing thoracic surgery are in the lateral decubitus position, both forearms are usually readily available to the anesthesiol-

ogist. If the bleeding time is normal, platelet administration is not required. If the platelet count is decreased and/or the bleeding time is prolonged, platelet therapy will be required, perhaps along with other therapies (see Fig. 13–3). The platelet dose is one platelet pack unit per 10 kg body weight if the platelet count is less than 60,000/mm, and one platelet pack unit can be expected to increase the platelet count by 10,000/mm.[25] After administration, defects due to storage may prevent the tranfused platelets from functioning normally for several hours.[25]

Defects in the coagulation cascade leading to fibrin result in excessive bleeding (Fig. 13–3). The performance of an activated clotting time (ACT) or activated partial thromboplastin time (aPTT) screens effectively virtually all of the intrinsic system coagulation cascade (Factors XII, XI, IX, VIII, platelet factor 3). The prothrombin time (PT) tests the extrinsic system (Factor XII, platelet tissue factor and Factor VII, tissue factor) in the same way that the aPTT tests the intrinsic system.[26] The ACT, aPTT, and PT all test the final common pathway sequence of conversion of Factor X to activated Factor X, which in turn converts, along with Factor V, prothrombin to activated Factor II, which in turn converts fibrinogen to insoluble fibrin. Normal values for the ACT, aPTT, and PT are 90 to 120 sec, less than 35 sec, and 12 sec, respectively.[27] The whole blood coagulation time (WBCT), which, with less sensitivity and more variability, tests the intrinsic system and final common pathway, can be performed in the operating room by drawing 1 ml of venous blood into a test tube maintained at 37°C and tilting the tube 90° back and forth at 30 sec intervals, permitting the liquid blood to run down the side to produce maximal surface activation. Normal values for WBCT in the one tube are 2.5 to 4.5 min. A normal WBCT does not ensure a normal bleeding time.

Increased fibrinolysis is rarely a cause of excessive bleeding. If the condition is present, the fibrinogen level will be markedly decreased, the production of fibrin split products (FSP) will be increased, and the FSP test will confirm the diagnosis. A negative test for FSP indicates a low level of FSP either because of little fibrinolysis or because of depleted fibrin or fibrinogen. Increased FSP is treated by stopping the cause of FSP production, infusing clotting factors that have been consumed, and by allowing time for the hepatic and reticuloendothelial clearance of FSP.

Table 13–5. Nonroutine Measures To Aid Intraoperative Blood Transfusion

1. Preoperative blood donation by the patients for their own intraoperative use.
2. Intraoperative transfusion of the patient's own shed blood aspirated from surgical field.
3. Preoperative normovolemic hemodilution.

2. Hemostatic Defects Due to Massive Blood Transfusion

Secondary disorders of hemostasis remain one of the persistent problems in the area of massive transfusion (Table 13–6). Factors V and VIII and platelets may be deficient in stored whole blood. These factor levels decrease 50 to 80 per cent after 21 days of storage; the remaining levels, 20 to 50 per cent of normal, are above or near the minimal hemostatic level for Factor V (20 per cent) and for Factor VIII (30 per cent). Thus, with transfusion of whole blood, deficiencies in these two factors are unlikely to be a primary cause of bleeding. However, if blood loss greater than 50 per cent of the blood volume is replaced with non–plasma products (packed red blood cells, non-coagulation factor–containing protein fluids, crystalloid fluids), then the level of Factors V and VIII may decrease well below minimum hemostatic levels. An abnormal aPTT will indicate a deficiency of Factors V and VIII.[28, 29]

In contrast to the relatively slow decay of coagulation factors, the number of stored platelets rapidly decays over 48 to 72 hours. Transfusion of 10 and 20 units of whole blood can be expected to decrease the platelet count to 100,000 and 50,000/mm,[25] respectively. When dilutional thrombocytopenia is the cause of a bleeding disorder, and there is also a moderate deficiency in either Factor V or Factor VIII, which is insufficient to cause bleeding on its own, the moderate deficiency in coagulation factor may possibly aggravate the thrombocytopenia-induced bleeding. Thus, when combat casualties who are bleeding have received more than 20 units of stored blood and have abnormal aPTT and PT times, infusion of 500 to 1000 ml of fresh frozen plasma (which contains Factors V and VIII but no platelets) restores the aPTT and PT times to normal but without significant correction of the bleeding disorder. Subsequent administration of platelets results in correction of these bleeding disorders.[30] During acute massive hemorrhage, it is always difficult to distinguish the amount of continued bleeding that results from the precipitating loss of vascular integrity from the subsequent bleeding caused

Table 13–6. Hemostatic Defects Due To Massive Transfusion of Stored Bank Blood

1. Decreased platelets—definite occurrence.
2. Decreased factors V and VIII—possible occurrence.
3. Decreased Ca^{++}—unlikely occurrence.

by the transfusion of massive amounts of stored blood.

Rapid infusion of citrated blood will decrease ionized calcium. This decrease is transient and rapidly reversed as the infused citrate is metabolized. Ionized calcium is a factor involved in the intrinsic coagulation cascade and final common pathway. Since the myocardial depressant effects of a decrease in ionized calcium occur long before the effects on the coagulation mechanism, and the myocardial depression is treated with calcium chloride, the anticoagulation effects of hypocalcemia are rarely seen.[27]

3. Management of Massive Transfusion

The proper management of massive transfusion logically follows from the problems that massive transfusion can cause (Fig. 13–4). First, it is important to send "stay ahead" orders to the blood bank for typing and crossing additional units of blood; the greatest problem in massive transfusion is the logistical one of always having compatible blood and blood products to infuse continuously. For example, if 8 units are available and 4 are used, and no end to the bleeding is in sight, 4 more units should be typed and crossed at the time the fifth unit is being used. If fully typed and cross-matched blood is not available, then the preferred order of using less well-prepared blood is type specific (for ABO-Rh types this must be known beforehand) partially crossmatched blood (sometimes referred to as an incomplete or immediate phase crossmatch, which eliminates ABO type compatibilities), type specific (ABO-Rh) uncrossmatched blood, and type O Rh-negative (universal donor) uncrossmatched blood (which should be used as packed red blood cells, since the plasma of type O blood may have anti-A and anti-B antibodies). All infused blood should be warmed and passed through a micropore filter.

Many diagnostic tests should be done following every 5 units of transfused blood (Fig. 13–4). Routine hemostatic tests should be platelet count, ACT or aPTT, and PT. Physiologic studies, such as arterial blood gases, hematocrit, hemoglobin, electrolytes, calcium and bicarbonate levels, should be obtained every 5 units. Calcium chloride, in a 500-mg intravenous bolus, should be administered after every 5 units, and sodium bicarbonate should be administered according to the arterial blood gases. Several activities should occur after every 10 units of transfused blood (Fig. 13–4). These

Management of Massive Transfusion

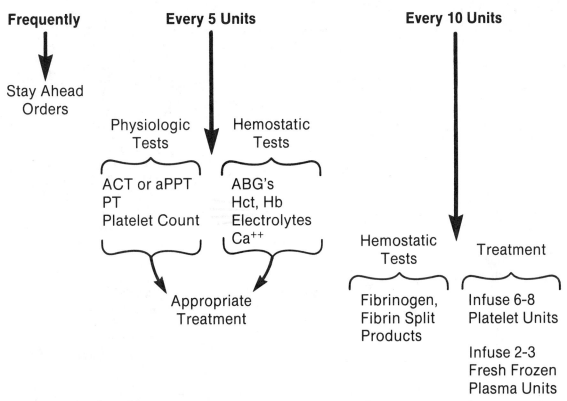

Figure 13-4. The management of massive transfusion involves several diagnostic and therapeutic activities that must be performed on a regular basis. The diagnostic activities are performed after approximately every five units of transfused blood, and the therapeutic activities are performed after approximately every ten units of transfused blood. (ACT = activated clotting time; aPTT = activated partial thromboplastin time; PT = prothrombin time; ABG = arterial blood gases; Hct = hematocrit; Hb = hemoglobin.)

consist of measuring fibrinogen levels and fibrin split products, and infusing fresh frozen plasma and 1 platelet pack/10 kg. Thus, massive transfusion is a busy time and requires staying ahead with prepared blood, monitoring the hemostatic and physiologic effects of the massive transfusion, and treating the hemostatic and physiologic derangements.

IV. TREATMENT OF NON–BLOOD LOSS DELETERIOUS HEMODYNAMIC CHANGES

It is possible for any or all of the factors that determine myocardial oxygen supply and demand to change a great deal during anesthesia and surgery. Fortunately, the availability of a wide range of therapeutic maneuvers and options usually allows the anesthesiologist to re-

turn any or all of the determinants of myocardial oxygen supply and demand to normal or to any particular desired value. Figure 13–5 shows most of the commonly used options for each hemodynamic aberration. The precise therapeutic modality chosen depends, of course, on the abnormality producing the deleterious hemodynamic change. For example, the heart rate may be too rapid because anesthesia is too light (which could be treated with fentanyl, deepening inhalation anesthesia, or infusing a beta-blocker) or the patient is hypovolemic (which should be treated by increasing vascular volume).

It is very unusual for just one of the determinants of myocardial oxygen supply and demand to change alone without change in any of the other determinants of myocardial oxygen supply and demand. The combination of a specific pattern of change in multiple hemodynamic

Hemodynamic Variable	Change	Therapy

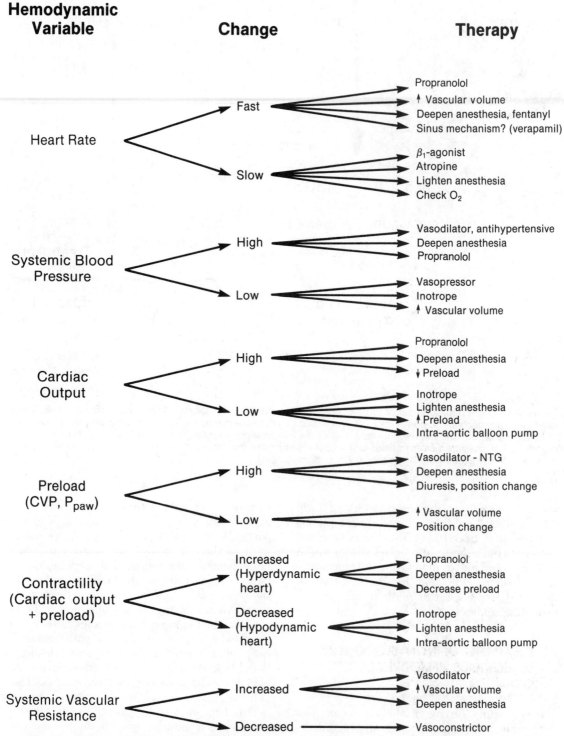

Figure 13–5. This figure lists the important hemodynamic variables that may change during anesthesia and the surgical procedure (left-hand column). These hemodynamic variables may change in either direction (middle column), and there are multiple therapeutic options for treating any change in any hemodynamic variable in any direction (right-hand column). See the text for a full explanation.

variables (constituting a hemodynamic syndrome or profile) within a specific clinical context usually makes the diagnosis. The most important and common hemodynamic syndromes that the anesthesiologist must be familiar with are caused by inadequate and excessive anesthesia, hyper- and hypovolemia, sepsis, cardiac failure due to increased afterload, and cardiac failure due to myocardial ischemia (Table 13–7).

In order to expand the hemodynamic profile enough so that a specific pattern becomes recognizable (and distinct from the other hemodynamic syndromes), it is sometimes necessary to use pulmonary artery catheter monitoring (which allows calculation of cardiac output, preload, contractility, and systemic vascular resistance) (see Table 13–7 and chapter 7). For example, the pulmonary artery wedge pressure distinguishes hypovolemia from cardiac failure due to myocardial infarction (when all other hemodynamic variables are not dramatically different) (compare row 3 with row 5, Table 13–7), whereas the cardiac output distinguishes sepsis from excessive anesthesia (when all other hemodynamic variables are not dramatically different) (compare row 6 with row 7, Table 13–7). The abnormal hemodynamic profile in the context of a specific history allows for diagnosis of the cause of the abnormal hemodynamic profile and the right therapeutic modalities to be chosen.

A. Coronary Artery Disease and Good Ventricular Function

The first three rows of Table 13–7 represent a progression of events, beginning with inadequate anesthesia and ending with cardiac failure secondary to myocardial ischemia, that might occur in a patient with coronary artery disease and good ventricular function. In this type of patient, angina pectoris is a primary symptom, hypertension is frequently present, the cardiac index is normal, the ejection fraction is greater than 0.5, left ventricular end-diastolic pressure is less than 12 mm Hg, there are no ventricular wall motion abnormalities, and the cardiovascular system is capable of a hyperdynamic response to sympathetic stimulation. Also, inadequate anesthesia causes all of the determinants of myocardial oxygen consumption to increase; that is, heart rate, preload and afterload, and contractility (row 1, Table 13–7). These early changes may be aborted by providing adequate anesthesia early on, perhaps along with nitroglycerin vasodilatation and beta-blockade. If the left ventricle experiences excessive afterload, it may become ischemic and begin to fail, as demonstrated by a decreased cardiac output despite an increased pulmonary artery wedge pressure (row 2 in Table 13–7). These intermediate changes may be reversed by dilating the arteriolar side of the circulation with nitro-

Table 13–7. Typical Common Hemodynamic Syndromes and Their Treatment

Condition	HR	P_{sa}	P_{cv}	P_{pa}	P_{paw}	Q	SVR	Treatment
Inadequate anesthesia	↑	↑	↑	↑	↑	↑	↑	Deepen anesthesia Propranolol? Vasodilator?
Cardiac failure; 2° to increased afterload	↑	↑↑	↑, N	↑	↑	↓, N	↑↑	Nitroprusside Give volume Inotrope?
Cardiac failure; 2° to myocardial ischemia	↑	↓	↓, N	↑	↑↑	↓↓	↑	Inotrope Nitroglycerin Plus volume
Hypervolemia	↓	↑	↑	↑	↑	↑	N	Restrict volume Diuretic
Hypovolemia	↑	↓	↓	↓	↓	↓	↑	Give volume
Sepsis	↓	↓	↓, N	↓, N	N	↑	↓↓	Vasoconstriction
Excessive anesthesia	↓	↓↓	↓	↓	↓	↓	↓	Lighten anesthesia Give volume Vasoconstriction

HR = heart rate; P_{sa} = systemic artery pressure; P_{cv} = central venous pressure; P_{pa} = pulmonary artery pressure; P_{paw} = pulmonary artery wedge pressure; Q = cardiac output; SVR = systemic vascular resistance; ↑ = increased; ↑↑ = very increased; ↓ = decreased; ↓↓ = very decreased; N = normal.

prusside. If the stress on the left ventricle remains unrelieved, the left ventricle then may become further ischemic and fail even more as evidenced by a further decrease in cardiac output, despite a further increase in pulmonary artery wedge pressure, and because the cardiac output is now so low there is also the beginning of systemic hypotension (row 3, Table 13–7). Under these late and severe circumstances, the heart must be aided with an inotropic drug. It should be remembered that whenever vasodilators are used, but particularly with the decreased preload effect of nitroglycerin infusion, concomitant volume infusion may often be required to maintain systemic and cardiac filling pressures at normal levels. This scenario emphasizes the importance of adequate anesthesia in patients with coronary artery disease and hyperdynamic ventricles.

B. Coronary Artery Disease and Poor Ventricular Function

The patient with coronary artery disease and poor ventricular function may have a history of or electrocardiographic evidence of previous myocardial infarction and symptoms of congestive heart failure. There is little or no cardiac reserve, the cardiac index is less than 2 L/min/m^2, the ejection fraction is less than 0.4, left ventricular end-diastolic pressure is often greater than 18 mm Hg, there may be hypokinetic or dyskinetic segments of the ventricular wall, and the heart does not tolerate loss of sympathetic input. In this patient, deep anesthesia and beta-blocking drugs should be avoided and cardiac function maintained by using narcotic anesthesia, nitroglycerin preload and afterload reduction, inotropic drugs if cardiac failure supervenes, and maintenance of preinduction filling pressures. It should be remembered that in order to maintain preinduction filling pressures in patients with poorly functioning ventricles, nitroglycerin increases the oxygen supply/demand ratio, in part, by decreasing preload (diastolic wall tension). Therefore, nitroglycerin infusion often needs to be accompanied by volume infusion in order to restore simultaneously toward normal both cardiac output and preload.

C. Arrhythmias

Finally, it should be pointed out that thoracic surgery patients are exposed to a great deal of manipulation of the heart and mediastinum; these manipulations are associated with a high incidence of supraventricular tachyarrhythmias and ventricular ectopy. Neck dissections may stimulate the carotid sinus reflex, resulting in bradycardia and hypotension. Usually, informing the surgeon of the occurrence of these arrhythmias and terminating the mechanical stimulus causes the cardiac rhythm to revert back to normal. However, on occasion the arrhythmias may persist, and it may be necessary to use one or more of the treatment modalities listed in Table 13–8. Of the halogenated anesthetics, halothane is most arrhythmogenic and isoflurane the least arrhythmogenic.

V. SPECIAL PROBLEMS RELATED TO ESOPHAGEAL SURGERY

A. Nutritional Status

Patients with esophageal diseases (strictures, tumors) present with dysphagia. The resultant dysphagia-induced poor nutrition leads to many secondary metabolic and functional changes that have important anesthetic implications (Table 13–9).[31] Dehydration due to poor fluid intake may be present, rendering the patient more susceptible to anesthesia-induced hemodynamic suppression. Dehydration may also cause prerenal failure as manifested by decreased urine output and increased blood urea nitrogen and creatinine. Hypoalbuminemia renders the patient more susceptible to an exaggerated response to drugs that are normally protein bound (thiopental, muscle relaxants, local anesthetics). Decreased plasma oncotic pressure will also make the patient more susceptible to pulmonary edema. Low levels of hemoglobin, due to poor iron intake or chronic bleeding from the site of the tumor, decrease the oxygen transport potential and often result in preoperative elevated cardiac output and a right-shifted oxygen-hemoglobin dissociation curve; subsequent decreased cardiac output due to anesthesia and left-shifting of the oxygen-hemoglobin dissociation curve due to hyperventilation may result in tissue hypoperfusion and hypoxia. Electrolytes may be altered secondary to starvation, commonly producing either hypokalemia or hypomagnesemia. Hypokalemia may be accentuated by unintentional hyperventilation or metabolic alkalosis (as may be caused by citrated blood, administration of sodium bicarbonate, loss of gastric acid, diuretics), which may cause cardiac arrhythmias, especially

Table 13–8. Arrhythmia Treatment Summary

Rhythm	First Treatment Choice	Second Treatment Choice	Third Treatment Choice
Ventricular fibrillation Ventricular tachycardia	Electrical defibrillation: 200 watt/sec (3 watt/sec/kg) with increased energy as required	Lidocaine (Xylocaine) 1.0 to 1.5 mg/kg initial IV bolus, infusion 1 to 4 mg/min (2 g/500 ml D_5W)	Propranolol (Inderal) 0.5 mg q 2 min up to 5 mg Fourth choice: Refractory ventricular fibrillation Bretylium 5 mg/kg qs 50 to 100 ml D_5W up to 30 mg/kg total dose
Premature ventricular contractions	Lidocaine (Xylocaine) 1.0 to 1.5 mg/kg initial bolus followed by infusion 1 to 4 mg/min	Propranolol (Inderal) 0.5 mg q 2 min up to 5 mg	Procainamide (Pronestyl) 100 mg q 5 min up to 1000 mg; may infuse 1 to 4 mg/min
Atrial fibrillation Atrial flutter	Digitalis (Lanoxin) 0.25 to 0.5 mg IV Ouabain 0.1 to 0.2 mg IV	Propranolol (Inderal) 0.5 mg q 2 min up to 5 mg	Cardioversion-external-synchronized-flutter: 50 watt/sec; fibrillation: 200 watt/sec; internal: 5 to 30 watt/sec-synchronized
Paroxysmal atrial tachycardia	Edrophonium 2 mg → 10 mg; can be used to improve response by increasing parasympathetic tone Carotid sinus massage: Care must be exercised with carotid vascular disease	Neosynephrine 50 to 100 μg/dose: ↑ BP and convert through carotid sinus reflex	Verapamil 5 to 10 mg IV Fourth choice: Propranolol (Inderal) 0.5 mg q 2 min up to 5 mg Fifth choice: Cardioversion, as in atrial flutter above
Sinus tachycardia	Eliminate underlying cause (e.g., fever, pain) Usually no specific treatment required. If ↑ HR → ischemia, go to second treatment	Propranolol (Inderal) 0.5 mg q 2 min up to 5 mg	
Sinus bradycardia	Eliminate underlying cause (e.g., fever, pain) Usually no specific treatment required. If hypotension or ventricular escape beats present go to second treatment	Atropine 0.3 to 2.0 mg	Ephedrine 5 to 10 mg Fourth choice: atrial pacing if heart exposed

Table 13–9. Poor Nutrition Problems Caused by Dysphagia and Their Anesthetic Implications

Dysphagia-induced Nutrition Problem	Anesthetic Implication
Dehydration	Hemodynamic instability, prerenal failure.
Hypoalbuminemia	Exaggerated response to drugs, increased susceptibility to pulmonary edema.
Decreased hemoglobin	Decreased O_2 transport, tissue hypoxia.
Hypomagnesemia	Arrhythmias, altered neuromuscular transmission.
Malnutrition	Depressed immune responses, sepsis, decreased muscle power, poor postoperative respiratory effort.

in a digitalized patient. Low levels of magnesium may cause alterations in the electrocardiogram and in neuromuscular transmission. Malnutrition also suppresses the immune response and impedes wound healing; these latter two abnormalities may increase the risk of wound infection. Malnutrition also decreases muscle power, and a poorly nourished patient is more likely to develop postoperative respiratory complications.

All these metabolic and functional abnormalities can now be corrected by total parenteral nutrition prior to surgery.[32] Consequently, parenteral nutrition is now frequently employed preoperatively; however, it is important for the anesthesiologist to realize that parenteral nutrition may pose two common special problems during anesthesia and surgery (Table 13–10).

Table 13–10. Intraoperative Problems That Can Be Caused by Preoperative Total Parenteral Nutrition

1. Hypoglycemia (reactive insulin secretion).
2. Hypercarbia (increased CO_2 production due to lipogenesis).

First, the risk of intraoperative hypoglycemia is increased in these patients.[33] The islet cells of the pancreas are stimulated during the infusion of dextrose-rich solutions, and these patients may have high levels of endogenous insulin. If the dextrose-rich infusion is stopped when the patient arrives in the operating room, and the islet cells continue to secrete insulin, hypoglycemia may develop intraoperatively within 45 to 60 minutes. If the hypoglycemic episode is prolonged, it may result in delayed awakening or coma in the postoperative period. This problem can be avoided either by infusing the parenteral nutrition solution throughout the intraoperative period at half the presurgical flow rate or by substituting 10 per cent dextrose in water at the same infusion rate.[31] Either technique prevents the intraoperative hypoglycemia, but both techniques require perioperative monitoring of the blood sugar.

Second, the preoperative administration of large amounts of glucose-rich parenteral nutritional solutions may result in lipogenesis.[34] Lipogenesis results in increased carbon dioxide production, which is removed in the awake patient by a spontaneous increase in ventilation. However, when these patients are paralyzed and mechanically ventilated intraoperatively, the use of a normal minute ventilation may result in severe hypercarbia. This can be prevented by hyperventilation, sometimes in excess of twice the normal minute ventilation. Postoperatively, the increase in CO_2 production (due to lipogenesis) may be a critical factor inhibiting the weaning of a patient from mechanical ventilatory support. Decreasing the glucose load or changing to fat emulsions, which causes a respiratory quotient of 0.7, may be useful in these circumstances (see chapter 3).[34]

B. Perioperative Regurgitation and Aspiration

Patients with esophageal disease are prone to regurgitation and aspiration. In very debilitated patients with poor laryngeal reflexes, regurgitation may lead to chronic aspiration, atelec- tasis, and pneumonia. In patients with an esophageal obstruction it may take many hours for the esophagus above the stricture to empty, and having the patient fast overnight prior to surgery does not guarantee an empty pouch above the stricture or obstruction. Consequently, if there is any question about the proximal esophageal pouch, it should be emptied by passing a large nasogastric tube and suctioning prior to induction of anesthesia. In spite of these attempts, the pouch may not be completely empty, and it is reasonable to consider these patients as having a full stomach. Patients with a hiatal hernia may have an obliterated esophagogastric angle and physiologically incompetent or dysfunctioning lower esophageal sphincter (often indicated by history of reflux).[35] They are also thus prone to regurgitation and aspiration during induction of anesthesia. With these considerations in mind, intubation should be performed either in an awake patient with sedation and topical anesthesia or by rapid-sequence induction. A nasogastric tube should be available toward the end of the operation for threading through any esophageal anastomosis and into the stomach, if the surgeon wishes. Its purpose is to prevent gastric distension and to indicate whether bleeding is continuing from the stomach; it provides no guarantee against aspiration of gastric contents into the lungs. Patients without significant pulmonary disease can be allowed to breathe spontaneously after an uncomplicated procedure but they should not be extubated until alert and sitting upright; this is because there may be no mechanical barrier to reflux and aspiration into the lungs postoperatively.

C. Preoperative Chemotherapy

Patients with esophageal cancer are often treated with chemotherapeutic drugs prior to surgery. The anticancer effect of these antibiotics is produced by formation of relatively stable complexes with DNA, which inhibits DNA and/or RNA function and synthesis.[36] These drugs affect not only the cancer cells but also rapidly growing normal cells (erythropoiesis, leukocyte and platelet production, and gastrointestinal tract lining). Commonly used chemotherapeutic drugs in carcinoma of the esophagus belong to the antibiotic group, which includes doxorubicin, bleomycin, and mitomycin C.

Toxicity secondary to doxorubicin includes severe cardiomyopathy, seen in 1.8 per cent of patients treated. When cardiomyopathy develops, it has been shown to be irreversible in 60 per cent of the patients, with death occurring within 3 weeks of the onset of the symptoms.[37] The left ventricular failure that occurs with doxorubicin is refractory to inotropic drugs. Electrocardiogram abnormalities are also part of doxorubicin toxicity, but they resolve 1 to 2 months after cessation of therapy.[38]

Bleomycin's action is similar to the effect of radiation, and bleomycin and radiation may act synergistically during simultaneous therapy.[39] Pulmonary toxicity is the most life-threatening drug-limiting effect, reported in 15 to 25 per cent of patients.[40, 41] Predisposing factors include age greater than 20 years, dose greater than 400 units, underlying pulmonary disease, and prior radiation therapy. Signs and symptoms of pulmonary toxicity are cough, dyspnea, and basal rales. The disease may manifest itself with minimal radiologic changes and normal resting P_aO_2, or it may progress to severe hypoxemia at rest, with radiologic changes similar to severe adult respiratory distress syndrome. A controversial factor that may predispose patients to pulmonary toxicity is the administration of oxygen in high concentrations.[42, 43]

Mitomycin C is also highly toxic and can cause pulmonary fibrosis and nephrotoxicity.[44] Thus, patients receiving mitomycin C should have their pulmonary and renal status fully evaluated in the preoperative period.

VI. TRANSPORT OF PATIENT[45]

Some thoracic surgery patients can be extubated while on the operating room table. These patients include those who had normal cardiopulmonary function preoperatively, underwent relatively short, physiologically nonintrusive surgery, and have an adequate postoperative vital capacity, peak inspiratory force, and spontaneous minute ventilation. These extubated patients should be sent to the postanesthesia recovery room for close observation for a period of time. However, in many thoracic surgery patients it is obvious, based on either the preoperative condition of the patient or the nature of the surgical procedure, that a period of postoperative mechanical ventilation and intensive care will be required; it is most cost effective to send these intubated patients directly to the intensive care unit (ICU). In these patients, preparation for transport to the intensive care

unit should be begun toward the end of the procedure.

A. Preparation of Patient for Transport

Once stability of the cardiovascular, respiratory, and hemostatic systems has been achieved, and the surgical wounds are being closed, preparations for transport to the ICU should be under way. The pretransport preparation checklist is shown in Table 13–11. Advance notice to the postoperative ICU should be given 30 to 45 minutes before leaving the operating suite. A suggested advance information sheet is provided in Table 13–12.

1. Respiration

If the patient is going to be intubated and/or mechanically ventilated postoperatively, the double-lumen tube must be changed to a single-lumen tube (except in rare situations in which differential lung ventilation is going to be used postoperatively [see chapter 19]). As the end of the operation approaches, the patient should be given narcotics and left paralyzed. After the patient is turned into the supine position, both lumens of the double-lumen tube, the oropharynx and nasogastric tube should be suctioned, and the patient is then ventilated with 100 per cent oxygen. The double-lumen tube should be visualized entering the larynx by direct laryngoscopy, and, while continuing to directly visualize the larynx, the double-lumen tube should be removed and the single-lumen tube inserted. Following single-lumen tube insertion, confirmation of proper single-lumen tube placement, and securement of the single-lumen tube with tape, the patient should be mechanically ventilated for several minutes while other measures are being done (see the following). It should be realized that an esophageal intubation following right pneumonectomy or transposition of the stomach into the chest may be particularly difficult to diagnose (left-sided or midline breath sounds will be heard, respectively, and left or midline chest movements seen, respectively, regardless of whether the tube is in the trachea or esophagus), and if the single-lumen tube cannot be seen to enter the trachea directly, use of capnography should be considered. Exhaled gas from the trachea will contain a normal concentration of carbon dioxide, whereas exhaled gas from the esophagus and stomach will have a minimal concentration of

Table 13–11. Pretransport Preparation Checklist

A. Respiratory system
   1. Double-lumen tube changed to single-lumen tube
   2. Arterial blood gases on $F_IO_2 = 1.0$
   3. Manual transport positive-pressure ventilation system ready
   4. Stethoscope in place
   5. Anesthesia mask present
   6. Laryngoscope present
B. Chest tube and drainage system
   1. Collection compartment below level of patient
   2. Blood and air leak not excessive
   3. Mediastinum midline
C. Circulatory system
   1. Hemodynamically stable
   2. EKG on oscilloscope
   3. Mean arterial pressure on manometer, or phasic waveform on oscilloscope
   4. Vascular catheters untangled, labeled; injection ports identified; heparin lock and flush on noninfusing lines; adequate fluid for infusing lines; drug infusions labeled and in pump meters
   5. Coagulation status satisfactory
D. Anesthesia requirements
   1. Narcotized
   2. Paralyzed
E. Miscellaneous
   1. ICU bed present
   2. Sufficient personnel available
   3. ICU notified
   4. Elevator called for
   5. Records collected
   6. All patient lines that have an operating room connection (intravascular, Foley, nasogastric, chest catheters, other monitoring lines, ventilation system) should be transferred to a transport system connection.

carbon dioxide. After 5 to 10 minutes of ventilation with 100 per cent oxygen via the single-lumen tube, arterial blood gases should be obtained and the values known before departure. A simple fool-proof manual system for providing controlled positive-pressure ventilation with an inspired oxygen concentration of 100 per cent during transport should be standing by. The transport ventilating system should allow PEEP to be provided to the patient. A sufficient supply of oxygen should be available,

remembering that a completely full E tank of oxygen contains enough gas to supply 10 to 12 L/min for approximately 50 minutes. Monitoring of ventilation should be provided both by observation of chest movements and by esophageal stethoscope breath sounds. The anesthesiologist should take along an appropriately sized anesthesia mask (to provide positive-pressure ventilation in case of inadvertent extubation), a laryngoscope (to reintubate), and some essential drugs for cardiovascular resuscitation.

Table 13–12. Advance Information Sheet for ICU

A. Respiratory system
   1. Endotracheal tube: route, size
   2. Ventilator settings: F_IO_2, tidal volume and/or peak inspiratory pressure, rate, PEEP
   3. T-piece: F_IO_2
   4. Extubated: mask F_IO_2
   5. Request immediate chest x-ray: yes, no
B. Monitoring system
   1. Arterial line: location
   2. Central venous pressure: location
   3. Pulmonary artery catheter: location
C. Intravenous catheters
   1. Site 1: location, fluid, drug
   2. Site 2: location, fluid, drug
D. Laboratory studies pending
E. Estimated time of arrival

2. Chest Tube and Drainage System[46]

The chest tube and drainage system must be functioning properly prior to transport. Two tubes are usually required to drain both air and fluid from the pleural space; one tube is placed at the anterior apex to favor the escape of air when the subject is sitting upright, and one tube is placed at the posterior base to drain accumulating fluid when the subject is supine. They are usually inserted through separate incisions just before the chest is closed. As the last stitch closing the pleural cavity is being tied, the lungs should be held fully inflated to reverse any remaining atelectasis and to help evacuate the pleural space of air and fluid.

Modern chest tube drainage systems have three compartments (Fig. 13–6). The first compartment is a simple graduated collection chamber where the amount of draining blood and fluid can be measured accurately (Fig. 13–6, right panel). The second compartment is an underwater seal that serves as a simple, but very reliable, one-way valve, which allows air to escape from the pleural space to the drainage system but not to enter the pleural space from the drainage system during the next inspiration. If the inlet drainage limb to the underwater seal compartment is put just a short distance (1 to 2 cm) below the level of the water, there is minimal resistance to the escape of air, but a huge inspiratory effort would be needed to break the seal by drawing water from the bottle up the drain and into the chest (Fig. 13–6, middle panel). The third compartment controls the amount of negative pressure that the suction can generate. The inlet drainage limb to the suction control compartment is exposed to the outlet suction above a level of water. The level of the water in the outlet limb of the suction control compartment is vented to atmosphere. If the negative pressure above the water level exceeds the height of the water level, air will come in from the suction control atmospheric vent, bubble through the water, and neutralize the excessive negative pressure above the water level (Fig. 13–6, left panel).

If functioning lung tissue remains on the operated side (resection less than a pneumonectomy, all nonpulmonary surgery), the drains should be joined to the inlet of an underwater seal as soon as the pleural cavity has been closed to prevent the lung from collapsing again (owing to accumulation of air in pleural space) while the remaining layers of the chest wall are sutured. If separate bottles are used for the drainage system (Fig. 13–6, upper panel), the

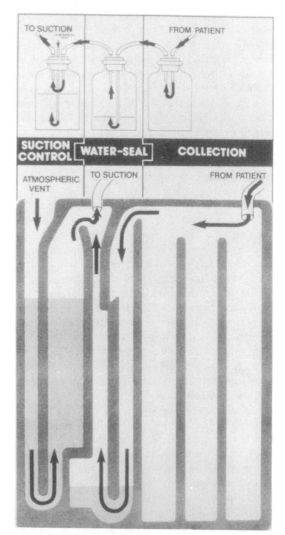

Figure 13–6. This schematic diagram of a modern chest tube drainage system shows that the chest tube drainage system is made up of three compartments. The first compartment is a collection chamber for fluids (blood, pus) from within the chest. The second compartment contains the origin of the chest tube suction and a water seal valve that prevents gas or fluid from being drawn, by a forceful spontaneous inspiration, into the chest. The third compartment controls, via an atmospheric vent, the degree of negative pressure that can be developed by chest tube drainage system suction. See the text for a further explanation.

collection compartment bottle should be below the level of the patient at all times to prevent the entry of fluid from the collection compartment and chest tube per se back into the chest. Modern disposable systems have hooks on them that can be easily attached to the lower part of the transport bed. Simple clamping of the drains is dangerous owing to the possible development of tension pneumothorax.

Air is expelled through the drain during expiration if the patient is breathing spontaneously, and the volume escaping increases during coughing. The drain will bubble continuously if there is a large leak, particularly if suction is used, and, if both blood and air are escaping simultaneously, a prohibitive amount of froth may appear; the froth can be controlled by adding an anti-foaming agent (such as a few drops of alcohol). If there is no air leak, the fluid level will move gently in the drainage tubing during quiet spontaneous respiration but will cease to swing when the lung is fully expanded and apposed to the chest wall, or if the drain is blocked. Frequent (every half hour) stripping or manually massaging the chest tubes if blood is being drained is important because once clots have begun to collect within the chest, chest tube function deteriorates, and the likelihood of the need for re-exploration for hemopneumothorax increases.

Following a pneumonectomy, but before transport, the position (laterality) of the mediastinum should be ascertained.[47] This can be done in two ways: clinical examination and measurement of pressure in the hemithorax. Clinical data consist of determining the position of the trachea and inspecting the anterior-posterior chest roentgenogram. Perhaps more practical and accurate is the measurement of pressure in the empty hemithorax by manometer. If the pressure in the empty hemithorax is significantly positive then it is likely the mediastinum is shifted into the contralateral hemithorax, and if the pressure in the empty hemithorax is significantly negative, then it is likely the mediastinum is shifted into the ipsilateral hemithorax. To get the mediastinum in the midline, air can be injected into or aspirated from the empty hemithorax, as dictated by the ongoing pressure manometer readings.

Closing the chest without drainage following pneumonectomy makes it more difficult to recognize serious postoperative hemorrhage. Consequently, a single basal chest drain is usually used and is joined to an underwater seal bottle without suction (suction would cause a mediastinal shift to the ipsilateral side and, perhaps, cardiovascular collapse). It is left unclamped until the patient is lying on his back and breathing spontaneously. Some air usually escapes through the drain when the patient is turned from the lateral to the supine position, or if coughing occurs, when spontaneous ventilation is being re-established. This air should be allowed to escape so that pressure does not build up within the space and cause surgical emphysema around the drain or the wound site. The mediastinum should be central at the end of the operation if this routine is followed, and once this has been confirmed, the tube is clamped and remains so while the patient is returned for postoperative supervision. Thereafter it is unclamped for 1 to 2 minutes every hour for the first 12 to 24 hours so that the excess fluid may drain, thereby preventing unwanted mediastinal shift.

3. Circulation

For the patient to be a candidate for leaving the operating room, the cardiovascular system must be stable. Vascular volume status should be optimal for that particular patient, as judged by the urine output, systemic pressure, left- or right-sided filling pressures or both, and cardiac output, if available. All vascular catheters should be identified by label, and should be free and untangled with at least one injection port conveniently placed. Adequate fluid for all vascular lines should be available. Drugs being administered by continuous infusion should be reviewed, and the administration rates and cardiovascular responses confirmed to be appropriate. The cardiac rate, rhythm, and mean arterial pressure should be monitored during transport. Essential cardiovascular resuscitation drugs should be taken along.

4. Coagulation

If massive transfusion was required intraoperatively, the coagulation status should be normal, or as nearly normal as possible at the time of transport. All products to treat coagulation abnormalities should have been administered if possible. Blood specimens should be sent to the laboratory from the operating room for the determination of coagulation status (ACT, aPTT, PT, fibrinogen), platelet count, hematocrit, serum potassium, and arterial blood gases. The results of these determinations will therefore be available to the ICU personnel within moments of the patient's arrival in the ICU.

5. Miscellaneous

A fully functional ICU bed should be available for direct patient transfer. All records should be collected in order for them to be transported with the patient. Sufficient personnel to effect a smooth transport should be gathered. Prior to moving the patient all possible connections of the patient to the operating room must be disengaged, such as pressure lines to transducers, electrocardiogram leads to the room monitor, chest tube and Foley catheters to the operating room table, and intravenous lines to operating room poles, and must be transferred to their appropriate places on the transport bed. If an elevator is to be used, it should be called for so that it is there waiting for the transport team.

B. The Transport[41]

Preferably, the patient should only be moved once, and that is directly from the operating room table to the ICU bed. The move should be performed smoothly and gently to minimize vascular volume shifts or changes in cardiac function. A carefully coordinated move by a sufficient number of personnel should prevent accidents such as disconnected intravascular lines and various tubes being pulled out or malpositioned. The anesthesiologist should only be responsible for ventilation and monitoring, not moving, fetching, or adjusting parts of the bed.

Monitoring during transport should include at least an esophageal stethoscope for respiratory and cardiovascular sounds and an oscillographic display of the electrocardiogram. In addition, if an arterial line is in situ, mean arterial pressure should be monitored, at a minimum, with a sterile anaeroid gauge directly connected to the arterial line by a 50 cm segment of sterile intravenous tubing. Still better, and presently practiced more commonly, is an oscillographic display of the electrocardiogram and arterial pressure waveform on a portable monitor for continuous observation during transport. A defibrillator should also accompany the very critically ill patient. The longer and more complex the route to the ICU, the more care must be exercised in planning and execution of this transport. If an elevator separates the operating room from the ICU, it should be equipped with a separate reserve oxygen system, electrical power outlet, phone communication system, and if possible, suction equipment (physicians responsible for transport should ask themselves what they would want available in an elevator that is jammed for 2 hours).

C. Arrival In Intensive Care Unit[41]

Upon arrival in the ICU, the pretransport operating room take-down should be reversed and a quick ICU arrival hook-up performed. Priorities should be the same as in a cardiac resuscitation; establishment of the airway, adequate gas exchange, and circulation. Ventilatory function is assessed as the patient's airway is connected to a ventilator, set initially with an F_IO_2 of 100 per cent. Other initial ventilator settings such as tidal volume, respiratory rate, and PEEP level should duplicate those found optimal in the operating room (see chapter 19). The chest must be seen and heard to move bilaterally. Vital signs of immediate importance are cardiac rate and rhythm (electrocardiogram) and mean arterial and cardiac filling pressures. Infusion rates of potent drugs are verified, and desired cardiovascular responses are confirmed.

Tasks of lesser importance can be performed as time permits. Laboratory and other diagnostic procedures should be performed as soon as practical (chest film, arterial blood gases, electrolytes, hematocrit, 12-lead electrocardiogram, and coagulation screen if indicated). Before the anesthesiologist leaves the ICU, he or she should ascertain the present status of the patient, confirm cardiovascular and respiratory stability, be assured that no problems of an acute nature exist, and confirm that the ICU nurses are satisfied with the patient's status. A brief early postoperative note as well as a copy of the anesthetic record should be placed in the patient's chart.

REFERENCES

1. Gold MI, Helrich M: Pulmonary mechanics during general anesthesia: V. Status asthmaticus. Anesthesiology 32:422–428, 1970.
2. Rossing TH, Fanta CH, Goldstein DH, et al: Emergency therapy of asthma: Comparison of the acute effect of parenteral and inhaled sympathomimetics and infused aminophylline. Am Rev Resp Dis 127:365, 1980.
3. Littenberg B, Gluck EH: A controlled trial of methylprednisolone in the emergency treatment of acute asthma. N Engl J Med 314:150–152, 1986.
4. Pietak S, Weenig CS, Hickey RF, et al: Anesthetic effects on ventilation in patients with chronic obstructive pulmonary disease. Anesthesiology 72:160, 1975.
5. Little AG, Lagmuir VK, Singer AH, Skinner DB: Hemodynamic pulmonary edema in dogs' lungs after contralateral pneumonectomy and mediastinal lymphatic interruption. Lung 162:139–145, 1984.
6. Zeldin RA, Normandin D, Landtwing D, Peters RM: Postpneumonectomy pulmonary edema. J Thor Cardiovasc Surg 87:359–365, 1984.

7. Lee E, Little AG, Hsu WH, Skinner DB: Effect of pneumonectomy on extravascular lung water in dogs. J Surg Res 38:568–573, 1985.
8. Zapol W: Commentary on postpneumonectomy pulmonary edema. Intell Anesth 2:15, 1985.
9. Sibbald WJ, Driedger AA, Myers ML, Short AIK, Wells GA: Biventricular function in the adult respiratory distress syndrome: Chest 84:126–134, 1983.
10. Sykes MK: Indications for blood transfusion. Can Anaesth Soc J 22:3–11, 1975.
11. Pineda AA, Taswell HF, Brzica SM: Delayed hemolytic transfusion reaction; an immunologic hazard of blood transfusion. Transfusion 18:1–7, 1978.
12. Anonymous: The bleeding time and the hematocrit (Editorial). Lancet 1:997–998, 1984.
13. Gillies IDS: Anaemia and anaesthesia. Br J Anaesth 46:589–602, 1974.
14. Roth JA, Gollub EA, Grimm BA, Eilber MD, Morton DL: Effects of operation on immune response in cancer patients. Sequential evaluation of in vitro lymphocyte function. Surgery 79:46–51, 1976.
15. Burrows L, Tartter PI: Effect of blood transfusions on chronic malignancy recurrence rate. Lancet 2:662, 1982.
16. Agarwal M, Blumber N: Colon cancer patients transfused perioperatively have an increased incidence of recurrence (Abstract). Transfusion 24:421, 1983.
17. Tartter PI, Papatestas AE, Lesnick G, Burrows L, Aufses AH Jr: Perioperative blood transfusion has prognostic significance for breast cancer. Surgery 97:225–230, 1985.
18. Tartter PI, Burrows L, Kirschner P: Perioperative blood transfusion adversely affects prognosis after resection of stage 1(N_0) non–oat cell lung cancer. J Thor Cardiovasc Surg 88:659–662, 1984.
19. Hyman N, Foster RS Jr, DeMeules JE, Costanza MC: Blood transfusion and survival after lung cancer. Am J Surg 149:502–507, 1985.
20. Peterffy A, Henze A: Haemorrhagic complications during pulmonary resection. Scand J Thor Cardiovasc Surg 17:283–287, 1983.
21. Bregman D, Parodi EN, Hutchinson JE: Intraoperative autotransfusion during emergency thoracic and elective open heart surgery. Ann Thorac Surg 18:590, 1974.
22. Horsey PJ: Blood transfusion. In Atkinson RS, Hewer CLA (eds): Recent Advances in Anaesthesia and Analgesia. New York, Churchill-Livingstone, 1982, chapter 14, pp 89–103.
23. McKittrick JE: Bank autologous blood in elective surgery. Am J Surg 128:137, 1974.
24. Anonymous: Haemoglobin and the ischaemic foot (Editorial). Lancet 2:184–185, 1979.
25. Fischbach DP, Fogdall RP: Coagulation: The Essentials. Baltimore, Williams & Wilkins Co, 1981.
26. Ellison N, Ominsky AJ: Clinical considerations for the anesthesiologist whose patient is on anticoagulant therapy. Anesthesiology 39:328–336, 1973.
27. Ellison N: Coagulation evaluation and management. In Ream AK, Fogdall RP (eds): Acute Cardiovascular Management. Philadelphia, JB Lippincott Co, 1982, chapter 24, pp 773–805.
28. Bowie EJW, Thompson HJ Jr, Didisheim P, et al: Mayo Clinic Laboratory Manual of Hemostasis. Philadelphia, WB Saunders Co, 1971.
29. Miller RD: Problems in massive transfusion. Anesthesiology 39:82–93, 1973.
30. Miller RD, Robbins TO, Tong MJ, et al: Coagulation defects associated with massive blood transfusion. Ann Surg 174:794–801, 1971.
31. Rao TLK, El-Etr AA: Esophageal and mediastinal surgery. In Kaplan JA (ed): Thoracic Anesthesia. New York, Churchill-Livingstone, 1983, chapter 14, pp 447–474.
32. Ruberg RL, Dudrick SJ: Intravenous hyperalimentation in head and neck tumor surgery: Indications and precautions. Br J Plast Surg 30:151–153, 1977.
33. Reinhardt GF, DeOrio AJ, Kaminski MV Jr: Total parenteral nutrition. Surg Clin North Am 57:1283–1301, 1977.
34. Askanazi J, Carpentier YA, Elwyn DH, et al: Influence of total parenteral nutrition on fuel utilization in injury and sepsis. Ann Surg 191:40–46, 1980.
35. Lowery BD, Vaccaro P, Anderson E, et al: The operative management of symptomatic esophageal reflux. Ohio State Med J 28:446–450, 1980.
36. Umezawa H: Principles of antitumor antibiotic therapy. In Holland JF, Frei 'R III (eds): Cancer Medicine. Philadelphia, Lea and Febiger, 1973, pp 817–826.
37. Gottlieb JA, Lefrak EA, O'Bryan RM, et al: Fatal adriamycin cardiomyopathy: Prevention by dose limitation. Proc Am Assoc Cancer Res 14:88–97, 1973.
38. Lefrak EA, Pitha J, Rosenheim S, et al: Adriamycin (NSC-12317) cardiomyopathy. Cancer Chemother Rep 6:203–208, 1975.
39. Jorgensen SJ: Time-dose relationships in combined bleomycin therapy and radiotherapy. Eur J Cancer 8:531–534, 1972.
40. Samuels MS, Johnson DE, Holoye PY, et al: Large-dose bleomycin therapy and pulmonary toxicity: A possible role of prior radiotherapy. JAMA 235:1117–1120, 1976.
41. Rudders RA, Mensley GT: Bleomycin pulmonary toxicity. Chest 63:626–628, 1976.
42. Goldiner PL, Carlon CC, Cvitkovic E, et al: Factors influencing postoperative morbidity and mortality in patients treated with bleomycin. Br Med J 1:1664–1667, 1978.
43. Matalon S, Harper WV, Nickerson PA, et al: Intravenous bleomycin does not alter the toxic effects of hyperoxia in rabbits. Anesthesiology 64:614–619, 1986.
44. Selvin BL: Cancer chemotherapy: Implications for the anesthesiologist. Anesth Analg 60:425–434, 1981.
45. Fogdall RP: The post-bypass period. In Ream AK, Fogdall RP (eds): Acute Cardiovascular Management. Philadelphia, JB Lippincott Co, 1982, chapter 15, pp 456–480.
46. Gothard JWW, Branthwaite MA: Anaesthesia for Thoracic Surgery. Oxford, Blackwell Scientific Publications, 1982, pp 97–98.
47. Gothard JWW, Branthwaite MA: Anaesthesia for Thoracic Surgery. Oxford, Blackwell Scientific Publications, 1982, p 124.

IV

**INTRAOPERATIVE
CONSIDERATIONS FOR SPECIAL
THORACIC SURGERY CASES**

Anesthesia for Special Elective Diagnostic Procedures

14

I. INTRODUCTION

There are a number of very common invasive diagnostic procedures used to evaluate thoracic surgery patients. These diagnostic procedures all have special anesthetic implications and problems. Bronchoscopy requires that the airway be shared between the anesthesiologist and the endoscopist, which causes special problems for ventilation and anesthetic technique. Mediastinoscopy can cause compression of important vessels and hemorrhage, and the anesthesiologist's attention must be focused on recognizing these complications. In addition, these patients must not be allowed to strain or cough. Thoracoscopy sometimes involves double-lumen tube intubation and one-lung ventilation. Esophagoscopy itself is relatively straightforward, but these patients are often debilitated and have a high risk of aspiration, and patient movement can cause an esophageal tear. This chapter considers these four common major diagnostic techniques in the order just mentioned.

II. BRONCHOSCOPY

Bronchoscopy is the most common invasive procedure used for the diagnosis and treatment

of chest diseases. There are three general diagnostic indications for bronchoscopy.[1] First, bronchoscopy is indicated to investigate the cause of medically resistant chronic chest symptoms and signs (cough, pain, wheeze, atelectasis, pneumonia). Second, bronchoscopy is indicated to determine the site, extent, and cause of acute changes such as hemoptysis, acute inhalation injury, and regional abnormality on the chest x-ray. Third, bronchoscopy is an essential tool in the evaluation of patients for thoracic surgery (to evaluate the tracheobronchial tree for tumors, to rule out metastases, to obtain tissue and specimens [cytology, biopsies, cultures], to determine presence and exact level of tracheobronchial esophageal fistula, to palpate the carinal and subcarinal areas). The therapeutic indications are to aid in the treatment of acute respiratory failure (remove secretions, reverse atelectasis, drain abscess, position endotracheal tubes), to aid in laser resection of bronchogenic carcinoma, and to allow for removal of foreign bodies. This chapter discusses anesthesia for diagnostic bronchoscopy. The anesthetic management of the various therapeutic bronchoscopies are discussed elsewhere (laser resection of tumors in chapter 15, removal of foreign bodies in chapter 16, treatment of acute respiratory failure and aid in mechanical ventilation in chapter 19).

There are three types of bronchoscopes in current use, and they consist of the flexible fiberoptic, rigid ventilating, and rigid Venturi (Sanders injector) types. The manner in which patients are ventilated with these bronchoscopes differs considerably, and the different ventilatory considerations have important implications for anesthetic technique (see Table 14–1). Flexible fiberoptic bronchoscopy may be performed with local or general anesthesia, whereas rigid ventilating and Venturi bronchoscopy is best performed under general anesthesia. Since the inspired oxygen and inhalational anesthetic concentration is known with a rigid ventilating bronchoscope but not known with a rigid Venturi bronchoscope, rigid ventilating bronchoscopy can be performed with either inhalational (including nitrous oxide) or intravenous general anesthesia, whereas rigid Venturi bronchoscopy is best performed with intravenous general anesthesia and 100 per cent oxygen. Since minute ventilation is constant with either fiberoptic or rigid Venturi bronchoscopy (no need to interrupt ventilation) but not with rigid ventilating bronchoscopy (need to interrupt ventilation when the eyepiece is removed), the former two can be comfortably used for long procedures, whereas the latter should be used for relatively short procedures. In view of these differences in ventilatory and anesthetic technique, the different bronchoscopes will be discussed separately.

A. Fiberoptic Bronchoscope

1. Indications

Use of the flexible fiberoptic bronchoscope is especially indicated for bronchoscopy whenever there are mechanical problems with the neck that would make rigid bronchoscopy especially difficult, whenever upper lobe and peripheral lung lesions need to be visualized and are

beyond the reach and capability of a rigid bronchoscope (the fiberoptic bronchoscope can examine the third to possibly the fourth order of bronchi), and whenever there is a need to find the site of limited and perhaps distal hemoptysis, to aid in the treatment of respiratory failure, to obtain very localized cultures, biopsies and cytology, and to perform selective bronchography.[1-5]

2. Ventilatory Considerations

In a nonintubated patient flexible fiberoptic bronchoscopes with outside diameters of 5.0, 5.7, and 6.0 mm occupy 6, 10, and 11 per cent, respectively, of the cross-sectional area of an average 70 kg adult trachea (which has a diameter of 18 mm). Consequently, spontaneous ventilation and removal of carbon dioxide is not usually significantly impaired in a nonintubated, nonbronchospastic, spontaneously ventilating patient undergoing fiberoptic bronchoscopy under local anesthesia. However, since the suction port is capable of removing large amounts of air (14.2 L/min at 760 mm Hg through a 2 mm suction port), which may cause atelectasis (especially if the bronchoscope becomes wedged during suctioning), oxygen supplementation is highly desirable.[6, 7] This can be accomplished by having the patient breathe through nasal cannulas or, more preferably, through a facial mask (which provides a higher F_1O_2) that has a hole cut in it to allow for insertion of the fiberoptic bronchoscope.

In an intubated patient (which would usually be the case if general anesthesia were used), the fiberoptic bronchoscope occupies a very significant amount of the cross-sectional area of the endotracheal tube. Figure 14–1 shows the reduction in effective size of any sized endotracheal tube with a 5.0, 5.7, and 6.0 mm outside diameter fiberoptic bronchoscopy.[8] For example, a 5.7 mm outside diameter fiberoptic bron-

Table 14–1. Ventilation Characteristics and Anesthetic Implications of the Three Different Types of Bronchoscopes

Type of Bronchoscope	F_1O_2	Concentration of Inhalation Anesthesia	Constancy of Minute Ventilation	Suitable Duration of Procedure	Preferred Type of Anesthesia
Flexible fiberoptic	Known	Known	Constant	Long	Local or general anesthesia
Rigid ventilating	Known	Known	Inconstant	Short (15 to 20 min)	Inhalational or intravenous general anesthesia
Rigid Venturi	Unknown	Unknown	Constant	Long	Intravenous general anesthesia

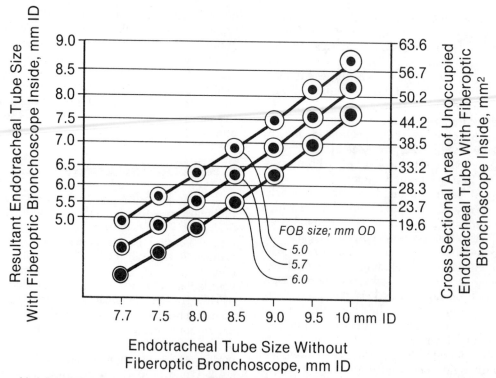

Figure 14–1. This diagram relates the size of an endotracheal tube without an indwelling fiberoptic bronchoscope (x-axis) to the resultant functional size that the endotracheal tube would have with an indwelling fiberoptic bronchoscope (left-hand y-axis) (three fiberoptic bronchoscope sizes are shown: 5.0, 5.7, and 6.0 mm outside diameter). The cross-sectional area of unoccupied endotracheal tube in mm² that is responsible for the resultant functional size is shown on the right-hand y-axis. (The diagram is a modification [with permission] of Figure 7 of reference 8.)

choscope occupies 41 and 52 per cent of the cross-sectional areas of 9 and 8 mm internal diameter endotracheal tubes, respectively, which reduces the functional internal diameters of these endotracheal tubes to 7.0 and 5.5 mm, respectively.[8] In view of the greatly reduced surface area available for ventilation under these circumstances, it is obvious that ventilation must either be controlled or vigorously assisted with positive-pressure ventilation. This may be easily accomplished by passing the fiberoptic bronchoscope through a self-sealing rubber diaphragm in the elbow connector to the endotracheal tube; tidal ventilation then occurs around the fiberoptic bronchoscope but within the endotracheal tube (Fig. 14–2). However, it must be realized that if the fiberoptic bronchoscope occupies too much of the cross-sectional area of the endotracheal tube, tidal gas may enter the lungs under positive pressure, but the elastic recoil of the lung may not force the tidal gas out of the lungs, and distal gas trapping, high distal PEEP, and barotrauma may result. Consequently, a low inspiratory-to-expiratory time

ratio is desirable. In light of these considerations, it is apparent that an endotracheal tube with an internal diameter of 8.0 to 8.5 mm or larger should be used with any adult-sized fiberoptic bronchoscope.[8] If a smaller endotracheal tube must be used (e.g., 7.0 mm internal diameter), then use of helium/oxygen mixtures should be considered (see chapter 3).[9] In addition, periods of hyperventilation with 100 per cent oxygen without the fiberoptic bronchoscope in place may need to be alternated with short periods of fiberoptic bronchoscopy.

3. Anesthetic Technique

a. LOCAL ANESTHESIA

Patients with reactive airways may need preoperative bronchodilatation (B_2-agonists, aminophylline, steroids; see chapter 13 and Fig. 13–1). In addition, atropine premedication[10, 11] is useful to decrease the volume of secretions and to cause some bronchodilatation. Diazepam and barbiturates are useful to decrease anxiety and systemic toxicity of local anesthetics.

Fiberoptic Bronchoscope
Endotracheal Tube Ventilating System

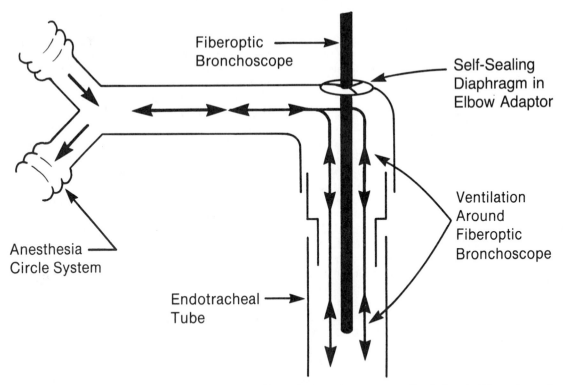

Figure 14–2. *This schematic diagram shows that a fiberoptic bronchoscope is ordinarily inserted through a self-sealing diaphragm in the elbow connector to an endotracheal tube. Inspired gas under positive pressure from the anesthesia circle machine goes around the outside of the fiberoptic bronchoscope but within the lumen of the endotracheal tube. Exhaled gas is via the same route into the anesthesia circle system. The seal of the diaphragm in the elbow connector around the fiberoptic bronchoscope insures the ability to continue positive pressure ventilation while the fiberoptic bronchoscope is in use.*

The fiberoptic bronchoscope is relatively easily and atraumatically passed through the nose into the trachea when the patient has had adequate topical anesthesia and sedation. The naris selected is the one that the patient can breathe through most easily (presumably, this is the naris that is the larger or less obstructed one). There are several local anesthetic techniques that clearly facilitate nasotracheal fiberoptic bronchoscopy; all techniques or combination of techniques must anesthetize the nose, pharynx, larynx, and trachea (Table 14–2).

The nose may be anesthetized by spraying either 0.5 per cent tetracaine with epinephrine or 4 per cent lidocaine with epinephrine, by topically applying cocaine by cotton-tipped

Table 14–2. *Local Anesthetic Techniques for Nasotracheal Fiberoptic Bronchoscopy*

1. Cocaine (10 per cent) to nasal mucosa.
2. Soft nasopharyngeal airways liberally coated with lidocaine ointment.
3. Local anesthetic spray to nasopharyngeal, oropharyngeal, laryngeal and tracheal mucosal surfaces.
   a. Tetracaine 0.5 per cent with epinephrine.
   b. Lidocaine 4 per cent.
4. Superior laryngeal nerve block.
   a. Externally by needle.
   b. Internally by swab soaked in local anesthetic.
5. Transtracheal block
6. Local anesthetic spray down suction channel of fiberoptic bronchoscope.

wooden pledgets (total dose over 15 min in a 70 kg patient not to exceed 300 to 400 mg [3 to 4 ml of 10 per cent solution]), or by passing progressively larger soft nasopharyngeal airways that are liberally coated with lidocaine. The first two nasal techniques both anesthetize the nose and shrink the nasal mucosa by active vasoconstriction, whereas the last technique anesthetizes the nose and dilates the nasal cavity by mechanical means.

The pharynx may be anesthetized by spraying local anesthetic through the oral cavity over the tongue and pharynx or by gargling viscous lidocaine. The larynx may be anesthetized by continuing the local anesthetic spray via the mouth and nose, by superior laryngeal nerve blocks with 2 ml of 2 per cent lidocaine, or by transtracheal block with 4 ml of 4 per cent lidocaine during exhalation. The superior laryngeal nerve block technique consists of needle application of local anesthetic to the thyrohyoid membrane between the superior lateral cornu of the thyroid cartilage and the inferior lateral margin of the cornu of the hyoid bone (Fig. 14–3).[12, 13] An internal superior laryngeal nerve block technique consists of painting the pyriform fossae with sponges that are soaked with local anesthetic. Superior laryngeal nerve block anesthetizes the lower pharynx, laryngeal epiglottis, vallecula, vestibule, aryepiglottic fold, and posterior rima glottis.

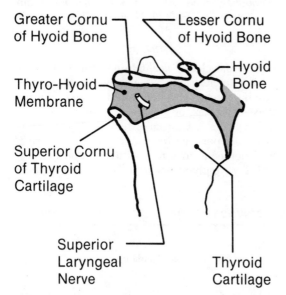

Greater Cornu of Hyoid Bone

Lesser Cornu of Hyoid Bone

Hyoid Bone

Thyro-Hyoid Membrane

Superior Cornu of Thyroid Cartilage

Superior Laryngeal Nerve

Thyroid Cartilage

Figure 14–3. This schematic diagram shows the point of emergence of the superior laryngeal nerve through the thyrohyoid membrane between the superior lateral cornu of the thyroid cartilage and the inferior aspect of the hyoid bone. Local anesthetic injected at this point will cause a superior laryngeal nerve block.

The trachea may be anesthetized by the local anesthetic spray as the patient breathes the nebulized material, by the transtracheal block, or by local anesthetic sprayed down the suction channel of the fiberoptic bronchoscope. Once the fiberoptic bronchoscope is introduced into the trachea, topicalization of the distal tracheobronchial tree can be accomplished by continuing to spray local anesthetic down the suction channel of the fiberoptic bronchoscope. Transtracheal block is the least performed maneuver because of the impressive anterior and posterior mucosal bruise that can be caused by the block and regularly observed with the fiberoptic bronchoscope following the block (personal observation).

As can be seen from the preceding list of techniques, the one that can anesthetize everything (naris, pharynx, largynx, trachea) is simply spraying local anesthetic through the nose and the oral cavity. In the author's experience, 0.5 per cent tetracaine with epinephrine provides a more complete block than 4 per cent lidocaine. A very simple but effective system that produces a very dense cloud or mist of local anesthetic is shown in Figure 14–4. In the author's experience, this system has made nebulization of local anesthetic to all the mucosal surfaces the single most effective local anesthetic maneuver and can provide adequate anesthesia by itself alone. It is extremely important for the anesthetist to be unhurried and complete (10-sec spraying periods should be alternated with 10- to 20-sec rest periods); this approach usually requires at least 15 min to result in adequate anesthesia. The total dose of tetracaine over 15 min in a 70-kg patient should not exceed 100 mg (20 ml of 0.5 per cent solution), and the total dose of lidocaine over 15 min in a 70-kg patient should not exceed 400 mg (10 ml of 4 per cent solution).

It cannot be stressed enough that tracheal intubation with a fiberoptic bronchoscope is a difficult procedure if anesthesia is inadequate (the operator will have a violent moving field of vision), whereas the procedure is relatively easy if the patient is adequately anesthetized (the operator has a quiet field). Consequently the author uses, in addition to the local anesthetic spray of all the mucosal surfaces (Fig. 14–4), cocaine to the nose or soft nasopharyngeal airways coated with lidocaine ointment (if the nose is going to be used), pharyngeal gargle of viscous lidocaine, and, perhaps, bilateral superior laryngeal nerve blocks.

It is apparent from Table 14–2 that there are several other permutations of local anesthetic

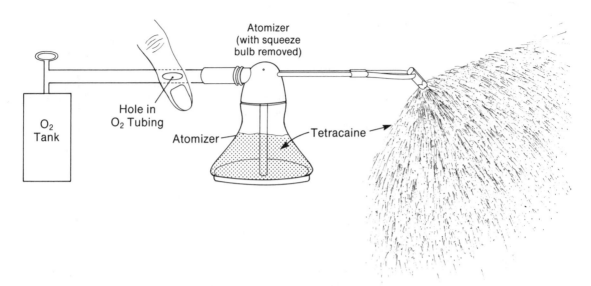

Figure 14–4. This schematic diagram shows the system for creating a fine mist of local anesthetic. Oxygen green tubing is connected to an oxygen tank. A hole is cut in the oxygen green tubing near the nebulization chamber. When oxygen is flowing in the green tubing and a finger is placed over the hole, a fine dense mist from the nebulization chamber results. The size and velocity of spread of the mist is proportional to the oxygen flow rate.

techniques that may be used to anesthetize all of the upper airway mucosal surfaces. However, no matter which technique or combination of techniques is used, unless the anesthetist is thorough and patient and allows for a sufficient amount of time (approximately 20 min) to achieve adequate anesthesia, any approach may result in spotty anesthesia. With all techniques, intravenous lidocaine is useful in depressing the cough reflex as well as decreasing the incidence of arrhythmias.[14-16]

b. GENERAL ANESTHESIA

It is important to realize at the outset that the amount of general anesthesia required for bronchoscopy can be greatly diminished if some topical local anesthesia is used. Again, the single most effective maneuver that one can do to anesthetize the entire upper respiratory passages is to nebulize local anesthetic to all the upper airway mucosal surfaces. Two types of general anesthesia, or a combination of the two, may be used with a fiberoptic bronchoscope. Either an oxygen-nitrous oxide, intravenous barbiturate/narcotic, short-acting muscle relaxant (succinylcholine drip, atracurium or vecuronium) and/or a halogenated drug anesthesia technique may be used. The factors that determine the choice between the two techniques are extensively discussed in chapter 8. It is important to emphasize that with either type of general anesthetic adequate anesthesia to prevent laryngospasm and bronchospasm is of par-

amount importance. Administration of intravenous lidocaine will significantly depress the cough reflex and decrease the incidence of premature ventricular contractions during either type of general anesthesia.[14-16] Postoperatively, the patients should breathe an elevated F_IO_2 for several hours (see complications).[10, 17]

4. Complications

Intraoperative laryngospasm and bronchospasm due to inadequate anesthesia are the most common intraoperative emergencies during fiberoptic bronchoscopy.[18, 19] Intraoperative hypoxemia is also common[6, 7, 17, 18] and can be a result of either poor ventilation (due to bronchospasm or using a fiberoptic bronchoscope that is too large) or atelectasis (due to suctioning from a wedged position). Major cardiac arrhythmias may develop in as many as 11 per cent of patients during fiberoptic bronchoscopy, and the occurrence of the arrhythmias is often associated with the presence of a $P_aO_2 < 60$ mm Hg.[20] If hypoxemia is corrected, the arrhythmias are usually self-limiting and do not need to be treated. Deleterious hemodynamic effects of PEEP and parenchymal barotrauma may result intraoperatively if the cross-sectional area of the endotracheal tube is reduced greatly enough by the fiberoptic bronchoscope, thereby preventing the escape of expired gases. A chest x-ray should be obtained postoperatively to rule out mediastinal emphysema and pneumothorax if high airway pressures were noted during the procedure.[3, 8] Bleeding is an infrequent complication of fiberoptic bronchoscopy (may follow transbronchial biopsy).[21]

Hypoxemia develops during fiberoptic bronchoscopy in both healthy volunteers and sick patients, with an average decline of the P_aO_2 by 20 mm Hg, and lasts for 1 to 4 hours following the procedure.[17, 22-24] Hypoxemia occurring after fiberoptic bronchoscopy is mainly due to atelectasis caused by suctioning while the bronchoscope was in a wedged position. Consequently, in patients with an endotracheal tube, the anesthesiologist should sigh the patient with positive pressure at the end of the procedure. In addition, patients may develop increased airway obstruction after fiberoptic bronchoscopy,[17] probably secondary to direct mechanical activation of cough and irritative reflexes in the airway and possibly by direct trauma-induced mucosal edema.[10]

B. Rigid Ventilating Bronchoscope

1. Indications

There are several relative indications for the use of a rigid bronchoscope. First, it is the instrument of choice for foreign body removal (see chapter 16). Second, massive hemoptysis (500 ml per 24 hours) must be assessed with an open tube bronchoscope (see chapter 16). Adequate suctioning, removal of blood clots with a large forceps, and packing of a major bleeding site can be much more readily accomplished with a rigid rather than a fiberoptic bronchoscope. In addition, control of the airway can be maintained during all these therapeutic maneuvers. On rare occasion, it may be necessary to position the bronchoscope in one mainstem bronchus to provide ventilation to one lung (and seal off the bleeding lung) while the patient is taken to the operating room. Third, constricting and/or bleeding lesions may be by-passed by an open tube bronchoscope if the airway becomes seriously compromised. Fourth, the open tube bronchoscope allows a large biopsy of a main bronchial neoplasm to be taken. Fifth, the rigid bronchoscope allows the surgeon to palpate the carina preoperatively to assess operability and to identify extension of subcarinal disease. Finally, the rigid bronchoscope is necessary for small children (see chapter 17).

2. Ventilatory Considerations

The rigid ventilating bronchoscope may be attached directly to an anesthesia machine circuit via a sidearm adapter (Fig. 14–5). Consequently, inspired oxygen and anesthetic gas concentrations are known and can be administered with conventional or high-frequency positive-pressure ventilation. Although spontaneous ventilation may be allowed, the dangers of inadequate ventilation due to bronchospasm and a tight chest wall (too light anesthesia), or hypoventilation (too deep anesthesia) and tracheobronchial tree damage due to unexpected coughing usually cause the risk/benefit ratio of spontaneous ventilation to be high. Consequently, these patients should usually be paralyzed, and ventilation should be controlled with positive pressure. Since the usual rigid Negus bronchoscope has an external diameter of 11 mm, there is usually a variable leak around the distal end of the bronchoscope (with the proximal eye piece in place), but this may be compensated for by using a high gas flow rate (greater than 10 L/min) (first choice) or by packing the pharynx with saline-soaked gauze (second choice). It is possible to provide effective ventilation in the vast majority of patients with this system. However, the proximal eye piece must be removed during suctioning, foreign body manipulations, or the taking of biopsies. Since ventilation must be interrupted when the surgeon removes the occluding eye piece (all the inspired gas including the inhalational anesthetics, which can sedate the endoscopist, go into the room out the open proximal end), a high F_IO_2 should be used if the surgeon requires removal of the eye piece for a considerable period of time. One to two minutes maximum of apnea may be allowed at any one time before ventilation must be resumed, with a shorter time allowed for obese patients and patients with lung disease.[25] In view of the leak around the bronchoscope and the frequent periods of apnea necessitated by removal of the eye piece, a rigid ventilating bronchoscope must be viewed as an inherently unstable system that should not be used for prolonged procedures (greater than 20 to 30 min).

3. Anesthetic Technique

a. LOCAL ANESTHESIA

Passing a rigid bronchoscope into the trachea requires a considerable amount of pressure, mucosal stimulation, and extreme neck extension that is not required for fiberoptic bronchoscopy. In addition, there is no guarantee in an awake patient that the patient will not suddenly move at a critical point due to some noxious or unpleasant stimulus. Consequently,

Rigid Ventilating Bronchoscope

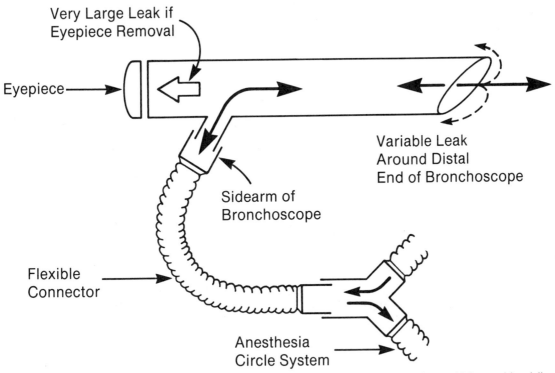

Figure 14–5. This schematic diagram shows a rigid ventilating bronchoscope system, which consists of the anesthesia circle system attached to a flexible connector that is attached to the sidearm of the bronchoscope. With the proximal eye-piece in place, most of the inspired gas goes into the patient. However, since the bronchoscope cannot fully fill the area of the trachea, there is a variable leak around the distal end of the bronchoscope. Exhaled gases are through the anesthesia circle system. When the eye-piece is removed there is a very large leak out the proximal end of the bronchoscope.

rigid bronchoscopy is usually performed under general anesthesia. If local anesthesia must be used, the premedication and various local blocks, as previously described for fiberoptic bronchoscopy and used collectively, will usually render rigid bronchoscopy tolerable.

b. GENERAL ANESTHESIA

Bronchospastic and asthmatic patients must have good pharmacologic control of bronchomotor tone prior to rigid bronchoscopy. General anesthesia for rigid bronchoscopy should also be preceded by some topical local anesthesia of the larynx. Thus, less general anesthesia will be required, permitting easier, more rapid awakening and return of laryngeal reflexes. Both nitrous oxide/intravenous anesthesia/short-acting muscle relaxant and halogenated drug/short-acting muscle relaxant anesthesia may be used with ventilating bronchoscopes. Intravenous and intratracheal lido-

caine with either type of general anesthetic minimizes straining, coughing, and arrhythmias.[14-16] Of course, the choice of anesthesia will also be based on the overall medical status of the patient and the skill and speed of the surgeon.

4. Complications

Experiencing the passing of a rigid bronchoscope can be very unpleasant for an awake patient. The rigid bronchoscope may fracture teeth and it is occasionally necessary to use extreme extension of the neck to insert the bronchoscope, which may cause vasovagal reactions. Massive hemorrhage from directly traumatized lesions may occur.[19, 21] The tip of the rigid bronchoscope can perforate the mucosa, causing pneumomediastinum and subcutaneous emphysema. Since a large leak may occur around the distal end of the bronchoscope, which may prevent adequate ventilation, and since periods of apnea may be required, there is an increased risk of hypoxemia and hypercarbia.[19, 21] In view of the inherent intense stimulation associated with the procedure, arrhythmias (especially if either hypoxemia, hypercarbia, inadequate anesthesia, or halothane anesthesia are present) may occur.[19, 21]

C. Rigid Venturi Bronchoscopy

1. Indications

The indications for the rigid Venturi bronchoscope are the same as those for the rigid ventilating bronchoscope. However, since the rigid Venturi bronchoscope provides more even ventilation for extended periods of time (see the following), it may be the rigid bronchoscope of choice when a prolonged procedure is anticipated. Since ventilation need not be interrupted, the Venturi technique provides the

surgeon with an unhurried viewing period. This may be particularly important when the procedure may involve photography, manipulations by several junior persons with extensive teaching done, and combined rigid and fiberoptic bronchoscopy.

2. Ventilatory Considerations

The rigid Venturi-effect bronchoscope relies on an intermittent (10 to 20/min) high-pressure oxygen jet to entrain air and ventilate the lungs with an air-oxygen mixture (Fig. 14–6). The Venturi jet is delivered via a reducing valve (Sanders injector) to a 1.0- to 1.5-inch, 18- or 16-gauge needle that is inside and parallel to the lumen of the bronchoscope. The high velocity of the Venturi jet exiting from the end of the needle creates a negative pressure just outside the open end of the needle that draws environmental air into the jet stream. The Venturi jet plus the entrained air creates a positive

Rigid Venturi Bronchoscope

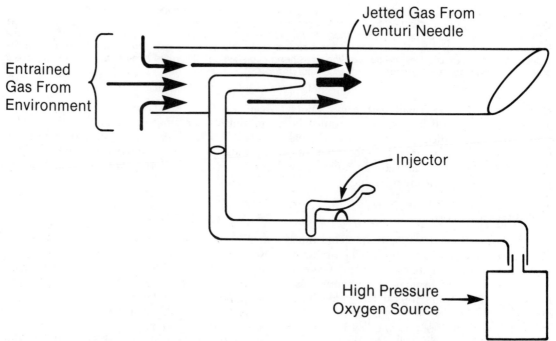

Figure 14–6. This schematic diagram of a rigid Venturi bronchoscope shows that the jet of gas exiting from a Venturi needle placed within the lumen and parallel to the long axis of the bronchoscope entrains gas from the environment. The jetted gas comes from a high pressure source and an intermittent (12/min) injector. The flow of gas from the tube into the patient is equal to the volume of gas through the jet plus the air entrained.

intraluminal tracheal pressure and a tidal volume. At any given reducing valve pressure, the exact amount of tracheal pressure and tidal volume depends on the driving pressure from the reducing valve, the size of the needle, and the diameter, length, and type of bronchoscope. With the usual Venturi bronchoscope (Negus) and an 18-gauge needle orifice, a 50 psi source causes a flow of 160 L/min and a peak airway pressure of 27 cm H_2O.[26] The jet reducing-valve pressure can be adjusted according to the tracheal pressure and observed chest movements; usually a tracheal pressure of 30 cm H_2O results in normocarbia. In comparison with the intermittent gas exchange often required by the rigid ventilating bronchoscope, the rigid Venturi bronchoscope provides more constant and adequate ventilation.[27] Recently, high-frequency jet ventilation at rates of 150 to 300 breaths/min (using a commercial high-frequency ventilator) through the rigid Venturi bronchoscope has resulted in adequate gas exchange.[28]

3. Anesthetic Technique

a. LOCAL ANESTHESIA

The rigid Venturi bronchoscope entails the same difficulties as the rigid ventilating bronchoscope when used with just local anesthesia. Consequently, the rigid Venturi bronchoscope is also used most commonly with general anesthesia. If local anesthesia must be used, the premedication and the regional blocks, as described under fiberoptic bronchoscopy and used collectively, will usually render rigid bronchoscopy tolerable.

b. GENERAL ANESTHESIA

As with the rigid ventilating bronchoscope, use of topical local anesthetics to the upper airway greatly reduces the amount of general anesthesia required for the rigid Venturi bronchoscope. Since the Venturi principle renders the inspired oxygen concentration and inhalational anesthetic concentration uncertain, an oxygen-narcotic-thiopental-muscle relaxant general anesthetic is most often used for bronchoscopy with a Venturi bronchoscope. Paralysis is a helpful part of the Venturi technique since a compliant thorax with minimal resistance is necessary to ensure adequate ventilation. Intravenous and intratracheal lidocaine is a helpful adjunct to depress the cough reflex and arrhythmias.[14-16]

4. Complications

The rigid Venturi bronchoscope can cause the same direct trauma complications as the rigid ventilating bronchoscope. In addition, there are several potential special disadvantages in using the rigid Venturi bronchoscope. First, there is no continuous documentation of delivered oxygen and inhaled anesthetic drug concentration. Second, the high gas flow rates due to the jet ventilation may cause blood or tumor particles to be accidentally blown down into more peripheral bronchi. Third, care must be taken not to generate excessive carinal airway pressures in children owing to a tight glottic fit, which may prevent escape of gas (exhalation) around the bronchoscope.

III. MEDIASTINOSCOPY

A. Indications

Mediastinoscopy is commonly performed prior to thoracotomy in order to establish a diagnosis and/or to determine resectability of a lung carcinoma. Following a suprasternal notch incision, a tunnel is created (through the pretracheal fascia) by blunt dissection along the anterior and lateral walls of the trachea into the mediastinum, behind (posterior to) the aortic arch down to the subcarinal area (Fig. 14–7). This procedure allows for direct inspection and biopsy of the superior mediastinal lymph nodes, which lie posterior to the aortic arch (the anterior and lateral paramainstem bronchial, anterior subcarinal, anterior, and lateral paratracheal lymph nodes) (Fig. 14–7). Contralateral positive nodes (to a lung carcinoma) are considered an absolute contraindication to thoracotomy, whereas if only ipsilateral nodes are involved, thoracotomy may be performed depending on the expected resectability of the tumor. Tumors of the thymus and anterior mediastinum are not examined by the usual diagnostic mediastinoscopic approach because they are anterior to the great vessels; thus, an anterior mediastinotomy is required to examine this area (this procedure utilizes a second rib interspace incision and is a much less complicated procedure than mediastinoscopy). Previous mediastinoscopy is an absolute contraindication to a repeat procedure because scarring eliminates the plane of dissection. Relative contraindications to mediastinoscopy include superior vena cava syndrome, severe tracheal

Mediastinoscopy

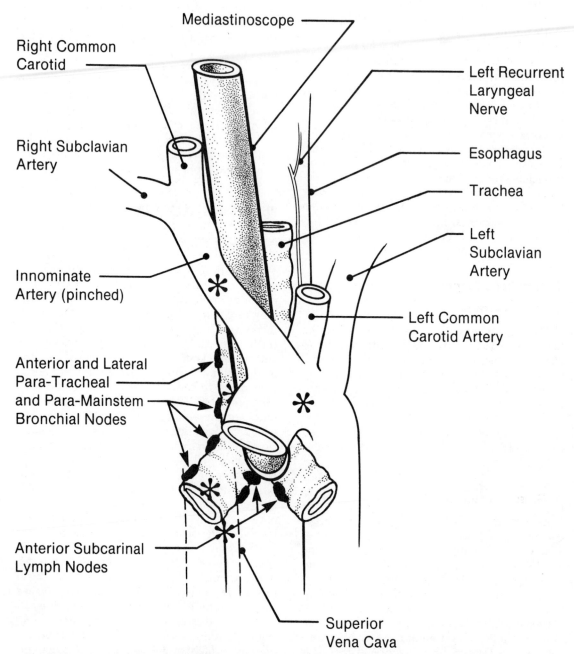

Figure 14–7. This schematic diagram shows the placement of a mediastinoscope into the superior mediastinum. The mediastinoscope passes in front of the trachea but behind the thoracic aorta. This location of the mediastinoscope allows for sampling of anterior and lateral paramainstem bronchial lymph nodes, anterior subcarinal lymph nodes, and anterior and lateral paratracheal lymph nodes. Anatomical structures that can be compressed by the mediastinoscope (see areas marked by an *) and that can cause major complications are the thoracic aorta (rupture, reflex bradycardia), innominate artery (decreased right carotid blood flow can cause cerebral vascular symptoms, and decreased right subclavian flow can cause loss of right radial pulse), trachea (inability to ventilate), and vena cava (risk of hemorrhage with superior vena cava syndrome).

deviation, cerebrovascular disease, and thoracic aortic aneurysm.[29] With the advent of computed tomography, the role of mediastinoscopy may diminish considerably in the future.

B. Anesthetic Technique

In addition to the usual preanesthetic evaluation of patients, one should specifically look for the signs and symptoms of the relative contraindications to mediastinoscopy, such as obstruction or distortion of the upper airway and superior vena caval obstruction, signs and symptoms of impaired cerebral circulation (which may be compounded during mediastinoscopy by compression of carotid vessels), and evidence of the myasthenic syndrome due to lung carcinoma. Since there is the potential risk of hemorrhage, a large-bore intravenous catheter should be inserted and blood should be immediately available during mediastinoscopy. If the superior vena cava is obstructed, a lower extremity intravenous catheter is highly desirable.

Although mediastinoscopy can be performed under local anesthesia,[30, 31] general anesthesia with controlled positive-pressure ventilation is preferred because it allows the surgeon more flexibility in his dissection, minimizes the potential for air embolus (see the following), and facilitates management of major complications such as massive hemorrhage.[32] However, local anesthesia may be considered for patients with active cerebrovascular disease in order to monitor cerebral function continuously in the awake state.

Following the intravenous induction of general anesthesia and paralysis with either succinylcholine, atracurium, or vecuronium, lidocaine is sprayed directly on the trachea and given intravenously in order to minimize coughing during orotracheal intubation and during the procedure itself. A nonkinking tube should be considered in cases in which tracheomalacia is a possibility. A short-acting muscle relaxant (succinylcholine drip, atracurium, vecuronium) is also used during the procedure to prevent coughing, venous engorgement from straining, and movement during the procedure. The head-up position minimizes the venous engorgement but maximizes venous air embolism. The choice of anesthetic agent used is determined by the patient's overall medical condition (see chapter 8). During mediastinoscopy the anesthesiologist's attention is primarily focused on detecting the occurrence of the complications of mediastinoscopy. This is performed by palpating the right radial pulse (vessels most commonly compressed are the innominate and right subclavian and carotid arteries) and by observing for reflex bradycardia (compression of the aorta), arrhythmias (mechanical stimulation of the aorta, ventricles), hypovolemia, tension pneumothorax, and compression of trachea (see the following). Blood pressure and oxygen saturation should be measured using the left arm; if an arterial line is placed, the right wrist may be preferable because it can immediately signal when compression of the innominate artery has occurred. Immediately following the procedure patients can usually be extubated. The patients should be nursed in a head-up position to minimize venous engorgement.

The anesthetic considerations for anterior mediastinotomy are very similar to those for mediastinoscopy except that the incision is larger, the incidence of complications is lower because structures can be visualized and controlled more readily, the position of the head is unimportant, and the blood pressure can be measured on either arm because there is little chance of compression of the innominate artery.

C. Complications

Although overall mortality from this procedure is low (0.1 per cent),[33] serious complications can occur that the anesthesiologist must be prepared to diagnose and to treat (Table 14–3). In a series of 6490 patients undergoing mediastinoscopy, the major complications reported (numbers of patients in parentheses) consisted of hemorrhage (48), pneumothorax (43), recurrent laryngeal nerve injury (22), infection (22), tumor implantation in the wound (8), phrenic nerve injury (3), esophageal injury (1), chylothorax (1), air embolism (1), and tran-

***Table 14–3. Major Complications
of Mediastinoscopy***

1. Hemorrhage
2. Pneumothorax
3. Recurrent laryngeal nerve injury
4. Air embolism
5. Compression of vessels
   a. Aorta → reflex bradycardia
   b. Innominate artery
      Right carotid → hemiparesis
      Right subclavian → loss of right radial pulse
6. Compression of trachea
7. Infection, tumor spread

sient hemiparesis (1).[33] The overall complication rate in various studies has been 1.5 to 3.0 per cent.[33-39] At the time of occurrence, most of these complications required a specific anesthetic management response.

Significant (occasionally massive) hemorrhage has been the most frequent major problem encountered during mediastinoscopy. If it occurs, thoracotomy must be performed immediately; while these rapid preparations are in progress, the surgeon should attempt to control hemorrhage by compressing the bleeding site with a sponge forceps or a small pack, although the relative inaccessibility of the operative field may make this maneuver difficult or ineffective. The anesthesiologist should (1) rapidly begin volume replacement through one (or more) large-bore intravenous cannulae that have been placed prior to the induction of anesthesia; (2) send for blood that was reserved for the patient preoperatively; (3) support the circulation pharmacologically until volume replacement is achieved; (4) assure adequate oxygenation and ventilation; (5) administer atropine for reflex bradycardia from aortic compression (if it occurs); and (6) discontinue or reduce the dose of all anesthetic drugs until normovolemia is reestablished. Rarely, it may be necessary to induce deliberate hypotension to control bleeding in this setting.[35] Should hemorrhage originate from a superior vena cava tear, volume replacement and drug treatment may be lost into the surgical field unless they are administered via a peripheral intravenous line placed rapidly in the lower extremity.[35]

Pneumothorax is another relatively frequently encountered complication of mediastinoscopy. It is usually not apparent until the postoperative period, and the majority of patients do not require chest tube decompression.[33] All patients should be monitored for signs of pneumothorax in the postoperative period, and a chest roentgenogram obtained when doubt exists. Pneumothorax that occurs intraoperatively, as evidenced by increased peak inspiratory pressure, tracheal shift, distant breath sounds, hypotension, and cyanosis, requires immediate treatment by chest tube decompression.[40]

When mediastinoscopy causes a recurrent laryngeal nerve injury (Fig. 14–7) it is permanent in approximately 50 per cent of patients.[33] If injury to the recurrent laryngeal nerve is suspected, the vocal cords should be visualized while the patient is spontaneously breathing (usually at the time of extubation). If the vocal cords are nonmoving and/or are in a midline position, consideration has to be given to the problem of postoperative laryngeal obstruction.

During mediastinoscopy the mediastinoscope tip is located intrathoracically and therefore directly exposed to pleural pressure. Venous air embolism (when venous bleeding is present) can occur much more easily if patients are breathing spontaneously because of the development of negative intrathoracic pressure during inspiration; therefore, controlled positive-pressure ventilation during this procedure minimizes the risk of air embolism.

The mediastinoscope can exert pressure against the innominate artery and result in diminished blood flow to the right carotid and right subclavian arteries (Fig. 14–7). This phenomenon may be of special significance in patients with pre-existing compromised cerebral circulation. Compression of the right carotid artery has been proposed as the cause of a left hemiparesis that occurred in one patient and that subsequently cleared 48 hours after the procedure.[33] In another patient compression of the right subclavian artery caused the loss of the pulse and blood pressure in the right arm and was misdiagnosed as an intraoperative cardiac arrest.[41] In another study, blood pressure in the right arm was significantly decreased for periods of 15 to 360 sec in four of seven patients who underwent mediastinoscopy.[42] This last report, therefore, recommended that blood pressure be measured in the left arm and that the right radial artery be continuously monitored by palpation or finger plethysmography during mediastinoscopy. A right radial arterial line, of course, would very sensitively and continuously monitor the occurrence of innominate or right subclavian artery compression. An oxygen saturation monitor would do this task less sensitively. Any decrease in right radial artery pressure requires repositioning of the mediastinoscope, especially in patients with cerebral vascular insufficiency. Avoiding excessive extension of the neck, which might contribute to pinching of neck vessels, is also important in this group of patients.

Autonomic reflexes may occur as a result of compression or stretching of the trachea, vagus nerve, or great vessels. Sudden changes in pulse and/or blood pressure during mediastinoscopy may initially be empirically treated by repositioning of the mediastinoscope. Atropine is given for persistent bradycardia.

IV. THORACOSCOPY

A. Indications

Thoracoscopy (pleuroscopy) permits a valuable examination of the thorax and is most commonly performed to aid in the diagnosis of pleural and parenchymal disease, to help establish the staging of suspected neoplasms, and to determine the etiology of recurrent pleural effusions.[43-47] It is most often done after thoracocentesis or closed chest pleural or lung biopsy has been performed and a diagnosis has still not been established. Thoracoscopy is done by making a small incision in the lateral thoracic wall (usually at the level of the sixth intercostal space) and then introducing a thoracoscope, laparoscope, or mediastinoscope into the pleural cavity. The procedure allows for complete inspection of the pleural space of a hemithorax. Fluid and biopsies can usually be obtained easily through the incision, although a few surgeons prefer to use a separate incision for additional instruments such as biopsy forceps.

B. Anesthetic Technique

Thoracoscopy can be done with either local, regional, or general anesthesia. The choice of anesthesia is determined by considering: (1) the expected scope and length of the procedure; (2) the gentleness and technical abilities of the surgeon; (3) the expertise of the anesthesiologist; and (4) the physical condition and psychologic state of the patient.

Local anesthetic infiltration of the lateral thoracic wall and parietal pleura is the simplest way to provide anesthesia for the patient,[48] although some patients may experience considerable discomfort when this method is used. Partial collapse of the lung on the operated side occurs when air enters the pleural cavity. This allows for good visualization of the pleural space by the surgeon. It is both hazardous and unnecessary to insufflate gases under pressure into the hemithorax in question in order to increase visualization of the pleural space. Surprisingly, even though many of these patients suffer from advanced pulmonary disease, changes in P_aO_2, P_aCO_2, and cardiac rhythm are usually minimal during the procedure when it is performed under local anesthesia and the patient is breathing spontaneously.[49, 50] However, it is prudent

to use a high F_IO_2 to overcome the loss in lung volume caused by the unavoidable pneumothorax.

Intercostal nerve blocks performed at the level of the incision and at two interspaces above and below may provide more complete analgesia for thoracoscopy, especially if they are placed far enough posteriorly to anesthetize the parietal pleura. The addition of an ipsilateral stellate ganglion block helps to prevent the cough reflex that is sometimes elicited during visualization and manipulation of the hilum.

When general anesthesia is performed for thoracoscopy, a standard endotracheal tube may be used. However, positive-pressure ventilation seriously interferes with visualization of thoracic contents, and thoracoscopy is therefore a relative indication for one-lung anesthesia.[51] Because the procedure is usually short and the ipsilateral lung needs to be deflated for only a brief period, blood gases are not routinely monitored during the procedure. However, for patients with marginal pulmonary status in whom the period of one-lung anesthesia lasts for more than a few minutes, the usual monitoring precautions should be taken, as discussed in chapter 7.

C. Complications

Complications are very rare during this simple procedure, although it is possible that any structure that the surgeon has to manipulate may be damaged. A few critically ill spontaneously breathing patients may experience impaired gas exchange during the procedure. Although some air may transiently remain in the pleural space following the procedure, this situation rarely requires chest tube insertion.

V. ESOPHAGOSCOPY

A. Indications

The major indication for esophagoscopy is the demonstration of an esophageal lesion following contrast studies that needs either etiologic or anatomic clarification.[52] Such lesions include all strictures, intraluminal filling defects, mucosal abnormalities, and upper gastrointestinal bleeding. In most of these situations biopsies and cytologic brushings will also need to be obtained. Candidates for esophagoscopy include patients who have symptoms of difficulty in swallowing and those with esophageal reflux. Finally, therapeutic esophagoscopy is required for removal of foreign bodies, dilatation of strictures, placement of plastic prosthesis across a malignant stricture, the injection of sclerosing agents into esophageal varices, and coagulation of bleeding lesions.

Table 14–4 compares the advantages and disadvantages of fiberoptic esophagoscopy and open-tube rigid esophagoscopy.[52] Generally, fiberoptic esophagoscopy lends itself to greater patient comfort, the ability to examine the entire upper gastrointestinal tract, and greater safety. Consequently, flexible fiberoptic esophagoscopy is usually carried out under local anesthesia. Disadvantages of the fiberoptic instrument are the inability to achieve deep biopsies and inadequate instrumentation for foreign body removal.

Specific indications for the use of open-tube esophagoscopy include removal of a foreign body and determination of the source of massive esophageal bleeding. Although open-tube esophagoscopy can be carried out under topical anesthesia, it is more radily accomplished under general endotracheal anesthesia.[53] Open-tube esophagoscopy is to be avoided in the patient with a large thoracic aneurysm, as instrumentation may cause rupture. The procedure is also contraindicated in patients with acute pharyngitis, as infection may be aggravated.

B. Anesthetic Technique

Topical anesthesia of the oropharynx for fiberoptic esophagoscopy can be achieved by having the patient gargle viscous lidocaine followed by a tetracaine or lidocaine spray. The patient is further sedated before the examination with small doses of a sedative and/or narcotic.

General anesthesia is usually required for rigid esophagoscopy. Patients presenting for esophagoscopy are often debilitated or dehydrated as a result of their dysphagia (see chapters 5 and 13), and many are elderly, so that coexistent disease is common. These patients also can be anemic and hypoproteinemic and can be especially prone to regurgitation and aspiration.

Atropine premedication is useful in decreasing secretions and in preventing a vagal reaction to gastric distension. Oropharyngeal topical anesthesia (with lidocaine gargle and spray) is

Table 14–4. Fiberoptic versus Open Tube Esophagoscopy

Advantages	Disadvantages
Fiberoptic Esophagoscopy	
1. Patient comfort	1. Expensive equipment required
2. Ability to examine entire upper gastrointestinal tract	2. Greater occurrence of mechanical failure
3. General anesthesia not required	3. Dilation not possible
4. Greater safety	4. Smaller biopsies
Open Tube Esophagoscope	
1. Deeper biopsy possible	1. Patient discomfort
2. Greater aspiration capacity	2. Safety
3. Dilation feasible	3. Less readily done on outpatient basis
4. Foreign body removal	
5. Ease of sterilization	

useful in minimizing the amount of general anesthesia required. Preoxygenation is followed by intravenous induction using cricoid pressure to control reflux of esophageal contents. Following intravenous induction of anesthesia and paralysis, a small-sized endotracheal tube should be inserted to prevent anterior compression of the esophagus (as a large sized endotracheal tube might do) and thereby allow more room for esophageal instrumentation and passage of the esophagoscope. The endotracheal tube should be positioned to the left side of the patient's mouth so that the esophagoscope can be introduced through the right side of the mouth. The connecting tubing should be fastened over the front of the patient's chest to allow the surgeon easy access to the mouth. The patient's eyes should be protected since they are likely to be concealed by a drape around the head. Full relaxation should be maintained at least until the esophagoscope has been passed through the cricopharyngeal sphincter and, if this passage proves difficult, it may be necessary to deflate the cuff on the endotracheal tube for a few moments to provide a little more room for the esophagoscope. Although spontaneous ventilation can be permitted once the esophagoscope is through the cricopharyngeal sphincter, it is preferable to retain control of ventilation and maintain paralysis to prevent any coughing or bucking during the procedure, which may cause the esophagoscope to damage or tear the esophagus. Certainly, full relaxation should be maintained throughout the procedure if repeated instrumentation through the cricopharyngeus is required. Arrhythmias may occur as the esophagoscope passes behind the heart, but they are rarely a source of real concern and are usually only transitory.

Recovery of consciousness should be supervised with the patient on his side, slightly head-down on a gurney that can be tipped. A postoperative chest x-ray should be obtained to rule out signs of esophageal tear, such as surgical emphysema, pneumoperitoneum, pneumothorax, or pneumomediastinum. Emergency thoracotomy is required if esophageal rupture is suspected.

C. Complications

The complications of esophagoscopy include perforation, hemorrhage, and cardiopulmonary complications.[54, 55] The most frequent site of perforation is the hypopharynx, which carries a mortality rate ranging from 34 to 84 per cent.[56-58] Biopsies that are taken too deeply (i.e., full thickness) can also result in perforations. Hemorrhage may occur from esophageal varices, lacerations at the gastroesophageal junction induced by forceful wretching, and from biopsy. Cardiopulmonary problems are due to aspiration, pneumonia, cardiac arrhythmias, and myocardial infarction. Septicemia may occur in immunosuppressed patients, and prophylactic antibiotics are indicated in this group.

REFERENCES

1. Landa JF: Indications for bronchoscopy. Chest 73:686–690, 1978.
2. Barrett CR: Flexible fiberoptic bronchoscopy in the critically ill patient. Chest 73:746–749, 1978.
3. Raj PP, Forestner J, Watson RD, et al: Techniques for fiberoptic laryngoscopy in anesthesia. Anesth Analg 53:708–714, 1974.
4. Snider GL: When not to use the bronchoscope for hemoptysis. Chest 76:1–2, 1979.
5. Simelaro JP, Marks B, Meals R, et al: Selective bronchography following fiberoptic bronchoscopy. Chest 70:240–241, 1976.
6. Lampton LM: Bronchoscopy: Caution! JAMA 73:138, 1978.
7. Miller EJ: Hypoxemia during fiberoptic bronchoscopy. Chest 75:103, 1979.
8. Lindholm CE, Ollman B, Snyder JV, et al: Cardiorespiratory effect of flexible fiberoptic bronchoscopy in critically ill patients. Chest 74:362–368, 1978.
9. Pingleton SK, Bone CR, Ruth WC: Helium-oxygen mixtures during bronchoscopy. Crit Care Med 8:50–53, 1980.
10. Neuhaus A, Markowitz D, Rotman HH, et al: The effects of fiberoptic bronchoscopy with and without atropine premedication on pulmonary function in humans. Ann Thorac Surg 25:393–398, 1978.
11. Belen J, Neuhaus A, Markowitz D, et al: Modification of the effect of fiberoptic bronchoscopy on pulmonary mechanics. Chest 79:516–519, 1981.
12. Cooper M, Watson RL: An improved regional anesthetic technique for peroral endoscopy. Anesthesiology 43:273–374, 1975.
13. Gotta AW, Sullivan CA: Anaesthesia of the upper airway using topical anaesthetic and superior laryngeal nerve block. Br J Anaesth 53:1055–1057, 1981.
14. Christensen V, Ladegaard-Pedersen HJ, Skovsted P: Intravenous lidocaine as a suppressant of persistent cough caused by bronchoscopy. Acta Anaesth Scand (Suppl) 67:84–86, 1978.
15. Elguindi AS, Harrison GN, Abdulla AM, et al: Cardiac rhythm disturbances during fiberoptic bronchoscopy: A prospective study. J Thorac Cardiovasc Surg 77:557–561, 1979.
16. Luck JC, Messeder OH, Rubenstein MJ: Arrhythmias from fiberoptic bronchoscopy. Chest 74:139–143, 1978.
17. Salisbury BG, Metzger CF, Altose MD, et al: Effect of fiberoptic bronchoscopy on respiratory performance in patients with chronic airway obstruction. Thorax 30:441–446, 1975.
18. Suratt PM, Smiddy JF, Gruber B: Deaths and complications associated with fiberoptic bronchoscopy. Chest 69:747–751, 1976.
19. Lukomsky GI, Ovchinnikov AA, Bilal A: Complications of bronchoscopy: Comparison of rigid bronchoscopy under general anesthesia and flexible fiberoptic bronchoscopy under topical anesthesia. Chest 79:316–321, 1981.
20. Shrader DL, Lakshminarayan S: The effect of fiberoptic bronchoscopy on cardiac rhythm. Chest 73:821–824, 1978.
21. Zavala DC: Flexible Fiberoptic Bronchoscopy: A Training Handbook. Iowa City, The University of Iowa Publications Department, 1978.
22. Zavala DC: Complications following fiberoptic bronchoscopy, the "good news" and the "bad news." Chest 73:783–785, 1978.
23. Albertini RE, Harrell JH, Kurihara N, et al: Arterial hypoxemia induced by fiberoptic bronchoscopy. JAMA 230:1666–1667, 1974.
24. Dubrawsky C, Awe RJ, Jenkins DE: The effect of bronchofiberoptic examination on oxygen status. Chest 67:137–140, 1975.
25. Fraioli RL, Sheffer LA, Steffenson JL: Pulmonary and cardiovascular effect of apneic oxygenation in man. Anesthesiology 39:588–596, 1973.
26. Sanders RD: Two ventilating attachments for bronchoscopes. Del Med J 39:170–175, 192, 1967.
27. Giesecke AH, Gerbershagen HU, Dortman C, et al: Comparison of the ventilating and injection bronchoscopes. Anesthesiology 38:298–303, 1978.
28. Vourc'h G, Fischler M, Michon F, et al: High-frequency jet ventilation v. manual jet ventilation during bronchoscopy in patients with tracheo-bronchial stenosis. Br J Anaesth 55:969–972, 1983.
29. Preciano MC, Duvall AJ, Koop SH: Mediastinoscopy. A review of 450 cases. Laryngoscope 83:1300–1310, 1973.
30. Ward PH, Stephenson SE Jr, Harris PF: Mediastinoscopy: A valuable diagnostic procedure for the evaluation of lesions of the mediastinum. South Med J 60:51–56, 1967.
31. Morton JR, Guinn GA: Mediastinoscopy using local anesthesia. Am J Surg 122:696–698, 1971.

32. Fassoulaki A: Anesthesia for mediastinoscopy. Anaesthesia 34:75–76, 1978.
33. Ashbaugh DG: Mediastinoscopy. Arch Surg 100:568–573, 1970.
34. Weissberg D, Herczed E: Perforation of thoracic aortic aneurysm—a complication of mediastinoscopy. Chest 78:119–120, 1980.
35. Roberts JT, Gissen AJ: Management of complications encountered during anesthesia for mediastinoscopy. Anesth Rev 6:31–35, 1979.
36. Lee CM, Grossman LB: Laceration of the left pulmonary artery during mediastinoscopy. Anesth Analg 56:226–227, 1977.
37. Foster ED, Munro DD, Dobell ARC: Mediastinoscopy. Ann Thorac Surg 13:273–286, 1972.
38. Trinkle JK, Bryant LR, Hiller AJ: Mediastinoscopy—experience with 300 consecutive cases. J Thorac Cardiovasc Surg 60:297–300, 1970.
39. Barash PG, Tsai B, Kitahata LM: Acute tracheal collapse following mediastinoscopy. Anesthesiology 44:67–68, 1976.
40. Furgang FA, Saidman LJ: Bilateral tension pneumothorax associated with mediastinoscopy. J Thorac Cardiovasc Surg 63:329–333, 1972.
41. Lee J, Salvatore A: Innominate artery compression simulating cardiac arrest during mediastinoscopy: A case report. Anesth Analg 55:748–749, 1976.
42. Petty C: Right radial artery pressure during mediastinoscopy. Anesth Analg 58:428–430, 1979.
43. Rodgers BM, Ryckman FC, Moazam F, et al: Thoracoscopy for intrathoracic tumors. Ann Thorac Surg 31:414–420, 1981.
44. Canto A, Blasco E, Casillas M, et al: Thoracoscopy in the diagnosis of pleural effusion. Thorax 32:550–554, 1977.
45. Bloomberg AE: Thoracoscopy in perspective. Surg Gynecol Obstet 147:433–443, 1978.
46. Lewis RJ, Kunderman PJ, Sisler GE et al: Direct diagnostic thoracoscopy. Ann Thorac Surg 21:536–540, 1976.
47. Miller JI, Hatcher CR: Thoracoscopy: A useful tool in the diagnosis of thoracic disease. Ann Thorac Surg 26:68–72, 1978.
48. Morton JR, Guinn GA: Thoracoscopy using local anesthesia. Am J Surg 122:696–698, 1971.
49. Faurschou P, Madsen F, Viskum K: Thoracoscopy: Influence of the procedure on some respiratory and cardiac values. Thorax 38:341–343, 1983.
50. Oldenburg FA, Newhouse MT: Thoracoscopy. Chest 75:45–50, 1979.
51. Friedel H: Importance of bronchiological examination in cases of pleural diseases. Bronches 20:77–82, 1970.
52. Faber LP, Franklin JL: Endoscopic examinations. In Shields TW (ed): Thoracic Surgery. Philadelphia, Lea & Febiger, 1983, chapter 14, pp 203–229.
53. Anonymous Leading Article. Analgesia for endoscopy. Lancet ii, 1125, 1976.
54. Mandelstam P, et al: Complications associated with esophagogastroduodenoscopy and with esophageal dilation. Gastrointest Endosc 23:16, 1976.
55. McNab Jones RF: Summary of hazards of endoscopy. Proc R Soc Med 69:670–672, 1976.
56. Steyn JH, Brunner PL: Perforation of cervical oesophagus at oesophagoscopy. Scott Med J 7:494–497, 1962.
57. Wooloch Y, Zer M, Dintsman M, et al: Iatrogenic perforations of the esophagus. Arch Surg 108:357–360, 1974.
58. Aniansson G, Hallen O: Perforation of the esophagus. Acta Otolaryngol 59:554–558, 1965.

Anesthesia for Special Elective Therapeutic Procedures

15

I. INTRODUCTION

This chapter describes the anesthetic management of special elective thoracic surgery procedures. Each of these special thoracic surgery procedures involves anesthetic considerations that are distinct from those in all other types of thoracic surgery. The presentation of the special cases is organized according to anatomic location; the chapter considers diseases and problems of the proximal airway to the alveolar space, involvement of the great thoracic vessels, and, finally, thymectomy for myasthenia gravis and one-lung ventilation in morbidly obese patients. The major anesthetic considerations for esophageal surgery (problems associated with malnutrition, hyperalimentation, and risk of aspiration) are presented in chapters 5 and 13. Thoracic surgery procedures that do not have special anesthetic considerations (beyond such usual considerations as one-lung ventilation and massive blood loss, which have already been presented [see Section II]) are not discussed here.

II. LASER RESECTION OF MAJOR AIRWAY OBSTRUCTING TUMORS

A. General Considerations

Malignant tumors (bronchogenic and metastatic) of the tracheobronchial tree progressively obstruct major conducting airways, resulting in slow asphyxiation of the patient. Treatment with external radiation therapy and chemotherapy requires several weeks to result in temporary resolution of the obstructive lesions, and sometimes the progressive obstruction cannot be reversed by this means. Fortunately, in recent years the technology to permit passage of laser energy to ablate and cause necrosis of these previously inoperable airway tumor obstructions has been developed. Creating a channel

343

through a completely obstructing lesion or widening an existing channel by a partially obstructing lesion has resulted in a great improvement in symptoms, increase in P_aO_2, and improvement in the appearance of chest roentgenogram and ventilation-perfusion scans.[1-4] Partially obstructing lesions with a visible free bronchial wall and visible lumen are technically much easier to approach. This is because a laser beam can hit a free margin tangentially, whereas a laser beam must hit a fully obstructing lesion perpendicularly (blind penetration of the mass), which, therefore, involves a much greater risk of hemorrhage. Thus, the best results have been obtained with partially obstructing lesions, and in a high percentage of cases (greater than 85 per cent) the relief is immediate and dramatic and is associated with a low incidence of bleeding.[2, 3] When the obstructing lesion is complete, the improvement is more limited, occurs in a lesser percentage of patients (30 to 50 per cent), and is associated with a higher incidence of bleeding.[2, 3, 5] The most dramatic improvement is seen in those patients with obstructions of the trachea and mainstem bronchi because most of the lung benefits from improvement in ventilation, whereas ablation or creation of a channel through a peripheral lesion can only be expected to cause a limited increase in ventilation-perfusion ratio of the small amount of lung distal to the lesion.[3]

Use of the laser beam itself (as opposed to the ventilating system; see following sections) involves several risks. Airway and endotracheal tube fires are the most feared hazard during laser surgery of the airway.[6, 7] The intense heat field surrounding the laser beam can dry out and ignite most materials. The risk of fire depends on the nature of the material, the gaseous milieu, the beam wattage, and the mode of operation. All endotracheal tubes (rubber or plastic) can be ignited by a laser beam in 50 to 100 per cent oxygen, and, therefore, an F_IO_2 of less than 0.5 in nitrogen should be used during the firing of the laser beam.[5, 8-11] The surgeon also has a responsibility for preventing airway fires. The laser should not be used as a cautery. The surgeon should use the laser intermittently, at moderate wattage (45 W), and in a noncontinuous mode (durations less than 0.5 to 1 sec).[9] This will help prevent excessive heat field buildup and tissue desiccation and will decrease tissue penetration, which decreases the risk of hemorrhage and damage to underlying or adjacent normal tissue.

The hazards of laser surgery also include inadvertent exposure of operating personnel to laser beam energy. The eye is most susceptible to injury. All operating room personnel must wear appropriate safety glasses during laser use. The patient's eyes must be taped closed and be well covered with aluminum foil during the procedure.

Finally, the target site must be still. The consequences of missing the target are great, namely, destruction of normal tissue and hemorrhage. Occasionally, it may be expected that a distal abscess may be encountered following relief of a total obstruction; this complication requires aggressive evacuation of pus and support of ventilation. The overall perioperative mortality for palliative procedures is presently about 1 to 2 per cent, but some earlier series have reported mortality as high as 10 per cent.[2, 12-14]

B. The Various Types of Laser and Adjunctive Therapies

1. Neodymium-Yttrium-Aluminum-Garnet (Nd-YAG) Laser Resection

a. GENERAL CONSIDERATIONS

For several reasons the Nd-YAG is by far the most commonly used laser to resect obstructing tracheobronchial tree tumors.[1-4] First, since tissue is destroyed by a coagulation-vaporization sequence, bleeding is minimal and remaining tissue margins do not become edematous or scar. Second, the Nd-YAG laser is capable of destroying a large amount of tissue because it has good tissue penetration (is poorly absorbed by hemoglobin). Third, the transmission characteristics of the Nd-YAG laser system are suitable for tracheobronchial tree tumors. The Nd-YAG laser has a wave length (1064 nm) that is readily conducted through a flexible quartz monofilament and that can be readily passed down either a fiberoptic or a rigid bronchoscope. Since the laser beam is invisible, a companion light beam that projects a visible spot is simultaneously transmitted down the fiber to allow for accurate aiming. The aiming spot is in the same position and is the same size as the invisible laser beam. This pilot light permits accurate aiming with a laser fiber-to-target beam distance of only 5 to 10 mm. At this distance, the laser beam divergence is less than 10°, with an area of photovaporization 1 to

2 mm in diameter and up to 4 mm in depth. A continuous 3 L/min flow of air is passed simultaneously through a coaxial Teflon sheath to keep the fiber tip cool and free of debris. Fourth, since the Nd-YAG laser can be used with a fiberoptic bronchoscope, it is suitable for resection of airway lesions beyond the direct range of a rigid bronchoscope, such as upper lobe and peripheral lesions; nevertheless, lesions in such remote locations should be approached with great caution.

b. ANESTHETIC CONSIDERATIONS

The anesthetic technique used depends greatly on the ventilation/bronchoscopy technique (see below). However, in all cases complete stillness is mandatory to provide accurate aiming of the laser beam toward the lesion. Consequently, if local anesthesia is used it must be complete and solid and usually requires that a fiberoptic bronchscope (as opposed to a rigid bronchoscope) and supplemental intravenous sedation be used.[1–3]

Since the nature of this procedure requires instrumentation of the airway, general anesthesia is most commonly used to provide a still target area. Certainly, neuromuscular blockade will guarantee stillness but it also requires intermittent positive-pressure breathing (IPPB). Neuromuscular blockade may result in bits of tissue and blood being blown around and down the airways; if this complication occurs, spontaneous ventilation is obviously preferable. However, if spontaneous ventilation is allowed, it must be realized that the window of anesthetic depth between a nonmoving patient and an adequately spontaneously ventilating patient may be narrow and difficult to find. If spontaneous ventilation is allowed, it is important to have syringes of a ultra-short-acting barbiturate and lidocaine in the intravenous line so that anesthetic response to any sudden patient reaction to surgical stimulation may be immediate. Usually a reaction to the stimulation is first signaled by an invagination of the posterior membranous part of the trachea and a simultaneous feeling of outward tension on the bronchoscopy/ventilation system as the patient begins to bronchoconstrict.

c. VENTILATION/BRONCHOSCOPY SYSTEMS

There are several ventilatory procedures that must be followed with use of any ventila-

tion/bronchoscopy system. First, arterial oxygenation should be continuously monitored using a pulse oximeter. Second, if the pulse oximeter shows decreasing values (less than 90 per cent in previously fully saturated patients) the laser resection should be interrupted, and ventilation with high concentrations of oxygen should be resumed until an adequate oxygen saturation is obtained. During 100 per cent oxygen breathing, obstructed airways should be lavaged and aspirated via a fiberoptic bronchoscope. If periods of desaturation are persistent, the surgeon must be asked to resect smaller amounts of tissue, resect for shorter periods of time, control bleeding better, remove more necrotic tissue with forceps, and minimize suction. During actual laser resections the inspired oxygen concentration should always be less than 50 per cent, with the balance being nitrogen (nitrous oxide supports combustion of oxygen). Third, a fiberoptic bronchoscope must be used to reach upper lobe and peripheral lesions. A fiberoptic bronchoscope can be passed down a rigid bronchoscope; thus, the two bronchoscopes do not have mutually exclusive uses.

The simplest of all ventilation/bronchoscopy systems is to pass a fiberoptic bronchoscope alone under local anesthesia into the tracheobronchial tree.[1, 2] The patient then spontaneously breathes supplemental oxygen around the fiberoptic bronchoscope. The operator must always be cognizant that the patient may move even though liberal amounts of local anesthesia and sedation were used.

The fiberoptic bronchoscope can be passed through an indwelling endotracheal tube[5, 10] (see Fig. 14–2). Use of an endotracheal tube to introduce the fiberoptic bronchoscope almost always requires general anesthesia. As described in chapter 14, the endotracheal tube must be larger than 8 mm in internal diameter, since positive-pressure ventilation must occur around the fiberoptic bronchoscope but within the endotracheal tube lumen (see Figs. 14–1 and 14–2); adequate spontaneous ventilation through this restricted surface area is not possible in most patients. The fiberoptic bronchoscope must be passed through a self-sealing diaphragm to allow administration of positive-pressure ventilation. However, even with positive-pressure ventilation, hypercarbia may be a problem, and in one series hypoventilation (P_aCO_2 45 to 60 mm Hg) occurred in 30 of 32 procedures done in this fashion.[5]

Most laser resections are now performed using a rigid open-tube bronchoscope[3, 4, 11] (see Fig. 14–5). There are two reasons for this preference. First, there is no doubt that from the standpoint of the operator's comfort and facility of manipulation of the laser beam, the rigid scope is the first choice compared with the fiberoptic bronchoscope. The reasons the laser beam can be manipulated better with the rigid bronchoscope consist of better field of vision, better suction, easy cleaning of the telescope, easy removal of tumor fragments by forceps, and the possibility of application of adrenaline-cottonoids for hemostasis. In addition, the rigid bronchoscope can be used to establish an airway. This is not the case when a fiberoptic bronchoscope is used, and the procedure is much more tedious. Second, the open-tube technique minimizes the possibility of endobronchial and endotracheal tube fires. In distinction to the flammable coating of the fiberoptic bronchoscope, "steel does not burn."[3]

It must be realized that the rigid bronchoscope cannot visualize upper lobe lesions and, if the bronchoscope is used below the tracheal carina, it must have side holes to ventilate the other lung. If the bronchoscope does not have side holes, there must be some additional method of ventilating the other lung, such as jet ventilation, high-frequency ventilation, or high-flow apneic ventilation. However, and fortunately, a fiberoptic bronchoscope can be easily introduced through a tracheally positioned (above the carina) rigid bronchoscope to reach airways below the tracheal carina; in this instance ventilation is around the fiberoptic bronchoscope but within the walls of the rigid bronchoscope. Passage of the fiberoptic bronchoscope through the rigid bronchoscope is easily accomplished since the internal diameter of adult rigid bronchoscopes in general use today is 10.5 mm. As described in chapter 14, ventilation through a rigid bronchoscope can be with intermittent positive-pressure breathing, spontaneous ventilation, jet ventilation, or high-frequency ventilation.

d. Suggested Anesthesia and Ventilation Technique for Laser Resection of Airway Tumors

The following is the author's anesthetic management of laser resection cases involving the use of a rigid bronchoscope (Table 15–1). Anesthesia is induced with a short-acting barbiturate. Controlled positive-pressure breathing by mask is instituted, and isoflurane is adminis-

Table 15–1. Suggested Anesthesia and Ventilation Technique for Laser Resection of Airway Tumors

1. Preoxygenation, pulse oximetry
2. Short-acting barbiturates
3. Isoflurane via mask IPPB → surgical anesthesia
4. Laryngoscopy, spray tracheobronchial tree with local anesthetic
5. Isoflurane via mask IPPB
6. Insert rigid bronchoscope
7. Pack nose and mouth
8. Short-acting barbiturate and lidocaine in-line to control any small sudden reaction to stimulation
9. Spontaneous versus controlled ventilation (see text)
10. No paralysis versus paralysis (see text)
11. F_IO_2 <0.5 in N_2 during laser firing (no N_2O)
12. If % saturation ↓ excessively
    A. Ventilate with 100% O_2
    B. Control bleeding
    C. Suction blood
    D. Remove necrotic tissue
13. Extubate if at all possible

tered until surgical levels of anesthesia are achieved (10 to 15 min). Isoflurane is chosen because these patients may become hypercarbic and acidotic; compared with halothane, isoflurane minimizes the risk of arrhythmias. Laryngoscopy is then performed (usually without paralysis), and the tracheobronchial tree is sprayed with local anesthetic. Controlled ventilation via mask with 100 per cent oxygen and isoflurane is resumed for a short period of time; then the surgeon and assistants sequentially insert a mouth guard, the rigid bronchoscope, Vaseline-gauze packing into the nose, saline-wetted gauze into the mouth, and a transparent dressing over the mouth and around half the bronchoscope. The gauze and transparent dressing greatly decrease the leak around the bronchoscope (see Fig. 14–5). After passage of the bronchoscope, the anesthesia/ventilation system is then connected to the side arm of the bronchoscope. A large syringe of both an ultra-short-acting barbiturate and lidocaine is placed in the intravenous line. If any tensing on the bronchoscope or movement of the tracheobronchial tree (particularly invagination of the posterior membranous part) is observed, small doses of the short-acting barbiturate (50 to 100 mg) and lidocaine (1 mg/kg) are administered. If the endoscopist thinks that spontaneous ventilation is indicated or is essential for the bronchoscopic procedure, spontaneous ventilation is allowed to return at this point. If spontaneous ventilation is not an issue, ventilation is usually controlled with intermittent positive-pressure breathing, and relaxants may be administered to appropriately facilitate this mode of ventilation. A pulse oximeter is always used, 100 per cent oxygen is used during nonresection periods, and less than 50 per cent oxygen in nitrogen is used during resection periods. Since the laser resection of the tumor usually makes ventilation and gas exchange better, every effort is made to extubate the patient after resection. If the patient can be extubated, there is a strong tendency to treat laser resection bronchoscopy as an outpatient procedure. Approaching the procedure on an outpatient basis minimizes the financial impact and maximizes the amount of good quality postresection lifetime.

2. Hematoporphyrin Derivative/Laser Beam Photodynamic Therapy of Bronchogenic Carcinoma

During the last several years it has become apparent that complete remission and, in some cases, apparent cure of bronchogenic carcinomas can be obtained by use of hematoporphyrin derivative/laser beam photodynamic therapy of bronchogenic carcinoma.[15-18] Phototherapy in the presence of a sensitizer, hematoporphyrin derivative produces cytotoxicity through two distinct mechanisms: One is energy dependent, and the other is power dependent. The energy-dependent mechanism is the result of selective photon absorption by the tumor and selective energy transfer to the tumor by hematoporphyrin derivative. When tumor cells have been sensitized in this manner, a laser beam, which can have a low energy level, then produces activated oxygen in the tumor cells; this results in photodynamic chemical reactions that impair tumor cell membrane function and cause tumor cell death within 24 to 48 hours. In contrast, the power-dependent mechanism has the direct thermal laser beam effect of causing coagulation, vaporization, and cutting and excision. The cellular death in this instance is related to the power of the light and is independent of photochemical reactions mediated by the hematoporphyrin derivative. Normal tissue is not harmed by the photodynamic therapy.

The patients receive hematoporphyrin derivative intravenously 3 to 5 days before light irradiation. The laser is carried by a medical-grade quartz optical fiber, which can be passed through either a flexible fiberoptic bronchoscope or a rigid open-tube bronchoscope. The same anesthesia technique and ventilation considerations that apply to Nd-YAG laser therapy apply here. In the only two reported studies to

date, the optical fiber has been introduced through a flexible fiberoptic bronchoscope, and both local and general anesthesia techniques have been used.

In contradistinction to the palliative nature of Nd-YAG laser therapy, photodynamic therapy can be curative of small young lesions. Patients best suited for this approach are those with small carcinomas in situ or early invasive carcinoma lesions and for whom an operation is not feasible either physiologically or technically. In addition, it may be used for patients who have failed to respond to standard therapy and have residual local disease. Photodynamic therapy may be also used in patients in whom it is desirable to reduce the extent of surgical resection; with preoperative photodynamic therapy, selected patients are able to undergo sleeve lobectomy rather than pneumonectomy. Finally, it is possible that the technique can be used in a palliative way to open obstructed bronchi, but this hypothesis has not been tested. An early danger of this technique is bleeding within a large mass, and a late danger is obstruction of the tracheobronchial tree with necrotic tissue.

3. The Carbon Dioxide Laser

a. GENERAL CONSIDERATIONS

The carbon dioxide laser is absorbed by tissues to a much greater extent than the Nd-YAG laser. Consequently, if cutting or vaporization with a shallow depth of penetration with minimal scattering is required the CO_2 laser is the tool of choice. Therefore, the CO_2 laser is most commonly used for removal of lesions that can be directly visualized in the laryngeal and supralaryngeal areas.

b. ANESTHESIC CONSIDERATIONS

The removal of laryngeal lesions by a CO_2 laser requires rigid instrumentation.[18] If the lesion is subglottic, a bronchoscope must be used. The anesthesic considerations for these kinds of cases are similar to those for procedures utilizing the Nd-YAG laser. If the lesion is supraglottic, an endotracheal tube can be used to ventilate the patient. However, the chance that a laser beam could strike and ignite the oxygen-containing endotracheal tube and result in a catastrophic intraluminal blowtorch-type airway fire is much greater. Consequently, the endotracheal tube needs to be meticulously protected from the laser. This may be done by wrapping the endotracheal tube circumferentially with metallic tape above and below the endotracheal tube cuff. Protection of the cuff of the endotracheal tube is provided by placing saline-saturated sponges above the endotracheal tube in the subglottic larynx and filling the cuff with saline. Finally, an operating platform (a flat circular metal instrument) can be inserted into the subglottic larynx above the level of the packed sponges to act as a "catcher's mitt" to further protect the sponges, endotracheal tube and cuff, and tissues of the subglottic larynx from laser beam irradiation.[18]

Alternatively, a cuffless flexible metal tube has been developed.[19] Depending on the site of surgery, a cuff seal may be obtained by saline-soaked pharyngeal packs (surgery on the nose, tongue, palate, oral cavity) or subglottic saline-soaked swabs attached to wires (surgery on the larynx, trachea). Cuffed (to be filled with saline), metal-impregnated, laser beam–resistant tubes are available commercially, but they are for single use only, are expensive, and retain some vulnerability to the carbon dioxide laser beam (the tube can be damaged after approximately 10 hits). The metal-impregnated tube offers no resistance at all to the Nd-YAG laser beam.

4. Adjunctive Endobronchial Radiotherapy

a. GENERAL CONSIDERATIONS

The advent of the laser has made it possible to reopen airways that had been completely or partially obstructed by recurrent carcinoma. However, the limitations of the laser are now being appreciated. Since only the intraluminal extent of the tumor can be treated, recurrences of tumor are rather frequent, even expected, and they necessitate repeat laser treatments at a potentially higher risk of hemorrhage each time.[4, 11, 20–22] Thus, laser therapy has a relatively short duration of therapeutic effect. In addition, laser therapy is limited to treatment of endobronchial tumors and is not suitable for treatment of bronchial obstruction due to extrinsic (peribronchial) malignant disease. To circumvent some of these problems and attempt to offer palliation to patients not suitable for laser therapy, insertion of temporary endobronchial catheters for endobronchial radiotherapy has been tried and appears promising. Endobronchial radiotherapy places a radioactive source near the tumor and delivers a relatively high dose (compared with external radiation) without damage to normal tissue.[23–25]

When this approach was first tried, and only a relatively low-intensity radioactive source was available, a flexible fiberoptic bronchoscope was first inserted through the self-sealing diaphragm of the elbow connector to an endotracheal tube, usually under general anesthesia.[23, 24] If complete bronchial obstruction was encountered, the Nd-YAG laser fiber was passed through the biopsy channel of the fiberoptic bronchoscope and used to reopen the airway. Immediately after completion of the Nd-YAG laser therapy, the endobronchial radiotherapy catheters were inserted percutaneously into the trachea via cricothyroid membrane puncture (see below) and positioned under the direct vision of the fiberoptic bronchoscope. If only partial obstruction of the bronchial airway was observed, the endobronchial radiotherapy catheter was inserted into the trachea via cricothyroid membrane puncture (see below) right away for endobronchial irradiation. Similarly, distal segmental obstructions were also treated with a distally positioned endobronchial catheter instead of the laser. All patients were extubated at the completion of the catheter insertion procedure; this is not surprising in view of previous Nd-YAG laser experience providing symptomatic respiratory relief that is sometimes immediate and dramatic. The symptomatic relief due to the reopening of a large segment of the lung was accompanied by improvements in pulmonary function test results, arterial blood gas values, and ventilation-perfusion lung scans.

The endobronchial radiotherapy catheter had a percutaneous subglottic placement because the catheter had to be left in situ for 1 to 4 days, the subglottic placement diminished irritative cough reflexes and reduced the risk of catheter dislodgment, and it allowed the patient to eat normally while being treated with radiation for several days.[23] The subglottic placement was effected either by a small incision over the cricoid thyroid membrane followed by direct placement of the catheter into the trachea or by percutaneously passing a 12 French introducer through the cricothyroid membrane and using the introducer as a sheath through which the endobronchial catheter can be passed.[23]

The endobronchial radiation catheter was placed in the correct position within the tracheobronchial tree under direct vision with the fiberoptic bronchoscope. When the endobronchial radiotherapy catheter is in the correct position, the catheter can be loaded with the radiation (iridium-192 seeds) so that the length of the radiation source is 2 cm more than the length of the obstruction. The radius of the cylindric volume treated with radiation is 5.0 mm for endobronchial lesions and 7.5 to 15.0 mm for peribronchial disease. Once treatment is complete, the endobronchial catheter is removed. The tiny cricothyroid incision heals readily, and persistent air leaks have not been a problem.

Recently, the technology has improved so that the radioactivity can be delivered to the tumor in a matter of minutes by use of a high-intensity radioactivity remote afterloader.[24, 25] This device consists of a lead safe containing a high-intensity radioactive source. The source is attached to the end of a long radioactivity-transferring cable (4 mm in diameter) (Gamma Med[24] or Selectron[25] catheters), which can be advanced into the appropriate treatment position through a fiberoptic bronchoscope.

These two studies have used two different ways to deliver a short course of high-intensity radiation. In the first study,[24] the position of the treatment cable was determined as follows. An endotracheal and/or endobronchial tube was advanced to a position close to the tumor. A fiberoptic bronchoscope was passed through the endotracheal/endobronchial tube and measured the proximal and distal limits of the tumor. The radioactivity-transferring catheter was inserted into the endotracheal/endobronchial tube and positioned against the distal end of the tumor. After roentgenographic verification of the proper position of the endotracheal/endobronchial tube and the radioactivity-transferring cable, the length of the tumor and dosage of radioactivity to be used was entered into the computer and the treatment was begun. The cable remained in each position for a few seconds, as determined by the computer, and then was retracted proximally in 0.5- to 1.0-cm steps to the next position until the treatment was completed. The total treatment time is usually approximately 3 to 5 min. In the second study,[25] a transnasal fiberoptic bronchoscope, passed under local anesthesia, directed the radioactivity-transferring catheter into a position 1 cm from the tumor. With the cable in this position high-intensity radiation was administered for 12 to 27 min. Since the procedure is so short and physiologically unintrusive, it can be done on an outpatient basis.

b. ANESTHETIC CONSIDERATIONS

The major anesthetic consideration for these cases is the same as that for laser resection with a fiberoptic bronchoscope through an endotracheal tube, namely, a narrowed airway (due to both the fiberoptic bronchoscope and the radiotherapy cable) with which to ventilate the patient. The endotracheal tube is inserted using topical anesthesia and intravenous sedation. The techniques discussed above for intubation with the patient awake are applicable for this procedure. Use of a spiral-wire endotracheal tube is advisable, since it visualizes well on the roentgenographic films needed to confirm proper placement. The endotracheal tube cuff is not inflated, and the patient breathes around and through the tube. For bronchial lesions a smaller tube is required and, again, the cuff is not inflated, and the "intubated" lung breathes through and around the endobronchial tube while the "unintubated" lung breathes independently around the tube. In one advanced case,[23] a lung abscess was encountered distal to a total obstruction after using the laser to vaporize the total occlusion. Aspiration of purulent material into the contralateral lung followed, necessitating evacuation of pus with a rigid bronchoscope, immediate reintubation with a double-lumen tube, and differential lung ventilation for 1 week while the abscess and aspiration pneumonia were treated aggressively. While the patient was intubated, an endobronchial catheter was inserted through the double-lumen tube into the right mainstem bronchus for radiotherapy.

III. TRACHEAL RESECTION

A. General Considerations

Tracheal resection is indicated, if technically feasible, in patients who have tracheal obstruction due to a primary tracheal tumor (the majority are carcinomas) or prior tracheal trauma (e.g., stenosis due to prolonged intubation). Unfortunately, primary tracheal tumors are frequently diagnosed late because they are not readily apparent on the plain chest film, and in many cases the slowly progressive symptoms of upper airway obstruction are misdiagnosed as asthma or chronic bronchitis for long periods of time. Generally, the airway must be narrowed to 5 to 6 mm in cross sectional diameter before signs and symptoms become clinically evident. For patients who have operable tumors, approximately 80 per cent have a segmental resection (which may include carina or larynx) with primary anastomosis, 10 per cent have segmental resection with prosthetic reconstruction, and 10 per cent have insertion of a T-tube stent. Adjuncts to surgical extirpation include pre- and postoperative external radiation, internal radioactive seed radiation (transferred by endobronchial catheter as described above or directly placed by thoracotomy), and preoperative laser debulking therapy.

Median sternotomy with or without a cervical collar incision[26] or a right posterior lateral thoracotomy[27] provides adequate exposure for most cases. Exposure of the carina and main bronchi through a median sternotomy requires a transpericardial approach. The anterior pericardium is divided vertically to permit circumferential mobilization of the ascending aortic arch, which is then retracted laterally to the left. The superior vena cava is displaced laterally to the right, and the right main pulmonary artery is exposed and displaced inferiorly (see Figs. 2–25 and 14–7). The posterior pericardium, which is displayed by these latter maneuvers, is then divided vertically, and the entire mediastinum, trachea, and carina are clearly exposed and accessible. Occasionally, additional posterolateral thoracotomy may be necessary to gain additional exposure. Whenever a primary anastomosis is performed the anesthesiologist may be asked to flex the patient's head in order to reduce the tension on the anastomosis; if undesirable tension is still present, it may be expected that further cervical incisions and proximal laryngeal release or thoracotomy and distal mainstem bronchi release, or both, will have to be done.

Many previous technical limitations to the performance of tracheal surgery can now be overcome by careful preoperative delineation of the site and degree of obstruction, close intraoperative communication between the surgeon and anesthesiologist, improved anesthetic management techniques, and meticulous postoperative care. All of these components contribute to the ability to provide adequate ventilation throughout the perioperative period. Although the results of this complicated surgery on primary tracheal tumors depend on tumor cell type, location, and method of resection, it is generally accepted that in the few institutions with a reasonable degree of surgical experience worthwhile survival can be obtained in the majority of patients. The next section discusses the care of patients undergoing tracheal resection and describes several different methods of airway management.[28–47]

B. Anesthetic Considerations

Unless airway obstruction is imminent, pulmonary function should routinely be studied preoperatively. The presence of preoperative lung disease that is severe enough to indicate postoperative ventilatory support is a relative contraindication to tracheal resection, since the trauma of positive airway pressure and an endotracheal tube cuff at the tracheal suture line may cause wound dehiscence.[31] Obtaining a history of position-dependent airway obstruction is important because the induction of anesthesia should be accomplished with such patients in a position that does not cause airway obstruction. Preoperative evaluation should also include tracheal tomograms, computed tomography (to define the exact position of the lesion), bronchoscopy (usually deferred until the time of operation in order not to precipitate airway obstruction due to edema or hemorrhage), flow-volume loops (upper airway obstructions have characteristic shapes to the loop; extrathoracic obstructions cause an inspiratory limb plateau, and intrathoracic obstructions cause an expiratory limb plateau [Fig. 15–1]), and arterial blood gas determinations. Steroids may be given when tracheal edema is a contributing factor to the decreased size of the airway lumen.

During surgery all patients should have an arterial catheter placed in order to facilitate frequent determination of arterial blood gases. It should be placed in the left radial artery since the innominate artery (which supplies the right radial artery) crosses the trachea and may be compressed during surgery (see Figs. 2–25 and 14–7). Other appropriate monitoring, as described in chapter 7, should be placed prior to the induction of anesthesia. A variety of methods for providing adequate oxygenation and carbon dioxide elimination have been utilized during tracheal resection and are described in Table 15–2. These can be divided into five approaches: (1) standard orotracheal intubation, (2) insertion of a tube into the opened trachea distal to the area of resection, (3) high-frequency jet ventilation through the stenotic area, (4) high-frequency positive-pressure ventilation (HFPPV), and (5) cardiopulmonary bypass.

The first technique utilizes a standard but uncut long orotracheal tube; this is placed above the tracheal lesion after the induction of general anesthesia and is merely insinuated, by the surgeon, past (distal to) the area of stenosis or mass.[33, 34] As the trachea and carina are being

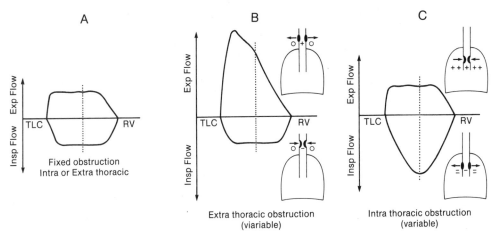

Figure 15–1. Maximal inspiratory and expiratory flow-volume curves in (A) fixed obstruction (intrathoracic or extrathoracic), in which airway diameter does not change with either inspiration or expiration, (B) extrathoracic variable obstruction, and (C) intrathoracic variable obstruction. The dotted line indicates 50 per cent of the vital capacity (VC); the ratio of expired to inspired flow at this point is the mid-VC ratio and is normally 0.9 to 1.0. A, With a fixed obstruction, both expiratory (exp) and inspiratory (insp) flows are equally altered and the mid-VC ratio remains normal. B, With a variable extrathoracic obstruction, forced expiration results in a slightly positive (+) intratracheal pressure that is greater than the pressure around the airway (atmospheric or 0), resulting in a decrease of the obstruction (airway dilates). During forced inspiration when pressure around the airway (0) exceeds the intratracheal pressure (−), the obstruction is increased (airway narrows). Since the expiratory curve is normal and the inspiratory curve is altered, the mid-VC ratio is much greater than normal. C, With a variable intrathoracic obstruction, forced expiration results in a very positive (+ +) pleural pressure that is greater than the slightly positive (+) intratracheal pressure, resulting in an increase of the obstruction (airway narrows). During forced inspiration, the intratracheal pressure (–) is greater than the pleural pressure (––), thus decreasing the obstruction (airway dilates). Since the inspiratory curve is normal and the expiratory curve is attenuated, the mid-VC ratio is much less than normal. A normal flow-volume curve is a composite of the inspiratory curve in B and the expiratory curve in C. (TLC = total lung capacity; RV = residual volume.)

dissected, gentle ventilation by hand facilitates exposure. Although this method is relatively easy to employ, a large tube may traumatize the lesion and cause bleeding or dislodgment of tissue, resulting in further airway obstruction. Furthermore, the technique is limited to cases with a relatively mild stenosis, and the presence of an endotracheal tube in the surgical field makes the tracheal anastomosis more difficult to complete.

To overcome these problems, endotracheal or endobronchial tubes have been inserted into the opened trachea distal to the site of resection (second approach).[31, 35–41] With this second approach, initially either a small endotracheal tube is passed distal to the obstruction or a standard endotracheal tube is placed proximal to it (Figs. 15–2A, 15–3A, and 15–4A). All further tracheal and endobronchial intubations are performed with armored tubes passed into the airway, which is surgically opened distal to the lesion. The surgeon must have a complete set of sizes of endotracheal tubes to choose from, since either mainstem bronchus or any lobar bronchus may need to be intubated.

With a high tracheal lesion, a cervical incision, possibly combined with a median sternotomy, provides adequate surgical exposure. An opening is made in the trachea distal to the area to be resected, and a sterile endotracheal tube is inserted by the surgeon into the distal trachea[31, 35, 36] (Fig. 15–2B). This second endotracheal tube is connected to a Y-piece and a second set of anesthetic hoses and is handed off to the anesthesiologist in order to continue ventilation. After excision of the tracheal lesion and placement of the posterior tracheal sutures, the second (distal) endotracheal tube is removed from the trachea, the original (first) endotracheal tube is advanced past the anastomosis line and reconnected to the anesthetic circuit, and the anastomosis is completed (Fig. 15–2C and D).

With a low tracheal lesion, a right thoracotomy provides the necessary surgical exposure. If there is sufficient trachea distal to the area of resection, a Foley catheter with the tip cut off just distal to the balloon may be used as a single-lumen endotracheal tube; it is inserted by the surgeon and secured just above the

Table 15–2. Approaches to Airway Management During Tracheal Resection

General Approach	Year	Surgical Approach	Technique	Remarks
I. Orotracheal Intubation				
A. Belsey[33]	1950	Right thoracotomy	Orotracheal tube	First description of this type of management—tube advanced distally as resection carried out
B. Kamvyssi-Dea et al[34]	1975	Right thoracotomy	Orotracheal tube	Tube advanced distally as resection carried out
II. Insertion of Tube into Opened Trachea Distal to Area of Resection				
A. Geffin et al[31]	1969	Cervical incision for high lesion; right thoracotomy for low lesion	Endotracheal tube / Endobronchial tube	Excellent review article described experience with 31 patients; stressed avoiding tracheostomy and cardiopulmonary by-pass for this procedure
B. Debrand et al[35]	1979	Cervical incision	4-mm endotracheal tube into distal trachea	Patient 4 months old
C. Boyan et al[36]	1976	Median sternotomy	Cuffed endotracheal tube into distal tracheal stump	Stressed preoperative forced vital capacity loop of airflow versus volume to confirm diagnosis of airway obstruction
D. Abou-Madi et al[37]	1979	Median sternotomy	28 Foley catheter into distal tracheal stump	End cut off just distal to balloon allowed bilateral lung ventilation through short tracheal stump
E. Lippmann et al[38]	1977	Right thoracotomy	Left endobronchial tube	Tube quickly inserted following intraoperative tracheal resection
F. Akdikmen et al[39]	1965	Right thoracotomy	Right endobronchial tube	Patient died postoperatively; authors suggested use of cardiopulmonary by-pass for this procedure
G. Dodge et al[40]	1977	Right thoracotomy	Right and left endobronchial tubes	Two anesthesia circuits used
H. Theman et al[32]	1976	Right thoracotomy	Right and left endobronchial tubes	Two ventilation systems used; selective occlusion of contralateral pulmonary artery during one-lung ventilation
III. High-Frequency Jet Ventilation				
A. Lee et al[41]	1974	Median sternotomy	8 French suction catheter passed through stenotic area; bronchoscope injector	Patient 8 years old
B. McNaughton et al[42]	1975	Not stated	No. 12 catheter; jet ventilation	No significant effects on the circulation noted
C. Baraka[43]	1977	Right thoracotomy	5-mm cuffed endotracheal tube; jet ventilation	Tube pushed (from above) past lesion during anastomoses
D. Ellis et al[44]	1976	Not stated	1.52-mm diameter manometer line; bronchoscope injector	Patient 13 years old
IV. High-Frequency Positive-Pressure Ventilation (HFPPV)				
A. Eriksson et al[30]	1975	Cervical incision	No. 14 catheter; rate 60/min	First report of HFPPV for tracheal resection
B. El-Baz et al[29]	1982	Cervical incision	2-mm catheter; rate 150/min	Used with uncuffed tracheal T-tube stent
C. El-Baz et al[28]	1982	Right thoracotomy	2-mm catheter; rate 150/min	Two patients for carinal resection and one for tracheal resection; only left lung ventilated
V. Cardiopulmonary Bypass				
A. Woods et al[46]	1961	Right thoracotomy	Cardiopulmonary by-pass	First reported case; instituted after chest was open
B. Coles et al[47]	1976	Right thoracotomy	Cardiopulmonary by-pass	By-pass instituted under local anesthesia prior to operation

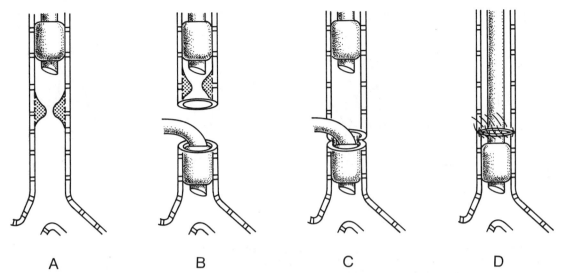

Figure 15–2. Airway management and surgical procedure for resection of a high tracheal lesion. A, Initial intubation above the lesion. B, Second endotracheal intubation distal to the lesion after the trachea has been opened. C, Placement of sutures for the posterior anastomosis. D, The second endotracheal tube has been removed, and the original endotracheal tube has been advanced distal to the anterior anastomosis. (Redrawn with permission from Geffin B, Bland J, Grillo HC: Anesthetic management of tracheal resection and reconstruction. Anesth Analg 48:884, 1969.)

carina, avoiding endobronchial intubation and the need for one-lung anesthesia.[37] Otherwise, if there is not enough distance between the tracheal lesion and the carina to provide placement of even this homemade endotracheal tube, endobronchial intubation and one-lung ventilation are necessary[38–40] (Fig. 15–3B). If

oxygenation or ventilation is inadequate, it may be possible to decrease blood flow to the atelectatic lung by tightening reversible snares around the pulmonary artery of the nonventilated lung.[31, 32] However, this maneuver may be technically difficult, and an alternative technique is to pass a second endobronchial tube

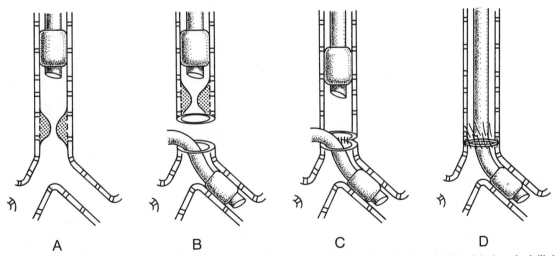

Figure 15–3. Airway management and surgical procedure for resection of a low tracheal lesion. A, Initial intubation above the lesion. B, Left endobronchial intubation distal to the lesion after the trachea has been opened. C, Placement of sutures for the posterior anastomosis. D, The endobronchial tube has been removed, and the original endotracheal tube has been advanced distal to the anterior anastomosis into an endobronchial position. (Redrawn with permission from Geffin B, Bland J, Grillo HC: Anesthetic management of tracheal resection and reconstruction. Anesth Analg 48:884, 1969.)

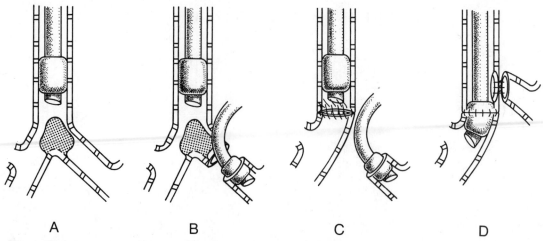

Figure 15–4. *Airway management and surgical procedure for resection of a carinal lesion. A, Initial intubation above the lesion. B, Left endobronchial intubation distal to the lesion after the left mainstem bronchus has been severed. C, The trachea is anastomosed to the right mainstem bronchus. D, The left endobronchial tube has been removed in order to allow for anastomosis between the trachea and the left mainstem bronchus. Ventilation during (D) is accomplished via the original endotracheal tube. (Redrawn with permission from Geffin B, Bland J, Grillo HC: Anesthetic management of tracheal resection and reconstruction. Anesth Analg 48:884, 1969.)*

into the other bronchus to provide ventilation to both lungs[40] (see below). As with the technique for the high tracheal lesion, after the posterior anastomosis is completed, the endobronchial tube(s) is removed and the original endotracheal tube is pushed past the site of resection; in this situation, however, it is likely that an endobronchial intubation may again be required to complete the anastomosis (Fig. 15–3C and D).

Several methods have been described for managing the airway during carinal resection.[31,32] While the affected segment is being resected, left lung ventilation may be carried out via an endobronchial intubation of the left mainstem bronchus below this lesion[31] (Fig. 15–4B). After the right mainstem bronchus and trachea have been reattached, the left endobronchial tube is removed, and the original endotracheal tube is advanced distal to the suture line. The right lung is then ventilated via this tube, while the left main bronchus is reanastomosed to the trachea at a different point of origin (Fig. 15–4C and D). Again, blood flow to the nonventilated lung can be reduced by tightening ties placed around the appropriate pulmonary artery. An alternate method of ventilation during carinal resection is to perform endobronchial intubation of both severed bronchi, a technique that enables two-lung ventilation for a much longer period during the procedure.[32] This latter technique requires the use of two ventilating systems. As the posterior anastomosis is being

made, ventilation is achieved through both of the distal mainstem bronchi. During repair of the anterior wall, ventilation is done via the original endotracheal tube (above the anastomosis site). The air leak that initially occurs through the anastomosis site diminishes progressively as the anterior sutures are placed. If the anastomosis site leak is excessive, the endotracheal tube can be pushed into an endobronchial position until the placement of additional sutures reduces the leak.

It is apparent that the above conventional techniques of airway management for tracheal resection are fraught with hazard. During operation a slight head-down tilt helps to minimize aspiration of blood and secretions. Intermittent sighs help prevent bronchiolar obstruction and atelectasis. A high inspired oxygen concentration is employed, since an oxygen-filled functional residual capacity (FRC) permits a few extra minutes to correct relatively common episodes of airway obstruction and/or tube displacement. Ventilation is continuously monitored by auscultation and observation of the chest, measurement of compliance (peak inspiratory pressure), and arterial blood gas determinations. Several different sizes of armored endotracheal tubes must be available for use throughout the procedure. Finally, close comminication must exist between the surgery and anesthesia teams. Disadvantages of these complex airway techniques include soilage of the lung with blood and debris, the presence of tubes in the surgical field, and the occasional necessity of utilizing one-lung (or less) ventilation.

In an effort to overcome these problems, a third approach to airway management during tracheal resection consists of high-flow jet ventilation through small-bore endotracheal tubes or catheters[41-45] (see Fig. 12–2). With this technique a small-bore uncuffed catheter is placed through the stenotic area, and ventilation is accomplished by exposing the lung to rapid, intermittent, high-flow, fresh gas from the catheter. Oxygen jets entrain ambient air, which, in turn, provides the volume necessary for adequate ventilation. Using this technique, acceptable blood gas values have been maintained and there have been no deleterious effects on the circulation. With only a small catheter in the field the surgeon can more easily perform the tracheal resection and anastomosis. The disadvantages of this technique, however, include possible inadequate escape of air around the jet catheter during exhalation when the catheter is passed through a tight stenotic area, plugging of the catheter with blood, displacement of the catheter, aspiration of blood, and technical difficulties with high-pressure injectors.

Recently, the above technique of jet ventilation for tracheal stenosis has been modified with good success.[45] A small cuffed endotracheal tube (6-mm internal diameter) is placed above the stenosis, and jet ventilation around the mass is begun. When the lesion has been excised, the small jet ventilation endotracheal tube is passed into a mainstem bronchus, and jet ventilation of just the one lung is continued. When the anastomosis has been completed around the small endotracheal tube, the endotracheal tube is brought back above the anastomotic line.

The fourth approach to airway management during tracheal resection utilizes high-frequency positive-pressure ventilation (HFPPV)[30] (see Fig. 12–2). This technique utilizes small tidal volumes (50 to 250 ml) delivered via a small catheter at relatively rapid rates (50 to 150/min). Advantages of using HFPPV for tracheal resection include a relatively unobstructed surgical field, no interruption of ventilation during operation, minimized contamination of the lungs from blood and debris by a continuous outflow of gas, minimized lung and mediastinal movement, and production of continuous positive airway pressure lessens the risk of alveolar collapse. This technique has been used by others successfully,

for both tracheal[28, 29] and carinal resections.[28] During carinal operations HFPPV to the left lung alone generally provided adequate oxygenation and ventilation, although a system of two catheters and bilateral HFPPV could be used if necessary.[30]

The fifth approach to airway management during tracheal resection, especially in cases of carinal resection, has been the institution of cardiopulmonary bypass either at the time of resection[46] or prior to the start of surgery.[47] Following resection, anesthesia can be continued by conventional techniques using a standard endotracheal tube. Although many surgical teams perform difficult tracheal resections with the cardiopulmonary bypass team standing by, the risk of intrapulmonary hemorrhage due to heparinization precludes its use in most cases.[31]

Helium-oxygen breathing mixtures can significantly decrease the resistance to gas flow through stenotic areas and may be considered preoperatively for some of these patients.[47] However, the use of helium-oxygen mixtures prevents the use of high inspired oxygen concentration during anesthesia, and it is therefore not often recommended.[31]

Postoperatively, most patients are kept in a position of head flexion in order to reduce tension on the suture line. If ventilatory support is necessary postoperatively, the endotracheal tube must be positioned so that the cuff does not rest on any suture line. Early extubation is highly desirable in order to minimize the compromise of blood flow to the trachea, which might be caused by an inflated tracheal cuff. Chest physiotherapy to remove secretions should not be too vigorous and may need augmentation by fiberoptic bronchoscopy. Systemic antibiotics and steroids are not routinely given unless infection or excessive edema, respectively, is strongly anticipated. If massive bleeding into the airway or chest occurs postoperatively, it is likely due to erosion into the pulmonary artery or aorta (high incidence following insertion of a tracheal prosthesis) and is usually not treatable.

IV. GIANT BULLOUS EMPHYSEMA AND AIR CYSTS

A. General Considerations

A bulla is defined as an air-filled, thin-walled space within the lung that results from the destruction of alveolar tissue. The walls of bullae are formed by connective tissue septa, compressed lung parenchyma, or pleura. A bulla usually represents a local end-stage area of emphysematous destruction. As a separate but related entity, air cysts in the lung have their own epithelial margins, and they may also be associated with chronic obstructive lung disease[48] or found in the absence of other pulmonary pathology.[49]

Bullectomy is the surgical resection of one or more bullae and is performed only in selected patients. Indications for bullectomy in chronic obstructive pulmonary disease patients include intolerable breathlessness even after full medical therapy, rapidly enlarging bullae, or the repeated occurrence of pneumothorax.[50] Patients with otherwise healthy lungs may undergo removal of a giant air cyst or bulla if it compresses a large area of normal lung and causes functional impairment. The compression of a large area of lung can be visualized on the chest roentgenogram (as well as on an angiogram) as the crowding together of pulmonary vessels. A strong case for functional impairment can be made if radioisotope studies show that the compressed area has good perfusion and some, but reduced, ventilation[51, 52] (see chapter 5 and Fig. 5–9).

The long-term results of bullectomy for giant bullae in emphysema are encouraging.[53] In 27 emphysematous patients who had either unilateral (10 patients) or bilateral (17 patients) bullae that occupied over 50 per cent of the hemithorax, bullectomy significantly decreased dyspnea, they were no longer functionally disabled, and mean survival time was greater than 7 years. The postoperative spirographic improvement depended on the type of bullae; resection of bullae with open communication with the bronchial tree resulted predominantly in improvement of forced expiratory flow in one second (FEV_1) as a percentage of vital capacity, whereas resection of closed bullae resulted predominantly in an increase in vital capacity. The long-term prognosis after surgical treatment of bullous emphysema is, of course, diminished in patients who have chronic purulent bronchitis preoperatively and/or do not abandon smoking.

B. Anesthetic Considerations

Anesthesia for the removal of bullae involves several specific ventilation hazards (Table 15–3). First, most of these patients have severe generalized chronic lung disease with little or no ventilatory reserve. Thus, ventilation (which

Table 15–3. Ventilation Hazards During Bullectomy

I. Rest of lung is diseased
II. Bullae may increase in size owing to:
   A. IPPB
   B. N_2O
   C. One-way check-valve
III. Bulla may rupture → pneumothorax

needs to be controlled once the chest is opened) of one severely diseased lung (the one without the giant bulla) may be hazardous and runs the risks of hypoxemia, hypercarbia, and pneumothorax on the ventilated side. If the ventilated lung also contains a bulla, the risks are obviously even greater. In addition, since general anesthesia is necessary for the procedure, it is likely that many patients with severe lung disease will be committed to at least a short period of postoperative mechanical ventilatory support. Second, when a bulla or air cyst is in communication with a bronchus, positive-pressure ventilation may cause it to increase in size.[54] If a significant portion of the tidal volume enters the bullous cavity, alveolar dead space ventilation will be greatly increased, and unless there is an equivalent increase in minute ventilation, the rest of the lung may be inadequately ventilated. This complication is most likely to occur when the chest is opened because the chest wall no longer limits the expansion of the bulla. Third, because of the rapidity with which closed air spaces take up nitrous oxide and expand in size,[55] this agent is best avoided (especially in patients whose bullae are thought to have poor communication with the bronchial system).[56] Fourth, if a check-valve is present in the airway that communicates with the cavity, overinflation and air trapping may occur within the cavity. Fifth, and most important, positive pressure within the bulla might cause it to rupture, creating a pneumothorax, which would likely be under tension if the chest were closed (especially in patients whose bullae are thought to have good communication with the bronchial system).[54] Tension pneumothorax in these patients is usually a catastrophic event owing to the impairment of venous return and cardiac output as well as further compromise of ventilation. Insertion of a chest tube at this point would create, in effect, a large bronchopleural cutaneous fistula that could divert much of the ventilation out through the chest tube. Recently, high-frequency ventilation with low tidal volumes and airway pressure has been used successfully to avoid positive-pressure rupture of a bulla.[57]

The cornerstone of the anesthetic management of patients with giant bullae or cysts is the insertion of a double-lumen tube to allow differential treatment of the two lungs. Thus, in patients with unilateral disease, the double-lumen tube can allow adequate ventilation of the nondiseased side while at the same time preventing rupture of the diseased side. In patients with bilateral disease the double-lumen tube still allows differential lung treatment to maximize gas exchange as well as providing an increased capability to deal with the complications of a ruptured bulla. For example, a double-lumen tube allows all possible permutations of high-frequency ventilation, continuous positive airway pressure, positive end-expiratory pressure (PEEP), and zero end-expiratory pressure to the two lungs, depending on the pathology in each lung (see Differential Lung Ventilation, chapter 19). In addition, as each bulla is resected, the double-lumen tube allows ventilation to the operated lung to be reestablished for short periods, enabling the surgeon to identify and suture any air leaks that may be present.

A double-lumen endotracheal tube can be inserted with the patient either awake and the airway topically anesthetized (for those with histories of repeated pneumothorax and/or bilateral bullae) or under general anesthesia (for the majority of patients) in order to isolate the affected lung and provide positive-pressure ventilation to the contralateral lung.[58, 59] While the depth of general anesthesia is being increased, spontaneous ventilation may be maintained (most indicated in patients with a history of repeated pneumothorax or bilateral bullae), but it should be realized that spontaneously breathing patients with significant pulmonary disease under general anesthesia probably will not be able to ventilate themselves adequately. Alternatively, and preferably in the majority of patients, the patient can be anesthetized and both lungs ventilated using a limited amount of positive airway pressure; gentle ventilation by hand is the best way to assure low airway pressures.

If limited positive-pressure ventilation is chosen, it is important that the anesthesiologist be able to diagnose and treat a pneumothorax rapidly. External stethoscopes should be attached over each hemithorax at the points where breath sounds are maximal in order to monitor for pneumothorax on each side.[60] However, it should be realized that advanced bullous disease may completely prevent breath sounds from being heard externally at all. In addition to a decrease in breath sounds, a pneumothorax or check-valve mechanism in a cyst may be signaled by an increase in airway pressure, tracheal shift to the opposite side, or hypotension out of proportion to the depth of anesthesia. Equipment for chest tube placement must be immediately available for these patients. However, chest tube placement for a ruptured bulla poses two problems. First, rupture of only one of several bullae present in a lung may result in a somewhat localized pneumothorax that is decompressed only by precise localization of the chest tube. Second, as discussed above, a large bronchopleural cutaneous fistula may be created when the chest tube is placed, making ventilation difficult (see Bronchopleural Fistula, chapter 16).

Theoretically, following bullectomy, the patient's pulmonary status should be improved since the "healthy" lung tissue that was previously compressed by the bullae should now be able to expand. However, in the author's experience the weaning and extubation process may take up to several days in some patients with advanced disease. When mechanical ventilation is required postoperatively, positive airway pressure should again be minimized in order to decrease the possibility of producing a pneumothorax from rupture of suture lines and/or residual bullae.[61]

When bilateral bullectomy is done because of extensive disease in both lungs, a sternal splitting incision with the patient supine is usually employed.[62] However, sequential posterolateral thoracotomies may be planned if it is desired to see how the patient responds to the first bullectomy. With bilateral bullectomy, the same anesthetic principles apply as with unilateral bullectomy. A double-lumen endotracheal tube is again the cornerstone of management, allowing differential lung treatment throughout the operation. If sequential posterolateral thoracotomies are planned, provision for gaining access to the closed chest should be made in the way the skin is prepared and the patient is draped, in case suspicion of a pneumothorax in the closed chest arises.

V. PULMONARY RESECTION IN PATIENTS AFTER PNEUMONECTOMY

A. General Considerations

Patients who have had a pneumonectomy may have a new lesion appear in the remaining lung; the density, if it persists and increases in size, is almost always malignant. Pneumonectomy has been generally considered in the past to be a contraindication to further pulmonary resection. However, six case reports involving eight patients[63-68] and one recent series of 15 patients[69] have provided evidence that limited pulmonary resection after pneumonectomy is feasible with a low operative mortality. The long-term results show that resection of these "secondary" tumors can result in a reasonably prolonged and worthwhile survival in some patients.

B. Anesthetic Considerations

These cases must be done with a single-lumen endotracheal tube. Fluid balance must be carefully regulated because the size of the pulmonary vascular bed will be decreased further from an already small size and the risk of pulmonary hypertension will be increased by the resection. Thus, all aspects of postoperative care, such as maintenance of fluid balance (risk of pulmonary edema and pulmonary hypertension), positive-pressure ventilation (risk of right-sided heart failure), and adequate evacuation of the pleural space (risk of lung compression), must be undertaken with increased care because of the patient's increased sensitivity to derangements in any of these factors.

VI. UNILATERAL BRONCHOPULMONARY LAVAGE[70]

A. General Considerations

Unilateral bronchopulmonary lavage or massive irrigation of the tracheobronchial tree of one lung has been employed with good success in patients with pulmonary alveolar proteinosis as a means of removing the enormous accumulations of alveolar lipoproteinaceous material that these patients characteristically have.[71-78] The lipoproteinaceous material is thought to be surfactant,[79] and the abnormal accumulation is due to failure of clearance mechanisms rather than enhanced formation.[80] The abnormal accumulation of alveolar lipoproteinaceous material is bilateral and symmetric and causes the classic chest roentgenographic picture of air space consolidation with patchy, poorly defined shadows throughout the lung[81]; the roentgenographic picture parallels the course of the disease. The air space consolidation causes progressive hypoxemia and shortness of breath

(first on exertion and then finally at rest),[81, 82] and the lungs have a low compliance. The diagnosis of alveolar proteinosis is made by correlating the above clinical, roentgenologic, and laboratory data with the results of a lung biopsy. The indications for lavage consist of P_aO_2 less than 60 mm Hg at rest or hypoxemic limitation of normal activity.[83, 84] Infrequently, lung lavage may be performed in patients with asthma, cystic fibrosis, and radioactive dust inhalation.[71, 76, 85, 86]

Unilateral lung lavage is performed under general anesthesia with a double-lumen endotracheal tube, allowing lavage of one lung while the other lung is ventilated (Fig. 15–5). In patients with alveolar proteinosis, lavage is performed on one lung and then after a few days rest on the other lung. Following lung lavage, these patients usually have marked subjective improvement, which correlates with increases in P_aO_2 during rest and exercise, vital capacity and diffusion capacity, and clearing of the chest roentgenogram.[87, 88] Some patients require lavage every few months, whereas others remain in remission for several years, and the disease may even eventually completely remit.[87, 88]

B. Anesthetic Considerations[70]

This section discusses the technique for managing bronchopulmonary lavage in patients with pulmonary alveolar proteinosis. When the patient is admitted to the hospital, ventilation-perfusion scans of the lung are obtained. Ventilation can be maximized during lung lavage by performing the first lavage on the most severely affected lung, allowing the "better" lung to provide gas exchange. If the scan indicates relatively equal involvement (as is usually the case), the left lung is lavaged first, leaving the larger right lung to support gas exchange.

Unilateral lung lavage is performed in the operating room, where the appropriate amount and type of equipment and ancillary personnel are present to enhance safety. Patient safety is also enhanced if a relatively constant team, composed of members of the departments of anesthesia and pulmonary medicine, becomes familiar with the nuances and technique of unilateral lung lavage. Patients are usually cooperative and require only light premedication. Since many of these patients are hypoxemic at rest, they are given oxygen by face mask following premedication and during transport to the warmed operating room.

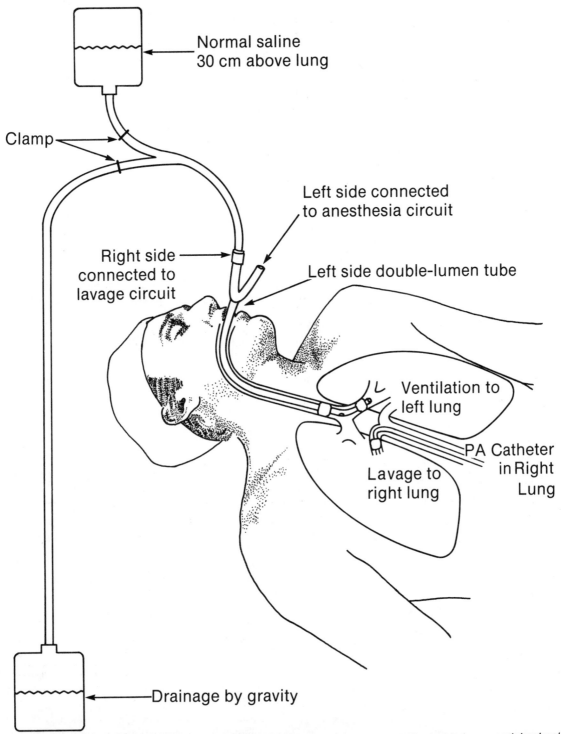

Normal saline
30 cm above lung

Clamp

Left side connected
to anesthesia circuit

Right side
connected to
lavage circuit

Left side double-lumen tube

Ventilation to
left lung

PA Catheter
in Right
Lung

Lavage to
right lung

Drainage by gravity

Figure 15–5. Technique for providing unilateral pulmonary lavage. A left clear plastic double-lumen endotracheal tube allows ventilation to the left lung during lavage of the right lung (and vice versa). Normal saline is infused and drained by gravity; clamps on the connection tubes determine direction of fluid flow. (Reproduced with permission from Alfery DD, Benumof JL, Spragg RG: Anesthesia for bronchopulmonary lavage. In Kaplan J (ed.): Thoracic Anesthesia. New York, Churchill Livingstone, 1982, chapter 12, pp. 403–420.)

The procedure takes several hours to complete, and lavage fluid temperature cannot always be precisely controlled, thus some patients require external warming (e.g., with heating blanket) to maintain normal body temperature. The monitoring system consists of a blood pressure cuff, electrocardiogram, precordial stethoscope, temperature probe, pulse oximeter, and peripheral arterial and central venous pressure catheters. Patients with compromised cardiovascular function are monitored with a pulmonary artery catheter in place of the central venous catheter.

After several minutes of preoxygenation (see below), general anesthesia is induced with 3 to 4 mg/kg of thiopental in divided doses and inhalation of either isoflurane or halothane in 100 per cent oxygen. Isoflurane is relatively indicated in patients in whom therapeutic levels of theophylline (and the risk of arrhythmias) are present. Neuromuscular blockade is monitored with a peripheral nerve stimulator and is induced with a nondepolarizing muscle relaxant. When a suitable level of anesthesia has been reached, the trachea is topically anesthetized with lidocaine and intubated with the largest size left-sided double-lumen endotracheal tube that can be passed atraumatically through the glottis (see chapter 9). A clear plastic disposable left-sided double-lumen tube is used because of the ease and certainty with which it is correctly positioned, the reliable left cuff seal obtained (the right endobronchial cuff is small and inflates asymmetrically), and the ability to continuously observe the tidal movements of respiratory gas moisture (ventilated lung) and the lavage drainage fluid for leaking air bubbles (lavaged lung). The largest size tube is used because the left endobronchial cuff will make contact over a greater bronchial mucosal area with less air in the left cuff (compared with a small double-lumen tube). In addition, a large tube facilitates suctioning, which is an important consideration at the end of the case when the lungs need to be made as clear as possible. Precise placement of the tube and detection of leaks are essential because of the serious hazard of spillage during the lavage procedure. The position of the double-lumen tube must be confirmed with a fiberoptic bronchoscope as described in chapter 9, and cuff seal must be demonstrated to hold against 50 cm H_2O pressure using the catheter-under-water technique described in chapter 9. The eyes should be protected with a lubricant and eye pads.

The question of patient position during unilateral lung lavage is important, for there are major advantages and disadvantages related to each position (Table 15-4). The lateral decubitus position with the lavaged lung dependent minimizes the possibility of accidental spillage of lavage fluid from the dependent lavaged lung to the nondependent ventilated lung. However, during periods of lavage fluid drainage, pulmonary blood flow, which is gravity dependent, would preferentially perfuse the nonventilated dependent lung, and the right-to-left transpulmonary shunt would be maximal. The lateral decubitus position with the lavaged lung nondependent minimizes blood flow to the nonventilated lung but, on the other hand, increases the possibility of accidental spillage of lavage fluid from the lavaged lung to the dependent ventilated lung. As a compromise, the supine position is used in order to balance the risk of aspiration against the risk of hypoxemia.

Following insertion and checking of the double-lumen endotracheal tube and positioning of the patient, baseline total and individual lung compliance should be measured. Airway pressure can be electronically transduced and continuously recorded on a paper write-out, and a Wright spirometer should be placed in the expiratory limb of the anesthesia circle system in order to accurately measure tidal volume. A volume ventilator that can deliver relatively high inflation pressures is required, since these patients have diseased and noncompliant lungs. Prelavage total dynamic compliance (chest wall and lung) of both lungs together (using 15 ml/kg of breath) and then of each lung separately (using 10 ml/kg of breath) is measured. Following measurement of total and individual lung compliance, and with the patient breathing 100 per cent oxygen, baseline arterial blood gases are measured.

Table 15-4. Unilateral Lung Lavage: Position of Patient

I. Lateral decubitus with lavaged lung nondependent
   Advantage: minimizes blood flow to the nonventilated lung
   Disadvantage: maximizes the possibility of spillage
II. Lateral decubitus with lavaged lung dependent
   Advantage: minimizes the possibility of spillage
   Disadvantage: maximizes blood flow to the nonventilated lung
III. Supine position
   Balances spillage and blood flow distribution problems

The patients are completely preoxygenated prior to the induction of anesthesia and lavage for two reasons. First, as with the induction of general anesthesia in any patient, an oxygen-filled functional residual capacity greatly minimizes the risk of hypoxemia during the apneic period required for laryngoscopy and endotracheal intubation. This consideration has increased importance for patients with alveolar proteinosis since they are already severely hypoxemic. Second, preoxygenation eliminates nitrogen from the lung that is to be lavaged. Alveolar gas is then composed only of oxygen and carbon dioxide. During fluid filling, these gases will be absorbed, which allows the lavage fluid maximal access to the alveolar space. Failure to remove nitrogen from the lung prior to filling with lavage fluid may leave peripheral nitrogen bubbles in the alveoli and thus limit the effectiveness of the lavage.

Warmed isotonic saline is used as the lavage fluid and is infused by gravity from a height of 30 cm above the midaxillary line. After the lavage fluid ceases to flow (i.e., lung filling is complete), drainage is accomplished by clamping the inflow line and unclamping the drainage line, which runs to a collection bottle placed 20 cm below the midaxillary line (Fig. 15–5). The inflow and outflow fluid lines are connected to the appropriate endotracheal tube lumen by a Y-adapter. Each tidal lavage filling is accompanied by mechanical chest percussion and vibration to the lavaged hemithorax prior to drainage. The lavage fluid that is drained is typically light brown, and the sediment layers out at the bottom of the collection bottle after a short period of time. Filling and drainage of approximately 500- to 1000-ml aliquots are repeated until the lavage effluent clears (Fig. 15–5). Volumes delivered to and recovered from each tidal lavage are recorded. Total lavage fluid volumes of 10 to 20 L are usually employed.

Most patients studied have been hemodynamically stable throughout the entire lavage procedure. In particular, lavage itself has caused no significant changes in systemic and pulmonary artery pressures and cardiac output. In these patients, the parterial saturation as measured by oximetry has increased and decreased, with each lung filling and lung drainage, respectively. Arterial saturation increases during lung filling because blood flow to the nonventilated lung is decreased by the lavage fluid infusion pressure.[89] The opposite set of events (increased nonventilated lung blood flow, decreased arterial oxygen saturation) occurs during drainage.[89] An adequate degree of neuromuscular blockade must be maintained because unexpected vigorous coughing during the procedure could alter double-lumen endotracheal tube position.

If a small leak should occur during lavage, the following may be observed sequentially: (1) the appearance of bubbles in the lavage fluid draining from the lavaged lung, (2) rales and rhonchi in the ventilated lung, (3) a difference between lavage volumes administered and those drained from the lavaged lung (the former exceeds the latter), and (4) a fall in arterial oxygen saturation. If a small leak is suspected or detected by any of the above signs and the lavaged lung has been only minimally treated, the lavaged lung should be drained of all fluid, and the position of the double-lumen endotracheal tube, the adequacy of cuff seal, and separation of the lungs should be rechecked with a fiberoptic bronchoscope. Before beginning the lavage procedure again, and no matter what the double-lumen tube malposition was, the functional separation of the two lungs and adequacy of cuff seal should be tested and found adequate by using the previously described air bubble leak detection method.

Massive spillage of fluid from the lavaged lung to the ventilated lung is not a subtle event and results in a dramatic decrease in ventilated lung compliance and a rapid and large decrease in arterial oxygen saturation. Under these circumstances the lavage procedure must be terminated no matter how much treatment has been accomplished. The patient should be moved quickly to the lateral decubitus position with the lavaged side dependent, and the operating room table should be placed in a head-down position in order to facilitate removal of lavage fluid. Vigorous suctioning and inflation of both lungs should be carried out. The double-lumen tube should be changed to a standard single-lumen tube, and the patient should be additionally treated with a period of mechanical ventilatory support with positive end-expiratory pressure. Timing of further unilateral lung lavage attempts will be dictated by the patient's subsequent clinical course and gas exchange status.

After the effluent lavage fluid becomes clear, the procedure is terminated. The lavaged lung is thoroughly suctioned, and ventilation is begun. Since the compliance of the lavaged side will be much less than that of the ventilated side at this time, large tidal ventilations (sighs) (15 to 20 ml/kg) to that side alone (with the nonlavaged side temporarily nonventilated) are necessary to reexpand alveoli. Arterial blood oxygenation may decrease precipitously during this time, but this can be minimized by clamping the nonlavaged side after a large inspiration of 100 per cent oxygen.

After lavage the recovery procedure consists of repetitive periods of large tidal ventilations, suctioning and chest wall percussion to the previously lavaged side, conventional two-lung ventilation with PEEP, and bilateral suctioning and postural drainage while intermittently measuring combined (total) and individual lung dynamic compliance. As the compliance of the lavaged lung returns toward prelavage values, ventilation with an air-oxygen mixture may help lavaged lung alveoli with low ventilation-perfusion ratios to remain open. When the compliance of the hemithorax of the lavaged side returns to its prelavage value, the neuromuscular blockade is reversed. Mechanical ventilation and extubation guidelines are the same as for any patient with pulmonary disease (see chapter 19); most patients are able to be extubated while still in the operating room. If the patient is not considered a candidate for extubation, the double-lumen tube is changed to a single-lumen tube and the patient is mechanically ventilated with PEEP in a conventional manner.

In the immediate postlavage period, deep breathing (incentive spirometry), coughing exercises, chest percussion, and postural drainage are used to remove remaining fluid and secretiions and to reexpand the lavaged lung. After 3 to 5 days of recovery, the patient is returned to the operating room to have the opposite side lavaged. The anesthetic considerations for the second lavage are the same as those for the first lavage, although oxygenation is usually not nearly as severe a problem as during the first lavage because the treated and near now-normal lung will be used to support gas exchange.

There are two special problems associated with pulmonary lavage that may be encountered. First, a few critically ill patients may be unable to tolerate the conventional procedure. Second, unilateral lavage through a double-lumen tube is not possible in children and small adults.

There are three alternative (and more complicated) ways of accomplishing lung lavage in patients who simply cannot tolerate one-lung ventilation under any circumstance. First, extracorporeal membrane oxygenation (ECMO) has been utilized to provide support of gas exchange during standard unilateral lung lavage. Partial venoarterial cardiopulmonary bypass has been used for a few hours during unilateral or bilateral lung lavage,[90–92] but the distribution of oxygenated blood from the venoarterial by-pass can be markedly nonhomogeneous and dependent on the site of blood return[93, 94] and requires major arterial cannulation. Venovenous by-pass allows uniform arterial distribution and the safety of not requiring major arterial cannulation.[95, 96] In one of these latter cases[96] partial venovenous (femoral vein–inferior vena cava to internal jugular vein–superior vena cava connection) cardiopulmonary by-pass with a membrane oxygenator was especially successfully used to exchange respiratory gases during and after bilateral lung lavage in a patient with severe hypoxemia due to alveolar proteinosis (the patient had previously been unable to tolerate otherwise conventional unilateral lung lavage). During by-pass the lungs were mechanically ventilated. During right lung lavage, the mechanically ventilated left lung was incapable of any gas exchange ($P_aO_2 = P_{\bar{v}}O_2$ when by-pass was interrupted). After the first lavage, both lungs were mechanically ventilated with PEEP, and by-pass was continued for 12 hours, at which time the left lung was lavaged while by-pass was continued. Ten hours later the patient was successfully weaned from by-pass. The patient was then mechanically ventilated with PEEP for 24 hours and then extubated. At discharge the patient was markedly improved.[96]

The second way of accomplishing lung lavage in patients who cannot tolerate conventional unilateral lung lavage has been the use of lobar lavage via a fiberoptic bronchoscope inserted with topical anesthesia.[97, 98] With this technique, a cuffed fiberoptic bronchoscope is inserted into a lobar bronchus, and saline irrigation is carried out. The patient remains awake and breathes high-flow oxygen delivered via a face mask. One or two lobes may be done at a time, and lobar lavages may be repeated as many times as necessary. Ventilation-perfusion scans of the lung can be used to dictate which lobes are most severely affected and should thus be lavaged first. This technique has been used successfully, and it is thought that the relative ease with which it can be done makes it a preferable alternative to the use of an ECMO support system.[97]

Third, there are patients who cannot tolerate

the periods of lavage drainage when nonventilated lung blood flow markedly increases (because there is no alveolar pressure) and P_aO_2 decreases; however, they can tolerate the periods of lavage installation (when the pressure of the lavage fluid markedly decreases blood flow in the nonventilated, lavaged lung and increases P_aO_2).[71, 72, 77, 89, 99] In an effort to reduce this particular risk, pulmonary blood flow has been diverted away from the lavaged lung during drainage by inflation of a pulmonary artery catheter balloon in the main pulmonary artery of the side being lavaged.[89, 99] In these reports the pulmonary artery catheter was placed in the right main pulmonary artery (as determined by chest x-ray) and its balloon inflated during periods of right lung drainage until the phasic pulmonary artery trace just began to dampen; in every patient an increase in P_aO_2 and arterial oxygen saturation occurred. As measured by flow probes and transpulmonary shunt in dogs, the increase in P_aO_2 was due to the deflection of approximately 15 per cent of the cardiac output away from the right (nonventilated) lung. Because of the potential hazard of pulmonary artery rupture, and because of the impossibility of predicting which patients cannot selectively tolerate periods of lung drainage, this technique should be reserved as a second try in patients who had unacceptable oxygenation during lung drainage on a first try.

Lavage in the conventional manner is not possible in children (or small adults) in whom double-lumen endotracheal tubes are too large to be inserted. This problem routinely occurs in persons weighing less than 25 to 30 kg, since the smallest double-lumen endotracheal tube made is 28 French, with each lumen being slightly less than 4.5 mm. In this situation, partial cardiopulmonary by-pass has been successfully used to provide oxygenation during unilateral or bilateral lavage.[90, 100, 101] In one of these reports, the technique was used in two brothers aged 4 and 2.5 years.[100] Both these patients underwent whole-lung lavage, during which time blood was removed from both femoral veins, oxygenated, and then returned to the left femoral artery. Both patients were eventually discharged from the hospital, although they continued to require supplemental oxygen by face mask. In another report the technique was used to support gas exchange during whole-lung lavage in a ventilator-dependent, 3.7-kg, 8-month-old child.[101] The extracorporeal oxygenation system was again venoarterial (right internal jugular–right atrium

catheter to right axillary artery catheter). Marked improvement in pulmonary function was noted after lavage (total 420 ml/kg), by-pass was able to be discontinued 3 hours after lavage, and the patient was extubated 48 hours following lavage. In the last report,[100] partial venoarterial bypass with a bubble oxygenator permitted bilateral simultaneous lung lavage in two siblings aged 3 and 4 years. By-pass in these patients was carried out with femoral vein and femoral artery cannulation. During by-pass, radial artery P_aO_2 ranged between 25 and 30 mm Hg, which may, in part, have been related to continued cardiac output of desaturated blood into the proximal aorta. No neurologic sequelae were noted. Oxygenation and functional levels were improved following lavage. These various efforts to treat pulmonary alveolar proteinosis in children with bilateral lung lavage support by extracorporeal oxygenation must be regarded as successful, considering that in children the average survival from the time of severe symptoms without this kind of treatment is less than 1 year.

VII. TUMORS AT THE CONFLUENCE OF THE SUPERIOR, ANTERIOR, AND MIDDLE MEDIASTINA

A. General Considerations

The mediastinum is divided arbitrarily, for the purposes of description, into upper and lower parts at the upper level of the pericardium by a plane that extends from the sternal angle to the lower border of the fourth thoracic vertebra. The upper part is named the superior mediastinum, and the lower part is again subdivided into three parts: the anterior mediastinum, in front of the pericardium; the middle mediastinum, containing the heart and pericardium; and the posterior mediastinum, behind the pericardium. At the confluence of the superior, anterior, and middle mediastina are the middle portion of the superior vena cava, the tracheal bifurcation, the main pulmonary artery, the aortic arch, and parts of the cephalad surface of the heart (see Figs. 2–27 to 2–29 and 14–7). In adults, the majority of tumors in this region originate from involvement of the hilar lymph nodes with bronchial carcinoma or lymphoma, whereas in babies the masses are most often benign bronchial cysts, esophageal duplication, or teratoma. Tumors of this region can cause compression and obstruction of three of the vital mediastinal structures: the tracheo-bronchial tree in the region of the tracheal carina, the main pulmonary artery and atria, and the superior vena cava. The most common complication to occur during anesthesia for masses involving these three vital mediastinal structures is airway obstruction; this was a feature in 20 of 22 patients traced (1969–1983) and succinctly summarized.[102] Although airway obstruction has been predominant in terms of symptomatology, it is not uncommon for compression of two or three of these three major organs to be present in varying degrees in the same patient.[102] Each of these complications is life-threatening and can cause acute deterioration and death during anesthesia if not handled with the most extreme caution and expertise. Each of these three major complications and anesthetic management problems will be discussed separately.

B. Compression of the Tracheobronchial Tree

Most anterior mediastinal masses that cause airway obstruction are lymphomatous in origin. However, a number of benign conditions such as cystic hygroma, teratoma, and thymoma and thyroid tumors can occur in a similar fashion. A tissue diagnosis, therefore, must be made before radiation or chemotherapy can be undertaken. Thus, most patients with a mediastinal mass causing airway obstruction will first require anesthesia for a diagnostic procedure (cervical or scalene node biopsy, staging laparotomy for Hodgkin's disease). Not all patients who have developed severe intraoperative respiratory problems had respiratory symptoms and signs preoperatively.

1. Anesthetic Management

The anesthetic management of these patients is based on two overriding considerations. First, the obstruction of major airways by a tumor is usually life-threatening because the obstruction usually occurs around the bifurcation of the tracheobronchial tree and is, therefore, distal to the endotracheal tube. Inhalation induction precipitated obstruction in three cases, and in none of these did intubation completely relieve it. In one case, intubation made the obstruction complete until a long, thin tube was passed, producing partial improvement.[102] In another case,[103] ventilation was difficult until sponta-

neous ventilation returned with the tube still in place. In another case,[103] only a 4.5-mm rigid bronchoscope eventually secured a patent airway in an 11-year-old boy. In eight cases, intubation itself precipitated or exacerbated a partial mainstem bronchial obstruction.[103–106] The obstruction was thought to be relieved by the return of spontaneous respiration in some of the patients.[103–105] It may be that loss of chest wall tone and the distending forces of active inspiration following administration of muscle relaxants release extrinsic support of a critically narrowed airway. Alternatively, intubation in the presence of distortion or compression of the trachea may cause complete obstruction if the orifice of the tube impinges on the tracheal wall, or if the lumen of the tube is occluded where it passes a narrowed section or turns a sharp angle; such obstruction developed in five patients and was only relieved by a long, thin tube or a bronchoscope passed beyond the stenosis.[103, 106–109] In view of this reported seriousness of airway obstruction during general anesthesia, all possible attempts to do the procedure under local anesthesia should be undertaken.

Second, the response of lymphomatous tumors to radiation or chemotherapy is normally dramatic. Chest roentgenograms reveal a marked decrease in tumor size, and the symptoms are usually improved. Consequently, it behooves the treating physicians to use radio- or chemotherapy if at all possible (sometimes the cell type can be known with a reasonable degree of certainty without a biopsy) prior to general anesthesia.

The following management plan is based on the two above principles[100] (Table 15–5). If a patient with a mediastinal mass near the confluence of the superior, anterior, and middle mediastina exhibits dyspnea and/or intolerance of

Table 15–5. Important Management Principles for Tumors at the Confluence of the Superior, Anterior, and Middle Mediastina

1. Do all procedures under local anesthesia if at all possible
2. Use radiation and/or chemotherapy if at all possible prior to general anesthesia
3. If general anesthesia, then consider inspection of tracheobronchial tree with fiberoptic bronchoscope and intubate awake
4. If general anesthesia, then maintain spontaneous ventilation

the supine position and is scheduled for biopsy, it should be done under local anesthesia if at all possible. If the cell type is thought to be radiosensitive or chemosensitive, then appropriate types of therapy should be undertaken before any further surgery is performed. Following these types of therapy, the radiologic appearance of the tumor must be reviewed along with a dynamic evaluation of pulmonary function (see below).

If the patient does not have dyspnea or intolerance of the supine position (i.e., is asymptomatic), a series of noninvasive tests should be performed to evaluate the anatomic and functional position of the tumor. First, a flow-volume loop should be performed in the upright and supine positions. The flow-volume loop is an extremely sensitive tool for evaluating obstructive lesions of the major airways,[111] and can differentiate between extrathoracic and intrathoracic airway obstructions. With extrathoracic obstruction, the inspiratory limb of the flow-volume loop will show a plateau, and with intrathoracic airway obstruction the expiratory limb of the flow-volume loop will show a plateau (see Fig. 15–1). Second, the chest computed tomographic scan will best reveal the anatomic location of the tumor and, perhaps, show a static picture of airway obstruction. Third, echocardiography should be performed in both the upright and supine positions to determine the impact of the tumor on the geography of the heart. If any of these three tests have positive results, then local anesthesia should be used for biopsy even if the patient is asymptomatic. If all three of these major noninvasive diagnostic tests have negative results, the patient may be anesthetized with general anesthesia if necessary, but local anesthesia is still preferable. Again, once the biopsy has been taken and the tissue shown to be radio- or chemosensitive, appropriate therapies should be instituted and the patient should be reevaluated radiographically and functionally before further surgery is attempted.

If general anesthesia is to be used, the airway should be evaluated by fiberoptic bronchoscopy with topical anesthesia prior to the induction of general anesthesia.[110] The fiberoptic bronchoscope should be jacketed with an endotracheal tube, and after the fiberoptic bronchoscopy examination has been completed, the patient may be intubated. General anesthesia should be induced with the patient in the semi-Fowler's position, the patient should be allowed to breathe spontaneously throughout the proce-dure, and muscle relaxants should be avoided. Large swings in intrathoracic pressure, which may promote collapse of a weakened tracheobronchial tree, must be avoided. The operating room team should retain the capability of changing the patient's position rapidly to the lateral or prone position. A rigid ventilating bronchoscope should be on hand, and the appropriate personnel and equipment for cardiopulmonary by-pass also should be available.

These patients must be watched extremely closely in the first few postoperative hours. Airway obstruction requiring reintubation and mechanical ventilation has occurred, possibly secondary to an increase in tumor size due to tumor edema following instrumentation.

C. Compression of the Pulmonary Artery and Heart

This condition is rare, since the pulmonary trunk is more or less protected by the aortic arch and tracheobronchial tree; there are only three case reports in the literature.[112–114] However, in view of the lethal nature of this complication, it warrants discussion. Although experience with this problem is extremely limited, the cell type has been lymphomatous in nature in all three reports. Large mediastinal lymphomas have been associated with arrythmias under anesthesia owing to pericardial or myocardial involvement.

1. Anesthetic Management

Similar principles for compression of the tracheobronchial tree apply to compression of the pulmonary artery. Most patients have their first anesthetic experience because they require a diagnostic procedure (e.g., a biopsy). All diagnostic procedures should be performed under local anesthesia if at all possible. Since the symptoms usually worsen when the patient assumes the supine position, an unusual position may need to be utilized (see below). Lymphomatous tumors are usually radiosensitive.

These patients should be evaluated preoperatively in a manner similar to that for those with compression of the tracheobronchial tree. If there is absolutely no indication of the cell type, local anesthesia should be tried, if at all possible, to perform the biopsy. If the cell type is known or is highly suspected, preoperative irradiation should be seriously considered. If general anesthesia is required, the sitting, leaning forward, or even face-down position is advised, and spontaneous ventilation should be maintained throughout the procedure. Measures to maintain venous return, pulmonary artery pressure, and cardiac output, such as volume loading and use of ketamine, should be considered. Arrangements for extracorporeal oxygenation should be completed preoperatively. The anesthetist has to be aware of the danger of air embolism in a patient in the sitting position having a vertically nondependent surgical procedure.

D. Superior Vena Cava Syndrome

The superior vena cava syndrome is caused by mechanical obstruction of the superior vena cava. The causes of superior vena caval obstruction, in order of rapidly decreasing incidence, are bronchial carcinoma (87 per cent), malignant lymphoma (10 per cent), and benign causes (3 per cent), such as pulmonary artery, central venous, hyperalimentation, and pacemaker catheter–induced thrombosis of the superior vena cava,[115] idiopathic mediastinal fibrosis, mediastinal granuloma, and multinodular goiter.[116, 117] The classic features of the superior vena cava syndrome include dilated distended veins in the upper half of the body due to increased peripheral venous pressure (which can be as high as 40 mm Hg); edema of the head, neck, and upper extremities; dilated venous collateral channels in the chest wall; and cyanosis. Venous distension is most prominent in the recumbent position, but in most instances the veins do not collapse in the normal manner with the patient upright. The majority of patients have respiratory symptoms (shortness of breath, cough, orthopnea), which are due to obstruction of the airways by engorged veins and mucosal edema and are ominous signs. Similarly, a change in mentation, due to cerebral venous hypertension and edema, is an ominous sign. In some cases the superior vena cava becomes occluded quite slowly and the signs and symptoms may be insidious in onset. When the occlusion occurs relatively rapidly all clinical manifestations are more prominent; in this setting facial edema may be so severe that it prevents the patients from opening their eyes. Moreover, rapidly increasing venous pressure in the cerebral circulation may lead to neurologic impairment as cerebral perfusion pressure is decreased.

Most patients with superior vena cava syndrome due to a malignant process are treated with irradiation and chemotherapy (for patients with incomplete obstruction).[118] However, in patients with near-complete to complete obstruction (who usually have signs of cerebral venous hypertension and/or airway obstruction), or when irradiation or chemotherapy proves ineffective, surgical by-pass or resection of the lesion via median sternotomy is indicated.[118] These operations are usually technically quite difficult because tissue planes are poorly delineated, anatomy is grossly distorted, and varying degrees of fibrosis are present.

1. Anesthetic Management

The preoperative anesthetic evaluation of a patient for superior vena caval decompression should include careful assessment of the airway. The same degree of edema that is present externally in the face and neck can be expected to be present in the mouth, oropharynx, and hypopharynx. In addition, the airway may be compromised by external compression, fibrosis limiting normal movement, or recurrent laryngeal nerve involvement. If tracheal compression is suspected it should be evaluated by computed tomography.

Premedication for these patients is light or deleted when there is concern about the integrity of the airway. A drying agent is helpful if a difficult intubation is anticipated, and it should be administered to all patients having difficulty swallowing. The patient is transported to the operating room in the head-up position in order to minimize airway edema. A radial artery catheter is inserted in all patients and, depending on the medical condition of the patient, a central venous or pulmonary artery catheter is inserted via the femoral vein prior to the induction of anesthesia. On one occasion atrial pacing via a pulmonary artery catheter was utilized in a patient with suspected cardiac involvement from a mediastinal tumor who was experiencing significant bradycardia preoperatively. At least one large-bore intravenous cannula should be inserted in the leg or femoral vein prior to operation; the upper extremities are not used for intravenous infusions because of the long and unpredictable circulation time that results from the superior vena caval obstruction. The method chosen for induction of anesthesia and intubation is dependent upon the preoperative airway evaluation. If it is necessary for the patient to maintain the sitting position in order to achieve adequate ventilation prior to induction, intubation with the patient awake may be facilitated by using a fiberoptic laryngoscope[119] or bronchoscope.[120]

The most significant intraoperative problem encountered is bleeding. Substantial venous blood loss results from the abnormally high central venous pressure. Further, unexpected arterial bleeding may occur because of the difficulty of dissecting in a distorted surgical field. Cross matched blood should therefore be available in the operating room at the time of sternotomy.

Postoperatively, especially after diagnostic procedures such as mediastinoscopy and bronchoscopy, wherein the superior vena caval obstruction has not been relieved, acute severe respiratory failure requiring intubation and mechanical ventilation may occur.[117, 121-125] The mechanisms of the acute respiratory failure are obscure, but the most likely ones that are unique to the superior vena cava snydrome are acute laryngospasm and/or acute bronchospasm (both due to continued and, perhaps, increased obstruction of the superior vena cava), impaired respiratory muscle function (patients with malignant disease may have an abnormal response to muscle relaxants,[125] and increased airway obstruction by the tumor (due to tumor swelling). Consequently, these patients must be closely monitored in the first few postoperative hours.

VIII. REPAIR OF THORACIC AORTIC ANEURYSMS

Patients with thoracic aortic aneurysms may come to the operating room on either an elective or an emergency basis. Thoracic aortic aneurysms in patients who are hemodynamically stable and free of significant symptoms are repaired on an elective basis. Patients with thoracic aortic aneurysms that were caused by trauma, or those who are hemodynamically unstable with acute symptoms (e.g., chest pain) due to an acute dissection, come to the operating room on an emergency basis. Consequently, the anesthetic management of patients with thoracic aortic aneurysms could be logically discussed as either an elective therapeutic procedure or an emergency procedure.

The anesthetic management of patients with thoracic aortic aneurysms is discussed with special emergency procedures (see Thoracic Aortic Aneurysms and Dissections/Disruptions, chapter 16). The reason for this is twofold. First, patients requiring emergency repair of thoracic aortic aneurysms outnumber patients requiring elective repair.[126] Second, the emergency cases are more challenging, involve higher risks, and entail a greater number of anesthetic considerations. Indeed, there is a 16 per cent surgical mortality for emergency resection compared with a 5 per cent surgical mortality for elective resection. The discussion of the anesthetic management of patients with thoracic aortic aneurysms in chapter 16 includes all the anesthetic considerations that would apply to patients undergoing elective resection of thoracic aortic aneurysms.

IX. THYMECTOMY FOR MYASTHENIA GRAVIS

A. General Considerations

Myasthenia gravis is a disease of neuromuscular transmission characterized by weakness and easy fatigability of the voluntary muscles. If untreated, myasthenia gravis has a 40 per cent mortality in 10 years. Recent evidence indicates that the disease is caused by an autoimmune attack on the post-synaptic acetylcholine receptors in skeletal muscle. There appears to be a causal connection between the binding of antibody to receptors, a decrease in number of the receptors in motor endplates, and interference with neuromuscular transmission[127] (Fig. 15–6). The place of thymectomy in the treatment of myasthenia gravis is well established. It has been reported to result in remission or clinical improvement in at least 80 per cent of patients.[128]

The diagnosis can usually be established by the typical historical and neuromuscular examination findings.[129] The most frequent complaint of myasthenic patients is diplopia; ptosis, the second most common sign, may be missed if it is mild. Ptosis may be unilateral and characteristically may shift from side to side. Dysarthria is an early symptom of bulbar involvement, followed by difficulties in chewing and swallowing, leading to weight loss. In advanced myasthenia gravis, the most frequent bulbar sign is facial weakness. In 15 to 20 per cent of myasthenic patients the chief complaint is extremity weakness and easy fatigability; the arms are affected more frequently. Respiratory muscle weakness may prompt the patient to visit a physician, but this is rarely the first symptom.

Various tests can be used to confirm the diagnosis. Electromyography shows a decre-

Pharmacology of Myasthenia Gravis

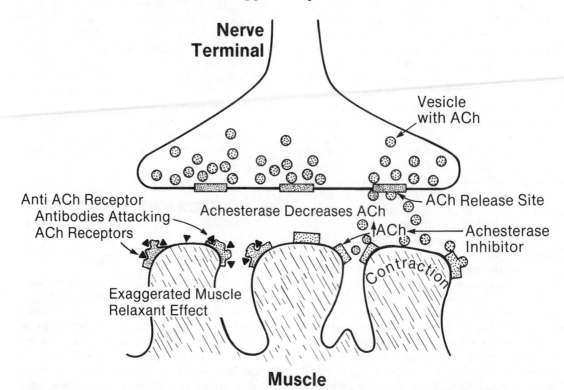

Figure 15–6. Schematic diagram of the motor end-plate. In myasthenia gravis, antibodies to the post-synaptic acetylcholine (Ach) receptors destroy and reduce the number of receptors; hence, the affected muscle fatigues easily. Muscle relaxants have a much more exaggerated effect because they easily bind the reduced number of receptors. Acetylcholinesterase (Achesterase) metabolizes Ach. Achesterase inhibitors increase the amount of end-plate Ach and increase Ach-receptor binding and thereby increase muscle strength.

mental response in repetitive nerve stimulation. Administration of edrophonium or neostigmine (Prostigmine) results in a transient increase in muscle strength. Computed tomography of the mediastinum is helpful in determining whether a thymoma is present (9 to 16 per cent of myasthenic patients). Finally, acetylcholine receptor antibody titers are elevated in a majority of patients.

There are five classifications of the clinical status of the patient:[129] I, ocular symptoms and signs only, without progression (these patients are not treated by thymectomy); IIA, generalized weakness, mild bulbar and skeletal symptoms; IIB, generalized weakness, moderate-to-severe bulbar and skeletal symptoms; III, acute fulminating weakness with severe bulbar involvement; IV, late onset or exacerbation, severe bulbar symptoms, and severe generalized weakness; and V, myasthenia gravis with muscular atrophy.

The nonoperative therapy of myasthenia gravis arises from the apparent autoimmune etiology of the known deficiency in acetylcho-

line receptors. The mainstay of treatment of patients with myasthenia gravis is use of the oral anticholinesterase pyridostigmine (Mestinon) (Table 15–6). The anticholinesterase maintains the local concentration of acetylcholine at the motor end-plate at a high level and increases the chance of acetylcholine binding to an acetylcholine receptor (Fig. 15–6). Occasional patients with myasthenia gravis may not respond to anticholinesterase drug therapy, which may be due to complete absence of postsynaptic acetylcholine receptors so that even the increased amount of acetylcholine present has no place to act. In addition, myasthenics on prolonged chronic anticholinesterase drug therapy may show decreased sensitivity to the drug. The therapeutic benefits of steroids (immunosuppression) and plasmapheresis (removal of anti–post-synaptic receptor antibody) are thought to be due to the autoimmune etiology of myasthenia gravis.

Exacerbation of myasthenia gravis can occur secondary to emotional and/or surgical stress with the subsequent development of a myasthenic crisis. During crisis, patients have decreased responsiveness to anticholinesterase. This situation must be differentiated from a cholinergic crisis, which is secondary to an anticholinesterase overdosage.[130] In both situations there is an increase in muscle weakness, which may involve the respiratory musculature and, thereby, necessitate respiratory support. A small dose of edrophonium (10 mg intravenously) will improve strength in a patient with myasthenic crisis, but will have little or a negative effect in a patient with cholinergic crisis. In both myasthenic and cholinergic crisis it is best to withhold anticholinesterase medications while providing mechanical supportive ventilation. The treatment of myasthenic crisis may also include plasmapheresis. In some situations a mixed crisis can arise with overtreatment of a patient with anticholinesterase drugs during a myasthenic crisis.

B. Anesthetic Considerations

1. Preoperative Considerations

Physical examination should include airway evaluation and tests of muscle strength and the ability to cough, chew, and swallow. Vital capacity, peak inspiratory force, and maximum breathing capacity should be measured in every patient. Those with impaired respiratory function need complete respiratory function tests performed, including analysis of arterial blood gases. A chest roentgenogram and computed tomogram should be reviewed to assess the presence and size of the thymic tumor. Myasthenic patients may also have associated myocardial degenerative changes, which make a preoperative electrocardiogram necessary. Thyroid abnormalities may be associated with myasthenia gravis, and patients need to be evaluated clinically and by laboratory tests for evidence of hypo- or hyperthyroidism. Nutritional status should be evaluated by measurement of serum electrolyte, albumin, globulin, and hemoglobin levels. Special attention must be given to serum glucose and electrolyte concentrations in pa-

tients maintained with steroid preparations, since prolonged therapy may induce fluid and electrolyte disturbances and hyperglycemia or glycosuria.

All nutritional deficiencies, dehydration, electrolyte imbalances, and respiratory tract infections must be treated preoperatively. Plasmapheresis is commonly used in the preoperative period to optimize the patient's physical status.

At present, it is recommended that anticholinesterase therapy at the regular dose be continued until the day of surgery. On the day of surgery, in mild cases, none or half the amount of the morning dose of pyridostigmine is administered, whereas in severe cases the full morning dose is prescribed. In patients receiving systemic steroids, suppression of the pituitary-adrenal axis should be considered and the regular dose of steroid should be maintained throughout the immediate perioperative period. Postoperatively the cortisone administration may be tapered from the second to approximately the fifth postoperative day.

In view of the propensity for stress to cause a myasthenic crisis, and because many of these patients demonstrate some emotional instability, special attention must be paid to the psychologic preparation of these patients. Premedication is indicated, but care should be taken not to depress an already weakened respiratory apparatus.

2. Intraoperative Considerations

Anesthesia may be induced with thiopental, followed by the administration of a halogenated drug. The surgical approach is through a median sternotomy, but in patients who have a nonmidline thymoma, a lateral thoracotomy may be necessary. If the incision is a median sternotomy, a single-lumen tube may be used, and if the incision is a lateral thoracotomy, a single- or double-lumen tube may be used.

Muscle relaxation is a special problem in these patients. Succinylcholine is associated with an early onset of a phase II block, which has a prolonged duration. All nondepolarizing

Table 15–6. Anticholinesterase Medications Available in the United States for the Treatment of Myasthenia Gravis

Drug	Trade Name	Oral Dose (mg)	Parenteral Dose (mg) IV	IM
Neostigmine	Prostigmine	15	0.5	0.5–1.0
Pyridostigmine	Mestinon	60	2	3–4
Ambenonium	Mytelase	6	Not available	

muscle relaxants have an unacceptable duration of action in these patients if administered in usual doses. Consequently, if relaxation is required small doses of nondepolarizing relaxants should be given. Atracurium in small doses (5 to 15 mg)[131] appears to be the drug of choice due to its short duration of action and method of elimination by spontaneous decomposition (Hoffman elimination). No matter what relaxant or how much was used, neuromuscular blockade must be monitored with a nerve stimulator. The time course of the neuromuscular blockade after these small doses of nondepolarizing muscle relaxants is similar to that observed after larger doses in nonmyasthenic subjects. At the end of the operation, the residual effects of the muscle relaxant can be effectively antagonized by neostigmine.

A scoring system to predict which patients will require postoperative ventilatory support has been devised.[132] The components of the scoring system consist of duration of myasthenia gravis equal to or greater than 6 years (equals 12 points); other concomitant respiratory disease present (equals 10 points); pyridostigmine requirement greater than 750 mg/day (equals 8 points); and a vital capacity less than 2.9 L (equals 4 points). A score of 10 points or more predicts the need for ventilatory support. The scoring system was derived in patients undergoing trans-sternal thymectomy with halogenated drug anesthesia without muscle relaxation; the predictive accuracy of this scoring system was 80 per cent.[132] However, in patients undergoing transcervical thymectomy with the same anesthetic, the predictive accuracy of the scoring system was only 13 per cent.[133] The variation in predictability of the scoring system may be due to differences in stress between the two surgical approaches.

Alternatively, postoperative mechanical ventilation of all patients with myasthenia gravis has also been recommended.[128] Extubation can be accomplished in an unhurried fashion and according to such objective criteria as vital capacity and peak inspiratory force. In addition, this approach allows time to restart the anticholinesterase therapy after clinical examination of the patient, especially with regard to bulbar and respiratory function, and testing of handgrip strength with a dynamometer. The aim of the immediate postoperative anticholinesterase therapy is to maintain adequate spontaneous respiratory exchange. If the spontaneous ventilation is adequate or if mechanical ventilation is instituted, the anticholinergics are not required in the postoperative period. However, if spontaneous respiratory exchange is not adequate, half the regular dose of anticholinesterases may be administered during the first 3 postoperative days. On the fourth postoperative day, regular doses of anticholinesterases may be started. If the patient cannot take oral medication, parenteral administration of neostigmine (0.5 to 1 mg intramuscularly) can be given every 2 to 3 hours until medication can be absorbed orally, at which time pyridostigmine can be restarted. Because the beneficial effects of thymectomy can be delayed for several weeks to several years postoperatively, it is necessary to reassess the doses for a prolonged postoperative period. Pain relief can be obtained by titrating small doses of commonly used narcotics to the desired end-point. All patients with myasthenia gravis should be monitored postoperatively in an intensive care unit setting.

The results of surgery are encouraging.[128] Approximately 12 per cent of patients will demonstrate a complete remission, 40 per cent demonstrate marked clinical improvement on a decreased anticholinesterase inhibitor dosage, 20 per cent demonstrate clinical improvement with no change of medications, and 6 per cent show no improvement with medication unchanged.

X. ONE-LUNG ANESTHESIA IN MORBIDLY OBESE PATIENTS

Gastric stapling has become an accepted treatment for refractory morbid obesity.[134, 135] Although the procedure is usually performed through an abdominal incision, a transthoracic transdiaphragmatic approach with the patient in the right lateral decubitus position recently has been described and provides an improved operative exposure. As with any intrathoracic procedure, the transthoracic transdiaphragmatic surgical exposure can be greatly increased by using one-lung ventilation. Morbidly obese patients have heavy chest walls that cause a reduction in functional residual capacity below the closing volume of the lung, low ventilation-perfusion relationships, and hypoxemia. Consequently, one-lung ventilation in morbidly obese patients may be thought to be associated with an increased risk of hypoxemia. However, in one study of eight morbidly obese patients undergoing one-lung ventilation, no particular intraoperative or postoperative problems were encountered.[135] The patients were ventilated with a tidal volume of 15 ml/kg of ideal weight and an F_IO_2 of 1.0; P_aO_2 ranged from 72 to 230 mm Hg during one-lung ventilation. The most probable reason good success was obtained during one-lung ventilation in these morbidly obese patients was that the lateral decubitus position allowed the panniculus to displace itself on the operating room table, thereby reducing abdominal pressure against the diaphragm (compared with the supine position) and allowing increased FRC and greater tidal diaphragmatic excursion.[137] Postoperative depression of P_aO_2 and depression of postoperative pulmonary function test studies were slightly greater in the one-lung ventilation patients compared with a similar group of patients undergoing only an abdominal incision approach. Thus, it is reasonable to conclude that morbidly obese patients can tolerate one-lung ventilation/anesthesia for transthoracic gastric stapling surgery with safety comparable to that for the abdominal approach.

REFERENCES

1. Dedhia HV, Leroy L, Jain PR, et al: Endoscopic laser therapy for respiratory distress due to obstructive airway tumors. Crit Care Med 13:464–467, 1985.
2. Gelb AF, Epstein JD: Laser in treatment of lung cancer. Chest 86:662–666, 1984.
3. Unger M: Bronchoscopic utilization of the Nd:YAG laser for obstructing lesions of the trachea and bronchi. Surg Clin North Am 64:931–938, 1984.
4. Parr GVS, Unger M, Trout RG, et al: One hundred neodymium-YAG laser ablations of obstructing tracheal neoplasms. Ann Thorac Surg 38:374–381, 1984.
5. Warner ME, Warner MA, Leonard PF: Anesthesia for neodymium-YAG (Nd-YAG) laser resection of major airway obstructing tumors. Anesthesiology 60:230–232, 1984.
6. Snow JC: Fire hazard during CO_2-laser microsurgery on larynx and trachea. Anesth Analg 55:146, 1976.
7. Hirshman CA, Smith J: Indirect ignition of the endotracheal tube during carbon dioxide laser surgery. Arch Otolaryngol 106:639, 1980.
8. Burgess GE, LeJeune FE: Endotracheal tube ignition during laser surgery. Otolaryngology 5:561, 1979.
9. Patel KF, Hicks JN: Prevention of fire hazards associated with the use of carbon dioxide lasers. Anesth Analg 60:885, 1981.
10. Brutinel WM, McDougall JC, Cortese DA: Bronchoscopic therapy with neodymium-yttrium-aluminum-garnet (Nd-YAG) laser during intravenous anesthesia. Chest 84:518–521, 1983.
11. Vourch G, Fischler M, Personne C, et al: Anesthetic management during Nd-YAG laser resection for major tracheobronchial obstructing tumors. Anesthesiology 61:150–151, 1984.
12. Arabian A, Spagnolo SV: Laser therapy in patients with primary lung cancer. Chest 86:519–523, 1984.
13. McDougall JC, Cortese DA: Neodymium-YAG laser therapy of malignant airway obstruction. Mayo Clin Proc 58:35–39, 1983.
14. McElvein RB, Zorn GL: Indications, results and complications of bronchoscopic carbon dioxide laser therapy. Ann Surg 199:522–525, 1984.
15. Cortese DA, Kinsey JH: Hematoporphyrin derivative phototherapy in the treatment of bronchogenic carcinoma. Chest 86:8–13, 1984.
16. Cortese DA, Kinsey JH: Bronchoscopic phototherapy using hematoporphyrin derivative. Surg Clin North Am 64:941–946, 1984.
17. Marcus CG: Photodynamic therapy: New method for eradicating endobronchial cancer. Can Med Assoc J 132:1363–1364, 1985.
18. Ossoff RH, Karlan MS: Instrumentation for CO_2 laser surgery of the larynx and tracheobronchial tree. Surg Clin North Am 64:973–980, 1984.
19. Hunton J, Oswal VH: Metal tube anaesthesia for ear, nose and throat carbon dioxide laser surgery. Anaesthesia 40:1210–1212, 1985.
20. Hetzel MR, Millard FJC, Ayesh R, et al: Laser treatment for carcinoma of the bronchus. Br Med J 136:12–16, 1983.
21. Gelb AF, Epstein JD: Nd:YAG laser in lung cancer. West J Med 140:393–397, 1984.
22. Toty L, Personne C, Colchen A, Vourch G: Bronchoscopic management of tracheal lesions using the neodymium yttrium aluminum garnet laser. Thorax 36:175–178, 1981.
23. Allen MD, Baldwin JC, Fish VJ, et al: Combined laser therapy and endobronchial radiotherapy for unresectable lung carcinoma with bronchial obstruction. Am J Surg 150:71–77, 1985.
24. Rooney S, Goldiner PL, Bains MS, et al: Anesthesia for the application of endotracheal and endobronchial radiation therapy. J Thorac Cardiovasc Surg 87:693–697, 1984.
25. Seagren SL, Harrell JH, Horn RA: High dose rate intraluminal irradiation in recurrent endobronchial carcinoma. Chest 86:810–814, 1985.
26. Pearson FG, Todd TRJ, Cooper JD: Experience with primary neoplasms of the trachea and carina. J Thorac Cardiovasc Surg 88:511–518, 1984.
27. Grillo HC: Carinal reconstruction. Ann Thorac Surg 34:357–373, 1982.
28. El-Baz N, Jensik R, Faber P, et al: One-lung high frequency ventilation for tracheoplasty and bronchoplasty: A new technique. Ann Thorac Surg 34:564–572, 1982.
29. El-Baz N, Holinger L, El-Ganzouri A, et al: High-frequency positive-pressure ventilation for tracheal reconstruction by tracheal T-tube. Anesth Analg 61:796–800, 1982.
30. Eriksson I, Nilsson LG, Nordstrom S, et al: High-frequency positive-pressure ventilation (HFPPV) during transthoracic resection of tracheal stenosis and during perioperative bronchoscopic examination. Acta Anaesthesiol Scand 19:113–119, 1975.
31. Geffin B, Bland J, Grillo HC: Anesthetic management of tracheal resection and reconstruction. Anesth Analg 48:884–894, 1969.
32. Theman TE, Kerr JH, Nelems JM, et al: Carinal resection. A report of two cases and a description of the anesthetic technique. J Thorac Cardiovasc Surg 71:314–320, 1976.
33. Belsey R: Resection and reconstruction of the intrathoracic trachea. Br J Surg 38:200–205, 1950.
34. Kamvyssi-Dea S, Kritikon P, Exarhos N, et al: Anaesthetic management of reconstruction of the lower part of the trachea. Br J Anaesth 47:82–84, 1975.
35. Debrand M, Tseuda K, Browning SK, et al: Anes-

thesia for extensive repair of congenital trachea stenosis in an infant. Anesth Analg 58:431–433, 1979.

36. Boyan PC, Privitera PA: Resection of stenotic trachea: A case presentation. Anesth Analg 55:191–194, 1976.

37. Abou-Madi MN, Cuadrado L, Domb B, et al: Anaesthesia of tracheal resection: A new way to manage the airway. Can Anaesth Soc J 26:26–28, 1979.

38. Lippman M, Mok MS: Tracheal cyclindroma: Anaesthetic management. Br J Anaesth 49:383–386, 1977.

39. Akdikmen S, Landmesser CM: Anesthesia for surgery of the intrathoracic portion of the trachea. Anesthesiology 26:117–119, 1965.

40. Dodge TL, Mahaffey JE, Thomas JD: The anesthetic management of a patient with an obstructing intratracheal mass: A case report. Anesth Analg 56:295–298, 1977.

41. Lee P, English ICW: Management of anesthesia during tracheal resection. Anaesthesia 29:305–306, 1974.

42. McNaughton FI: Catheter inflation ventilation in tracheal stenosis. Br J Anaesth 47:1225–1227, 1975.

43. Baraka A: Oxygen-jet ventilation during tracheal reconstruction in patients with tracheal stenosis. Anesth Analg 56:429–432, 1977.

44. Ellis RH, Hinds CJ, Gadd LT: Management of anaesthesia during tracheal resection. Anaesthesia 31:1076–1080, 1976.

45. Baraka A, Mansour R, Jaoude CA, et al: Entrainment of oxygen and halothane during jet ventilation in patients undergoing excision of tracheal and bronchial tumors. Anesth Analg 65:191–194, 1986.

46. Woods F, Neptune W, Palatchi A: Resection of the carina and mainstem bronchi with extracorporeal circulation. N Engl J Med 264:492–494, 1961.

47. Coles JC, Doctor A, Lefcoe M, et al: A method of anesthesia for imminent tracheal obstruction. Surgery 80:379–381, 1976.

48. Laurenzi G, Turino G, Fishman A: Bullous disease of the lung. Am J Med 32:361–378, 1962.

49. Baldwin EP, Harden KA, Greene DG, et al: Pulmonary air cysts of bullae. Medicine 29:169–194, 1950.

50. Foreman S, Weill H, Duke R, et al: Bullous disease of the lung: Physiologic improvement after surgery. Ann Intern Med 69:757–767, 1968.

51. Peters RM: Indications for operative treatment of bullous emphysema. Ann Thorac Surg 35:479, 1983.

52. Nakahara K, Nakaoka K, Ohno K, et al: Functional indications for bullectomy of giant bulla. Ann Thorac Surg 35:480–487, 1983.

53. Laros CD, Gelissen HJ, Bergstein PG, et al: Bullectomy for giant bullae in emphysema. J Thorac Cardiovasc Surg 91:63–70, 1986.

54. Ting EY, Klopstock R, Lyons HA: Mechanical properties of pulmonary cysts and bullae. Am Rev Respir Dis 87:538–544, 1963.

55. Eger EI II, Saidman LJ: Hazards of nitrous oxide anesthesia in bowel obstruction and pneumothorax. Anesthesiology 26:61–66, 1965.

56. Gold MI, Joseph SI: Bilateral tension pneumothorax following induction of anesthesia in two patients with chronic obstructive airway disease. Anesthesiology 38:93, 1973.

57. Normandale JP, Feneck RO: Bullous cystic lung disease. Anaesthesia 40:1182–1185, 1985.

58. Isenhower N, Cucehiara RF: Anesthesia for vanishing lung syndrome: Report of a case. Anesth Analg 55:750–752, 1976.

59. Mudge BJ, Kilaru P, Pandit U, et al: Anesthetic management for resection of a giant emphysematous bulla in a patient with bilateral bullous disease. Anesthesiol Rev 9:34–37, 1982.

60. Caseby NG: Anaesthesia for the patient with a coincidental giant lung bulla: A case report. Can Anaesth Soc J 28:272–276, 1981.

61. Tinker J, Vandam L, Cohn LH: Tension lung cyst as a complication of postoperative positive-pressure ventilation therapy. Chest 64:518–520, 1973.

62. Iwa T, Watanabe Y, Fukatani G: Simultaneous bilateral operations for bullous emphysema by median sternotomy. J Thorac Cardiovasc Surg 82:732–737, 1981.

63. Hughes R, Blades B: Multiple primary bronchogenic carcinoma. J Thorac Cardiovasc Surg 41:421, 1961.

64. Martini N, Melamed MR: Multiple primary lung cancers. J Thorac Cardiovasc Surg 70:606, 1975.

65. Neptune WB, Woods FM, Overholt RH: Reoperation for bronchogenic carcinoma. J Thorac Cardiovasc Surg 52:342, 1966.

66. Shields TW, Drake CT, Sherriack JC: Bilateral primary bronchogenic carcinoma. J Thorac Cardiovasc Surg 48:401, 1964.

67. Shields TW, Higgens GA Jr: Minimal pulmonary resection in treatment of carcinoma of the lung. Arch Surg 108:420, 1974.

68. Struve-Christensen E: Diagnosis and treatment of bilateral primary bronchogenic carcinoma. J Thorac Cardiovasc Surg 61:501, 1971.

69. Kittle CF, Faber LP, Jensik RJ, et al: Pulmonary resection in patients after pneumonectomy. Ann Thorac Surg 40:294–299, 1985.

70. Alfery DD, Benumof JL, Spragg RG: Anesthesia for bronchopulmonary lavage. In Kaplan J (ed): Thoracic Anesthesia. New York, Churchill Livingstone, 1982, chapter 12, pp 403–420.

71. Blenkarn GD, Lanning CF, Kylstra JA: Anaesthetic management of volume controlled unilateral lung lavage. Can Anaesth Soc J 22:154–163, 1975.

72. Busque L: Pulmonary lavage in the treatment of alveolar proteinosis. Can Anaesth Soc J 24:380–389, 1977.

73. Wasserman K, Cosfley B: Advances in the treatment of pulmonary alveolar proteinosis. Am Rev Respir Dis 111:361–363, 1975.

74. Ramirez RJ: Alveolar proteinosis: Importance of pulmonary lavage. Am Rev Respir Dis 103:666–678, 1971.

75. Wasserman K, Blank N, Fletcher G: Lung lavage (alveolar washing) in alveolar proteinosis. Am J Med 44:611–617, 1968.

76. Rogers RM, Tantam KR: Bronchopulmonary lavage: A "new" approach to old problems. Med Clin North Am 54:755–771, 1970.

77. Rogers RM, Szidon JP, Shelburne J, et al: Hemodynamic response of the circulation to bronchopulmonary lavage in man. N Engl J Med 296:1230–1233, 1972.

78. Smith JD, Miller JE, Safer P, et al: Intrathoracic pressure, pulmonary vascular presures and gas exchange during pulmonary lavage. Anesthesiology 33:401–405, 1970.

79. McClenahan JB, Mussenden R: Pulmonary alveolar proteinosis. Arch Intern Med 133:284–287, 1974.

80. Ramirez J, Harlan WJ Jr: Pulmonary alveolar proteinosis. Nature and origin of alveolar lipid. Am J Med 45:502–512, 1968.

81. Ramirez J: Pulmonary alveolar proteinosis. A roentgenologic analysis. Am J Roentgenol 92:571–577, 1964.

82. Martin RJ, Rogers RM, Myers NM: Pulmonary alveolar proteinosis: Shunt fraction and lactic acid dehydrogenase concentration as aids to diagnosis. Am Rev Respir Dis 117:1059–1062, 1978.

83. Rogers RM, Levin DC, Gray BA, et al: Physiological effects of bronchopulmonary lavage in alveolar proteinosis. Am Rev Respir Dis 118:255–264, 1978.

84. Smith LJ, Ankin MG, Katzenstein A, et al: Management of pulmonary alveolar proteinosis. Chest 78:765–770, 1980.

85. Rausch DC, Spock A, Kylstra JA: Lung lavage in cystic fibrosis. Am Rev Respir Dis 101:1006, 1970.

86. McClellan RO, Boyd HA, Benjamin RG, et al: Recovery of ^{239}Pu following bronchopulmonary lavage and DTPA treatment after an accidental inhalation exposure case. Health Phys 31:315–321, 1976.

87. Selecky PA, Wasserman K, Benfield JR, et al: The clinical and physiological effect of whole lung lavage in pulmonary alveolar proteinosis: A ten-year experience. Ann Thorac Surg 24:451–461, 1977.

88. Kariman K, Kylstra JA, Spock A: Pulmonary alveolar proteinosis: Prospective clinical experience in 23 patients for 15 years. Lung 162:223–231, 1984.

89. Alfery DD, Zamost BG, Benumof JL: Unilateral lung lavage: Blood flow manipulation by ipsilateral pulmonary artery balloon inflation. Anesthesiology 55:376–381, 1981.

90. Seard C, Wasserman K, Benfield JR, et al: Simultaneous bilateral lung lavage (alveolar washing) using partial cardiopulmonary bypass. Am Rev Respir Dis 101:877–884, 1970.

91. Freedman AP, Pelias A, Johnston RF, et al: Alveolar proteinosis lung lavage using partial cardiopulmonary bypass. Thorax 36:543–545, 1981.

92. Altose MD, Hicks RE, Edwards MW: Extracorporeal membrane oxygenation during bronchopulmonary lavage. Arch Surg 111:1148–1153, 1976.

93. Zapol WM, Snider MT, Schneider RC: Extracorporeal membrane oxygenation for acute respiratory failure. Anesthesiology 46:272–285, 1977.

94. McEnany MT, Zapol WM, Seebacher J, et al: Cannulation of the proximal aorta during long term membrane lung perfusion. J Thorac Cardiovasc Surg 70:631–643, 1975.

95. Cooper JD, Duffin J, Glynn MFX, et al: Combination of membrane oxygenator support and pulmonary lavage for acute respiratory failure. J Thorac Cardiovasc Surg 71:304–308, 1976.

96. Zapol WM, Wilson R, Hales C, et al: Venovenous bypass with a membrane lung to support bilateral lung lavage. JAMA 251:3269–3271, 1984.

97. Brach BB, Harrell JH, Moser KM: Alveolar proteinosis. Lobar lavage by fiberoptic bronchoscopic technique. Chest 69:224–227, 1976.

98. Vast C, Demonet B, Mouveroux J: Value of selective pulmonary lavage under fiberoptic control in alveolar proteinosis. Poumon Coeur 34:305–307, 1978.

99. Spragg RG, Benumof JL, Alfery DD: New methods for performance of unilateral lung lavage. Anesthesiology 57:535, 1982.

100. Lippmann K, Mok MS, Wasserman K: Anaesthetic management for children with alveolar proteinosis using extracorporeal circulation. Br J Anaesth 49:173, 1977.

101. Hiratzka LF, Swan DM, Rose EF, et al: Bilateral simultaneous lung lavage utilizing membrane oxygenator for pulmonary alveolar proteinosis in an 8-month-old infant. Ann Thorac Surg 35:313–317, 1983.

102. Mackie AM, Watson CB: Anaesthesia and mediastinal masses. A case report and review of the literature. Anaesthesia 39:899–903, 1984.

103. Bray RJ, Fernandes FJ: Mediastinal tumour causing airway obstruction in anaesthetised children. Anaesthesia 37:571–575, 1982.

104. Bittar D: Respiratory obstruction associated with induction of general anesthesia in a patient with mediastinal Hodgkin's disease. Anesth Analg 54:399–403, 1975.

105. Hall DK, Friedman M: Extracorporeal oxygenation for induction of anesthesia in a patient with an intrathoracic tumor. Anesthesiology 42:493–495, 1975.

106. Piro AJ, Weiss DR, Hellman S: Mediastinal Hodgkin's disease: A possible danger for intubation anesthesia. Int J Radiat Oncol Biol Phys 1:415–419, 1976.

107. Todres ID, Reppert SM, Walker PF, et al: Management of critical airway obstruction in a child with a mediastinal tumor. Anesthesiology 45:100–102, 1976.

108. Amaha K, Okutsu Y, Nakamuru Y: Major airway obstruction by mediastinal tumour. A case report. Br J Anaesth 45:1082–1084, 1973.

109. Shambaugh BE, Seed R, Korn A: Airway obstruction in substernal goitre. Clinical and therapeutic implications. J Chronic Dis 26:737–743, 1973.

110. Neuman GG, Weingarten AE, Abramowitz RM, et al: The anesthetic management of the patient with an anterior mediastinal mass. Anesthesiology 60:144–147, 1984.

111. Abramson AL, Goldstein M, Stenzler A, et al: The use of the tidal breathing flow volume loop in laryngotracheal disease of neonates and infants. Laryngoscope 92:922–926, 1982.

112. Keon TP: Death on induction of anesthesia for cervical node biopsy. Anesthesiology 55:471–472, 1981.

113. Hall KD, Friedman M: Extracorporeal oxygenation for induction of anesthesia in a patient with an intrathoracic tumor. Anesthesiology 42:493–495, 1975.

114. Levin H, Bursztein S, Heifetz M: Cardiac arrest in a child with an anterior mediastinal mass. Anesth Analg 64:1129–1130, 1985.

115. Gore JM, Matsumoto AH, Layden JJ, et al: Superior vena cava syndrome. Its association with indwelling balloon-tipped pulmonary artery catheters. Arch Intern Med 144:505–508, 1984.

116. Perez CA, Presant CA, Van Amburg AL: III. Management of superior vena cava syndrome. Semin Oncol 5:123, 1978.

117. Quong GG, Brigham BA: Anaesthetic complications of mediastinal masses and superior vena caval obstruction. Med J Aust 2:487–488, 1980.

118. Stanford W, Doty DB: The role of venography and surgery in the management of patients with superior vena cava obstruction. Ann Thorac Surg 41:158–163, 1986.

119. Shapiro HM, Sanford TJ, Schaldach AL: Fiberoptic stylet laryngoscope and sitting position for tracheal intubation in acute superior vena cava syndrome. Anesth Analg 63:161–162, 1984.

120. Rogers SN, Benumof JL: New and easy techniques for fiberoptic endoscopy-aided tracheal intubation. Anesthesiology 59:569–572, 1983.

121. Piro AJ, Weiss DR, Hellman S: Mediastinal Hodgkin's disease: A possible danger for intubation anesthesia. Int J Radiat Oncol Biol Phys 1:415, 1976.

122. Meeker WR Jr, Richardson JD, West WO, et al: Critical evaluation of laparotomy and splenectomy in Hodgkin's disease. Arch Surg 105:222, 1972.

123. Davenport D, Ferree C, Blake D, et al: Radiation therapy in the treatment of superior caval obstruction. Cancer 42:2600, 1978.
124. Steen SN, Kepes ER, Arkins RE: Superior vena cava obstruction during anaesthesia. NY State J Med 69:2906, 1969.
125. Croft PB: Abnormal responses to muscle relaxants in carcinomatous neuropathy. Br Med J 1:181, 1958.
126. Pressler V, McNamara JJ: Aneurysm of the thoracic aorta. J Thorac Cardiovasc Surg 89:50–53, 1985.
127. Oosterhuis H: Immunopathology. In Oosterhuis H (ed): Myasthenia Gravis. New York, Churchill Livingstone, 1984, pp 104–130.
128. Hankins JR, Mayer RF, Satterfield JR, et al: Thymectomy for myasthenia gravis: Fourteen-year experience. Ann Surg 201:618–625, 1985.
129. Osserman KE: Studies in myasthenia gravis—Review of a 20-year experience in over 1,200 patients. Mt Sinai J Med 38:538, 1971.
130. Osserman KE, Kaplan LI: Studies in myasthenia gravis: Use of edrophonium chloride in differentiating myasthenia from cholinergic weakness. Arch Neurol Psych 70:385, 1953.
131. Baraka A, Dajani A: Atracurium in myasthenics undergoing thymectomy. Anesth Analg 36:1127–1130, 1984.
132. Leventhal SR, Orkin FK, Hirsh RA: Predicting postoperative ventilatory need in myasthenia. Anesthesiology 53:26, 1980.
133. Eisenkraft JB, Papatestas AE, Kahn CH, et al: Predicting the need for postoperative mechanical ventilation in myasthenia gravis. Anesthesiology 65:79–82, 1986.
134. Buckwalter JA, Herbst LA: Complications of gastric bypass for morbid obesity. Am J Surg 139:55–60, 1980.
135. Pace WG, Martin EW Jr, Tetirick T, et al: Gastric partitioning for morbid obesity. Ann Surg 190:392–400, 1979.
136. Brodsky JB, Wyner J, Ehrenworth J, et al: One-lung anesthesia in morbidly obese patients. Anesthesiology 57:132–134, 1982.
137. Vaughan RW, Bauer S, Wise L: Effect of position (semi-recumbent versus supine) on postoperative oxygenation in morbidly obese subjects. Anesth Analg 58:345–347, 1979.

Anesthesia for Emergency Thoracic Surgery

16

I. INTRODUCTION

The vast majority of cases requiring emergency thoracic surgery consist of massive hemoptysis, thoracic aortic aneurysms and dissections/disruptions, bronchopleural fistula, lung abscess and empyema, chest trauma (chest wall fractures, pulmonary parenchymal contusions, tracheobronchial disruption, and esophageal and diaphragmatic trauma), and tracheobronchial tree foreign bodies. Since chest trauma can cause massive hemoptysis and thoracic aortic disruptions and necessitate emergency room thoracotomy, it is obvious that the above classification is an arbitrary one. However, since each of these indications for emergency thoracic

375

surgery commonly occurs independently of chest trauma, they warrant separate consideration.

II. MASSIVE HEMOPTYSIS

A. General Considerations

Massive hemoptysis is uncommon, occurring in less than 0.5 per cent of patients admitted to a large pulmonary medicine service.[1] It has been arbitrarily defined, on the basis of the amount of daily volume of blood expectorated, as 200 ml,[2] more than 300 ml,[3] more than 500 ml,[4] more than 600 ml in 24 to 48 hours,[1, 5-7] and (massive) more than 600 ml within 16 hours.[5] However, others have evaluated hemoptysis not in terms of rate of bleeding, but from the standpoint of its threat to vital functions. Thus, a life-threatening hemoptysis was one that caused acute airway obstruction or caused hypotension severe enough to require blood transfusion.[8] In all of these reports, massive hemoptysis often occurred abruptly, unexpectedly, and without prodromal symptoms. The differential diagnosis of massive hemoptysis is shown in Table 16–1.[9, 10] On occasion, aspirated and/or swallowed epistaxis and hematemesis can be mistaken for hemoptysis.

Greater than 90 per cent of reported cases of massive hemoptysis have had a chronic infectious etiology.[9] The reason for this is that chronic inflammation leads to profuse vascularization of the high-pressure bronchial artery system. Subsequently, any erosion or rupture of enlarged bronchial arteries will result in massive hemoptysis. Active tuberculosis is the most common, with bronchiectasis the second most common, infection causing massive hemoptysis.[10]

The majority of the remaining causes of hemoptysis are due to bleeding neoplasms. Although the cause of spontaneous bleeding with neoplasms is the same as with the infectious etiologies (erosion into bronchial arteries), in present-day clinical practice massive hemoptysis from neoplasms increasingly occurs during diagnostic fiberoptic bronchoscopic manipulations of exophytic airway tumors. Massive hemoptysis may also occur when the low-pressure pulmonary circulation is transected or ruptured, as may occur with accidental trauma with sharp or blunt objects and pulmonary artery catheter trauma. The likelihood of massive endobronchial hemorrhage following pulmonary artery catheterization is increased by subsequent heparinization.[11, 12] Thus, massive hemoptysis may arise from either the pulmonary or the systemic circulation.

Death from massive hemoptysis usually results from asphyxiation, rarely from exsanguination. However, the amount of blood that has actually been lost may be seriously underestimated based on the history, since at least some of the coughed-up blood is swallowed. In addition, the accurate measurement of expectorated blood is frequently difficult.

B. Surgical Considerations

In a series of 55 pulmonary resections performed for massive hemoptysis (600 ml/16 hours),[5] there was a mortality of 18 per cent reported; this was markedly better than with conservative treatment, which resulted in a mortality of 75 per cent in patients who bled 600 ml or more in 16 hours and of 54 per cent in those who bled 600 ml or more in 48 hours.[5, 6] However, routine use of surgery has been debated as other authors have found that somewhat lesser degrees of hemoptysis may be successfully managed conservatively regardless of the amount of bleeding in the first 24 hours.[2, 13, 14] Nevertheless, surgery (resection) is probably indicated in patients who require multiple transfusions, in those in whom bleeding results

Table 16–1. Causes of Massive Hemoptysis

I. Infection
    Tuberculosis
    Bronchiectasis
    Bronchitis
    Lung abscess
    Necrotizing pneumonia
II. Neoplasm
    Bronchogenic carcinoma
    Metastatic carcinoma
    Mediastinal tumor
    Endobronchial polyp
III. Cardiovascular disease
    Mitral stenosis
    Pulmonary arteriovenous malformation
    Pulmonary embolus
    Pulmonary vasculitis
IV. Miscellaneous causes
    Pulmonary artery catheterization
    Exploratory needling
    Cystic fibrosis
    Pulmonary contusion, laceration
    Reperfusion of pulmonary vasculature after
        pulmonary embolectomy and after
        cardiopulmonary bypass

in progressive impairment of pulmonary function (aspiration should be evaluated by frequent serial chest roentgenograms), and in those in whom hemoptysis persists for several days despite optimum medical management.[14] Contraindications to surgery include inoperable carcinoma of the lung, inability to localize the bleeding site, and the presence of severe bilateral pulmonary disease and systemic disease (debilitation). These patients are candidates for bronchial artery embolization (Fig. 16–1) (see below).

The chest x-ray may contain strong clues (evidence of tuberculosis or opacifications) as to where the bleeding is coming from. However, considering that blood can be, and probably has been, aspirated into the nonbleeding lung, it cannot be safely assumed that the chest x-ray pathologic findings correspond to the site of bleeding.[15]

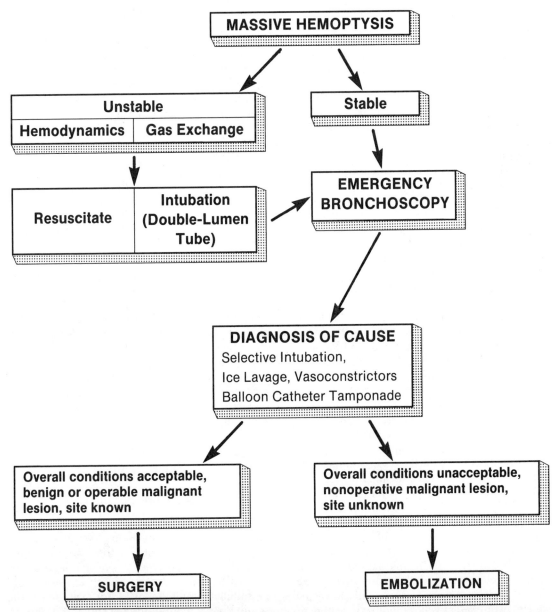

Figure 16–1. Treatment algorithm for massive hemoptysis. The most important function of emergency bronchoscopy is to establish or to diagnose the cause of bleeding. However, the amount and spread of bleeding can also be controlled during emergency bronchoscopy (see items under Diagnosis of Cause).

Bronchoscopy during active bleeding is the single most important technique for determining the cause and location of bleeding and should be performed in all patients; the procedure should be done in the operating room so that immediate resection can be performed (Fig. 16–1).[16] Most bronchoscopists will use a rigid bronchoscope because of the much greater suctioning and ventilating capability. However, the flexible fiberoptic bronchoscope may be used if there is no active bleeding and/or the site of bleeding is thought to be in the upper lobes. If localization is still uncertain after bronchoscopy and if the clinical situation permits, bronchial and pulmonary arteriography can be helpful. When bronchoscopy is coupled with selective angiography, a high rate of accurate localization can be achieved. When bronchoscopy has caused the bleeding (as in diagnostic procedures), the site of bleeding is known and the patient can proceed to surgery without delay.

The surgeon may be able to control bleeding and the spread of bleeding during bronchoscopy (Fig. 16–1). Topical iced saline and vasoconstrictors can be administered through the bronchoscope to control bleeding, provided the bleeding is not so massive as to preclude visualization of the origin.[7] Control of spread of blood from one lung to the other can be achieved by use of a bronchial blocker (balloon-tipped Fogarty catheter) in the main bronchus of the bleeding side or by use of a gauze packing of the bleeding segment or side.[16–20] During bronchoscopy, the surgeon should frequently restore adequate oxygenation and ventilation by intubating the uninvolved mainstem bronchus.

In some of the patients with a contraindication to resectional surgery, control of hemorrhage can be achieved by selective bronchial artery embolization using resorbable material.[22–25] The major risk of bronchial artery embolization is spinal cord injury due to spinal cord embolization via arterial collaterals to the spinal cord. The presence of spinal cord collaterals on scout arteriograms is an absolute contraindication to bronchial embolization.

In one patient with hemorrhage from the left lung, the combined occlusion of left pulmonary and bronchial arteries was used to control repeated hemorrhage.[25] In this patient, a Swan-Ganz catheter was guided by fluoroscopy into the left main pulmonary artery while bronchial arteries were selectively embolized. When recurrent hemorrhage occurred, the balloon in the pulmonary artery was inflated with 4 ml of saline. The decrease in pulmonary artery blood flow to the bleeding area was believed to be instrumental in stopping the second episode of hemorrhage.

Figure 16–1 summarizes most of the surgical considerations involving massive hemoptysis. The site of bleeding must be known, and in the vast majority of patients this will require bronchoscopy; the rigid bronchoscope is preferred. Unstable patients must be stabilized, and if they require intubation, a double-lumen tube is preferred (see Anesthetic Considerations below). During bronchoscopy, the surgeon may help to control bleeding by performing regional ice lavage, applying topical vasoconstrictors, and instituting tamponade of the bleeding region. If the patient can withstand surgery and has an operable lesion, surgery should be performed. If the patient cannot withstand surgery and/or has an inoperable lesion, bronchial embolization should be tried.

Recently, an approach to the clinical management of massive hemoptysis in patients with cystic fibrosis has been recommended. It is similar to the above algorithm but differs in one key respect; that is, embolization is the first choice, and surgery is a second choice of treatment.[27] The reason for the difference is that patients with cystic fibrosis have generalized lung disease, and preservation of tissue is a much more crucial issue. The site of bleeding is first identified by bronchoscopy, ideally under general anesthesia. Then selective bronchial arteriography is performed instead of surgery. If there are no collaterals to the spinal cord, then bronchial embolization is performed. If collaterals to the spinal cord are visualized, arterial embolization is abandoned and pulmonary resection is undertaken within the limits dictated by the patient's overall pulmonary function.

C. Anesthetic Considerations

1. Preoperative Considerations

The most important preoperative priorities are to prevent asphyxiation, localize site of bleeding, prevent contamination of normal lung if possible, and correct hypovolemia. It must be realized that many of these priorities should be fulfilled simultaneously. For example, at the same time a double-lumen tube is being inserted to prevent asphyxiation by drowning in blood, large-bore intravenous cannulae must be

ANESTHESIA FOR EMERGENCY THORACIC SURGERY • 379

inserted to begin to rapidly correct hypovolemia. Antibiotics should be administered preoperatively, and antituberculous drugs should be started in patients with tuberculosis.

a. PREVENT ASPHYXIATION

An increased F_IO_2 should be immediately administered as continuously as possible (oxygen administration may be interrupted by episodes of hemoptysis). Oxygenation and ventilation should be monitored, when possible, with arterial blood gas determinations. If the site of bleeding is known, the bleeding lung should be placed in a dependent position to prevent soiling of the nonbleeding lung. Patients who cannot cough out the blood effectively enough to prevent contamination of the nonbleeding lung must have the lungs separated as soon as possible. In the large majority of these patients, this can be done most expeditiously and effectively with a double-lumen tube; however, in the unusual case in which the bleeding is intermittent and a fiberoptic bronchoscope that was being used for diagnostic purposes is positioned near the site of bleeding, placement of a bronchial blocker is a viable alternative (see chapter 9). Rarely, insertion of a single-lumen tube down a mainstem bronchus must suffice as a life-saving measure when the other technically more difficult procedures cannot be accomplished (see chapter 9). Ventilatory support (intermittent positive-pressure breathing and positive end-expiratory pressure) must be provided as needed. Suctioning of the tracheobronchial tree must be aggressive.

b. PREVENT CONTAMINATION OF NORMAL LUNG

Coughing may increase bleeding. The advisability of using sedatives and cough suppressants is time dependent.[14] In the unintubated patient, the ability to cough may be life-saving, and suppressants should be avoided. The patient should be at strict bed rest in the semi-Fowler's position or with the radiologically normal lung in a nondependent position. In the intubated patient, suctioning can replace the cough mechanism, and suppression of cough may decrease bleeding. If possible, the initial intubation should be with a double-lumen tube. A coagulation profile should be drawn early; if any abnormalities are noted, they should be corrected. During and after bronchoscopy, the surgeon and internist can control bleeding by iced saline lavage, placement of topical vasoconstrictors, placement of a bronchial blocker or gauze packing, and use of bronchial artery embolization (see above).

c. CORRECT HYPOVOLEMIA

As soon as possible, large-bore intravenous cannulae should be inserted. The patient's blood should be typed and screened and cross matched for adequate amounts of blood products (whole blood, packed red blood cells, platelets, fresh frozen plasma). Transfusion should begin if appropriate. Finally, the appropriate monitoring (e.g., arterial line, central venous line) should be instituted.

2. Intraoperative Considerations

The patient with massive hemoptysis can come to the operating room without an endotracheal tube in place, with a single-lumen endotracheal tube in place, or with a double-lumen endotracheal tube in place (Fig. 16–2). In deciding what type of airway the patient needs, it is important to remember several general principles. First, the important advantages of a double-lumen tube include separation of the two lungs in order to prevent the spread of blood from one lung to the other lung; improved surgical exposure; the ability to ventilate, provide continuous positive airway pressure (CPAP), and sigh the operative lung when desired; and the ability to safely inspect an open bronchus during resection. Second, the potential disadvantages of a double-lumen tube include the increased technical difficulty in intubating a bloody trachea in a hypoxic patient and, if a large quantity of blood has already spread to the contralateral lung, it may be impossible to adequately ventilate and oxygenate the patient using only the now-soiled contralateral lung. Third, if a single-lumen tube is already placed or is inserted, the lungs can still be separated by a subsequent endobronchial intubation (right mainstem bronchus blindly and left mainstem bronchus with the aid of a fiberoptic bronchoscope) or by insertion of a bronchial blocker along the side of the single-lumen tube into the appropriate mainstem bronchus (see chapter 9).

If the patient with massive hemoptysis is without an indwelling endotracheal tube, preoxygenation should be instituted immediately. Adequate suctioning must be available. It may be necessary for the patient to be awake for intubation during massive, active, spontaneous

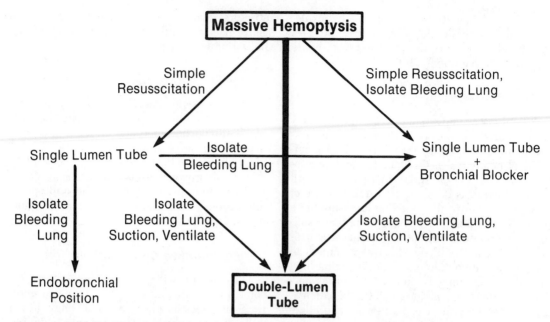

Figure 16–2. Endotracheal intubation options in massive hemoptysis and the sequence of conversion of one option to another. Double-lumen tubes are the intubation option of choice in the majority of patients.

bleeding in order to avoid the hazard of trying to visualize a blood-obscured airway in a paralyzed patient. Intubation performed in the semiupright position may minimize coughing that results in the presence of blood in the upper airway and, thereby, may provide a clearer field of vision.

If the patient without an indwelling endotracheal tube is to be put to sleep, aspiration precautions (e.g., cricoid pressure) should be utilized. Because these patients are likely to be hypovolemic, the induction of anesthesia should be accomplished with a small dose of short-acting barbiturate or ketamine or with narcotics followed in rapid sequence by relaxation. If the larynx can be visualized, insertion of a double-lumen tube is preferable to insertion of a single-lumen tube (see General Considerations above and Fig. 16–2). It should be remembered that if the patient is not actively bleeding but has a blood-filled cavity (i.e., a hemorrhagic lobe) this cavity will likely empty its contents into the dependent unsoiled lung when the patient is turned to the lateral decubitus position; therefore, this situation is a strong indication for placement of a double-lumen tube. If a single-lumen tube is inserted, serious consideration should be given to converting the single-lumen tube to an endobronchial position or using a bronchial blocker alongside it before turning the patient to the lateral decubitus position.

If a single-lumen tube is already in place, the same conversion considerations to bronchial blocker and endobronchial position apply (Fig. 16–2). In addition, consideration should be given to converting the single-lumen tube to a double-lumen tube (Fig. 16–2). If a double-lumen tube is in place, it should remain and be utilized (provided serious bilateral lung contamination has not occurred). In all situations, if active tuberculosis is present or suspected, contamination precautions should be utilized.

Once the airway has been established, the patient must be placed in the lateral decubitus position with the bleeding lung in the nondependent position. Use of this position, of course, emphasizes the importance of separating the lungs. Blood products must be administered according to the continued loss of blood, updated coagulation profiles, and hemodynamic monitoring findings. Insertion of an arterial line greatly facilitates monitoring of cardiovascular status and allows repetitive sampling for arterial blood gas analysis during the operation. The use of blood warmers is strongly recommended.

A unique management of a patient who required right upper lobectomy for massive hemorrhage has been described.[28] Following nasotracheal intubation with the patient awake and sitting upright, the standard endotracheal tube was pushed into a right endobronchial position. Inflation of the cuff of the endotracheal tube resulted in isolation of the right upper lobe bronchus from the rest of the lung, preventing further spillage of blood into nondiseased lung areas. General anesthesia was induced via a mask that fit over the endotracheal tube, the mouth, and the nose so that ventilation and oxygenation of the left lung and distal right lung could be accomplished. A tracheostomy was then performed, and the right endobronchial tube was replaced by a left-sided Carlens double-lumen endotracheal tube, which was passed in a 180° reversed position from its normal alignment. Inflation of the distal (endobronchial) cuff again prevented the spread of blood from the right upper lobe to the rest of the lung, and ventilation was more easily accomplished using the two catheter lumens of the tube. Although the indications for tracheostomy and failure to use a reversed left-sided double-lumen tube from the beginning were unclear in this patient, this case does illustrate the unique adaptation of a left-sided double-lumen tube for managing massive right upper lobe bleeding. For patients with massive bleeding the Robertshaw tube should be utilized because of its relative ease of placement and the larger lumens for suction and ventilation.

At the end of the case, the endotracheal tube should be left in place and the patient should be ventilated mechanically. Most of these patients will have impaired gas exchange postoperatively owing to preexisting lung disease, the probability that the nonbleeding lung has been soiled by the recent hemoptysis from the diseased lung, and the physiologic consequence of having just undergone a major anesthetic and surgical experience. Coagulation profiles, electrolyte concentrations, and acid-base status must be monitored in the immediate postoperative period, and abnormalities must be treated quickly.

III. THORACIC AORTIC ANEURYSMS AND DISSECTIONS/DISRUPTIONS

A. General Considerations

A true thoracic aortic aneurysm is a dilatation of all three layers of the aortic wall. Dissection of the thoracic aorta is a propagation of hematoma between the intima and the adventitia (i.e., in the media). Aortic dissection is caused by the sudden development of a tear in the aortic intima, opening the way for blood to enter the media of the aortic wall, thereby separating intima from the adventitia for variable distances along the length of the aorta. The most important forces acting to propagate the dissecting hematoma are the steepness of the ascending pressure pulse wave (dp/dt) and the aortic blood pressure. Spontaneous dissections occur in aneurysms, and traumatic dissections occur without being preceded or accompanied by an aneurysm.

1. Spontaneous Dissection of Thoracic Aortic Aneurysms

Spontaneously occurring aneurysms are usually repaired electively, and spontaneous acute dissection in a spontaneously occurring aneurysm usually requires emergency surgical repair.[29] Spontaneous dissection is approximately four times as common as a spontaneous rupture.[30] Spontaneous rupture is usually a fatal event.

There are two classifications of thoracic aortic dissections, and they are based on anatomic location. The DeBakey classification[31] consists of types I, II, and III (Fig. 16–3). Type I dissection begins in the ascending aorta and extends for varying distances past the aortic arch and below the diaphragm. Type II dissection also starts in the ascending aorta, but ends proximal to the left subclavian artery. Type III aortic dissection generally starts just distal to the left subclavian artery, extends for varying distances, and may even include the iliac arteries. Type I aortic dissection is the most common, occurring in approximately 70 per cent of all cases of spontaneous thoracic aortic dissection. The Stanford classification[32] consists of types A and B (Fig. 16–3). Type A encompasses Debakey types I and II, and type B consists of Debakey type III. The Stanford classification emphasizes the all-important point that Stanford type A and Debakey types I and II require immediate surgery.

There are numerous conditions that predispose to aneurysmal dilatation and spontaneous dissection of the thoracic aorta; all of these conditions cause degeneration of the aortic wall. Hypertension mechanically weakens the thoracic aortic wall because of chronic wall stress and shear forces. Similarly, the mechanical effect of a jet stream due to aortic valve stenosis and the proximal hypertension due to a coarctation of the aorta are associated with aneurysm of the thoracic aortic arch. Turner's syndrome, which is associated with coarctation of the aorta, is also associated with thoracic aortic aneu-

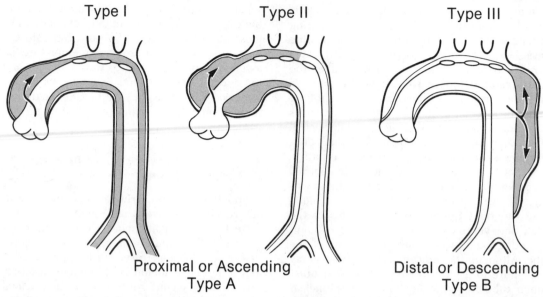

Figure 16–3. The classification of thoracic aortic dissections is based on anatomic location. The DeBakey classification consists of types I, II, and III, and the Stanford classification consists of types A and B. DeBakey types I and II and Stanford type A involve the ascending aorta and aortic arch, and DeBakey type III and Stanford type B originate distal to the left subclavian artery.

rysms. Inflammation of the aorta will weaken the wall, and, not surprisingly, giant cell aortitis and syphilitic aortitis are associated with thoracic aortic aneurysms. Marfan's and Ehlers-Danlos syndromes are associated with thoracic aortic aneurysms owing to hereditary defects in connective tissue strength. The hormonal changes of pregnancy can cause a loss of thoracic aortic wall structural integrity. Finally, although spontaneous internal tears are seldom seen through atheromatous lesions, thoracic aortic dissections can occur around atheromatous plaques following retrograde catheterization of the central arteries. Patients with thoracic aortic aneurysms have a high incidence of other arterial diseases, such as cerebrovascular and other vessel occlusive disease, abdominal aortic aneurysms, hypertension, and coronary artery disease.

2. Traumatic Disruption

Thoracic aortic injury caused by blunt objects results from differential rates of deceleration of the fixed aortic arch relative to the more mobile cardiac chambers and descending thoracic aorta. Consequently, traumatic disruption of the thoracic aorta usually occurs in the region of the ligamentum arteriosum, just distal to the left subclavian artery. A less common site is just above (cephalad to) the aortic valve. The

tear may involve the intima, intima and media, or the entire aortic wall.

Traumatic dissection and rupture of the thoracic aorta has been estimated to be associated with 10 to 16 per cent of all automobile accident fatalities.[32, 33] When a traumatic thoracic aortic tear occurs, 80 to 90 per cent of the patients die at the scene of the accicent.[32–34] Among the 10 to 20 per cent of patients who survive an initial traumatic thoracic aortic tear, the leak is temporarily controlled by the adventitia of the aorta. Even though the adventitia is strong, it is not capable of resisting the same bursting pressure as was the intact aorta and increases in blood pressure above normal limits must be avoided. Most of these patients will have associated injuries and a priority system must be established; often head and abdominal injuries take precedence. In the group of patients arriving at the hospital alive, as high as 80 per cent may survive postoperatively.[32, 35]

3. Signs and Symptoms of Any Type (Traumatic or Spontaneous) of Dissection

The most common presenting symptom is the sudden onset of severe, unremitting, tearing or ripping chest or back pain. In dissections involving the ascending aorta, aortic valvular insufficiency may be present due to stretching of the aortic annulus by the dissecting hematoma. Other presenting signs and symptoms of thoracic aortic dissection/disruption result from the anatomic course that the propagating hematoma takes.[36] As the medial hematoma dissects or as the intimal flap peels off, partial or complete obstruction of the lumen of an artery arising from the aorta can occur, and the signs and symptoms reflect the distribution of the obstructed artery. Involvement of the coronary arteries causes acute myocardial infarction and frequently sudden death. Involvement of the innominate and/or common carotid artery may cause syncope, confusion, stroke, or coma. Involvement of the innominate and/or subclavian artery can cause upper limb gangrene and paralysis. Involvement of the intercostal and/or lumbar arteries can cause spinal cord ischemia and paraplegia. Involvement of the renal, mesenteric, and common iliac arteries can cause oliguria, bowel ischemia, and lower leg gangrene and paralysis, respectively. Through-and-through rupture of the aorta can cause extravasation of blood into any adjacent region; consequently, blood may be found in the pericardial sac, pleural space, mediastinum, retroperitoneum, wall of the pulmonary trunk and/or main right and left pulmonary arteries (because of common adventitia with aorta), lung parenchyma, and esophagus.

B. Surgical Considerations

Since there are tremendous differences in mortality with surgical versus medical treatment of proximal aortic lesions,[36-38] the indications for surgery are based on the location of the dissection/disruption. Stanford type A and complicated Stanford type B lesions require immediate surgery. Complications of type B dissection consist of any of the following: failure to control hypertension, continued pain, expanding aortic diameter, development of neurologic deficit, evidence of compromise of a major subdiaphragmatic aortic branch vessel, and development of aortic valvular insufficiency.

On the basis of widespread experience, a consensus has emerged concerning major principles and management of suspected acute aortic dissection.[39-43] During the first few hours following admission, the patient's blood pressure should be stabilized with sodium nitroprusside (to systolic blood pressure of 100 to 110 mm Hg) and propranolol (to heart rate of 60 to 70 beats/min), and an upright chest radiograph with a nasogastric tube in place should be obtained. The chest radiograph criteria for proceeding to aortic angiography include the presence of any of the following: mediastinal widening, the loss of normal contour of the aortic knob, opacification of the aortopulmonary window, depression of the left main bronchus, deviation of the trachea or nasogastric tube to the right, and the apical cap sign.[44] Ratios of mediastinal width to chest width at the aortic knob greater than 0.28 have been found to be accurate predictors of thoracic aortic rupture.[45]

If the patient is stable, the patient should be transferred for aortography.[35] While the patient is in the aortography suite, use of pain medications or sedatives should be restricted. The persistence of pain despite an adequate decrease in arterial blood pressure is a sign of continuing hematoma formation. Similarly, depression of mental status is an ominous clinical finding, which may indicate involvement of the major extracranial cerebral vessels in the dissection of the hematoma. Both these valuable and important signs (pain and depressed mental status) are masked by overmedication with narcotics or sedatives. Small doses of a mild hypnotic agent such as diazepam should provide adequate relief of patient anxiety. Oxygen should be administered by face mask. If the patient is hemodynamically unstable, the patient should immediately be transferred to the operating room.

Based on the results of aortography, the lesion can be classified as Stanford type A or B. This information, coupled with the patient's in-hospital course and response to emergency therapy, dictates whether immediate surgery, further stabilization with later surgery, or no surgery will be required.

The surgical approach (Fig. 16–4) is dictated by several considerations. First, and foremost, is the site of the lesion. Proximal repairs (Stanford type A) require cardiopulmonary by-pass and a median sternotomy (approaches A and B of Fig. 16–4). Distal repairs (Stanford type B) utilize a left thoracotomy and usually some form of partial by-pass (approaches C and D of Fig. 16–4). With partial by-pass the organs proximal to the clamp area are perfused by the patient's heart and oxygenated by the patient's lungs, whereas the organs distal to the clamped area are perfused and oxygenated by a pump-oxygenator system. The second consideration is control of proximal hypertension during partial by-pass. Approach C decreases proximal hyper-

A. Ascending Aorta

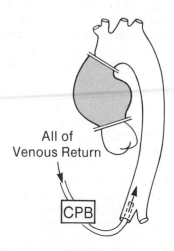

All of
Venous Return

CPB

B. Aortic Arch

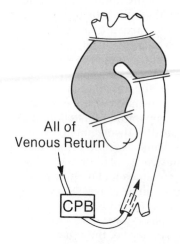

All of
Venous Return

CPB

C. Descending Thoracic Aorta (Shunt Method)

D. Descending Thoracic Aorta (Partial Bypass Method)

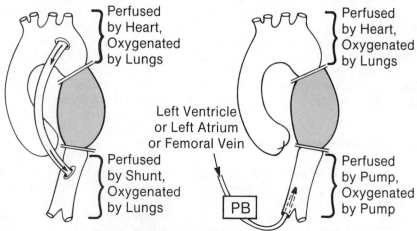

Perfused
by Heart,
Oxygenated
by Lungs

Perfused
by Shunt,
Oxygenated
by Lungs

Left Ventricle
or Left Atrium
or Femoral Vein

Perfused
by Heart,
Oxygenated
by Lungs

Perfused
by Pump,
Oxygenated
by Pump

PB

E. Descending Thoracic Aorta (Simple Clamp)

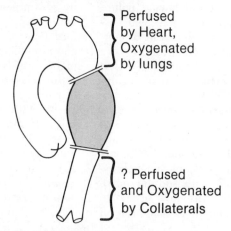

Perfused
by Heart,
Oxygenated
by lungs

? Perfused
and Oxygenated
by Collaterals

Figure 16–4. See legend on opposite page

tension by inserting a proximal-distal shunt (Gott, TDMAC-heparin shunt). The heparin-bonded shunt (systemic heparinization is not used) is inserted proximally in the ascending aorta, or apex of the left ventricle, or, if neither is available, the left subclavian artery, and distally into the aorta or femoral artery. Approach *D* decreases proximal hypertension by a left ventricular, or left atrial, or femoral vein–femoral artery partial by-pass. The left ventricular, or left atrial, or femoral vein drain decreases venous return to the left heart, thereby limiting left heart preload, cardiac output, and hypertension proximal to the descending thoracic aortic clamp. The third consideration is minimizing neurologic (spinal cord) damage. Approaches *C* and *D* provide some form of distal perfusion. However, there has been no difference in the incidence of paraplegia between these approaches (*C* and *D*) and simple aortic cross clamping (approach *E* of Fig. 16–4).[46, 47] The reason for this is that the most important common denominators for spinal cord injury are prolonged systemic hypotension, removal of long segments of aorta, and removal of aortic segments from which a collateral circulation to the spinal cord has not had time to develop; the presence of these denominators has little to do with the type of by-pass.[46, 47] The fourth consideration is maintenance of renal function, and partial by-passes are theoretically most protective. The fifth consideration is associated injuries. For example, systemic heparinization is contraindicated with closed-head injuries and would eliminate use of pump by-pass. Simple aortic cross clamping avoids heparinization and allows for more prompt management of other injuries owing to shorter surgical time, there are no cannulation site complications, and post-operative renal function is normal if clamping time is less than 30 min. Use of the TDMAC-heparin–bonded shunt also avoids the use of heparin.

C. Anesthetic Considerations

This disease has an extremely high early mortality, and the aim of preoperative medical management is to limit the extent of dissection or prevent frank aortic rupture. The time spent in establishing monitoring should be inversely proportional, and the speed of induction of anesthesia should be directly proportional, to the likelihood of further dissection/rupture and the hemodynamic stability of the patient. Proper judgment as to the appropriate balance between preoperative preparation and patient risk is extremely critical with this disease.

1. Preoperative Considerations

Preoperative anesthetic considerations consist of correction of hypovolemia, institution of monitoring, drug therapy, and laboratory analysis. The extent of correction of hypovolemia will depend on the need for speed of control of the thoracic aorta. At a minimum, adequate intravenous access must be ensured by at least two large-bore intravenous catheters connected to blood warmers, and the patient's blood must by typed and cross matched for adequate amounts of blood products (10 units of whole blood, platelets, fresh frozen plasma). Consideration should be given to use of autotransfusion (i.e., the cell saver). Monitoring should be instituted as permitted by the overall hemodynamic status of the patient. If possible, the V_5 or equivalent leads (CMV_5 or CB_5) should be used to monitor myocardial ischemia. A right radial intra-arterial catheter should be inserted because the left subclavian artery and, therefore, the left radial artery might be compromised by the aortic dissection. In addition, the left subclavian artery is more likely to be compromised by intraoperative clamping than the innominate artery. A second arterial line distal to the cross clamp (e.g., femoral artery, dorsalis pedis artery) may be useful for measuring distal perfusion pressure during cross clamping.[48] Urine output should be monitored with a urinary catheter. If time permits, a pulmonary artery catheter or central venous pressure catheter should be inserted. Prior to the induction of anesthesia, cerebral function should be simply noted by briefly talking with the patient and by observing the pupils. Drug therapy consists of controlling blood pressure with sodium nitroprusside and heart rate with propranolol. The sodium nitroprusside should be ti-

Figure 16–4. The repair of the various thoracic aortic dissections requires different surgical approaches. A, Complete cardiopulmonary bypass (CPB); cardioplegia for myocardial preservation. B, Cardiopulmonary bypass for cooling prior to cross clamping, then cessation of bypass with profound hypothermia during cross clamping. C, TDMAC-heparin shunt for descending aortic dissection. D, Left ventricular, atrial, or femoral vein–femoral artery partial bypass (PB) for descending aortic dissection. E, Simple aortic cross clamping for descending aortic dissection.

trated to an end-point of systemic arterial blood pressure of 100 to 110 mm Hg, and propranolol should be titrated to the end-point of a heart rate of 60 to 70 beats/min. Laboratory analysis should consist of complete blood count, determination of electrolytes and blood urea nitrogen/creatinine concentrations, clotting studies (prothrombin time [PT]/partial thromboplastin time [PTT]/bleeding time/platelet count), and a 12-lead electrocardiogram (EKG). Oxygen should be administered by a face mask throughout all these procedures.

2. Intraoperative Considerations

The important intraoperative considerations will be mentioned in approximately the order that they arise during the repair of the thoracic aortic aneurysm (Table 16–2). The aim of induction of anesthesia is to prevent both hypertension and hypotension. In patients with acute dissection the induction should be smooth and rapid but controlled. In these patients, anesthesia should be induced intravenously with small to moderate doses of narcotic, ketamine, or thiopental (or some combination of these drugs, depending on the starting blood pressure and the degree of hypovolemia thought to be present), followed by profound muscle relaxation, cricoid pressure, and rapid endotracheal intubation. For elective aneurysm repair, higher induction doses of narcotic are usually used and the induction pace can be more leisurely. Adjuncts for control of hypertension include administration of increasing sodium nitroprusside dose, intravenous lidocaine (Xylocaine) bolus administration, intravenous propranolol bolus administration, further intra-

Table 16–2. Important Anesthetic Considerations for Descending Thoracic Aortic Aneurysms/Disruptions

I. Control hemodynamic responses:
  A. Nitroprusside (systolic blood pressure 110 to 100 mm Hg)
  B. Propranolol or labetalol (heart rate 60 to 70 beats/min)
II. One-lung ventilation (collapse left lung, ventilate right lung)
III. Following clamping control proximal hypertension:
  A. Nitroprusside,
  B. Increase partial by-pass drainage,
  C. Decrease intravenous infusion
IV. Prior to and during unclamping avoid hypotension:
  A. Infuse volume,
  B. Taper nitroprusside,
  C. Discontinue by-passes,
  D. Bicarbonate as indicated,
  E. Restore coagulation

venous anesthetic drug administration, and the initiation of inhalation anesthesia. Adjuncts for control of hypotension consist of volume infusion and vasopressor drug administration. The goal of the maintenance of anesthesia is to control systemic blood pressure, which can be done in a variety of ways (halogenated drug anesthesia, high-dose narcotic anesthesia with sodium nitroprusside).

Unless there is a strong contraindication, these cases should be done with a double-lumen tube and collapse of the left lung and ventilation of the right lung (with patient in the right lateral decubitus position for left thoracotomy). There are three important reasons why one-lung ventilation and double-lumen tube intubation are particularly advantageous for these cases. First, as in many other thoracic surgery cases, surgical exposure is greatly improved and collapse of the adjacent left lung is particularly important during the difficult period of initial aortic mobilization. Second, initial surgical dissection can cause bleeding into the bronchi of the left (nondependent) lung because the aorta is often adherent to the adjacent lung tissue. The double-lumen tube protects the right (dependent) lung, which might otherwise be flooded by this blood traversing the carina. Third, collapse of the left lung protects the left lung from damage during periods of heparinization. If the left lung were being ventilated during this period, considerable retraction would have to be placed on it to allow for adequate surgical access. This, in a fully heparinized patient, could again initiate bleeding in the left lung.

One-lung ventilation, therefore, confers several benefits to the patient. However, it should be noted that these patients are likely to have a sodium nitroprusside infusion, which is a potent inhibitor of hypoxic pulmonary vasoconstriction in the collapsed left lung. Consequently, use of sodium nitroprusside during one-lung ventilation requires that arterial blood gas concentrations be monitored frequently (pulse oximetry is useful in this situation). If severe hypoxemia occurs, nondependent lung CPAP or temporary clamping of the left pulmonary artery to diminish the shunt flow through the left lung should be instituted (see chapter 11).

Blood loss may be considerable during the initial mobilization of the aorta, and adequate volume replacement is a high priority. Once the section of the aorta that is diseased has been freed and mobilized, arterial cross clamps will be placed proximal and distal to the lesion. Prior to placement of the cross clamps, a sample of unheparinized blood must be drawn from the patient to preclot the prosthetic graft and the patient must be adequately anticoagulated with intravenous heparin; the activated clotting time (ACT) should be approximately four times the control value.[49] From the point of view of both possible preclamp hypovolemia and postclamp hypoperfusion, the well-being of the kidneys must be monitored closely by the urine output. If oliguria or anuria is present, an osmotic diuretic should be administered.

Placement of an aortic cross clamp causes an increase in left ventricular afterload. If the ascending aorta or aortic arch is cross clamped, the heart must be fibrillated and cardiopulmonary by-pass must be used (Fig. 16–4, approach A or B). When the descending aorta is cross clamped, structures that are proximal to the cross clamp are still perfused by the heart, and structures distal to the cross clamp are either unperfused or perfused via a shunt or partial by-pass pump (Fig. 16–4, approaches C, D, and E). However, since the heart is now pumping into a markedly reduced vascular bed, hypertension proximal to the clamp occurs, which is dangerous because the proximal hypertension may cause the heart to become ischemic and/or excessively distended. Consequently, proximal hypertension must be controlled by infusing vasodilator drug, increasing the drainage of the heart by the partial by-pass (Fig. 16–4, approach D), and decreasing intravenous volume infusion (let the systemic blood pressure drift downward). Structures distal to the cross clamp, especially the kidneys and lower spinal cord, must also receive blood flow. In this regard a distal perfusion pressure of 50 to 70 mm Hg must be maintained.[50]

During the period of cross clamping, intraoperative monitoring of somatosensory evoked potentials as a guide to the state of spinal cord perfusion should be considered. An early warning of cord ischemia may allow for modification of surgical technique, such as reanastomosis of sacrificed intercostal artery or repositioning of hemostatic clamps, in an attempt to restore cord perfusion.

The intravascular volume management before unclamping is critical. Just as the placement of the cross clamp decreased the arterial space and vascular compliance, unclamping will have the opposite effect. To prepare for this sudden return to normal vascular size and compliance and to avoid precipitous hypotension, the anesthesiologist should begin transfusion to high-normal cardiac filling pressures as the final vascular anastomosis is performed. If hypoten-

sive agents have been necessary to treat proximal hypertension, careful drug infusion tapering should begin. Adequate amounts of blood and blood products should be available if further transfusion is necessary once the cross clamp is removed. Unclamping the descending thoracic aorta must be accompanied by simultaneous discontinuance of the distal perfusion mechanism. With unclamping, bleeding may occur along fresh suture lines and must be monitored and replaced. Metabolic acidosis after unclamping should be corrected as indicated by arterial blood gas tensions. Urine output should be monitored closely in order to detect oliguria early. After aortic unclamping, the coagulation status should be managed in the following sequence: reverse heparin with protamine; check ACT (or equivalent method to detect residual heparin effect); give additional protamine as indicated to return ACT to control level; perform coagulation tests (laboratory), including PT, PTT, and platelet count; and treat according to results of clotting studies. After aortic unclamping the goal of anesthesia should be to end the case so that the patient is paralyzed and adequately sedated. As the patient emerges from deeper levels of anesthesia, hypertension must be treated to prevent suture line stress. When the patient is in the supine position, the double-lumen tube should be converted to a single-lumen tube and the patient should be ventilated mechanically until all vital functions are adequate and have stabilized.

IV. BRONCHOPLEURAL FISTULA

A. General Considerations

A bronchopleural fistula may be caused by the rupture of a lung abscess, bronchus, bulla, cyst, or parenchymal tissue (as in the case of high levels of positive end-expiratory pressure [PEEP] during mechanical ventilation) into the pleural space; erosion of a bronchus can occur by a carcinoma or chronic inflammatory disease and by breakdown of a bronchial suture line following pulmonary resection.

B. Surgical Considerations

The diagnosis of bronchopleural fistula is usually made clinically. In early postpneumonectomy patients, the diagnosis is based upon sudden dyspnea, subcutaneous emphysema, contralateral deviation of the trachea, and disappearance of the fluid level on roentgenograms of the chest. In patients after lobectomy, persistent air leak, purulent drainage, and expectoration of purulent material are usually diagnostic. When the fistula appears after removal of the chest tube, the diagnosis of a bronchopleural fistula is made on the basis of fever, purulent sputum, and a new air fluid level in the pleural cavity on the roentgenogram of the chest. The diagnosis is confirmed by bronchoscopic examination in most, bronchography in a few, and sinograms (of the fistula) in an occasional patient.[51]

In postpneumonectomy patients, if the disruption occurs early, it is possible to resuture the stump. Late postpneumonectomy bronchial disruption associated with empyema has been managed by conservative drainage, but definitive operative closure is now considered the treatment of choice. Operations for late postpneumonectomy disruption consist of closure with pedicled flaps of muscle and omentum using a lateral thoracotomy and staple closure through an anterior transpericardial approach via median sternotomy.[52]

In non-postpneumonectomy cases, if the lung expands to fill the thoracic cavity, the leak can usually be controlled with chest tube drainage alone. However, if the fistula is large, and a large leak through a large persistent pleural space occurs, it is unlikely that the fistula will close, and surgical resection is usually necessary.[51] The most commonly performed operations are staged multiple rib resection thoracoplasties (to obliterate the pleural space), resuturing of bronchial stump, and suture of intercostal muscle pedicle over the open bronchial stump.[51] An empyema complicating a bronchopleural fistula should, if possible, be drained prior to surgery. This is done under local anesthesia with the patient in an upright position in order to minimize the possibility of contaminating healthy lung tissue with the cavity's purulent material.

Finally, a spontaneous pneumothorax (no prior lung resection involved) is pathophysiologically similar to a bronchopleural fistula. There are three situations in which definitive surgical treatment is indicated in treating a spontaneous pneumothorax. First, surgery is required when conventional tube drainage and suction have been unsuccessful in clearing the pleural space and when, in effect, a bronchopleural fistula has formed. Second, surgical intervention is usually indicated when a second ipsilateral or first contralateral spontaneous pneumothorax occurs. Third, considering that

a spontaneous pneumothorax has a recurrence rate of 10 to 25 per cent, if after the initial event the patient's life style is such that a recurrence might be life-threatening or highly inconvenient, definitive treatment is indicated. In younger patients with a simple pneumothorax, pleurectomy is the prophylactic procedure of choice and results in a low recurrence rate.[53, 54] In older patients with severe chronic airflow obstruction, chemical pleurodesis with talc, dextrose, or other irritant is safer, but also less effective.[55]

C. Anesthetic Considerations

There have been several medical (nonsurgical) approaches (use of various mechanical ventilation–chest tube drainage systems) to the treatment of patients with bronchopleural fistula that are important for the anesthesiologist and intensive care physician to know about[56-65] (see Fig. 12–3). In all of these approaches, initial adequate conventional positive-pressure ventilation through a single-lumen endotracheal tube was generally difficult to achieve because of loss of much of the tidal volume through the fistula. This, in turn, retarded healing and may have even made the fistula larger. One solution was to selectively intubate the bronchus of the contralateral normal lung and provide ventilation to only one lung, thereby allowing the fistula to heal in a relatively quiet environment[56] (see Fig. 12–3). However, this approach may not be applied to patients with a bronchopleural fistula who have associated pulmonary pathologic changes and are, therefore, unable to tolerate the large transpulmonary shunt inherent in this method of treatment. In addition, this type of patient may require PEEP during mechanical ventilation to maintain functional residual capacity (FRC), and unilateral PEEP may increase the shunt through the nonventilated lung.

It is difficult to apply PEEP effectively in the presence of a large bronchopleural fistula because a constant air leak is present.[59, 60] Furthermore, the suction chest drainage, which is normally present in these patients, may cause the ventilator to cycle if it is set in the assist mode.[59, 60] One solution to the problem of maintaining PEEP in the presence of a large bronchopleural fistula has been the application of positive intrapleural pressure equal to the end-expiratory pressure desired during mechanical ventilation[57] (see Fig. 12–3). This method is effective in maintaining PEEP and in preventing gas leak during exhalation, but it does not prevent an air leak during positive-pressure inspiration. Alternatively, the insertion of a unidirectional valve into the chest tube drainage apparatus solves the problems of avoiding an air leak during positive pressure inspiration and using PEEP.[58] The unidirectional chest tube valve is closed by the inspiratory phase of the ventilator and opens during expiration. A small tension pneumothorax is created with each mechanical inspiration, but it is immediately relieved when the chest tube valve opens. Deleterious cardiovascular effects have not been noted with this technique. However, the chest tube valve must frequently be checked because chest tube drainage fluids may cause the valve to either stick closed or remain permanently open.

One report describes a conservative approach to managing a bronchopleural fistula by decreasing airway pressure delivered to the diseased lung using differential lung ventilation.[61] A double-lumen endotracheal tube was placed in the patient, and independent volume settings for each lung were achieved by using two synchronized ventilators. The nondiseased lung was ventilated normally (tidal volume 800 ml, PEEP 12 cm H_2O, rate 10/min), while tidal volume was kept low in the diseased lung (tidal volume 150 ml, PEEP 5 cm H_2O, rate 10/min). Oxygenation and ventilation were improved over that provided by conventional mechanical ventilatory support, although the patient eventually expired. The authors stated that, in retrospect, they should not have ventilated the diseased lung at all; rather, a level of continuous positive airway pressure just below the critical opening pressure of the fistula might have been more beneficial.

High-frequency ventilation may be the treatment of choice for a large bronchopleural fistula (see chapter 12 and Fig. 12–3). The advantages of high-frequency ventilation for bronchopleural fistual include the following: (1) There is minimal loss of tidal volume through the bronchopleural fistula; (2) the fistula may heal more quickly; (3) the airway resistance (or lack of) and pulmonary compliance have minimal influence on ventilation; (4) low airway pressures result in minimal effects on cardiac output; and (5) spontaneous ventilatory efforts are usually abolished, thereby lowering oxygen consumption from respiratory muscles and eliminating the need for paralysis and excessive sedation.

The first report of the successful treatment of a bronchopleural fistula with high-frequency jet ventilation appeared in 1980.[62] This paper

described a patient in whom a bronchopleural fistula occurred along with an empyema several months after a right upper lobectomy. The patient was ventilated (rate 115/min) for several weeks until the fistula closed and weaning was possible. The use of dual-mode independent lung ventilation utilizing both conventional and high-frequency jet ventilation for the intraoperative repair of a bronchopleural fistula has also recently been reported.[63] This paper described a patient who was managed during thoracoplasty with a double-lumen endotracheal tube; the nondiseased lung was ventilated in a conventional manner (tidal volume 500 ml, rate 9/min), while the lung with the bronchopleural fistula received high-frequency jet ventilation (rate 150/min). This method was continued for 2 hours following successful repair of the bronchopleural fistula until extubation was accomplished. Finally, high-frequency jet ventilation has been used in the nonoperative management of a patient with bilateral bronchopleural fistula.[64] This report describes a patient who required high-frequency jet ventilation for almost 2 months; at the time of extubation small fistulae were still present but eventually healed. Thus, although the eventual role of high-frequency jet ventilation for treating bronchopleural fistula is not fully established,[65] it is emerging as the best nonsurgical method to treat this condition when mechanical ventilatory support is required and the proper equipment and personnel experienced with its use are available.

No matter which ventilation method and chest tube drainage system are used, the entire approach should be evaluated by continuously measuring the volume (flow) of gas passing from the chest tube by inserting a sterile "flow-tube" sensor into the chest tube drainage system.[66] The usual methods of visually assessing the amount of bubbling in the water-sealed chamber or subtracting the measured exhaled lung volume from the present inspired tidal breaths are only intermittent semiquantitative measures of lost volume, which are especially inaccurate if the patient is breathing spontaneously. In addition, flow through the fistula may frequently be changed during the patient's clinical course. Continuously measuring fistula flow allows on-line titration of tidal volume, PEEP, inspiratory occlusion of the chest tube, and balancing airway/chest tube PEEP.[66] In addition, the response time of the flow meter is short enough to separate fistula flow during the inspiratory phase of ventilation from that of exhalation in most patients.

Obviously from the above, and for the preoperative nonintubated patient, the ability to deliver positive-pressure ventilation adequately to a patient with a bronchopleural fistula and chest tube drainage, or to a patient with a bronchopleurocutaneous fistula, must be carefully considered preoperatively. If a fistula is obviously small, chronic, and uninfected, a standard endotracheal tube can likely be used safely. When in doubt, positive-pressure ventilation can be tested and, if found inadequate, the standard endotracheal tube can be replaced with a double-lumen endotracheal tube. If, after the chest is opened, an excessive leak is encountered when using a standard endotracheal tube, ventilation can be improved by lung packing and manual control of the air leak.[67]

For large fistulae or fistulae of unknown size, and for those in which an associated abscess of empyema is known or suspected to be present, intraoperative use of a double-lumen endotracheal tube has the great dual benefits of permitting positive-pressure ventilation of the normal lung without loss of the minute ventilation through the fistula and avoiding the great hazard of contamination of the uninfected lung with infected material when the patient is turned to the lateral decubitus position.[68–70] Indeed, in one series of 22 patients undergoing operations for bronchopleural fistula following pulmonary resection for tuberculosis or tuberculous empyema, management with a single-lumen endotracheal tube, despite intubation in the head-up position and frequent suctioning, resulted in extensive contamination of normal lung in two patients.[71] In one patient the operation had to be terminated, and in the other emergency bronchoscopy had to be performed. The use of a double-lumen endotracheal tube effectively isolates the leaking and, perhaps infected, lung cavity from the normal lung. For the patient who cannot have a double-lumen tube (e.g., small child, patients with inability to tolerate being taken off the ventilator, those with anatomic difficulties), bronchial blockade and endobronchial intubation are less satisfactory alternatives.

V. LUNG ABSCESSES AND EMPYEMA

A. General Considerations

Aspiration secondary to alcoholic stupor has classically been reported as the most common factor that precipitates lung abscess. Other historical factors that predispose patients to lung abscess formation consist of abuse of other drugs, prior pneumonia, lung carcinoma, immunosuppression with steroid drugs, diabetes mellitus, presence of distant septic focus (hematogenous spread), and chronic obstructive pulmonary disease.[72]

Empyema is the accumulation of pus in the pleural cavity. All of the above causes of a lung abscess may produce empyema, and a lung abscess per se may cause empyema. In particular, empyema may be caused by infection of residual clotted blood following a hemothorax (which was treated by chest tube placement) and following diagnostic thoracentesis, especially if there is a concurrent intra-abdominal injury or infection.[73] Both a lung abscess and an empyema may erode a bronchus and cause a bronchopleural fistula (see Chest Trauma and Fig. 16–5).

The symptoms of lung abscess and empyema are similar and include cough, purulent sputum production, fever, chest pain, and dyspnea. The most frequent physical findings include decreased breath sounds, rales, tachypnea, rhonchi, dullness on percussion, and tachycardia.[72, 74]

B. Surgical Considerations

Simple empyemas (without abscess) may be treated by repeat thoracentesis, tube thoracostomy, or open drainage with rib resection. In a recent study the incidences of success with these approaches were 11 per cent, 35 per cent, and 91 per cent for repeat thoracentesis, tube thoracostomy, and rib resection, respectively.[74] Of those who failed to be cured by repeat thoracentesis, some had successful tube drainage, and some had successful rib resection. Of those who failed with closed tube thoracostomy as the initial mode of therapy, some were successfully treated with multiple tube placements and repositioning for successful drainage, a few required decortication, a few required repeat decortication, and a few required rib resection. Of those who were treated with rib resection and drainage of empyema as the initial procedure, almost all were cured by this initial treatment. It was concluded that early open drainage and rib resection, especially for postoperative empyema and empyema that occurs in an immunocompromised patient, is the treatment of choice. Recently, good resolution of empyema has been outlined with irrigation of the empyema cavity with antibiotic-containing solution via a thoracoscope.[75, 76] This technique avoids rib resection.

Several surgical procedures have been used in the treatment of lung abscess.[72] Tube thoracostomy has occasionally helped heal a small abscess, especially in patients who have associated nonloculated empyema (i.e., the patient has simple associated empyema). Recently, good success has been obtained following radiologic and needle location of the abscess with percutaneous tube drainage.[77] If a loculated empyema cavity(s) develops, open drainage with decortication is indicated. In any patient who does not improve with any of these therapies, an open drainage procedure followed by either lobectomy or segmentectomy is required.[78, 79]

C. Anesthetic Considerations

If a surgical procedure is going to be done under general anesthesia in a patient with either a lung abscess or an empyema, then double-lumen tube intubation is absolutely indicated to prevent contamination of the uninfected lung by the infected lung. In addition, if an empyema is going to be treated with thoracoscopy, collapse of the diseased lung greatly aids access to the empyema.[75, 76] The seal of the endobronchial cuff should be tight and can be quantitated by the bubble-under-water technique described in chapter 9. The position of the tube should be determined by fiberoptic bronchoscopy. Both of these maneuvers (checking of tube by fiberoptic bronchoscopy and determination of pressure level of cuff seal) should be done before the patient is turned to the lateral decubitus position.

During the surgical procedure, the diseased side should be suctioned frequently. Whenever possible, but particularly at the end of the procedure, the diseased lung should be fully expanded manually. When the lung has been fully expanded, the surgeon should check carefully for the presence of a bronchopleural fistula.

VI. CHEST TRAUMA

A. General Considerations

Blunt thoracic injury is usually associated with other injuries to the head, abdomen, or limbs, and it is the associated injuries that often determine the prognosis for the patient. Associated head injury is often severe, and severe head injury is the single most common cause of death in patients with chest injury. The presence of associated abdominal injuries makes respiratory failure and the need for mechanical ventilation more likely. Orthopedic injuries cause patient discomfort and require immobility, which makes management of the chest injury technically difficult.

Overall, less than 15 per cent of all patients with chest trauma will require a thoracotomy. The management of those patients near death from chest trauma requiring immediate thoracotomy upon arrival at the hospital will be covered under Emergency Room Thoracotomy in the Management of Trauma. Patients requiring less urgent thoracotomy after chest trauma may have a variety of thoracic injuries. Figure 16–5 shows the variety of primary and secondary thoracic injuries, and the inter-relationships of the injuries, as a traumatic force penetrates inward. Most of the initial primary injuries can result in major chronic secondary complications.

1. Chest Wall Fractures (Flail Chest)

Flail chest may be defined as an abnormal movement of the chest wall occurring as a result of fractures of two or more ribs in two places on the same side. Each rib section between the two fracture sites essentially floats free. With spontaneous inspiration and the development of a more negative intrathoracic pressure, the injured segment moves inward upon the lung (paradoxic chest wall movement), preventing lung expansion and impairing oxygenation. The reverse occurs during a spontaneous exhalation. This injury most commonly involves the anterolateral aspect of the chest. The posterior wall is heavily fortified with muscle and, therefore, is rarely involved. The thoracic cage in older age groups is more calcified and brittle and, therefore, more susceptible to flail and other serious injuries. In contrast, the thoracic cage in pediatric patients is extremely elastic and resilient and affords much greater protection to underlying structures.

The major concerns with chest wall and sternal injuries are correction of inadequate gas exchange due to flail chest, the provision of adequate analgesia (to decrease splinting), and the diagnosis of possible underlying injury. Indications for institution of mechanical ventilation are severe hypoxemia, severe hypercarbia,

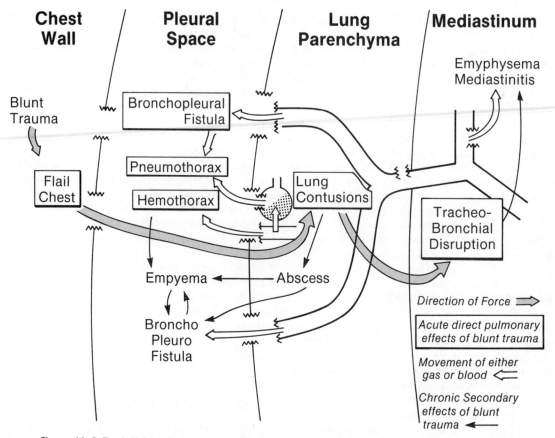

Figure 16–5. *The initial injuries due to chest trauma and the late complications of the initial injuries.*

clinically obvious excessive work of breathing (usually present with major flail and paradoxic chest wall movement), and severe associated injuries (e.g., parenchymal contusion and hemothorax). Associated injuries, especially parenchymal contusions, are likely to be present with sternal fractures and fractures of the upper ribs because these fractures require a large force in order to occur. Some patients can be effectively treated without intubation and mechanical ventilation if they are provided with adequate analgesia (see Anesthetic Considerations, page 396 and Chapter 20); in addition to increasing lung volume (by decreasing splinting), adequate analgesia decreases the respiratory rate, which, in turn, makes the overall flail of the chest much less pronounced.[80]

In summary, the approach to flail chest injuries should be flexible. In a prospective study of 36 patients with this injury[81] only 30 per cent required mechanical ventilation, even though 69 per cent developed pneumonia and about 30 per cent developed the adult respiratory distress syndrome. In the ventilated patients, the mean duration of ventilation was 10.5 days. The overall mortality was approximately 10 per cent. Depending upon the series, the mortality may vary between 6 and 50 per cent.[83, 84]

2. Pleural Space (Hemothorax, Pneumothorax) and Pulmonary Parenchyma (Contusions)

a. HEMOTHORAX[85, 86]

The hemithorax is a potential space that can easily accommodate 30 to 40 per cent of a patient's blood volume (greater than 2000 ml in a 70-kg adult). Consequently, patients with a massive hemothorax have severe hypotension.[87] In addition, as blood progressively accumulates in the pleural space, the underlying lung is compressed. The chest is dull to percussion, the breath sounds are diminished, and a shift in the mediastinum toward the uninvolved hemithorax (displaced apical cardiac impulse and trachea) may compress the uninvolved lung; the compression of the contralateral lung will exacerbate the ventilatory impairment. Thus, these patients also can have severe hypoxemia.[87]

b. PNEUMOTHORAX

Pneumothorax occurs secondary to blunt or penetrating trauma to the chest wall. With penetrating trauma the mechanism of air escape is obvious; the most common cause of penetrating pneumothorax is iatrogenic and is due to subclavian puncture, which has an overall incidence of pneumothorax of 2 per cent.[88] Penetrating knife wounds and gunshot wounds have close to a 100 per cent incidence of pneumothorax. With blunt trauma the mechanism of air escape may be tearing of the lung by the edge of a rib fracture or development of an alveolar bursting force during the trauma. With a pneumothorax ipsilateral breath sounds are decreased, and the chest is tympanic to percussion.

A tension pneumothorax occurs when air enters the pleural cavity during inspiration but, owing to a ball-valve action, cannot escape during exhalation. A tension pneumothorax can cause circulatory embarrassment because of decreased venous return and mediastinal shift and causes respiratory embarrassment via compression of ipsilateral lung by direct tension and contralateral lung by mediastinal shift.

An open pneumothorax communicates with the environment and has been referred to as a "sucking" chest wall defect. The sucking refers to air being drawn into the hemithorax from the environment during a spontaneous inspiration; the physiology of the situation is identical to the paradoxic respiration and mediastinal flap described in chapter 4.

C. PULMONARY CONTUSION

Pulmonary contusions occur either with penetrating lung injury or as the result of rapid deceleration forces (blunt injury), which cause the lung to forcibly impact upon the chest wall.[85, 86] Rib fractures occur in approximately 50 per cent of the cases of pulmonary contusion. Deceleration forces cause rupture of alveoli and vessels with hemorrhage, and increased endothelial and epithelial permeability causes interstitial and intra-alveolar edema. The edema phase develops progressively with time (hours) and with fluid administration and is accompanied by progressive chest x-ray changes and a decrease in P_aO_2. Consequently, the initial chest roentgenogram is often not a good indicator of the severity or extent of the contusion.

3. Tracheobronchial Disruptions

Tracheobronchial disruptions should be suspected in any patient with either penetrating or blunt trauma to the neck or chest, especially if accompanied by subcutaneous or mediastinal emphysema (escape of air into adjacent tissues), hemoptysis (bleeding within the bronchus), or pneumothorax and/or bronchopleural fistulae (escape of air into the pleural space). Although the trachea and major bronchi may be involved at any level (especially with penetrating trauma), greater than 80 per cent of injuries with blunt objects are within 2.5 cm of the carina (see below).[89–92] Penetrating trauma to the neck may cause combined tracheoesophageal injuries.[93]

Tracheobronchial disruptions due to blunt objects require a large force and are, therefore, often associated with trauma to adjacent structures.[94] In fact, in a recent series of tracheobronchial disruptions due to blunt trauma there was an average of 3.8 injuries per patient.[94] The major late complications of tracheobronchial disruption consist of bronchopleural fistula, empyema, and mediastinitis. Proximal tracheobronchial tree injuries, which cause dramatic clinical symptoms, are often recognized and treated earlier and, therefore, have a better outcome than distal injuries, which involve a smaller volume of air, go undetected longer, and have a higher incidence of major late complications.

There are three reasons why tracheobronchial disruptions anatomically localize around the carina.[95] First, anterior chest compression causes rapid lateral movement of the lungs, which creates a shearing force on the carina. Second, an increase in intrathoracic pressure with the glottis closed causes the greatest wall tension (and, therefore, risk of tear) to occur in the airways with the largest diameter (Laplace's relationship $T = P \times R$, in which T = tension, P = transmural pressure difference, and R = radius of curvature). Third, the fixation of the trachea above and below the carina predisposes the more mobile carina to shear forces.

4. Esophageal Disruptions[85, 86, 96]

Esophageal ruptures occur from internal trauma (following medical instrumentation, ingestion of penetrating or corrosive material, and use of esophageal obturator airway); as a result of external trauma (blunt and penetrating); spontaneously (postemetic); and as part of the natural history of a preexisting esophageal lesion (e.g., tumor and caustic burns).

Unrecognized and untreated traumatic esophageal injury has an extremely high late mortality (20 per cent) due to mediastinitis, empyema, and sepsis.[97, 98] In a recent series, all patients operated on within 24 hours of perforation survived, whereas there was a 33 per cent mortality when an operative delay of more than 24 hours occurred.[99] Unfortunately, esophageal injury may go unrecognized for hours to days in a multiply traumatized patient when attention is not focused on the esophagus. The diagnosis should be suspected in patients who have dysphagia, hematemesis, cervical or mediastinal emphysema, chest pain, and fever. If a chest tube has been inserted because of associated injuries, continuous bubbling may reflect an air leak from the esophagus and drainage of particulate matter should raise suspicion of an esophageal tear. The diagnosis can be confirmed with meglumine diatrizoate (Gastrografin) roentgenographically (esophagogram). Esophagoscopy is frequently unnecessary. If the tear is diagnosed early (less than 6 hours), primary repair is accomplished often with good results.

5. Diaphragmatic Disruptions

Diaphragmatic injuries can occur secondary to either penetrating or nonpenetrating (blunt) trauma.[100-102] Penetrating trauma as high as the fourth intercostal space can penetrate the diaphragm and cause intra-abdominal injury. Extreme forces are necessary to cause diaphragmatic rupture with blunt trauma and, therefore, there is a high incidence of associated injuries with blunt diaphragmatic trauma. Ninety-five per cent of diaphragmatic tears following a blunt trauma occur on the left side because of the protection afforded the right side by the liver.

There are several important pathophysiologic consequences of diaphragmatic tears. First, if the disruption is extensive, diaphragmatic movements will be ineffectual and the thoracic cage will behave as a flail chest. Second, abdominal pressure is greater than thoracic pressure and, therefore, there is always the potential for abdominal viscera to work their way into the thorax through the diaphragmatic defects. Small diaphragmatic tears are more likely to capture and strangulate abdominal organs. The organs that most commonly herniate (in decreasing frequency) are stomach, small bowel, spleen,

omentum, liver, and kidney.[103] Third, herniation of abdominal contents into the thorax can cause lung compression, mediastinal shift, and decreased venous return.

B. Surgical Considerations

1. Chest Wall Fractures (Flail Chest)

The treatment varies with the severity of the injury, ranging from simple supportive therapy, such as oxygen enrichment, physical therapy, and pain management, to full ventilatory support. The latter is now considered to be the most effective treatment for patients who develop acute or subacute respiratory failure. Other much less frequently used treatments consist of external stabilization of the flail segment by traction on the injured segment[104] and stabilization of the chest wall by intramedullary pinning of fractured ribs.[105]

2. Pleural Space (Hemothorax, Pneumothorax) and Pulmonary Parenchyma (Contusions)

a. HEMOTHORAX

About 500 ml of blood must accumulate in the chest cavity before it is detectable radiologically. Upright chest films are preferable, if possible. Tube thoracostomy allows immediate confirmation of the diagnosis. Hypovolemia from blood loss is the most common presenting problem in patients with significant hemothorax. Therefore, the immediate treatment should be directed toward restoring blood volume.

Thoracostomy tube insertion (usually in sixth intercostal space in the midaxillary line) alone is the only surgical treatment required in more than 80 per cent of patients with hemothorax.[106] In the majority of cases, the source of bleeding is the pulmonary vessels, which normally have low perfusion pressures. Although chest tube drainage is the first step in the treatment of hemothorax, one must remember that chest tube drainage can occasionally release a major vessel tamponade and cause rapid exsanguination. Patients who have responded adequately to volume replacement, have less than 150 ml/hour thoracostomy tube output after initial drainage, or have reexpanded the injured lung on chest x-ray without reaccumulation of hemothorax do not require emergency thoracotomy. On the other hand, bleeding from systemic vessels is usually much more persistent and voluminous and usually requires thoracotomy (for blood loss greater than 300 ml/hour for 4 hours).

Sometimes residual clot remains in the thorax following tube thoracostomy drainage of a hemothorax. The residual clotted blood remaining in the pleural cavity has the potential for causing empyema or pleural fibrosis with lung entrapment. Consequently, some authors recommended early thoracotomy to evacuate the residual blood and decorticate any early fibrosis process.[73]

b. PNEUMOTHORAX

Pneumothoraces of less than 20 per cent are usually not detectable clinically. Patients with larger pneumothoraces (20 to 40 per cent) usually complain of chest pain, which is accentuated by deep breathing. With even larger pneumothoraces (40 to 60 per cent), cyanosis may be evident and the trachea may be deviated. The presence of rib fractures or tissue emphysema should suggest the diagnosis. Radiologic examination is the best diagnostic aid available, and all films should be taken during expiration.

A simple closed pneumothorax (greater than 10 per cent on chest x-ray) requires only a chest tube; further surgical intervention is not required unless there are underlying injuries. Minor-sized penetrating defects can be sealed with Vaseline gauze, dressing, and tape and with chest tube evacuation of the pleural space. A suspected tension pneumothorax (by clinical signs or chest x-ray) requires immediate decompression; this should first be done by insertion of a needle in the second intercostal space in the midclavicular line. A tension pneumothorax is a dire emergency that may get worse, and valuable time should not be wasted seeking radiologic confirmation. If the diagnosis was correct, rapid improvement will be observed. The needle should be followed by chest tube insertion. Large-sized open defects often require debridement and primary closure.

c. PULMONARY CONTUSION

There are no special surgical considerations for pulmonary contusions (they are not resected). The contusion must be watched for the possible development of infection and abscess formation within the contusion.

3. Tracheobronchial Disruptions

A persistent pneumothorax and air leak after tube thoracostomy and the presence of subcutaneous and mediastinal emphysema is suggestive of a tracheobronchial tree disruption. The few cases that can be treated nonsurgically include small distal tears with minimal air leak, those in a major bronchus that are less than one third of the circumference and have no air leak, and small tracheal wounds with good apposition of the margins. Small to moderate-sized high cervical tracheal wounds may be treated by endotracheal intubation, with the cuff of the endotracheal tube placed below the wound site.[107] Tracheostomy is indicated when there is extensive injury to the cervical trachea and larynx or when endotracheal intubation cannot be performed.

Surgery is indicated for most tracheobronchial disruptions. Surgery should be preceded, if possible, by diagnostic bronchoscopy to identify the site and severity of lesion. The surgical approach is a right thoracotomy for right-sided and tracheal lesions and a left-sided thoracotomy for left-sided lesions. The procedures consist of primary suture repair if technically feasible and, if not, lung resection.[94] The long-term sequela of these injuries is airway stenosis.

4. Esophageal Disruptions

All traumatic (due to external causes), mitotic, and spontaneous esophageal tears must be treated surgically as soon as they are diagnosed; any delay results in a sharp increase in mortality. Surgical procedures consist of primary repair and drainage (adjacent wall tissue normal), pure drainage procedure (adjacent wall tissue injured), esophageal exclusion, and esophagogastrectomies.[99] Tears of the upper and middle thirds are repaired through a right thoracotomy, and tears of the lower third are repaired through a left thoracotomy. Unfortunately, extensive esophageal injuries often leak after repair and result in the late complications of tracheoesophageal fistula, mediastinal abscess, wound infection, and carotid artery blowout.[93]

Patients with a small well-contained perforation due to a medical instrument (internal trauma) can be treated nonoperatively with antibiotics and intravenous alimentation.[99] Nonoperative management is successful in these cases because the perforations are small and frequently patients undergoing medical instrumentation have esophageal disease with peri-esophageal inflammation and fibrosis that limit the spread of the mediastinal contamination.

5. Diaphragmatic Disruptions

Patients with massive herniation of intra-abdominal contents into the thorax with obvious embarrassment of pulmonary function require immediate operative intervention. If the diaphragmatic injury is not life-threatening, repair can be undertaken after diagnostic confirmation by chest radiography and diagnostic pneumo-peritoneum and hemodynamic stabilization. However, undue delay is associated with an increased incidence of organ strangulation and perforation. In fact, patients with a chronic diaphragmatic tear most often have symptoms of intestinal obstruction. The surgical approach may be either abdominal or thoracic, or both, depending on the presence of associated or concomitant injuries.[108, 109]

C. Anesthetic Considerations

1. Chest Wall Fractures (Flail Chest)

Patients with wall injuries that require surgical repair also require general anesthesia, intubation, and mechanical ventilation. Analgesia for continued mechanical ventilation is most effectively provided by continuous lumbar or thoracic epidural narcotics (see chapter 20).

2. Pleural Space (Hemothorax, Pneumothorax) and Pulmonary Parenchyma (Contusions)

a. HEMOTHORAX

Intravascular volume should be replaced through large-bore intravenous lines. Preoperatively, the potential for sudden massive blood loss with chest tube insertion should be remembered. Intraoperatively, the use of an autotransfuser should be strongly considered. Acute respiratory failure may occur prior to surgery and may require intubation and mechanical ventilation. A double-lumen tube should be considered if there is a large concomitant air leak out the chest tube (raising the possibility of a tracheobronchial tree disruption) or if there is hemoptysis or a significant amount of blood in the airway. Other specific anesthetic considerations depend upon associated injuries and the specific site of bleeding (which may not be diagnosed until later; for example, following arteriographic demonstration of an aortic disruption).

b. PNEUMOTHORAX

The only surgical response to a pneumothorax that requires general anesthesia is debridement and primary closure of a large open pneumothorax. Of course, if a pneumothorax is associated with other injuries, general anesthesia will likely be required for the treatment of the other injuries. In all cases involving a potential pneumothorax, the anesthesiologist must consider the possibility of converting a small, untreated, simple, closed pneumothorax to a large tension pneumothorax during the induction of anesthesia and the initiation of intermittent positive-pressure breathing. If chest tubes have been inserted, they must be monitored for continued function (i.e., if they fail to function properly, tension pneumothorax can still occur). The signs of the development of a tension pneumothorax consist of decreased breath sounds, decreased compliance, deteriorating arterial blood gas values, tracheal deviation, and cardiovascular collapse. As soon as a tension pneumothorax is suspected, a large-bore needle should be inserted into the pleural cavity, allowing air to drain freely. Nitrous oxide should be avoided if a pneumothorax is a possibility.[110]

c. PULMONARY CONTUSION

It is important to remember that the edema phase of a pulmonary contusion may coincide with the intraoperative period when fluid is necessarily administered. The edema phase will be accompanied by a progressive decrease in P_aO_2 and compliance and should be treated with PEEP and perhaps fluid restriction and diuretics. The type of fluid infused (colloid versus crystalloid) is not a critical matter since the permeability characteristics of the involved areas are grossly deranged and the area will become edematous regardless of the type of fluid infused.

3. Tracheobronchial Disruptions

Separation of the lungs is often required. Since positive-pressure ventilation may convert a simple mucosal tear to a major bronchopleural fistula or pneumothorax, spontaneous ventilation should be maintained during the induction of anesthesia, endotracheal intubation, and the maintenance of anesthesia if a single-lumen tube is used. Double-lumen tubes should be used for injuries located at or below the carina. Alternatively, small catheters can be passed below injuries near the carina for high-frequency ventilation and high-flow apneic ventilation (see chapter 12). Injuries above the carina are best handled by passing single-lumen or double-lumen tubes past the injury and ventilating one (or both) of the lungs. With high cervical tracheal transections it is advisable to use a fiberoptic bronchoscope as a stent across the transection. It should be remembered that tracheostomy under local anesthesia may be the safest way to establish the airway in severely traumatized patients, and that gentle positive-pressure ventilation will be necessary when the chest is opened. The anesthesiologist should have sterile endotracheal tubes of various sizes available for bronchial placement from within the chest during airway repair.

4. Esophageal Disruptions

Surgical exposure can be greatly facilitated by double-lumen tube insertion and use of one-lung ventilation. Further esophageal instrumentation, such as insertion of esophageal stethoscope and nasogastric tube, is contraindicated. At the end of the case, the surgeon may gently guide a nasogastric tube or esophageal stent past the injured area.

5. Diaphragmatic Disruptions

If the injury is approached by thoracotomy, then surgical exposure can be greatly facilitated by double-lumen tube insertion and use of one-lung ventilation. Dcompression of the stomach may significantly improve the hemodynamic and ventilatory status.

VII. EMERGENCY ROOM THORACOTOMY IN THE MANAGEMENT OF TRAUMA

A. General Considerations

The use of emergency room thoracotomy in the management of trauma has increased greatly in the last decade. Thoracotomy in the emergency room is used when the patient's condition is thought to be so dire that it precludes taking the time necessary to transfer the patient to the operating theater. Emergency room thoracotomy has been performed by surgeons as well as emergency room physicians in a wide variety of clinical conditions. As experience with the procedure accumulates, it has become apparent that the mode of injury (blunt versus penetrating trauma), site and extent of injury, the condition of the patient at the scene of injury (e.g., presence of vital signs, reactivity of pupils), and the rapidity of transport are the most important determinants of the outcome. The procedure is most useful in penetrating lung injuries (the lung hilum can be clamped so as to control lung bleeding and prevent pulmonary venous air embolism), is progressively less useful in penetrating cardiac injuries (pericardial tamponade can be relieved, cardiac bleeding can be controlled with digital pressure and internal defibrillation, and cardiac massage can be performed) and penetrating abdominal wounds (thoracic aorta can be occluded to provide proximal control of massive abdominal arterial bleeding), and is least successful in blunt thoracoabdominal injuries[111] (Table 16–3). If the patient is alive at the scene of injury, the ultimate survival of critically injured patients will be increased by minimizing the use of time-wasting field stabilization measures (e.g., starting many intravenous lines[112] and applying MAST suits[113]) and by transporting the patient

Table 16–3. Results of Immediate Emergency Room Thoracotomy[111]

Type of Injury	Number of Cases (Number of Reports)	Number of Thoracotomies (%)	Mortality (%)
Penetrating	1699 (7)	321 (19)	9
Penetrating cardiac	324 (14)	All	71
Penetrating abdominal	194 (6)	All	95
Blunt thoracoabdominal	252 (7)	All	96

as rapidly as possible to the hospital.[114] Lack of ventricular activity or a palpable pulse and the absence of reactive pupils at the scene of injury carry an almost uniformly fatal prognosis. Patients who are clinically dead at the scene of injury and who remain so throughout transport do not benefit from heroic emergency room thoracotomy.[115]

In penetrating injuries of the thorax, the lung is the most frequently injured organ.[116] The majority of these injuries may be treated with just tube thoracostomy[116] (see Chest Trauma). However, with penetrating thoracic battle injuries, the number of patients requiring thoracotomy is significantly increased.[117] Still, of those who require thoracotomy for penetrating injury, only a small fraction ever require thoracotomy in the emergency room. These patients are the ones who arrive in extremis, and thoracotomy performed in the emergency room may be life-saving[111, 118] (Table 16–3).

The prehospital mortality of penetrating cardiac wounds is high (38 to 83 per cent).[111, 118] Patients with penetrating cardiac injuries who survive the initial injury but show signs of acute decompensation on or just before arrival in the emergency room may also benefit from emergency room thoracotomy. The majority of these survivors have cardiac tamponade (as has been demonstated by previous immediate thoracotomy experience); simple pericardiocentesis is recommended only to transiently improve hemodynamic function, allowing the necessary time for transfer to the operating room. The more aggressive approach of performing thoracotomy in the emergency room has resulted in a significant decrease in the mortality due to this injury[119, 120] (Table 16–3).

Thoracotomy in the emergency room has been used for injured patients with arterial abdominal bleeding. The rationale for this practice is that proximal control of the bleeding by thoracic aortic cross clamping prior to release of the tamponading effects of blood in the intact abdominal cavity would increase survival following abdominal decompression. However, experience with patients with penetrating abdominal injuries subjected to emergency room thoracotomy discloses an extremely low survival rate[111, 118] (see Table 16–3). The difference between the relatively high success rate with lung injuries compared with that of abdominal injuries can probably be explained by two factors. First, emergency thoracotomy and aortic occlusion will not substantially affect the rate or volume of bleeding from major abdominal venous injuries. Such venous injuries include penetrating injuries to the liver, the vena cava, and major portal venous structures. The second factor is that many of these patients with penetrating abdominal injury did not have demonstrable vital signs before the performance of thoracotomy. The thoracotomy was undertaken as a "last-ditch," heroic attempt in the emergency room to save the patient. Thus, the trauma victim who has suffered a cardiac arrest from abdominal hemorrhage has a slim chance of recovery and, in most instances, is not a candidate for emergency room thoracotomy.[111, 118] Only patients in whom there is a strong suspicion of major intra-abdominal arterial injury, and who still have signs of life, are candidates to survive emergency room thoracotomy. The alive, but severely hypovolemic patient with penetrating abdominal injury and massively distended abdomen should go immediately to the operating room, where the surgeon may elect to perform a left anterior thoracotomy with aortic cross clamping in a thorough manner before opening the abdomen.

Patients with blunt injury severe enough to necessitate emergency room thoracotomy also demonstrate uniformly poor results[111, 116, 118] (see Table 16–3). The reasons for these dismal results probably include widespread damage, venous bleeding, and much higher incidence of head trauma.[121]

B. Surgical Considerations

A left anterolateral thoracotomy is most often performed for aortic cross clamping and left hilar clamping. The pericardial sac should be inspected and if the sac is bulging or dark blue, or if there are no signs of underlying cardiac activity, it should be immediately opened. Care should be taken during the opening of the pericardial sac to avoid injury to the coronary arteries. Once the pericardial sac has been opened, clots should be removed, bleeding should be controlled by digital pressure, and, if there is no cardiac activity, internal defibrillation and cardiac massage should be instituted. Finally, a left thoracotomy provides good access for descending thoracic aortic occlusion to provide proximal control of massive abdominal arterial injuries. A right lateral thoracotomy will be performed only for right-sided lesions (i.e., suspected right hilar damage).

C. Anesthetic Considerations

The patient must be intubated immediately and ventilated with 100 per cent oxygen. Multiple large-bore intravenous lines must be inserted, and intravascular volume repletion should be begun immediately. As soon as a peripheral pulse can be palpated, an arterial line should be inserted for pressure measurement and blood sampling. As intravascular volume is being repleted, a central venous catheter should be inserted to measure central venous pressure. Paralysis should be instituted if the patient is moving at all. No, or extremely small doses of, intravenous anesthetics should be administered. A Foley catheter should be inserted as soon as possible. The patient's blood should be typed and cross matched for appropriate number of units of blood. Use of the autotransfuser should be considered.

VIII. REMOVAL OF TRACHEOBRONCHIAL TREE FOREIGN BODIES

A. General Considerations

The majority of foreign bodies are inhaled by children under the age of 3 years.[122] The lack of molars at an early age enhances potential aspiration.[122] In addition, adults who have an acutely (alcoholism) or chronically (dementia) depressed sensorium also are at risk for foreign body inhalation. Acute total upper airway obstruction is the immediate hazard, but far more commonly the foreign body is inhaled deeper into the tracheobronchial tree, where it impacts and initiates a local inflammatory reaction. The subsequent local inflammatory reaction holds the foreign body more securely in place. Without removal, the foreign body ultimately causes distal collapse and infection. Organic material is more dangerous than inorganic material because it swells after inhalation and may fragment, even before attempts are made to remove it. Peanuts are particularly liable to swell and fragment, and they liberate an irritant oil that causes severe local inflammation. Sweets are also a special problem because they dissolve in the tracheobronchial secretions, forming a viscous hypertonic solution that predisposes to obstruction and collapse. In a recent large series of inhaled foreign bodies, 66 per cent were peanuts, 16 per cent vegetable derivatives, and 17 per cent inert objects.[121] The majority of foreign bodies lodge in the right lung because of the disposition of the right mainstem bronchus relative to the trachea, but approximately 20 to 44 per cent can be found on the left side.[122, 123]

B. Surgical Considerations

The history remains the most reliable indicator of aspiration of a foreign body. Paroxysmal cough and wheeze are the common symptoms in children, but dyspnea, stridor, fever, and vomiting also occur. A chest infection that fails to clear in spite of antibiotic treatment in an otherwise healthy child warrants chest radiography and diagnostic bronchoscopy to exclude the presence of an inhaled foreign body. This is particularly true in patients with recurrent one-sided infection and/or persistent unilateral wheezing without prior evidence of underlying allergic diathesis. Unfortunately, a specific history of inhalation is unavailable in approximately 20 per cent of all patients with this problem; these patients consist of some children, adults after alcoholic excess, adults with dementia, and patients under general anesthesia having dental surgery without endotracheal intubation.[123]

In approximately 70 to 80 per cent of the patients, the initial chest roentgenogram will be positive and show the foreign body, distal atelectasis, air trapping (foreign body acts as a one-way ball-valve in a bronchus) or mediastinal shift.[122, 123] In those with initially normal chest radiographs, approximately half will develop positive x-ray findings prior to the removal of the foreign body. Thus, approximately one eighth of patients will come to bronchoscopy on the basis of the history and physical examination alone and have a normal chest roentgenogram. If fluoroscopy is added to routine radiographic techniques, a much higher yield of positive findings on initial radiologic examination is obtained.[123] Positive fluoroscopic findings include a mediastinal shift away from the affected side consistent with air trapping on expiration.[122]

In summary, a history compatible with foreign body aspiration dictates diagnostic and therapeutic endoscopy with or without radiologic confirmation. In order to decrease the approximately one fourth failure rate of plain films in the first 24 hours, fluoroscopy must be strongly considered as an initial diagnostic technique in foreign body evaluation. In many instances, a 24-hour interval, a safety zone, can be observed prior to endoscopy. The safety zone assures adequate gastric emptying and unhurried and thorough preparation for the procedure. During this period of time, postural drainage, chest percussion and vibration, and administration of bronchial dilators (including corticosteroids) may be used; in an occasional patient these measures may result in a spontaneous extrusion of the foreign body. However, these maneuvers should not be regarded as a substitution for endoscopic removal[124] and, on rare occasions, have caused increased airway obstruction and cardiac arrest.[125–127]

If a foreign body is not readily removed at the first endoscopic procedure, chest physical therapy and bronchodilatation should be resumed. Vegetable foreign bodies, including nuts, show a potential for self-extrusion. In an effort to avoid thoracotomy, repeated endoscopy should be used when clinically indicated. However, bronchotomy, or even lobectomy, may be necessary if the foreign body becomes deeply embedded in a mass of inflammatory tissue or erodes through the wall of a bronchus.

As discussed under Laser Resection of Major Airway Obstructing Tumors (chapter 15), a rigid bronchoscope was considered preferable to a fiberoptic bronchoscope because it allowed better control of secretions and blood, permitted better removal of larger pieces of necrotic material, and provided a better view. Similarly, foreign bodies to the tracheobronchial tree should be removed with a rigid bronchoscope because it allows passage of much larger instruments and foreign bodies, and the open-ended rigid instrument also makes ventilation easier in small children.[128]

A large foreign body cannot be removed through a small bronchoscope and must, therefore, be grasped with forceps and extracted while the bronchoscope is withdrawn simultaneously. Repeated instrumentation may be necessary, and even in skilled hands this will traumatize the vocal cords and upper respiratory tract. An alternative solution that has been reported is to pass a Fogarty embolectomy catheter beyond the foreign body; the balloon is inflated and the catheter is withdrawn so that the foreign body is trapped against the tip of the bronchoscope and the entire assembly is removed together.[129]

If thoracotomy for bronchotomy is required, the usual method of localizing the foreign body is by palpating the object through the firm bronchial wall. However, the palpation may not be positive or precise. During thoracotomy a fiberoptic bronchoscope can be a useful guide for the rapid and precise determination of the site of bronchotomy.[128] The fiberoptic bronchoscope finds the object and shines its light upon it.[128] Dimming the lights of the operating room is helpful in order to better visualize the light at the end of the bronchoscope. A small well-placed bronchotomy will predictably result in lower morbidity. This technique should be considered for all patients undergoing open removal of a foreign body or bronchial tumor in whom the precise placement of the bronchotomy is in question.

C. Anesthetic Considerations
(Table 16–4)

If the child has nondistressed respiration and crying does not cause an embarrassment of respiration, the child can be heavily premedicated intramuscularly and brought to the operating room for a smooth inhalation induction. If the child has respiratory distress and/or crying causes wheezing and/or cyanosis, premedication should be withheld. In this type of patient, anesthesia should be induced with intramuscular ketamine in the operating room. Although an intramuscular injection may cause crying, it is only for a short period of time, especially if the child is held and comforted. Since bronchoscopy involves intense airway stimulation, atropine or glycopyrrolate should be included in the intramuscular injection to decrease vagal reactions and secretions. As soon as the child appears sedated, the induction of anesthesia can be continued by inhalation, and intravenous

---

Table 16–4. Important Anesthetic Considerations with Tracheobronchial Tree Foreign Bodies

1. Minimize preanesthetic crying-induced respiratory distress
2. Administer atropine prior to passage of bronchoscope
3. Provide depth of anesthesia to prevent reaction to bronchoscope
4. Administer lidocaine to decrease reaction to bronchoscope
5. Try to maintain spontaneous ventilation
6. Paralyze if excessive reaction to bronchoscope (straining, bucking, laryngospasm, bronchospasm)
7. Beware of mechanical problems when the foreign body is being removed (lodge in trachea, fragment)
8. Consider endotracheal intubation and/or administration of steroids postoperatively if bronchoscope was passed several times

access can be established as quickly as possible. When the patient is adequately anesthetized, the larynx and tracheobronchial tree are sprayed with 4 per cent lidocaine. The eyes are taped shut, and soft pads are placed over the globes. The patient is then positioned for endoscopy. Although succinylcholine is kept available, we prefer spontaneous respiration until at least the nature and location of the foreign body are known; avoidance of relaxants requires the anesthesiologist to achieve adequate levels of anesthesia so that the insertion of the bronchoscope does not cause laryngospasm, bronchospasm, and chest wall rigidity due to energetic active exhalation. Intravenous lidocaine may diminish any coughing or straining reaction to the insertion of the rigid bronchoscope. However, the inability to quickly reverse any of these aforementioned problems at any time during the case may require the use of relaxants (small succinylcholine bolus, succinylcholine drip, atracurium, vecuronium). During the actual bronchoscopy one overhead spotlight is directed onto the anesthesia machine and another is directed onto the patient's feet to assess perfusion and color without interfering with the surgeon's vision.

Following passage of the rigid bronchoscope and during removal of the foreign body, the anesthesiologist should be aware of several important mechanical problems related to the physical characteristics of the foreign body (softness, smoothness, size).[130] First, beans and nuts can fragment and obstruct both mainstem bronchi. If this is thought to be a possibility, removal of the foreign body with the patient in the lateral decubitus position (with the foreign body in a dependent position) should be considered; if this is not practical, a thoracic surgeon and thoracotomy instruments need to be available. Second, plastic and smooth inert objects (beads) may be hard to grasp, and during removal they can slip out of the grasp of the forceps and block larger and more proximal airways. If a large airway does become occluded, the object should be pushed back to its previous location to reestablish ventilation and reassess the situation. Emphasis is necessary on previous location, for inflammation in new areas of the lung may occur quickly following relocation. Third, if vocal cord motion during extraction causes significant obstruction, succinylcholine should be administered. Fourth, the foreign body may sometimes be larger than the bronchoscope, and the bronchoscope and the foreign body may need to be removed at the same time. Fifth, infection may already be well established, and

vigilance in suctioning infected secretions is important; rarely, an abscess may be present distal to the foreign body.

In all of these situations, if the bronchoscope is withdrawn and the foreign body is not seen, the pharynx should be quickly inspected. If the object is not visible, the bronchoscope should be quickly reintroduced to make certain that the object is not occluding the trachea because the narrowing of the airway at the glottis makes this a most probable location. The advantage of spontaneous respiration becomes manifest during this situation, for tracheal obstruction is instantly obvious (tracheal tug, intercostal retractions). If the trachea is occluded, the object is quickly pushed back to its previous location to reestablish ventilation, and the situation is reassessed.

If positive-pressure ventilation is used, it should be possible to maintain adequate gas exchange without excessive inflation pressures, even when a small bronchoscope is in use. However, extreme care must be taken to avoid overinflation of the lungs when either an instrument or the foreign body is blocking the bronchoscope, and ventilation may need to be interrupted from time to time to prevent the foreign body or its fragments from being blown deeper into the respiratory tract when they are loose within the bronchial lumen.

The patient should be supervised closely until fully conscious. Laryngeal stridor is relatively common, particularly after a difficult and prolonged procedure (with many passages of the bronchoscope through the vocal cords) in a small child. Consequently, use of steroids and bronchodilators in the postoperative period is common. In addition, after a traumatic endoscopy nasotracheal intubation is indicated with a tube 0.5 mm smaller than indicated by age; this is left in place until chest x-ray and "air leak" both confirm that swelling is decreased. Chest physiotherapy should be used in patients who have postoperative atelectasis and patients with pneumonia who require antibiotics. The patient is then extubated and may be placed in a croup tent for up to 24 hours, if necessary. Racemic epinephrine may also be useful after extubation.[131] Patients who are extubated in the operating room should breathe humidified oxygen by face mask or croup tent postoperatively.

REFERENCES

1. Garzon AA, Gourin A: Surgical management of massive hemoptysis. Ann Surg 187:267–271, 1978.
2. Yeoh CB, Hubaytar RT, Ford JM, et al: Treatment of

massive hemorrhage in pulmonary tuberculosis. J Thorac Cardiovasc Surg 54:503–510, 1967.

3. Stern RC, Wood RE, Boat TF, et al: Treatment and prognosis of massive hemoptysis in cystic fibrosis. Am Rev Respir Dis 117:825–828, 1978.

4. Ehrenhaft JL, Taber RE: Management of massive hemoptysis not due to pulmonary tuberculosis or neoplasm. J Thorac Cardiovasc Surg 30:275–287, 1955.

5. Crocco JA, Rooney JJ, Fankushen DS, et al: Massive hemoptysis. Arch Intern Med 121:495–498, 1968.

6. Gourin A, Garzon AA: Operative treatment of massive hemoptysis. Ann Thorac Surg 18:52–60, 1974.

7. Conlan AA, Hurwitz SS: Management of massive haemoptysis with the rigid bronchoscope and cold saline lavage. Thorax 35:901–904, 1980.

8. Thoms NW, Wilson RF, Puro HE, et al: Life-threatening hemoptysis in primary lung abscess. Ann Thorac Surg 14:347–358, 1972.

9. Wedel M: Massive hemoptysis. In Moser KM, Spragg RG (eds): Respiratory Emergencies. 2nd Ed. St. Louis, CV Mosby Co, 1982, chapter 11, pp 194–200.

10. Bone RC: Massive hemoptysis. In Sahn SA (ed): Pulmonary Emergencies. New York, Churchill Livingstone, 1982, chapter 8, pp 225–238, 1982.

11. Cervenko FW, Shelley SE, Spence DG, et al: Massive endobronchial hemorrhage during cardiopulmonary bypass: Treatable complication of balloon-tipped catheter damage to the pulmonary artery. Ann Thorac Surg 35:326–328, 1983.

12. Rice PL, Pifarre R, El-Etr A, et al: Management of endobronchial hemorrhage during cardiopulmonary bypass. J Thorac Cardiovasc Surg 81:800–801, 1981.

13. Yang CT, Berger HW: Conservative management of life-threatening hemoptysis. Mt Sinai J Med 45:329–333, 1978.

14. Bobrowitz ID, Ramakrishna S, Shim YS: Comparison of medical v. surgical treatment of major hemoptysis. Arch Intern Med 143:1343–1346, 1983.

15. Smiddy JF, Elliott RC: The evaluation of hemoptysis with fiberoptic bronchoscopy. Chest 64:158–162, 1973.

16. Simmons DH, Wolfe JD: Hemoptysis: Diagnosis and management. West J Med 127:383–390, 1977.

17. Feloney JP, Balchum OJ: Repeated massive hemoptysis: Successful control using multiple balloon-tipped catheters for endobronchial tamponade. Chest 74:683–685, 1978.

18. Gottlieb LS, Hillberg R: Endobronchial tamponade therapy for intractable hemoptysis. Chest 67:482–483, 1975.

19. Hilbert CA: Balloon catheter control of life-threatening hemoptysis. Chest 66:308–309, 1974.

20. Saw EC, Gottlieb LS, Yokoyama T, et al: Flexible fiberoptic bronchoscopy and endobronchial tamponade in the management of massive hemoptysis. Chest 70:589–591, 1976.

21. Fermon C, Oliverio R Jr, Wollman SB, et al: Anesthetic management of cystic fibrosis and massive pulmonary hemorrhage. NY State J Med 81:1223–1224, 1981.

22. Remy J, Arnaud A, Fardou H, et al: Treatment of hemoptysis by embolization of bronchial arteries. Radiology 122:33–37, 1977.

23. Bookstein JJ, Moser KM, Kalafer ME, et al: The role of bronchial arteriography and therapeutic embolization in hemoptysis. Chest 72:658–661, 1977.

24. Prioleau WH, Vujic I, Parker EF, et al: Control of

hemoptysis by bronchial artery embolization. Chest 78:878–879, 1980.

25. Wholey MH, Chamorro HA, Rao G, et al: Bronchial artery embolization for massive hemoptysis. JAMA 236:2501, 1976.

26. Bredin CP, Richardson PR, King TKC, et al: Treatment of massive hemoptysis by combined occlusion of pulmonary and bronchial arteries. Am Rev Respir Dis 117:969, 1977.

27. Trento A, Estner SM, Griffith BP, et al: Massive hemoptysis in patients with cystic fibrosis: Three cases and a protocol for clinical management. Ann Thorac Surg 39:254–256, 1985.

28. Carron H, Hill S: Anesthetic management of lobectomy for massive pulmonary hemorrhage. Anesthesiology 37:658, 1972.

29. Pressler V, McNamara JJ: Aneurysm of the thoracic aorta. J Thorac Cardiovasc Surg 89:50–53, 1985.

30. Sorenson HR, Olsen H: Ruptured and dissecting aneurysms of the aorta: Incidence and prospects of surgery. Acta Chir Scand 128:644, 1964.

31. Debakey ME, Henly WS, Cooley DA, Morris GC Jr, Crawford ES, Beall AC Jr: Surgical management of dissecting aneurysms of the aorta. J Thorac Cardiovasc Surg 49:30, 1965.

32. Daily PO, Trueblood HW, Stinson FB, Wuerflein RD, Shumway NE: Management of acute aortic dissections. Ann Thorac Surg 10:237, 1970.

33. Schmidt CA, Jacobson JG: Thoracic aortic injury. Arch Surg 119:1244–1246, 1984.

34. Greendyke RM: Traumatic rupture of the aorta. JAMA 195:119, 1966.

35. Stiles QR, Cohlmia GS, Smith JH, et al: Management of injuries of the thoracic and abdominal aorta. Am J Surg 150:132–140, 1985.

36. Doroghazi RM, Slater EE: Aortic Dissection. New York, McGraw-Hill Book Co, 1983.

37. Wheat MW Jr, Palmer RF, Bartley TD, Seelman RC: Treatment of dissecting aneurysm of the aorta without surgery. J Thorac Cardiovasc Surg 50:364–373, 1965.

38. Miller DC, Stinson EB, Oyer PE, et al: Operative treatment of aortic dissection. J Thorac Cardiovasc Surg 78:365, 1979.

39. Wolfe WG, Moran JF: The evolution of medical and surgical management of acute aortic dissection. Circulation 56:503–505, 1977.

40. Anagnostopoulos CE, Athanasuleas CL, Garrick TR, et al: Acute Aortic Dissections. Baltimore, University Park Press, 1975.

41. Wheat MW Jr: Treatment of dissecting aneurysms of the aorta. Ann Thorac Surg 12:582, 1971.

42. Appelbaum A, Karp RB, Kirklin JW: Ascending vs. descending aortic dissections. Ann Surg 183:296, 1976.

43. Kidd JN, Reul GJ Jr, Cooley DA, et al: Surgical treatment of aneurysms of the ascending aorta. Circulation 54 (Suppl II–111):118–122, 1976.

44. Woodring JH, Dillon ML: Collective review. Radiographic manifestations of mediastinal hemorrhage from blunt chest trauma. Ann Thorac Surg 37:171–178, 1984.

45. Kirshner R, Seltzer S, D'Orsi C, et al: Upper rib fracture and mediastinal widening: Indications for aortography. Ann Thorac Surg 35:450–454, 1983.

46. Najafi H, Javid H, Hunter J, Serry C, Monson D: Descending aortic aneurysmectomy without adjuncts to avoid ischemia. Ann Thorac Surg 30:326–332, 1980.

47. Debakey ME, McCollum CH, Graham JM: Surgical

treatment of aneurysms of the descending thoracic aorta: Long term results in five hundred patients. J Cardiovasc Surg 19:571, 1978.

48. Kopman EA, Ferguson TB: Intraoperative monitoring of femoral artery pressure during replacement of aneurysm of descending thoracic aorta. Anesth Analg 56:603–605, 1977.

49. Fischbach DP, Fogdall RP: Coagulation: The Essentials. Baltimore, Williams & Wilkins Co, 1981.

50. Dritz RA: Surgery on the aorta and peripheral arteries. In Ream AK, Fogdall RP (eds): Acute Cardiovascular Management: Anesthesia and Intensive Care. Philadelphia, JB Lippincott Co, 1982, chapter 22, pp 728–754.

51. Steiger Z, Wilson RF: Management of bronchopleural fistulas. Surg Gynecol Obstet 158:267–271, 1984.

52. Baldwin JC, Mark JBD: Treatment of bronchopleural fistula after pneumonectomy. J Thorac Cardiovasc Surg 90:813–817, 1985.

53. Gaensler EA: Partial pleurectomy for recurrent spontaneous pneumothorax. Surg Gynecol Obstet 102:293–308, 1956.

54. Raj Behl P, Holden MP: Pleurectomy for recurrent pneumothorax. Chest 84:785, 1983.

55. Riordan JF: Management of spontaneous pneumothorax. Br Med J 189:71, 1984.

56. Brown CR: Postpneumonectomy empyema and bronchopleural fistula—use of prolonged endobronchial intubation: A case report. Anesth Analg 52:439–441, 1973.

57. Downs JB, Chapman RL Jr: Treatment of bronchopleural fistula during continuous positive-pressure ventilation. Chest 69:363–366, 1976.

58. Gallagher TJ, Smith RA, Kirby RR, et al: Intermittent inspiratory chest tube occlusion to limit bronchopleural cutaneous air leaks. Crit Care Med 4:328–332, 1976.

59. Zimmerman JE, Colgan DL, Mills M: Management of bronchopleural fistula complicating therapy with positive end-expiratory pressure (PEEP). Chest 64:526–529, 1973.

60. Tilles RB, Don HF: Complications of high pleural suction in bronchopleural fistulas. Anesth Analg 43:486–487, 1975.

61. Rafferty TD, Palma J, Motoyama EK, et al: Management of a bronchopleural fistula with differential lung ventilation and positive end-expiratory pressure. Respir Care 25:654–657, 1980.

62. Carlon GC, Ray C Jr, Klain M, et al: High frequency positive pressure ventilation in management of a patient with bronchopleural fistula. Anesthesiology 52:160–162, 1980.

63. Benjaminsson E, Klain N: Intraoperative dual-mode independent lung ventilation of a patient with bronchopleural fistula. Anesth Analg 60:118–119, 1981.

64. Derderian SS, Rajagopal KR, Abbrecht PH, et al: High frequency positive pressure jet ventilation in bilateral bronchopleural fistulae. Crit Care Med 10:119–121, 1982.

65. Kirby RR: High-frequency positive-pressure ventilation (HFPPV): What role in ventilatory insufficiency? Anesthesiology 52:109–110, 1980.

66. Powner DJ, Cline CD, Rodman GH: Effect of chest-tube suction on gas flow through a bronchopleural fistula. Crit Care Med 13:99–101, 1985.

67. Baker WL, Faber LP, Osteermiller WE, et al: Management of bronchopleural fistulas. J Thorac Cardiovasc Surg 62:393–401, 1971.

68. Dennison PH, Lester ER: An anaesthetic technique

69. Francis JG, Smith KG: An anaesthetic technique for the repair of bronchopleural fistula. Br J Anaesth 33:655–659, 1961.

70. Parkhouse J: Anaesthetic aspects of bronchial fistula. Br J Anaesth 29:217–227, 1957.

71. Khurana JS, Sharma VN: Bronchopleural fistula management during general anaesthesia. Br J Anaesth 36:302–306, 1964.

72. Pohlson EC, McNamara JJ, Char C, et al: Lung abscess: A changing pattern of disease. Am J Surg 150:97–101, 1985.

73. Coselli JS, Mattox KL, Beall AC Jr: Reevaluation of early evacuation of clotted blood hemothorax. Am J Surg 148:786–790, 1984.

74. Lemmer JH, Botham MJ, Orringer MB: Modern management of adult thoracic empyema. J Thorac Cardiovasc Surg 90:849–855, 1985.

75. Hutter JA, Harari D, Braimbridge MV: The management of empyema thoracis by thoracoscopy and irrigation. Ann Thorac Surg 39:517–520, 1985.

76. Oakes DD, Sherck JP, Brodsky JB, Mark BD: Therapeutic thoracoscopy. J Thorac Cardiovasc Surg 87:269–273, 1984.

77. Yellin A, Yellin EO, Lieberman Y: Percutaneous tube drainage: The treatment of choice for refractory lung abscess. Ann Thorac Surg 39:266–270, 1985.

78. Blades BB, Higgins GA Jr: Pulmonary suppurations: Empyema, bronchiectasis, and lung abscess. In Effler DB (ed): Blade's Surgical Diseases of the Chest. 4th ed. St Louis, CV Mosby Co, 1978, pp 69–71.

79. Mitchell RS: Lung abscess. In Baum GL (ed): Textbook of Pulmonary Diseases. 2nd ed. Boston, Little, Brown & Co, 1974, pp 388–394.

80. Trinkle J, Richardson J, Franz JL, et al: Management of flail chest without mechanical ventilation. Ann Thorac Surg 19:355, 1975.

81. Shackford SR, Smith DE, Zarins CK, et al: The management of flail chest: A comparison of ventilatory and non-ventilatory treatment. Am J Surg 132:759–762, 1976.

82. Shackford SR, Virgilio RW: Selective use of ventilator therapy in flail chest injury. J Thorac Cardiovasc Surg 81:194–201, 1981.

83. Sankaran S, Wilson RF: Factors affecting prognosis in patients with flail chest. J Thorac Cardiovasc Surg 60:402–410, 1970.

84. Thomas AN, Baisdell FW, Lewis FR, et al: Operative stabilization for flail chest after blunt trauma. J Thorac Cardiovasc Surg 75:793–801, 1978.

85. Daughtry DC (ed): Thoracic Trauma. Boston, Little, Brown & Co, 1980.

86. Kish MM, Sloan H (eds): Blunt Chest Trauma: General Principles of Management. Boston, Little, Brown & Co, 1977.

87. Drummond DS, Craig RH: Traumatic hemothorax: Complications and management. Am Surg 33:403–408, 1967.

88. Defalque RJ: Subclavian venipuncture: A review. Anesth Analg 47:677–682, 1968.

89. Payne WS, DeRemee RA: Injuries of trachea and major bronchi. Postgrad Med 49:152–158, 1971.

90. Richards B, Cohn RB: Rupture of the thoracic trachea and major bronchi following closed injury to the chest. Am J Surg 90:253–261, 1955.

91. Shaw RR, Paulson DL, Kee JL: Traumatic tracheal rupture. J Thorac Cardiovasc Surg 42:281–297, 1961.

92. Carter R, Wareham EE, Brewer LA III: Rupture of

the bronchus following closed chest trauma. Am J Surg 104:177–195, 1962.

93. Feliciano DV, Bitondo CG, Mattox KL, et al: Combined tracheoesophageal injuries. Am J Surg 150:710–715, 1985.

94. Jones WS, Mavroudis C, Richardson JD, et al: Management of tracheobronchial tree disruption resulting from blunt trauma. Surgery 95:319–322, 1984.

95. Lloyd JR, Heydinger DK, Klassen DP, et al: Rupture of the main bronchi in closed chest injury. Arch Surg 77:597, 1958.

96. Worman LW, Hurley JD, Pemberton AH, et al: Rupture of the esophagus from external blunt trauma. Arch Surg 85:173–178, 1962.

97. Skinner DB, Little AG, DeMeester TR: Management of esophageal perforation. Am J Surg 139:760–764, 1980.

98. Goldstein LA, Thompson WR: Esophageal perforations: A 15-year experience. Am J Surg 143:495–503, 1982.

99. Ajalat GM, Mulder DG: Esophageal perforations. The need for an individualized approach. Arch Surg 119:1318–1320, 1984.

100. Wise L, Connors J, Hwang YH, Anderson C: Traumatic injuries to the diaphragm. J Trauma 13:946–950, 1973.

101. Brooks JW: Blunt traumatic rupture of the diaphragm. Ann Thorac Surg 26:199–203, 1978.

102. DeLaRocha AG, Creel RJ, Mulligan GWN, Burns CM: Diaphragmatic rupture due to blunt abdominal trauma. Surg Gynecol Obstet 154:175–180, 1982.

103. Sutton JP, Carlisle RB, Stephenson SE: Traumatic diaphragmatic hernia. Ann Thorac Surg 3:136–150, 1967.

104. Jones TB, Richardson EP: Traction on the sternum in the treatment of multiple fractured ribs. Surg Gynecol Obstet 42:283, 1926.

105. Moore BP: Operative stabilization of nonpenetrating chest injuries. J Thorac Cardiovasc Surg 70:619–630, 1975.

106. Symbas PN: Acute traumatic hemothorax. Ann Thorac Surg 26:195–196, 1978.

107. Symbas PN, Hatcher CR, Boehm GA: Acute penetrating tracheal trauma. Ann Thorac Surg 22:473–477, 1976.

108. Brooks JW, Seiler HH: Traumatic hernia of the diaphragm. In Daughtry DC (ed): Thoracic Trauma. Boston, Little, Brown & Co, 1980, pp 175–193.

109. Ebert PA: Physiologic principles in the management of the crushed-chest syndrome. Monogr Surg Sci 4:69–94, 1967.

110. Eger EI II, Saidman LJ: Hazards of nitrous oxide anesthesia in bowel obstruction and pneumothorax. Anesthesiology 26:61–66, 1965.

111. Bodai BI, Smith JP, Ward RE, O'Neill MB, Auborg R: Emergency thoracotomy in the management of trauma. A review. JAMA 249:1891–1896, 1983.

112. Smith JP, Bodai BI, Hill AS, et al: Prehospital stabilization of critically injured patients: A failed concept. J Trauma 25:65–70, 1985.

113. Holcroft JW, Link DP, Lantz BMT, et al: Venous return and the pneumatic antishock garment in hypovolemic baboons. J Trauma 24:928–937, 1984.

114. Bodai BI: Field treatment or immediate transport to the ER—Which saves lives? Hosp Physician, December 1984, pp 7–10.

115. Washington B, Wilson RF, Steiger Z, et al: Emergency thoracotomy: A four-year review. Ann Thorac Surg 40:188–191, 1985.

116. Wiser D, Bodai BI, Smith JP, et al: Emergency department thoracotomy: Indications and technique. Hosp Physician, January 1984, pp 84–70.

117. Zakharia AT: Thoracic battle injuries in the Lebanon war: Review of the early operative approach in 1,992 patients. Ann Thorac Surg 40:209–213, 1985.

118. Shimazu S, Shatney CH: Outcomes of trauma patients with no vital signs on hospital admission. J Trauma 23:213–216, 1983.

119. Evans J, Gray LA: Principles for the management of penetrating cardiac wounds. Ann Surg 189:777, 1979.

120. Ivatury RR, Shah PM, Ito K, et al: Emergency room thoracotomy for the resuscitation of patients with "fatal" penetrating injuries of the heart. Ann Thorac Surg 32:377–385, 1981.

121. Vij D Simoni E, Smith RF, Obeid FN, Horst HM, Tomlanovich MC, Enriquez E: Resuscitative thoracotomy for patients with traumatic injury. Surgery 94:554, 1983.

122. Black RE, Choi KJ, Syme WC, et al: Bronchoscopic removal of aspirated foreign bodies in children. Am J Surg 148:778–781, 1984.

123. Strome M: Tracheobronchial foreign bodies: An updated approach. Ann Otol Rhinol Laryngol 86:649–654, 1977.

124. Burrington JD, Cotton EK: Removal of foreign bodies from the tracheobronchial tree. J Pediatr Surg 7:119–122, 1972.

125. Law D, Kosloske A: Management of tracheobronchial foreign bodies in children: A reevaluation of postural drainage and bronchoscopy. Pediatrics 58:362–367, 1976.

126. Campbell D, Cotton EK, Lilly JR: A dual approach to tracheobronchial foreign bodies in children. Surgery 91:178–182, 1982.

127. Kosloske A: Tracheobronchial foreign bodies in children: Back to the bronchoscope and a balloon. Pediatrics 66:321–323, 1980.

128. Rubenstein RB, Bainbridge CW: Fiberoptic bronchoscopy for intraoperative localization of endobronchial lesions and foreign bodies. Chest 86:935–936, 1984.

129. Saw HS, Ganendran A, Somasundaram K: Fogarty catheter extraction of foreign bodies from tracheobronchial trees of small children. J Thorac Cardiovasc Surg 77:240–242, 1979.

130. Ward CF, Benumof JL: Anesthesia for airway foreign body extraction in children. Anesthesiol Rev, December 1977, pp 13–15.

131. Adair JC, Ring WH, Jordan WS, et al: Ten year experience with IPPB in the treatment of acute laryngotracheobronchitis. Anesth Analg 50:649–652, 1971.

Anesthesia for Pediatric Thoracic Surgery

17

I. INTRODUCTION

This chapter has two major sections. The first section highlights the important physiologic and anatomic problems that premature infants and neonates have that have special relevance to anesthesia for thoracic surgery (as opposed to a broader discussion of all anesthesia problems for all pediatric surgery). These problems consist of persistence of the fetal circulation; the respiratory distress syndrome; retrolental fibroplasia; periodic breathing and apnea; impaired thermoregulation; precarious fluid, electrolyte, and caloric balance; and altered airway anatomy. The second section discusses the major pediatric thoracic surgical cases, which consist of congenital diaphragmatic hernia, tracheoesophageal fistula, vascular rings, congenital lobar emphysema, conditions necessitating

bronchoscopy, and various pulmonary parenchymal problems requiring lung separation. Anesthesia for resection of mediastinal tumors, thymectomy for myasthenia gravis, and removal of foreign bodies are procedures that also frequently involve pediatric patients, but are discussed in chapters 15 and 16.

II. SPECIAL PROBLEMS RELATED TO PREMATURE AND NEWBORN INFANTS

The unique anesthetic problems with the pediatric patient occur primarily in the neonatal period and with the premature infant. These patients may have persistence of the fetal circulation, the respiratory distress syndrome, greatly increased sensitivity to increased arterial

The Fetal Circulation

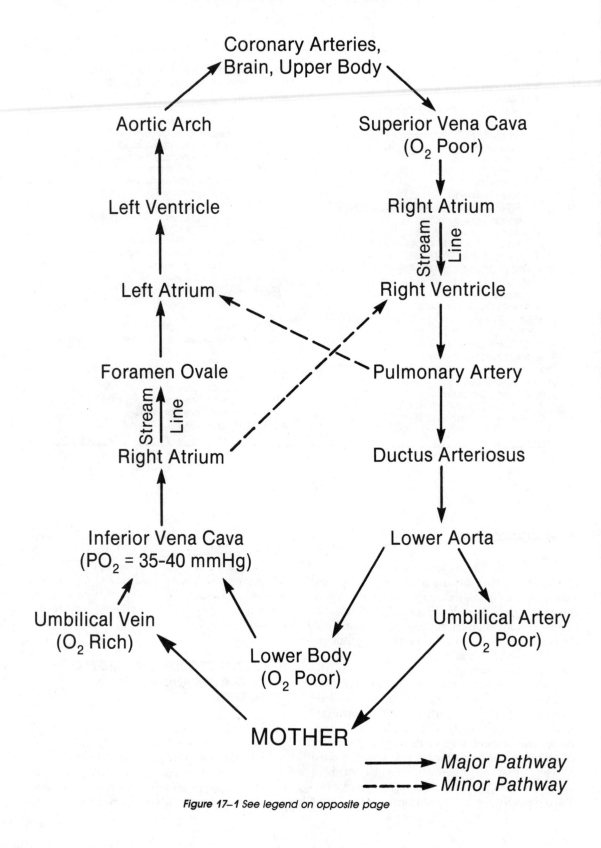

Figure 17–1 See legend on opposite page

oxygen tension, periodic breathing and apneic spells, difficulty in regulating temperature and the internal chemical and caloric status, and an airway anatomy different from that of the adult.

A. Persistence of the Fetal Circulation

In the fetal circulation well-oxygenated blood flows from the umbilical vein through the fetal liver and the ductus venosus to the inferior vena cava. The mixing of well-oxygenated umbilical vein blood with poorly oxygenated inferior vena cava blood results in an inferior vena cava oxygen tension of about 35 to 40 mm Hg (Fig. 17–1). Inferior vena cava blood then flows into the right atrium. Since fetal right atrial pressure is greater than left atrial pressure, the "trap door" flap of the foramen ovale in the atrial septum remains constantly open prior to birth; thus, the foramen ovale directs most of the relatively oxygen-rich inferior vena cava blood across to the left atrium. The relatively well-oxygenated blood that enters the left atrium from the right atrium goes into the left ventricle, is then ejected into the aorta, and perfuses the coronary arteries, the aortic arch, and the brain. Reversal of the right-left atrial pressure gradient following birth allows functional closure of the foramen ovale, even though it may not anatomically close for many years.

Venous blood from the superior vena cava with a relatively low oxygen tension enters the right atrium, mixes minimally with blood from the inferior vena cava, and crosses the tricuspid valve into the right ventricle. Right ventricular ejection of this low-oxygen-tension blood into the pulmonary circulation causes pulmonary vasoconstriction and elevation of pulmonary vascular resistance. The blood in the pulmonary artery subsequently follows the path of least resistance and passes from the pulmonary artery into the aorta via the ductus arteriosus to perfuse the lower portion of the systemic vascular

bed. A small amount of pulmonary circulation blood (10 per cent) mixes with bronchial artery blood to drain directly into the left side of the heart.

Persistence of the fetal circulation means that right-to-left shunting occurs through a patent ductus arteriosus and/or patent foramen ovale. Anything that increases pulmonary vascular resistance (hypoxia, hypercarbia, acidosis, stress, vasoactive drugs) and/or decreases systemic vascular resistance (inhalation anesthetics, vasodilators) will increase shunting through the ductus arteriosus. Hypoxemia, in particular, may also cause ductal dilatation. In addition, anything that increases pulmonary vascular resistance will increase right ventricular and right atrial pressures and increase right-to-left shunting through the patent foramen ovale. The shunting through the ductus arteriosus and foramen ovale results in a vicious cycle of increased hypoxemia, pulmonary vasoconstriction, pulmonary vascular resistance, shunting, and hypoxemia. It should be remembered that the foramen ovale is a potential site of a paradoxic air embolus should air enter the venous circulation, and for this reason it is essential to exclude all air from intravenous fluid administration sets.

The ductus arteriosus enters the aorta just distal to the left subclavian artery; however, there is enough mixing of ductal and left subclavian blood flow to make the left arm arterial oxygen tension significantly less than the preductal arterial oxygen tension. Consequently, preductal arterial oxygen tension must be obtained from the right radial artery and postductal arterial oxygen tension can be obtained from the umbilical artery. Simultaneous analysis of the pre- and postductal arterial oxygen tensions indicates the degree of ductal shunting. When the preductal arterial oxygen tension is at least 15 mm Hg higher than the postductal value, significant ductal shunting is present.[1] Indeed, a right-to-left shunt of 20 per cent is usually considered a "normal" amount of ductal shunt-

Figure 17–1. This schematic diagram shows the main central blood flow pathways in the fetal circulation. Oxygen-rich blood is delivered from the mother to the fetus via the umbilical vein. The oxygen-rich blood in the umbilical vein mixes with the oxygen-poor blood draining the lower fetal body in the inferior vena cava and increases the inferior vena cava oxygen tension up to 35 to 40 mm Hg. This now relatively oxygen-rich inferior vena cava blood flow streamlines through the right atrium into the foramen ovale into the left side of the circulation, where it perfuses the coronary arteries, brain, and upper body. These areas are drained by the superior vena cava, which contains oxygen-poor blood. Superior vena cava blood flow streamlines through the right atrium into the right ventricle, which then ejects the oxygen-poor blood into the pulmonary artery. The oxygen-poor blood causes pulmonary vasoconstriction, which directs the blood flow through the ductus arteriosus to the descending aorta to perfuse the lower body as well as to return to the mother via the umbilical artery. The dashed arrows represent minor blood flow pathways.

ing.[2] When the arterial oxygen tension in the preductal samples is below the value predicted for a 20 per cent shunt (see Fig. 3–30), preductal shunting (through the lungs and/or patent foramen ovale) is present. If the amount of preductal shunting is severe, it becomes impossible to detect ductal shunting.

Successful treatment of pulmonary vasoconstriction and ductal and foramen ovale shunting involves avoidance of the events that can increase pulmonary vascular resistance and/or decrease systemic vascular resistance. Metabolic acidosis is treated with sodium bicarbonate infusions. Endotracheal tube suctioning is minimized to avoid even transient changes in the alveolar and arterial oxygen partial pressure. The most consistently successful therapeutic modality is the alkalosis achieved with hyperventilation (if it can be achieved; V_D/V_T may be so high that the P_aCO_2 cannot be lowered less than 40 to 50 mm Hg).[3, 4] Frequently a threshold effect is observed such that the arterial oxygen tension does not rise until arterial pH reaches 7.55 to 7.60.[4] Generally, ventilatory rates of 60 to 120 breaths/min are necessary to achieve this level of hyperventilation. A number of pharmacologic pulmonary vasodilators have been tried, including morphine, prednisolone, chlorpromazine, tolazoline, bradykinin, and acetylcholine.[1, 5] No agent has consistently improved pulmonary hypertension, although tolazoline has been most frequently employed. If systemic hypotension occurs, volume repletion and/or dopamine infusion is indicated since a reduction in systemic pressure increases ductal shunting. Prostaglandin E_1 (PGE_1), which is a pulmonary and ductal dilator, has been used to decrease pulmonary vascular resistance in patients with persistent fetal circulation (the ductus is thought to be already fully patent in these patients and cannot dilate any more) and to dilate the ductus arteriosus in patients with ductal blood flow–dependent congenital heart defects (e.g., pulmonary atresia).[6]

The role of patent ductus arteriosus ligation in the infant with severe persistent fetal circulation is unclear. The patent ductus arteriosus, although a major source of right-to-left shunting and, therefore, of systemic hypoxemia and acidosis, is also a relief valve for the pressure-overloaded right ventricle. Ligation of the patent ductus arteriosus might cause acute right ventricular failure and, therefore, should not be performed on a routine basis.[5] Ligation of the ductus arteriosus is most commonly performed under local anesthesia, moderate levels of nar-

cosis, and neuromuscular blockade in the neonatal intensive care unit, which eliminates the precarious transportation of these very ill and tiny infants to the operating room.

B. Respiratory Distress Syndrome

The respiratory distress syndrome is a disease of atelectasis in premature infants caused by a failure of the type II alveolar cells to secrete a normal amount of surfactant. Surfactant acts to reduce surface tension in the alveolus, allowing for expansion during inhalation and preventing collapse during exhalation (see Fig. 3–16). When surfactant is absent or reduced in quantity, atelectasis and ventilation-perfusion abnormalities develop. The presence of the respiratory distress syndrome may cause increased pulmonary vascular resistance. Increased pulmonary vascular resistance may cause persistence of the fetal circulation.

The more severe the respiratory distress syndrome, the higher the pulmonary vascular resistance is in relation to the systemic vascular resistance. In severe forms of the respiratory distress syndrome, pulmonary resistance is higher than systemic resistance, and right-to-left shunting occurs through the ductus arteriosus, resulting in a lower arterial oxygen tension below the level of the ductus (Fig. 17–2). As the respiratory distress syndrome improves, pulmonary resistance falls below systemic levels, the shunt is reversed, and congestive heart failure may ensue and warrant closure of the ductus either pharmacologically or surgically.[7–9]

The primary aim of the treatment of the respiratory distress syndrome is to open atelectatic alveoli with positive-pressure ventilation and then to keep the alveoli open using positive end-expiratory pressure. Casual removal of the positive end-expiratory pressure during transport to and in the operating room may result in profound alveolar collapse and the development of marked hypoxia, acidosis, and hypercarbia. Consequently, the management of ventilation during anesthesia of a child with respiratory distress syndrome is critical; it is important to continue to provide the same ventilatory support during the operative period as was provided in the preoperative period. In many instances it may be simplest to bring the infant's own ventilator into the operating room to ventilate the patient during surgery and to use intravenous anesthesic agents and muscle relaxants.

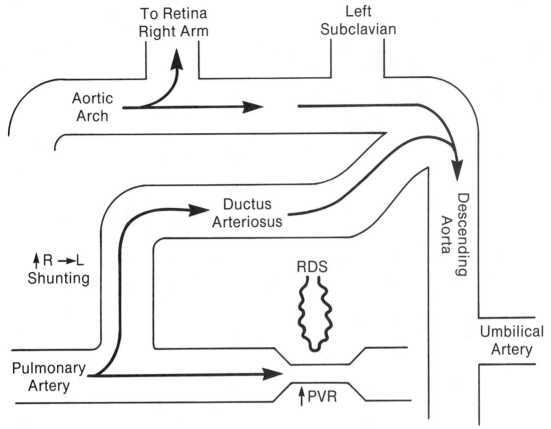

Figure 17–2. *The lack of surfactant in the respiratory distress syndrome (RDS) causes atelectasis and low ventilation-perfusion regions. The atelectatic and low ventilation-prefusion regions cause an increase in pulmonary vascular resistance (PVR), which directs pulmonary artery blood flow through the ductus arteriosus, thereby increasing right-to-left (R → L) shunting. The ductus arteriosus enters the descending thoracic aorta just distal to the left subclavian artery. Blood flow to the retina is preductal, and oxygen tension in preductal blood flow must be measured by a right arm arterial blood sample. Postductal oxygen tension can be measured from an umbilical artery blood sample.*

C. Retinopathy of Prematurity

Retinal damage due to inhaling an increased partial pressure of oxygen is unique to the premature newborn. The premature infant's retinal arteries react to increased partial pressure of oxygen with vasoconstriction, which induces retrolental fibroplasia that causes retinal detachment and destruction.[10] Premature infants are at risk and remain at risk for the retinopathy of prematurity until their retinal vasculature completes its growth at approximately 35 to 40 weeks of age after conception. If gestational age cannot be determined accurately, a birth weight of less than 1500 g seems to be the best indicator of risk for the retinopathy of prematurity.[11] There is no correlation between P_aO_2 levels and blindness risk.[12, 13]

However, in recent years it has become clear that factors other than high inspired oxygen concentration may be involved in the pathogenesis of the retinopathy of prematurity.[12] For example, the retinopathy of prematurity occurs in some babies who have never been treated with supplemental oxygen, the disease does not occur in all premature babies treated with high oxygen concentration, the incidence of prematurity appears to be rising at a time when there has been a pronounced improvement in the technical methods of oxygen delivery and monitoring. It may be that the apparent increase in incidence may be due to increased survival of very small infants [less than 1 kg]. Some other factors may be the absolute birth weight (risk is strongly inversely proportional to birth weight, indicating that this is a disease primarily caused by prematurity, with high inspired oxygen concentrations a secondary factor), maternal diabetes, frequent apneic spells, broncho-pulmonary dysplasia, degree of illness, need for blood transfusions, and sepsis.[14-16]

The anesthesiologist's responsibility is to maintain the arterial and/or transcutaneous oxygen tension between 60 and 80 mm Hg.[17] In patients without a ductus arteriosus the arterial and transcutaneous oxygen tension can be measured anywhere. In patients with a ductus arteriosus, the retinal arteries are supplied by pre–ductus arteriosus blood flow (Fig. 17–2). Consequently, in patients with a ductus arteriosus the arterial oxygen tension must be measured from the right radial artery and the transcutaneous oxygen tension must be measured from the right arm. The arterial and/or transcutaneous oxygen tension can be controlled by using nitrous oxide as a diluting gas or by using an air-oxygen blender to control the inspired oxygen concentration. Careful control of the inspired oxygen concentration and retinal artery oxygen tension is particularly important and difficult during thoracic surgery in which the patient may be either hypoxic or hyperoxic and may vary between these two states quickly, depending on whether or not the operative lung is compressed (retracted) or ventilated.

D. Periodic Breathing and Apnea

Premature infants often have short periods of apnea (10 sec) that are not associated with hypoxemia or bradycardia. Long periods of apnea (30 sec) that are associated with hypoxemia and bradycardia in the premature infant are distinctly abnormal and can be lethal (sudden infant death syndrome [SIDS]).[18] Indeed, irregular and periodic breathing is commonly seen in infants who have survived a "sudden infant death" episode (aborted SIDS), suggesting that immaturity of medullary and/or peripheral control of breathing (loss of responsiveness to hypoxemia and hypercarbia) is an important cause of this syndrome.[19] Theophylline and caffeine have been shown to increase the central chemoreceptor ventilatory response and decrease the number of apneic spells in premature babies.[20] In preparation for extubation after surgery, the breathing pattern of premature infants should be carefully observed for significant periodic breathing, the presence of which is a contraindication for the removal of the endotracheal tube. Immediately following extubation, an oral airway, if tolerated, may be especially helpful, since many infants (60 per cent) may

remain obligate nose breathers for as long as 2 months of age and may not open their mouths to breathe even if the nares are totally obstructed for any reason (e.g., secretions or edema).[21]

E. Thermoregulation

The relative surface area of the newborn is one ninth that of an adult, whereas the weight of a newborn is approximately 20 times less than that of an adult. Thus, the ratio of surface area to weight for infants is approximately two times greater than for adults. Consequently, an infant loses heat much more rapidly than an adult.

Hypothermia in the premature and newborn infant is a dangerous condition; there is a 90 per cent mortality in newborns whose temperatures are allowed to decrease below 32°C.[22] Hypothermia can cause a severe metabolic acidosis and cardiovascular depression. Oxygen consumption has been shown to double in the immediate postoperative period if the child is allowed to emerge from anesthesia in a hypothermic state.[23] Hypothermia below 35°C is a relative contraindication to extubation.

Hypothermia in the newborn and small child undergoing thoracic surgery is particularly likely to occur because there is a large surface area exposed to environmental air, allowing high evaporative and convective heat loss. It is far better to prevent this heat loss rather than to correct it after it occurs. Accepted techniques to maintain body temperature include raising the ambient temperature of the operating room to 30 to 34°C (neutral thermal environment); warming and humidifying anesthetic gases; using only warm scrub and irrigating solutions; using radiant heat lamps, portable heated isolettes, and thermal mattresses; and warming all intravenous fluids (Table 17–1). In most pediatric thoracic surgery cases most or all of these heat loss prevention measures should be used. Core temperature (either nasopharyngeal, esophageal, or rectal) should be measured in every case.

F. Vitamin, Caloric, Electrolyte, and Fluid Requirements

The newborn may be deficient in vitamin K_1 stores upon which the synthesis of coagulation factors II, VI, IX, and XI is dependent. There-

Table 17–1. Techniques to Prevent Heat Loss in Infants and Neonates

1. Use portable heated isolettes
2. Warm operating room to 30 to 40°C
3. Use thermal mattresses
4. Warm intravenous fluids
5. Use radiant heat lamps
6. Warm and humidify anesthetic gases
7. Warm scrub and irrigating solutions
8. Put hat on infant

fore, vitamin K_1 (0.5 to 1.0 mg) should be given intramuscularly or subcutaneously prior to surgery during the newborn period, especially if the child has never been fed. Hypoglycemia is common in the newborn period and is defined as a blood glucose level of less than 40 mg per cent during the first 72 hours of life, and less than 50 mg per cent after 72 hours of otherwise normal neonatal life. In low-birth-weight and premature infants hypoglycemia is defined as a blood glucose level of less than 30 mg per cent. Infants of diabetic mothers (high fetal insulin production) and infants experiencing perinatal distress of any kind can be hypoglycemic. The presence of any condition causing stress or a history of a diabetic mother should make the anesthesiologist aware of the possibility of hypoglycemia and the need to determine blood sugar levels in the perioperative period. Normal glucose requirements for premature and normal newborns are 4 mg/kg/min.

Neonatal hypocalcemia is related to low parathyroid hormone activity and decreased stores of available calcium.[24] A rapid infusion of 10 mg/kg of calcium chloride or 30 mg/kg of calcium gluconate is usually effective in reversing hypocalcemia. Sodium, potassium, and chloride requirements are all similar to those of adults at 1 to 3 mEq/kg/24 hours.

Using a solution of 5 per cent dextrose and 0.2 per cent saline with 20 mEq of KCl added per liter, maintenance fluids can be approximated by administration of 4 ml/kg/hour for the first 10 kg of body weight and an additional 2 ml/kg/hour for the second 10 kg of body weight.[25] If maintenance fluids are all that is required in a specific patient, it is advisable to calculate the preoperative fluid deficit and correct half of the deficit in the first hour, with further administration of fluid at 120 per cent of the baseline maintenance rate until the entire deficit is corrected. Generally, this simple approach is complicated by the trauma of surgery, requiring the intraoperative administration of substantially more fluid.[25] The increased re-

quirement may vary from 2 ml/kg/hour to 10 ml/kg/hour above the maintenance level and should consist of either a lactated Ringer's solution or saline. Blood should be infused if blood loss exceeds 15 per cent of the blood volume or reduces the hematocrit to less than 30.[26]

G. Airway Anatomy

Anatomically, the child, and especially the infant, has an airway that is different enough from that of the adult to make intubation more difficult (Fig. 17–3). The head and occiput are relatively larger than the rest of the body, which requires the neck to be flexed on the chest if the face is in a midline sagittal plane; this is why a newborn lies with the face turned to one side. However, if the child's head is put into a good "sniffing" position (neck flexed on chest and head extended on neck) by extending the head on the neck, the exposure of the larynx will be facilitated. Still, during and after intubation, the large occiput causes the head to be unstable, with a propensity to roll to one side or another; this can be remedied by placing the occiput inside a doughnut-shaped stabilizing sponge pillow.

There are other differences in the anatomy of the newborn airway compared with that of the adult airway. The narrowest portion of the infant's airway is the subglottic area at the level of the cricoid cartilage. Table 17–2 shows guidelines for selection of endotracheal tubes in terms of appropriate internal diameter.

In a normal newborn the neck is short in comparison to the adult. The larynx is more cephalad in the child, lying approximately at the level of C_2-C_3 as compared with C_5 in adults. The larynx-to-carina distance is only 4 cm in the infant, and consequently great care must be taken to pass the endotracheal tube beyond the vocal cords by only 1.5 to 2.0 cm in order to avoid bronchial cannulation. Table 17–3 shows guidelines for the proper depth of insertion of endotracheal tubes as judged from the level of the anterior gumline. The infant's epiglottis projects cephalad at approximately 45° from the anterior wall of the larynx, and it is relatively stiffer and longer than an adult epiglottis. Although this makes the epiglottis easier to visualize, it also makes the epiglottis more difficult to displace so that the laryngeal aperture may be visualized. For these reasons a Miller blade is preferable to a Mackintosh blade for intubation of infants. The tongue, like the

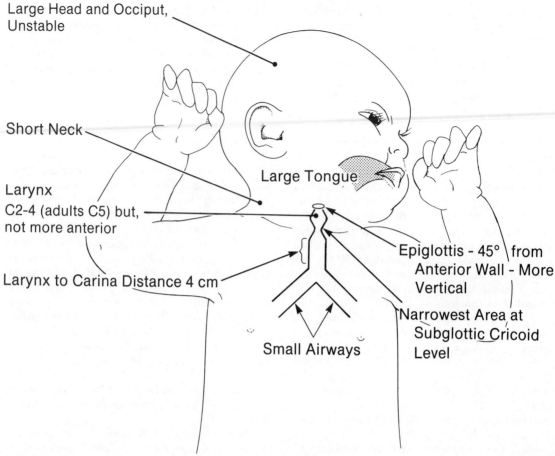

Figure 17–3. The head and airway anatomy of the infant differs from that of an adult in the ways that are listed in the figure.

Table 17–2. Guidelines for Selection of Endotracheal Tube in Terms of Appropriate Internal Diameter (ID)

Age	Internal Diameter (mm)
Premature or small for gestational age	2.5–3.0 mm
Normal term newborn	3.0–3.5 mm
6 months to 2 years	4.0–4.5 mm
Greater than 2 years	$\dfrac{age + 18}{4}$ = mm ID

may make the larynx seem to be more anterior compared with that of the adult, it is not. Finally, all of the air passages (nose, nasopharynx, trachea) are small; consequently, they may be easily obstructed and at this small size any

Table 17–3. Guidelines for Proper Depth of Insertion of Endotracheal Tubes in Pediatric Patients, from the Level of the Anterior Gumline

	Oral	Nasal
Newborn	9.5 cm	Crown-heel length × 0.21 cm
6 months	10.5–11 cm	Crown-heel length × 0.16 + 2.5 cm
Greater than 1 year	$\dfrac{age}{2}$ + 12 cm or $\dfrac{Height\ (in\ cm)}{10}$ + 5	Crown-heel length × 0.16 + 2.5 cm

head, is relatively larger in children than in adults and may cause obstruction during induction of anesthesia and ventilation by mask and may impair visualization of the larynx. Although the triad of more cephalad displacement of the larynx, increased difficulty in displacing the epiglottis, and the presence of a large tongue obstruction can cause a catastrophic increase in resistance to airflow.

III. CONGENITAL DIAPHRAGMATIC HERNIA

A. General Considerations

Abdominal contents can herniate through a defect in the diaphragm into the thoracic cavity (Figs. 17–4 and 17–5). The posterolateral defect of Bochdalek (at the vertebrocostal trigone) accounts for approximately 80 per cent of all diaphragmatic lesions,[27] with left-sided lesions eight times more common than right-sided lesions in newborns but with right-sided hernias twice as common as left-sided hernias after the neonatal period.[28] Fifteen to 20 per cent of diaphragmatic hernias occur through the esophageal hiatus, and 2 per cent of the hernias occur through the anterior foramen of Morgagni on either side of the sternum. The average incidence of congenital diaphragmatic hernia is approximately 1 in 5000.[29, 30] Associated anomalies are often present and include defects of the cardiovascular system (23 per cent), the gastrointestinal tract (malrotation in 40 per cent), the genitourinary system, and the central nervous system.[31] Patients without other congenital defects have a mortality of 25 per cent.[32] Patients with congenital heart disease in addition to congenital diaphragmatic hernia have a mortality in excess of 50 per cent.[23]

The major and always-present result of bowel contents being chronically in the chest during fetal development is chronic ipsilateral lung compression, which results in ipsilateral pulmonary hypoplasia. Shift of the mediastinal structures away from the hernia, causing chronic contralateral lung compression, may produce contralateral pulmonary hypoplasia. Consequently, significant diaphragmatic herniation presents as severe respiratory failure with hypoxemia, hypercarbia, and acidosis. Mediastinal distortion may impede venous return and cardiac output and cause a metabolic component to the acidosis. The increased pulmonary

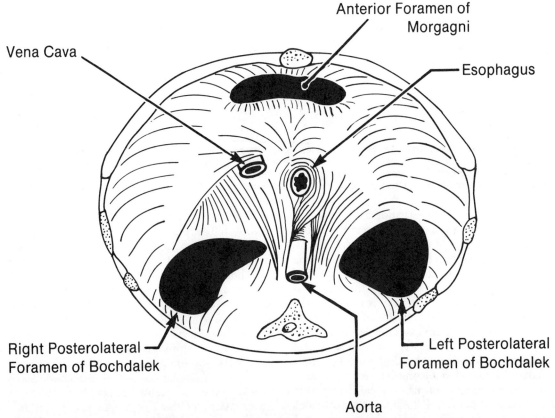

Figure 17–4. View of the diaphragm from a caudad direction showing potential sights of herniation of abdominal contents in congenital diaphragmatic hernia.

Physiologic Effects of Congenital Left Posterolateral Diaphramatic Hernia

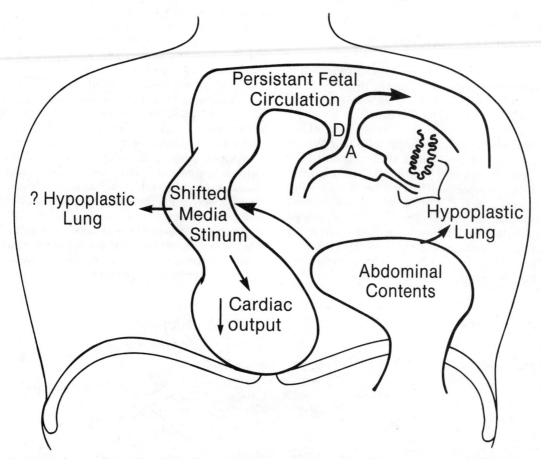

Figure 17–5. *The physiologic effects of congenital left posterolateral diaphragmatic hernia consist of causing the ipsilateral lung to be hypoplastic, shift in the mediastinum to the contralateral side, possibly causing a contralateral hypoplastic lung, persistence of the ductus arteriosus due to the high pulmonary vascular resistance caused by the hypoplastic lung, and possibly causing a decreased cardiac output due to the shifted mediastinum.*

vascular resistance of the hypoplastic lungs, as well as increased pulmonary vascular resistance due to hypoxemia, hypercarbia, and acidosis, may cause persistence of the fetal circulation with right-to-left shunting of desaturated blood at the level of the atrium and/or ductus arteriosus, which, if present, greatly compounds the degree of hypoxemia.[34, 35] Bochdalek hernias produce the most significant degree of respiratory compromise, whereas esophageal hiatus and foramen of Morgagni hernias are generally small in size, do not compromise pulmonary function as much, and may not be detected in the neonatal period. Patients with Bochdalek hernias are often in extremis and require intubation prior to arrival in the operating room.[36]

Eventration of the diaphragm is a congenital failure to develop the muscular part of the diaphragm. The lack of muscle allows the abdominal contents to billow the diaphragm into the thorax to a variable degree. The distinction between a hernia with a sac (which has no muscular elements) and an eventration (which does have a muscular or fibrous element) may not be significant in terms of symptoms produced. For example, cases of slight eventration may be asymptomatic, but severe cases occur in a fashion similar to that of left-sided Bochdalek congenital diaphragmatic hernias. Most eventrations of the diaphragm should be surgically corrected (diaphragmatic tightening procedure), whether they are symptomatic or not, because even slight chronic compression of the lung may cause infection.

B. Surgical Considerations

The diagnosis of congenital diaphragmatic hernia is usually straightforward. Approximately 30 per cent of the cases are associated with polyhydramnios.[37] Cyanosis is usually apparent soon after the umbilical cord is clamped. Signs of respiratory distress are common and severe and include tachypnea, nasal flaring, and both sternal and intercostal space inspiratory retraction. Frequently these infants require endotracheal intubation immediately or soon after birth. The abdominal contour is abnormally scaphoid, whereas the thorax may be barrel shaped. With a left posterolateral diaphragmatic hernia, the mediastinum may be shifted into the right hemithorax, both right and left breath sounds are poor, and cardiac sounds will best be heard in the right chest. Audible bowel sounds in the chest may or may not be present (there is no gas in the bowel at birth; gas formation takes several hours). A body radiograph usually confirms the diagnosis, showing intestinal loops in the hemithorax. The lung on the side of the hernia is compressed into the hilum, and the mediastinal contents are pushed to the opposite side. If a nasogastric tube had already been inserted, the chest radiograph might also show a decompressed stomach within the thoracic cavity.

The surgical tasks are to return the abdominal contents to the abdominal cavity, correct bowel malrotation, repair the diaphragmatic defect, and close the abdomen. Closure of the abdomen may prove to be difficult because the unstretched abdominal cavity is too small. In this situation, the surgeon may need to utilize a prosthetic material such as Gore-Tex to avoid excessive intra-abdominal pressure.[38] If the abdomen is closed under tension, the chance of recurrence is increased and the infant will likely require mechanical ventilation for several days until enlargement of the abdominal cavity allows the diaphragm to have its normal downward excursion. Most surgeons now use a transabdominal approach for repair of Bochdalek hernias, since this incision facilitates return of the bowel to the peritoneal cavity, correction of intestinal malrotation, repair of the diaphragm under direct vision, and stretching of the abdominal wall to accommodate the intestines if necessary.[39] A thoracic approach is often used for the operative repair of Morgagni hernias.

C. Anesthetic Considerations

Many of these infants have major cardiopulmonary problems (hypoplastic lungs, shifted mediastinum, possible persistent fetal circulation, respiratory distress syndrome, other congenital defects) and will not tolerate the induction of general anesthesia without a guaranteed airway. In addition, positive-pressure ventilation with a bag-and-mask system may inflate the stomach and further compromise pulmonary function. Consequently, critically ill neonates with congenital diaphragmatic hernia should be intubated when awake (Table 17–4).[27, 40–43] Those few infants who are too vigorous for this approach usually can be intubated without a relaxant after breathing halothane and oxygen spontaneously for a few minutes.

Table 17–4. Most Important Specific Anesthetic Considerations for Each of the Major Pediatric Thoracic Surgery Cases

I. Congenital posterolateral diaphragmatic hernia
  A. Awake intubation
  B. Avoid nitrous oxide
  C. Use small tidal volumes and rapid respiratory rates
  D. Do not attempt to inflate ipsilateral hypoplastic lung
  E. High index of suspicion for need for contralateral chest tube
  F. Patient may have high extracellular fluid requirements
  G. Postoperative mechanical ventilation
II. Esophageal atresia with tracheoesophageal fistula
  A. May need tip of endotracheal tube just above carina
  B. Maintain spontaneous ventilation, if possible
  C. Gentle positive pressure ventilation, if necessary
  D. Do not use esophageal stethoscope—use left axillary stethoscope
  E. Do not pass nasogastric tube—may need to measure length of proximal pouch
  F. Postoperative mechanical ventilation
III. Vascular rings
  A. May need right mainstem bronchial intubation
  B. May need to palpate upper extremity and head and neck pulses for surgeon
IV. Congenital lobar emphysema and cysts
  A. Nitrous oxide contraindicated
  B. Positive-pressure ventilation contraindicated until chest is open
  C. May need to separate the lungs
V. Unilateral infections (abscess, empyema)
  A. Separate the lungs (bronchial blocker, contralateral mainstem bronchus intubation)
VI. Bronchography
  A. May need to pass small contrast material catheter into one lung with the aid of a rigid or flexible bronchoscope or fluoroscopy
  B. Discuss with radiologist preferred pattern of ventilation
  C. May need to turn patient to various positions

Following intubation, moribund patients are given minimal intravenous anesthetics, initially 100 per cent oxygen, and a nondepolarizing muscle relaxant is added if the patient moves in response to the surgical stimulus. Peripheral perfusion should be supported with intravenous fluid and dopamine administration as necessary.[39] Halothane or narcotic, in addition to relaxant, is given to those infants who demonstrate cardiovascular stability; the amount given depends on the clinical status of the patient. Nitrous oxide should be avoided since it may distend the gut, further compromising lung function prior to hernia reduction and subsequent abdominal closure.[44]

In premature infants at risk of retrolental fibroplasia, air or nitrogen is added to lower the arterial oxygen tension to approximately 80 mm Hg.[17] To achieve this arterial oxygen tension end-point, it is highly desirable to have an arterial line. It should be remembered that the right radial artery must be used to estimate pre–ductus arteriosus (retinal artery) oxygen tension. An umbilical artery catheter measures post–ductus arteriosus oxygen tension.

Positive-pressure ventilation is administered by hand with small tidal volumes and rapid rates (60 to 120 breaths/min) in an attempt to keep the monitored inflating airway pressures under 20 to 30 cm H_2O.[27, 41, 42, 45] Hyperventilation (preductal P_aCO_2 = 25 to 30 mm Hg and postductal P_aCO_2 = 30 to 35 mm Hg) is recommended to lower pulmonary vascular resistance and minimize right-to-left shunting through the ductus arteriosus.[3] Attempts to inflate the hypoplastic ipsilateral lung should be avoided since the pressure required to even minimally expand the hypoplastic lung is higher than the pressure required to rupture the normal lung.[46] Consequently, it is not surprising to find that pneumothorax occurs more frequently on the side opposite the hernia.[41] Any sudden severe deterioration in heart rate, blood pressure, arterial oxygen tension, or lung compliance is strongly suggestive of such an event; time should not be wasted with radiographic confirmation of a pneumothorax, and a chest tube should be placed immediately.[47, 48] Indeed, some authors recommend inserting a contralateral chest tube prophylactically prior to surgery.[46, 49]

There are several other important anesthetic concerns. Metabolic acidosis should be treated with infusions of sodium bicarbonate (mEq

HCO_3^- = body weight [kg] × base deficit × 0.25). A nasogastric tube should always be passed to decompress the stomach. Normothermia must be maintained and hyperoxemia avoided (see Special Problems Related to Premature and Newborn Infants). Since a large extracellular fluid third space may develop owing to the trauma of handling the bowel, the volume status of these very sick infants may be borderline and hypovolemia may need to be treated vigorously with colloid and/or blood infusion. Frequently, total fluids administered may equal 25 to 50 ml/kg during the case.

The postoperative period is stormy much more often than not in these patients because of an abdomen that is under tension, the presence of pulmonary hypoplasia, the presence of associated congenital defects, and the persistence of the fetal circulation; artificial ventilation is typically required for at least several days. Consequently, intraoperative narcotics and relaxants are not reversed. Attempts should be made to keep the preductal arterial oxygen tension between 60 and 80 mm Hg and the arterial carbon dioxide tension between 35 and 40 mm Hg, if possible. Careful attention should be given to volume status, as well as the nutritional state of the patient. A gastrostomy is often placed at the time of surgery so that feeding may take place during recovery. The hypoplastic ipsilateral lung should not be expected to fill the hemithorax. The mediastinum usually returns to the midline slowly.[39]

Patients with persistent fetal circulation are often difficult to wean from ventilators. Pulmonary vasoconstriction, with resultant right-to-left shunting, can be triggered by minimal changes in inspired oxygen concentration, decreases in arterial oxygen tension, increases in acidosis, or sudden changes in pulmonary blood volume. Successful treatment of pulmonary vasoconstriction involves avoidance of these events. Although a number of pharmacologic pulmonary vasodilators have been tried, no drug has consistently improved pulmonary hypertension (see Persistence of the Fetal Circulation).[1, 4, 50] Other major considerations in the postoperative period consist of ligation of a patent ductus arteriosus, poor or absent function of the ipsilateral diaphragm, recurrence of the hernia (10 to 22 per cent, most of which require reoperation),[51, 52] risk of pneumothorax (7 to 20 per cent),[53, 54] and provision of adequate nutrition.

IV. ESOPHAGEAL ATRESIA AND TRACHEOESOPHAGEAL FISTULA

A. General Considerations

There are many different types and permutations of esophageal atresia and tracheoesophageal fistula, and these lesions are perhaps best described by their particular individual anatomies and without reference to use of letters and/or numbers. Esophageal atresia with distal (to the esophageal atresia) tracheoesophageal fistula is by far the most common of these, occurring in 80 to 90 per cent of cases[55-60] (Fig.

17–6). The distal fistula between the trachea and esophagus is usually located one or two tracheal rings above the carina on the posterior aspect of the trachea. Seven to nine per cent have esophageal atresia without tracheoesophageal fistula (Fig. 17–6). The remaining types (as many as 95)[61] are rare. The incidence of esophageal atresia and tracheoesophageal fistula is approximately 1 in 3000 births.[62]

The two most important determinants of survival in patients with tracheoesophageal fistula are prematurity and associated congenital anomalies. In the absence of prematurity and severe associated congenital anomalies survival currently approaches 100 per cent.[56, 63, 64] Pre-

A   **B**

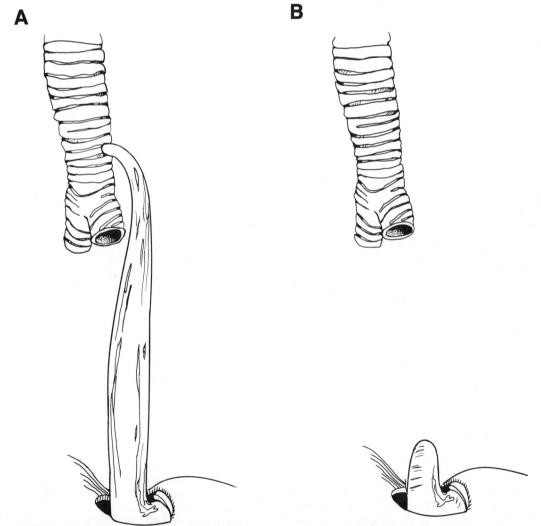

Figure 17–6. *The most common cases of esophageal atresia and tracheoesophageal fistula consist of (A) esophageal atresia with distal tracheoesophageal fistula (80 to 90 per cent), and (B) esophageal atresia without fistula (7 to 9 per cent).*

maturity with pulmonary hypoplasia and pneumonia, which accounts for at least 25 per cent of the tracheoesophageal fistula population,[64–69] is associated with a 15 to 90 per cent mortality.[64, 68–71] The incidence of associated congenital anomalies in tracheoesophageal fistula cases is 30 to 50 per cent, and in these patients the mortality approaches 50 per cent.[55, 58, 72, 73]

The cardiovascular anomalies are most troublesome and, in order of decreasing incidence of occurrence, are ventricular septal defect, patent ductus arteriosus, tetralogy of Fallot, atrial septal defect, and coarctation of aorta.[58, 72] The associated gastrointestinal anomalies are next most important with reference to mortality and consist of imperforate anus, midgut malrotation, duodenal atresia, pyloric stenosis, Meckel's diverticulum, and ectopic or annular pancreas.[74] Other defects involve the vertebrae and renal systems and together with the above anomalies constitute the VATER association[61–63] (V = vertebral and ventricular septal defect; A = anal defect; T = tracheoesophageal fistulae; E = esophageal atresia; and R = renal dysplasia).

B. Surgical Considerations

Atresia of the esophagus may be suspected prior to delivery if polyhydramnios is present.[75] If polyhydramnios is present, the diagnosis can be made shortly after delivery by failing to pass a radiopaque nasogastric tube into the infant's stomach. If the diagnosis is not suspected or made after delivery, the presence of excessive foamy oral secretions in the first few postnatal hours may suggest the diagnosis.[64] However, in most cases the diagnosis is usually delayed until coughing, choking, and regurgitation occur during the first or subsequent feedings. Following the first (or later) feeding, the respiratory rate increases and respirations become labored (presumably due to pulmonary aspiration). The urgency in making the diagnosis is to prevent further pulmonary aspiration. In addition, with a tracheoesophageal fistula, the abdomen usually becomes distended and tympanic and occasionally the distension can interfere with breathing.

The diagnosis is confirmed by trying to pass a radiopaque nasogastric catheter into the stomach. If the catheter stops abruptly in the proximal esophageal segment (at a distance of approximately 10 to 12 cm from the nares) the diagnosis is virtually assured.[72] Posterior and lateral chest radiographs are taken to determine the position of the nasoesophageal tube tip. The radiograph should include the entire abdomen so that presence or absence of air in the stomach and intestines can be determined. When the upper esophagus is atretic (tube tip will not pass into the stomach), air in the stomach is pathognomonic of a fistula between the trachea or esophagus. Absence of air in the gastrointestinal tract usually indicates the presence of esophageal atresia without tracheoesophageal fistula.

Tracheoesophageal fistula without atresia (H-type fistula) may not cause significant symptoms until adolescence or adulthood.[76] The diagnosis should be suspected with a history of recurrent pneumonia.[77] The diagnosis requires bronchoscopy or bronchography, and occasionally it is not possible to demonstrate the lesion prior to surgery. A diagnostic aid is the demonstration of elevated intragastric oxygen concentration during ventilation with 100 per cent oxygen.[78] The diagnosis should be considered in any patient who develops gastric distension while intubated and receiving positive-pressure ventilation.[76]

In infants, gastrostomy is almost always the first procedure to be done. In infants with extreme immaturity or severe lung disease, thoracotomy may be postponed until improvement in respiratory function has occurred and there has been a gain in weight to over 1800 g.[56, 64, 79] With the availability of hyperalimentation both of these goals are obtainable. Of course, such a delay is only feasible if the infant's course is not complicated by repeated aspiration of gastric contents.[56, 80] For definitive repair, a right thoracotomy is utilized and the dissection will be extrapleural. Important surgical tasks include ligation of the fistula between the trachea and esophagus and esophageal anastomosis. If the esophageal segments cannot be mobilized sufficiently to perform the anastomosis without tension on the suture line, the upper pouch will be preserved until further attempts at anastomosis are repeated during a subsequent thoracotomy.

Depending on the anatomy involved, gastrostomy is carried out in the operating room under either general (unusual) or local (usual) anesthesia (1 per cent lidocaine 2 to 4 mg/kg). The infant should be maintained in a head-up position to minimize the possibility of aspiration, and atropine (0.01 mg/kg) is administered intravenously upon arrival in the operating room. Esophageal stethoscopes and temperature probes are avoided for obvious reasons during gastrostomy, as well as during subsequent procedures. Appropriate oxygen is given as necessary, and careful attention is paid to maintenance of body temperature and proper fluid, electrolyte, and glucose administration.

C. Anesthetic Considerations

Premature infants with severe lung disease may require endotracheal intubation and mechanical ventilation prior to gastrostomy. Recently, two reports describe the development of massive life-threatening air leak out the gastrostomy tube as soon as the gastrostomy tube was put in.[81, 82] In one case the leak was successfully dealt with by putting the gastrostomy tube under a 25 cm H_2O seal,[81] and in the other case it was successfully dealt with by inflating a Fogarty embolectomy catheter balloon in the distal esophagus (placed via the gastrostomy tube with the aid of fluoroscopy).[82]

Definitive repair follows the gastrostomy. The infant should have already been premedicated with atropine (0.01 mg/kg intravenously) at the time of gastrostomy. After suctioning the esosphageal pouch and gastrostomy, venting the gastrostomy to the atmosphere, and providing preoxygenation, tracheal intubation is usually done with the infant awake (some anomalies permit general anesthesia with positive-pressure ventilation). The appropriate-sized endotracheal tube (usually 3.0 mm) is passed beyond the vocal cords while breath sounds are monitored on both sides of the chest.

In patients in whom intermittent positive-pressure ventilation may likely become necessary before ligation of the fistula (those with known large fistulae, pulmonary infiltrates and poor compliance, or other congenital anomalies), and assuming the fistula is above the carina, it may be important to take the trouble to position the endotracheal tube just above the carina (but below the fistula) to avoid either a large air leak out the gastrostomy or gaseous distension of the stomach. The endotracheal tube is advanced gently into the right mainstem bronchus (breath sounds heard only over right lung) and then withdrawn slowly to a position just above the carina (withdrawal is terminated the moment breath sounds are heard equally on both sides).[83] Although intubation of the fistula itself is a rare event, rotating the tube so that the bevel faces posteriorly may diminish this possibility even further (the fistula is on the posterior aspect of the trachea). Intubation of the fistula itself is recognized when the endotracheal tube is within the trachea and positive-pressure ventilation of the lungs is impossible, while, at the same time, the stomach becomes distended or the gastrostomy tube leaks air. Some leakage of air through the tracheoesophageal fistula may occur even with the endotracheal tube tip below the level of the fistula, and the amount of leakage may be large if the tracheoesophageal fistula is large. Tube position must be reconfirmed after positioning the child in the left lateral decubitus position; the best way to continuously monitor breath sounds during the case is with a precordial stethoscope in the left axilla. It should be realized that, with the endotracheal tube so close to the carina, intraoperative manipulation of the mediastinum may easily cause the endotracheal tube to become malpositioned.

Anesthesia is induced with nitrous oxide, oxygen, and small amounts of halothane with spontaneous ventilation. If halothane is not tolerated, a nitrous oxide, narcotic, or ketamine technique can be used. If possible, the infant should be allowed to breathe spontaneously until the fistula is ligated (Table 17–4). This may be important in some patients (e.g., those who do not have a gastrostomy tube) as severe gastric distension can impede ventilation (compress the lung) and circulation (decrease venous return), leading to cardiopulmonary arrest[70] and gastric rupture.[84] However, it should be realized that in most patients with a gastrostomy that is vented to atmospheric pressure the danger of gastric distension is minimized and it is usually possible to assist ventilation with gentle positive pressure. Similarly, positive-pressure ventilation should be cautiously attempted before administering muscle relaxants. If gastric distension occurs with positive-pressure ventilation, the function of the gastrostomy tube should be checked, nitrous oxide should be discontinued, and perhaps spontaneous breathing can be resumed.

During the procedure, air entry into the dependent lung should be monitored continuously by a stethoscope secured in the dependent axilla. Since secretions and obstruction of the endotracheal tube can be a problem at any time, suction apparatus and catheters should be readily available for suctioning. Airway obstruction may also result from surgical manipulation of the trachea; the surgeon must be informed when this occurs. Occasionally the small endotracheal tube can become occluded by thick secretions, which requires prompt passage of a suction catheter and, if that fails to clear the tube, a marked stylet.

The integrity of the fistula repair can be assured by the surgeon placing a small amount of saline into the wound and the anesthesiologist applying 20 cm H_2O constant positive-pressure ventilation to the airway and looking for any leak in the tracheal-suture line. If, after ligation of the fistula, primary repair of the esophageal atresia is undertaken with anastomosis of the proximal and distal segments, the surgeon may ask the anesthesiologist to pass a small suction catheter into the proximal segment until it can be felt near the end of the atretic esophageal pouch. When the catheter is palpable near the end of the pouch, and with the infant's head in a neutral or slightly flexed position, the anesthesiologist can mark on the catheter with a suture or umbilical tape the level of the infant's upper alveolar ridge. The catheter is then withdrawn and carefully measured to determine the maximum safe distance that catheters should be inserted for postoperative oropharyngeal suctioning without causing disruption of the esophageal anastomosis. Extension of the neck after repair is avoided for the same reason.

Most infants undergoing repairs for esophageal atresia and tracheoesophageal fistula are left intubated for several hours to several days after surgery. Weaning from the ventilator begins as soon as possible after blood gas values and radiologic findings indicate improvement in atelectasis or pneumonia. Feedings are usually started via gastrostomy on the third postoperative day. Unless the esophageal anastomosis is tenuous, oral glucose feedings are begun on the sixth to seventh postoperative day after an esophagogram is performed to document patency of the esophageal lumen.[53]

V. LIGATION OF PATENT DUCTUS ARTERIOSUS IN PREMATURE INFANTS

A. General Considerations

The vasoconstrictor response of the ductus arteriosus to an increase in the partial pressure of oxygen in the early neonatal period is proportional to gestational age; the lower the gestational age the greater is the likelihood of the ductus remaining open, and the greater the gestational age the greater is the likelihood of ductal closure. Forty per cent of infants weighing less than 1750 g at birth will have clinical

evidence of patency of the ductus; whereas, in those weighing less than 1200 g, the incidence rises to 80 per cent.[85] Initial therapy of patent ductus arteriosus is medical and consists of fluid restriction and administration of diuretics and, perhaps, digoxin in an attempt to decrease the effects of volume overload on the cardiovascular system.[86] If this usual medical therapy fails to close the ductus, then indomethacin, a prostaglandin synthetase inhibitor, should be administered in an attempt to produce pharmacologic closure of the ductus.[86] Surgical closure is indicated if the patient still has significant shunting (see Surgical Considerations below) after the usual medical and indomethacin therapies have been tried. However, routine surgical closure of patent ductus arteriosus in premature infants was recently found to be superior to chemical closure with indomethacin; there was a 15 per cent overall morbidity and a 17 per cent mortality for operative closure compared with a 51 per cent morbidity and a 40 per cent mortality for chemical closure.[87]

B. Surgical Considerations

There are two main well-established indications for ligation of a patent ductus arteriosus in the premature infant (as the only surgical procedure). First, ligation is indicated to decrease severe right-to-left shunting in premature infants with persistent fetal circulation. Second, ligation is indicated to decrease severe left-to-right shunting in patients with improving respiratory distress syndrome. These cases are usually done in the neonatal intensive care unit to avoid the perils of transporting these critically ill, tiny infants to the operating room. A left or anterior thoracotomy is utilized.[88]

C. Anesthetic Considerations

The vast majority of these patients will already be intubated and mechanically ventilated, and some will have already been treated with nondepolarizing muscle relaxants. These infants will almost always have monitoring and intravenous catheters in place. Anesthetic management is usually a continuance of preoperative supportive measures; these consist of avoidance of hypoxemia and hyperoxemia and maintenance of normothermia, fluid and electrolyte and caloric balance, and adequate gas exchange.

If the patients are not paralyzed, they should be. Anesthesia may be local, or local plus a moderate dose of narcotic, and if the operation is performed in the operating room, local anesthesia plus low concentration of inhalation agent/air/oxygen may be used. Although blood loss is usually minimal, it should be remembered that the ductus is friable and mobilization of the structure in order to ligate it may result in tearing and sudden massive blood loss; the anesthesiologist must be in a position to deal with massive blood loss (must have adequate vascular access).

VI. VASCULAR RINGS

A. General Considerations

A double aortic arch, a right aortic arch along with a left-sided ligamentum arteriosum, a left pulmonary artery sling, and an anomalous origin of the innominate artery (the "innominate artery compression syndrome") are vascular abnormalities that can cause a significant tracheobronchial tree obstruction (usually near the carina) and esophageal obstruction that requires surgery for relief. The first two anomalies are true "vascular rings," in that they form a continuous circle around the trachea and esophagus and compress them.

B. Surgical Considerations

Vascular rings usually cause symptoms in early childhood. The symptoms are referable to compression of the tracheobronchial tree or esophagus, or both. Chest computed tomography usually demonstrates these obstructions well. In addition, the diagnosis can also be established by a chest radiograph with barium swallow, the barium-filled esophagus being indented posteriorly by the vascular structure. Bronchoscopy with or without bronchography will clearly demonstrate the flattened and obstructed trachea just above the carina.

Operation is usually performed through a left thoracotomy. The tracheal compression caused by the vascular ring can be relieved by division of the ring at the appropriate point, care being required to preserve the vessels needed for circulation to the head and lower body. Palpation of appropriate pulses will aid this vascular preservation. Correction of the innominate artery syndrome requires only that the innominate artery be pulled forward away from the trachea that it is compressing. The artery is usually sutured to the posterior periostium of

the sternum to hold it away from the trachea. The results of operation are excellent in most cases.

The pulmonary arterial sling may require the use of cardiopulmonary bypass for correction. In this anomaly, the left pulmonary artery passes to the right of the trachea before crossing back posteriorly to the left lung. This "sling" thus pulls on and compresses the trachea and right mainstem bronchus at the carina. Correction requires division of the left pulmonary artery, removal of the left pulmonary artery from behind the trachea, and reanastomosis of the vessel to the main pulmonary artery just distal to the pulmonary valve.

C. Anesthetic Considerations

Fortunately, ventilation usually improves once the endotracheal tube is in proper position. The trachea is usually compressed just above the carina, so the tube must often be inserted more deeply into the trachea. Occasionally, a direct right mainstem bronchial intubation is required; in this situation, a side hole cut near the end of the endotracheal tube will allow ventilation of the left lung (Table 17–4). The surgeon will need to partially collapse the left lung to gain exposure of the vascular structures. Comparison of palpable pulses in the head and arms may assist the surgeon in identifying the proper location for division of the ring (Table 17–4). Postoperative relief of tracheal obstruction is usually clearly evident and dramatic. Occasionally, however, substantial tracheomalacia may have been caused by the chronic presence of the compressing vessel. In these children respiratory symptoms may persist postoperatively and may become more severe when the child is agitated since the trachea is more likely to collapse during forceful inspiration.

VII. CONGENITAL PARENCHYMAL LESIONS: LOBAR EMPHYSEMA, CYSTS, SEQUESTRATIONS, AND CYSTIC ADENOMATOID MALFORMATIONS

A. General Considerations

1. Congenital Lobar Emphysema

Congenital lobar emphysema is a pathologic accumulation of air in one lobe of the lung, usually an upper lobe or the right middle lobe.

The etiology of this condition is unknown in over half of the reported cases.[89-93] In those cases with a defined etiology, extrinsic bronchial compression (vessels or enlarged lymph nodes) or intrinsic bronchial obstruction (bronchial cartilaginous dysplasia, bronchial stenosis, or redundant bronchial mucosa) is most commonly cited. Bronchial cartilaginous dysplasia is the most common cause (25 per cent) of all cases, and the abnormality may involve the mainstem, lobar, or sublobar bronchi; the softened cartilage collapses on expiration, trapping air beyond the collapse.

2. Congenital Bronchogenic Cysts

Congenital bronchogenic cysts are derived from abnormal budding of the primitive tracheobronchial tree.[94] When the abnormal bronchial budding occurs at the level of the carina or first-order bronchi, the cyst assumes a mediastinal or subcarinal location (30 per cent). When the distal tracheobronchial tree is the origin of the abnormal budding, an intraparenchymal bronchogenic cyst results (70 per cent). Congenital bronchogenic lung cysts are usually less hyperinflated but, unfortunately, they may be more infected as a result of decreased bronchial communication. With congenital lung cysts, the remaining lung may be somewhat hypoplastic, resembling the situation found in congenital diaphragmatic hernia. Further, a congenital cyst may be supplied by an anomalous systemic vessel, which may represent a form of pulmonary sequestration.

3. Pulmonary Sequestration

Pulmonary sequestration is characterized by the presence of lung tissue that lacks bronchial communication with the normal tracheobronchial tree and a blood supply that is derived from a systemic arterial source.[94] Sequestrations can be extralobar (with its own separate visceral pleura) or intralobar (incorporated within the normal visceral pleural investment).

4. Cystic Adenomatoid Malformations

If the bronchial buds and alveolar mesenchyma fail to join at 16 to 20 weeks of gestation, uncontrolled overgrowth of the bronchioles, especially the terminal branches, occurs and is characteristic of cystic adenomatoid malformations.[94] The noncommunicating alveolar ducts and air sacs develop from the surrounding mesenchyma and contribute the alveolar component to this congenital anomaly. Cystic adenomatoid malformations are thus true hamartomas. Since the amount of bronchiolar and alveolar components can vary within the mass, the tumors can range from solid masses without cysts to mixed solid and cystic masses within the lungs.

There is a high incidence of congenital heart disease in patients with these congenital pulmonary parenchymal problems.[95-98] Although both cardiac and pulmonary lesions may be severe, pulmonary hyperinflation or infection is generally the more disruptive situation, and its correction is usually required before cardiac surgery can be contemplated.[99]

B. Surgical Considerations

1. Congenital Lobar Emphysema

The clinical presentation of clinical lobar emphysema is quite variable. The usual age of presentation is from birth to 4 months,[100] although an occasional child may present after 12 months.[99] The symptoms are similar to those of a pneumothorax, although in congenital lobar emphysema the air is not extrapleural. The direct compression of surrounding lung and compression of the contralateral lung by mediastinal shift results in dyspnea and cyanosis being the most frequent symptoms. Because of the mediastinal shift, there may also be severe cardiovascular compromise (decreased venous return, systemic hypotension).

Findings on a chest radiograph include a unilateral radiolucency from lobar distension, compression atelectasis of surrounding lung, mediastinal shift away from the affected side, and a flattening of the ipsilateral diaphragm. The presence of bronchovascular markings may help to differentiate congenital lobar emphysema from congenital lung cysts (with which it is most often confused).

Once the diagnosis is made, lobectomy is considered mandatory. Conservative therapy such as needle aspiration, placement of chest tubes, and administration of oxygen and antibiotics simply does not work and has been associated with over a 50 per cent mortality, whereas operative mortality is 3 to 7 per cent.[101] Long-term follow-up of children who have undergone pulmonary resection for congenital lobar emphysema problems in infancy shows minimal physiologic difference from unaffected individuals.[102]

2. Congenital Bronchogenic Cysts

Mediastinal cysts usually become evident clinically because they cause partial respiratory tract obstruction and distal pulmonary infection. Noncommunicating mediastinal cysts appear as soft tissue masses on chest roentgenograms. The presence of air or air fluid levels within a mediastinal cyst suggests some sort of tracheobronchial (or enteric) communication. In infants whose mediastinal bronchogenic cysts cause partial bronchial obstruction with distal air trapping, the radiographic picture can be similar to that in congenital lobar emphysema. Since only half of these infants with bronchogenic cysts who have lobar emphysema have mediastinal masses visible on their initial chest radiographs, the surgeon must consider the possibility of an unrecognized bronchogenic cyst whenever an exploratory thoracotomy is undertaken for congenital lobar emphysema.

When the bronchogenic cyst is intraparenchymal, it usually shows air fluid levels due to a partially obstructed tracheobronchial tree communication. Infection often supervenes, and cysts may be indistinguishable from cavitating pneumonia or lung abscesses.[103] Intraparenchymal bronchogenic cysts must be resected and, in cases in which there is superimposed infection of the surrounding normal lung, antibiotic administration to control the inflammatory process should precede operative intervention. With congenital lung cysts, anomalous systemic vessels from the hilum (or other places) must be identified; failure to do so has resulted in exsanguination.[25]

3. Pulmonary Sequestration

Extralobar sequestrations are often recognized by 1 year of age as incidental findings on chest radiographs. Respiratory insufficiency, associated cardiovascular or thoracic anomalies, and feeding problems are the most common symptoms stimulating evaluation. In 90 per cent of extralobar cases, the sequestration resides in the posterior left costophrenic sulcus adjacent to the esophagus.[104] The systemic arterial supply must be identified.

Intralobar sequestrations are evident relatively late compared with extralobar sequestrations. Few intralobar sequestrations are recognized prior to 1 year of age. The most frequent symptom is persistent or recurrent pneumonia within the same bronchopulmonary segment. Angiography is diagnostic of the pulmonary sequestration because it can define the anomalous systemic blood supply to the sequestered segment; the location and number of systemic vessels perfusing the anomaly and the venous drainage present must be clearly identified.

Pulmonary sequestrations should be resected. In patients with intralobar sequestrations complicated by pneumonia, infection should be controlled prior to thoracotomy with appropriate antibiotics. Lobectomy is the preferred procedure in most patients. In both intra- and extralobar forms, a careful search of the thorax must be undertaken prior to resection to identify and control the aberrant systemic artery or arteries.

4. Cystic Adenomatoid Malformations

The most common presentation of cystic adenomatoid malformation is progressive respiratory distress in a newborn infant that is associated with a complex cystic, solid, partially air-filled pulmonary mass on chest radiograph. Typically the mass displaces the mediastinum to the contralateral side, causing contralateral atelectasis, which intensifies the respiratory insufficiency. Radiographically the abnormality produced can be indistinguishable from a congenital posterolateral diaphragmatic hernia.[105, 106] Cystic adenomatoid malformations can also cause recurrent infections and become abscessed because the cystic cavities have poor bronchopulmonary drainage.

The treatment of cystic adenomatoid malformations is pulmonary resection, almost always a lobectomy. The malformation may have an abnormal systemic arterial supply from an infradiaphragmatic aortic branch. This vascular supply, similar to that of an intralobar sequestration, should be routinely searched for.

C. Anesthetic Considerations

1. Congenital Lobar Emphysema

Atropine should be administered prior to the induction of anesthesia. A gentle induction of anesthesia is performed with spontaneous ventilation of a volatile agent and 100 per cent oxygen.[100] Alternatively, intramuscular ketamine (6 to 8 mg/kg) may be used, followed by spontaneous ventilation of a volatile drug.[100] Struggling must be avoided to prevent further air trapping. However, the volatile drug must be administered with care because, if the mediastinum is distorted, the volatile drug may cause cardiovascular depression, which is unresponsive to volume infusion. Nitrous oxide and positive-pressure ventilation are contraindicated because of the danger of further expanding the emphysematous lobe (Table 17–4).[44, 99] The trachea is intubated without the use of muscle relaxants, and spontaneous ventilation is allowed until the chest is opened. Occasionally, it may be useful to intubate the contralateral mainstem bronchus in order to prevent further expansion of the lobe as well as facilitate surgical exposure (see Thoracic Surgical Procedures Requiring One-Lung Ventilation below). If the patient demonstrates cardiovascular depression after the induction of anesthesia, it is helpful if the incision is infiltrated with local anesthetic in order to lighten the level of anesthesia. Once the chest is opened, the emphysematous lobe usually herniates through the incision, which eliminates compression of the ipsilateral normal lung and mediastinal shift. Occasionally, emergency thoracostomy may be required during the induction of anesthesia to let the lobe expand out of the hemithorax. Controlled ventilation is instituted at this point and may be facilitated by muscle relaxants if desired. Postoperatively, the previously compressed ipsilateral lung may not always expand immediately.[100]

2. Congenital Bronchogenic Cysts

The anesthetic management of congenital bronchogenic cysts shares many of the same features as the management of congenital lobar emphysema (for example, the need to avoid nitrous oxide and preserve spontaneous ventilation) (Table 17–4). The two lungs may need to be separated if the cyst is infected (see Thoracic Surgical Procedures Requiring One-Lung Ventilation below). The management of mediastinal cysts has been considered in chapter 14.

3. Pulmonary Sequestrations

If the sequestration is infected, the lungs may need to be separated (see Thoracic Surgical Procedures Requiring One-Lung Ventilation below). Otherwise the anesthetic considerations are similar to those for other types of resections.

4. Cystic Adenomatoid Malformations

If the malformation is abscessed, then separation of the two lungs becomes extremely important (see Thoracic Surgical Procedures

Requiring One-Lung Ventilation below). Otherwise the anesthetic considerations are similar to those for other types of resections and include massive hemorrhage if a systemic arterial supply is not identified.

VIII. THORACIC SURGICAL PROCEDURES REQUIRING ONE-LUNG VENTILATION

The indications for one-lung ventilation in pediatric patients are the same as for adults. However, the most common indication for lung separation is the presence of infection in one lung, which could potentially contaminate the other lung. The infections consist of lung abscess, empyema, and hydatid cysts. Lung abscess may be caused by foreign bodies, infection within true congenital lung cysts, lung sequestration, and hypoplastic lobes and may occur following pneumonia. Other indications for lung separation consist of bronchiectasis and bronchopleural fistula. There are basically three ways to separate the two lungs in pediatric patients, and the methods consist of use of a bronchial blocker such as a Fogarty embolectomy catheter, mainstem bronchial intubation, and a combination of the two. Finally, use of the prone position may minimize the risk of cross contamination. See chapter 11 for the ventilatory management of one-lung ventilation (use 100 per cent oxygen, decrease the two-lung tidal volume by 20 per cent, increase the two-lung respiratory rate by 20 per cent).

A. Bronchial Blocker

A 3-Fr. gauge Fogarty embolectomy catheter is a balloon-tipped catheter with a capacity of 0.5 ml. A fully inflated balloon has a length of 10 mm and a width of 7.5 mm. When the patient is sufficiently deeply anesthetized, the tracheobronchial tree can be sprayed with local anesthetic, and either a rigid (3.2 to 3.6 mm outside diameter) or a fiberoptic (3.2 to 3.6 mm outside diameter)[107, 108] bronchoscope is passed into the appropriate mainstem bronchus (Fig. 17–7). Under direct vision the Fogarty embolectomy catheter can be placed in the appropriate mainstem bronchus, and the Fogarty catheter is inflated with 0.5 ml of sterile normal saline. If a rigid bronchoscope is used, the patient can be ventilated via the sidearm. The bronchoscope is then removed, and the patient is ventilated and oxygenated. A single-lumen tube (3.5 to 4.5 mm outside diameter) is then placed in the trachea. The bronchial blocker may also be guided into place with fluoroscopy[109] (Fig. 17–7).

Alternatively, and if the patient is large enough, a single-lumen tube (4.5 to 6.0 mm outside diameter) may be placed first and connected to an elbow adapter with a self-sealing diaphragm (Fig. 17–7). The pediatric fiberoptic bronchoscope (3.2 to 3.6 mm outside diameter) is then passed through the self-sealing diaphragm and identifies the carina. Then, depending on the size of the endotracheal tube used, the Fogarty embolectomy catheter can be passed alongside or within the endotracheal tube (also through the self-sealing diaphragm) into the proper mainstem bronchial position (Fig. 17–7).

The position of the single-lumen endotracheal tube and bronchial blocker should be confirmed with a chest x-ray. The bronchial blocker can be readily appreciated on chest radiograph if a radiopaque material is instilled into the blocking balloon.

It is important to realize that the bronchial blocker may back out of the mainstem bronchus at any time. Slight dislodgment may be indicated by the appearance of infected secretions. Complete dislodgment into the carinal area results in inability to ventilate either of the lungs due to blockage of the main airway by the inflated balloon. Under these circumstances the balloon must be immediately deflated to allow ventilation of both lungs. In addition, with dislodgment of the bronchial blocker the separation of the two lungs is lost; to prevent bilateral flooding of infected material, the surgeon may need to manually seal off the area in question with either a rubber snare or a bronchial clamp. These potentially catastrophic events may especially happen following external handling of the mainstem bronchus in question by the surgeon.

Insertion of Bronchial Blocker

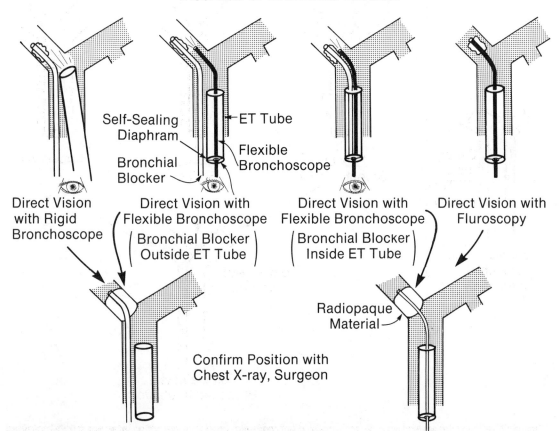

Figure 17–7. Insertion of a bronchial blocker may be accomplished by a number of methods depending on the age of the patient and the size of endotracheal tube that can be used.

B. Mainstem Bronchial Intubation

The mainstem bronchus of the healthy lung is the bronchus that requires intubation. When the left lung is diseased and the right mainstem bronchus is to be intubated, insertion of a single-lumen tube deep within the tracheobronchial tree will result in right mainstem bronchial intubation in a high percentage of cases (Fig. 17–8). The single-lumen endotracheal tube can then be withdrawn slowly until breath sounds are heard over all of the right hemithorax. When the right lung is diseased and the left mainstem bronchus requires intubation, use of a fiberoptic bronchoscope, fluoroscopy, or a curved stylet will be necessary (Fig. 17–8). With a fiberoptic bronchoscope or fluoroscopy,[109] precise positioning is possible. If a curved stylet is used the tube may need to be withdrawn until breath sounds are heard over

the entire left hemithorax. Following any method of insertion, the position of the mainstem bronchial endotracheal tube should be further confirmed by chest radiograph. With either mainstem bronchial intubation, the surgeon can further check the position of the tube at the time of thoracotomy.

C. Bronchial Blockade Plus Mainstem Bronchial Intubation

To more securely guarantee lung separation, a bronchial blocker can be used in conjunction with mainstem bronchial intubation.[107] A bronchial blocker must first be placed under bronchoscopic (either rigid or fiberoptic, see above) or fluoroscopic control (Fig. 17–7) and the mainstem bronchial intubation under fiberoptic bronchoscopic and/or fluoroscopic control (Fig.

Mainstem Bronchial Intubation

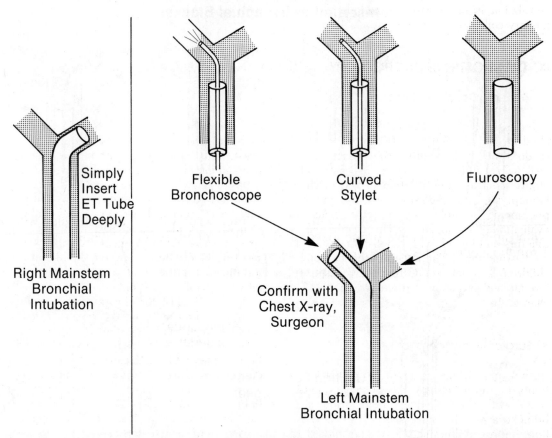

Figure 17–8. There are several ways to accomplish a left mainstem bronchial intubation, whereas a right mainstem bronchial intubation can almost always be achieved by simply inserting the endotracheal tube deep within the tracheobronchial tree.

17–8). When the bronchial blocker is used with a mainstem bronchial intubation a curved stylet is relatively contraindicated because if the single-lumen endotracheal tube enters the mainstem bronchus in which the bronchial blocker sits, ventilation will not be possible and it may cause malpositioning of the bronchial blocker. Finally, the position of the bronchial balloon and mainstem bronchial ventilating catheter should be confirmed with chest radiograph preoperatively and by the surgeon intraoperatively as described above.

D. Prone Positioning

The prone position may be used in patients who have lateral and posterior lesions. Following anesthesia induction and intubation, the children are placed in the prone position, with head slightly lower than the chest, thereby allowing secretions and blood to drain forward without spillage into the contralateral lung. The surgeon may find access to the lung facilitated, ventilation is more easily provided, and pulmonary collapse has not been a problem.

IX. DIAGNOSTIC BRONCHOSCOPY

A. General Considerations

Indications for diagnostic bronchoscopy in children include determination of the cause of stridor, such as laryngotracheal malacia, laryngeal webs, and postintubation or post-tracheotomy stenosis; identification of the origin of hemoptysis; the investigation of persistent pneumonia or atelectasis; and the diagnostic evaluation of a suspected tracheoesophageal fistula (in combination with esophagoscopy) and a mediastinal mass. Therapeutic bronchoscopy in children is usually done to remove aspirated foreign bodies and was discussed in detail in chapter 16.

B. Surgical Considerations

The surgical management of pediatric patients for bronchoscopy has improved significantly with the introduction of various-sized bronchoscopes that have a miniature lens system, improved illumination, and a standard 15-mm connector for the anesthesia circuit. With bronchoscopes larger than 3 mm, small biopsy forceps or grasping forceps can be passed through the instrument channel while ventilation is maintained with the telescope in place.[110]

C. Anesthetic Considerations

If an intravenous line is not present, anesthesia can be induced by intramuscular injection of ketamine or by inhalation of halothane/nitrous oxide/oxygen. Alternatively, if an intravenous line is in place, anesthesia can be induced with intravenous thiopental or ketamine and maintained by inhalation. Atropine (0.02 mg/kg) should be administered intravenously at the time of induction of anesthesia for its effect on secretions and vagal tone.

When the patient is adequately anesthetized, laryngoscopy is performed and the trachea is sprayed with lidocaine (3 to 4 mg/kg). Nitrous oxide is discontinued if previously used, and anesthesia is continued with halothane and oxygen by mask for another 2 to 3 minutes. Lidocaine (1.0 mg/kg) may be infused during this time. The bronchoscope is then inserted (may need to be facilitated by the administration of succinylcholine), and the anesthesia circuit is attached to the standard 15-mm side arm connector. Since this is almost a closed system (some gas leakage may occur around the outside of the bronchoscope), ventilation can be controlled (see Fig. 14–5). Controlled ventilation is desirable in most patients because the work of spontaneously breathing through the small, high-resistance, pediatric bronchoscopes is great, and the patients must be well anesthetized and, therefore, will have decreased central drive to spontaneously breathe. If the gas leak around the bronchoscope during positive-pressure ventilation is large, this can usually be remedied by pharyngeal packing with saline-soaked gauze and/or by gentle compression of the cricoid cartilage between the thumb and forefinger against the bronchoscope. With either controlled or spontaneous ventilation, if chest wall rigidity, forceful exhalation, or bronchospasm occurs during the case (usually the result of inadequate anesthesia), muscle relaxation may be needed quickly, but should not be achieved with multiple small doses of succinylcholine since severe bradycardia may occur after the second or third dose. Rather, the first bolus of succinylcholine should be followed by a 1 to 2 mg/ml succinylcholine drip to maintain 50 per cent twitch depression on the nerve stimulator. Alternatively, vecuronium or atracurium may be used, if appropriate, for the anticipated length of the procedure. Muscle relaxation, of course, necessitates controlled positive-pressure ventilation.

It must be stressed that anesthesia and ventilation must be adequate and suctioning limited to only short periods of time followed by lung inflation.[111] The combination of hypoventilation and prolonged suctioning, both of which may lead to hypoxia, and the presence of light anesthesia may result in cardiac arrhythmias. These arrhythmias are usually resolved with manual hyperventilation, adequate oxygenation, and deepened levels of anesthesia. If these measures are unsuccessful, lidocaine (1 mg/kg) is given intravenously to control cardiac irritability.

Bronchoscopic or laryngoscopic instrumentation of the upper airway always carries with it the possibility of significant laryngeal or subglottic edema, especially in smaller infants and children. Management of this complication includes postoperative humidification of inspired gases, adequate hydration, intermittent positive-pressure breathing of racemic epinephrine (0.5 ml of racemic epinephrine diluted with 3.5 ml of normal saline) every 2 to 3 hours, and dexamethasone (0.1 to 0.3 mg/kg intravenously).[112]

Although rarely performed in the pediatric population, flexible fiberoptic bronchoscopy can be done with the patient awake or lightly sedated.[113] If the patient's trachea is already intubated or general anesthesia is required for the procedure, the bronchoscope can be passed through an endotracheal tube. The smallest endotracheal tube that can be used with a 3.2-mm bronchoscope is 4.5 mm. The flexible fiberoptic bronchoscope must be introduced through a self-sealing diaphragm in the elbow connector to the endotracheal tube in order to maintain an airtight closed system.[114] Anesthesia technique is as described for rigid bronchoscopy except that ventilation must be controlled because of the increased resistance to airflow in the space around the bronchoscope but within the lumen of the endotracheal tube.

In very small children, in whom a 4- to 5-mm endotracheal tube is too large, the flexible fiberoptic bronchoscope must be passed without the aid of an endotracheal tube conduit. In this situation, the fiberoptic bronchoscope can only remain in the tracheobronchial tree for a short period of time. Pulse oximetry is helpful in this situation, and the end-point for withdrawal of the fiberoptic bronchoscope and resumption of ventilation via anesthesia mask is when the arterial saturation of oxygen begins to decrease.

X. BRONCHOGRAPHY

Bronchography may be necessary to define the extent of certain parenchymal diseases of the lung, such as segmental bronchiectasis. In order to selectively place the contrast material into the lung region in question, the contrast material must be introduced via a catheter placed in the lung region. The catheter can be placed in the lung region via a rigid bronchoscope or, depending on the age of the patient and the size of endotracheal tube that can be used, can be passed alongside or within an endotracheal tube and guided into the lung region by a flexible fiberoptic bronchosope within the endotracheal tube. This procedure is usually done in the radiology department, and the patient may need to be turned to several positions in order to obtain adequate films. Anesthesia for bronchography is similar to that for bronchoscopy, using either an intravenous induction and halothane/oxygen maintenance or an inhalation induction as described above. If an endotracheal tube is used instead of a bronchoscope to pass the contrast catheter, and the contrast catheter is passed within the endotracheal tube, the elbow connector to the endotracheal tube should have a self-sealing diaphragm through which the contrast catheter can be passed and a self-sealing positive-pressure system maintained.

The anesthesiologist should consult with the radiologist as to whether spontaneous or controlled ventilation is preferred. Spontaneous ventilation allows the contrast medium to be drawn gradually into the bronchi, giving dense and even distribution; whereas forceful positive-pressure ventilation may disperse the contrast medium too readily into the alveoli, so that the bronchial tree is poorly delineated and obscured by densities at the periphery. Perhaps the best compromise is gentle controlled ventilation during short periods of paralysis. Anesthesia should be sufficiently deep to prevent coughing when the contrast material is introduced, because coughing may spread the material and result in poor-quality radiographs.

The patient is turned to the lateral decubitus position to favor filling of an upper lobe. A slight head-up tilt helps filling of both the middle and lower lobes. After the necessary radiographs are obtained, as much of the contrast material as possible is suctioned from the bronchial tree. The endotracheal tube should be left in place until there is an active cough reflex.

REFERENCES

1. Dibbins AW, Wiener ES: Mortality from neonatal diaphragmatic hernia. J Pediatr Surg 9:653, 1974.
2. Nelson NM, Prod'Hom LS, Cherry RB, et al: Pulmonary function in the newborn infant: The alveolar-arterial oxygen gradient. J Appl Physiol 18:534, 1963.
3. Peckham GJ, Fox WW: Physiologic factors affecting pulmonary artery pressure in infants with persistent pulmonary hypertension. J Pediatr 93:1005, 1978.
4. Drummond WH, Gregory GA, Heymann MA, Phibbs RA: The independent effects of hyperventilation, tolazoline, and dopamine on infants with persistent pulmonary hypertension. J Pediatr 98:603, 1981.
5. Collins D, Pomerance JJ, Travis KW, et al: New approach to congenital posterolateral diaphragmatic hernia. J Pediatr Surg 12:149, 1977.
6. Graham TP Jr, Atwood GF, Boucek RJ: Pharmacological dilatation of the ductus arteriosus with prostaglandin E$_1$ in infants with congenital heart disease. South Med J 71:1238–1246, 1978.
7. Heymann MA, Rudolph AM, Silverman NH: Closure of the ductus arteriosus in premature infants by inhibition of prostaglandin synthesis. N Engl J Med 295:530, 1976.
8. Friedman WF: Pharmacologic closure of patent ductus arteriosus in the premature infant. N Engl J Med 295:526, 1976.
9. Nadas AS: Patent ductus revisited (editorial). N Engl J Med 295:563, 1976.
10. Payne JW, Patz A: Current status of retrolental fibroplasia. The retinopathy of prematurity. Ann Clin Res 11:205–221, 1979.
11. Kinsey VE, Arnold HJ, Kalina RE, et al: P$_a$O$_2$ levels and retrolental fibroplasia: A report of the cooperative study. Pediatrics 60:655–668, 1977.
12. Silverman WA: Retinopathy of prematurity: Oxygen dogma challenged. Arch Dis Child 57:731–733, 1982.
13. Lucey JF: Retrolental fibroplasia may not be preventable. J R Soc Med 75:496–497, 1982.
14. Purohit DM, Ellison C, Zierler S, et al: Risk factors for retrolental fibroplasia: Experience with 3,025 premature infants. Pediatrics 76:339–344, 1985.
15. Phelps DL: Retinopathy of prematurity: An estimate of vision loss in the United States—1979. Pediatrics 67:924–926, 1981.
16. Gunn TR, Easdown J, Outerbridge EW, et al: Risk factors in retrolental fibroplasia. Pediatrics 65:1096–1100, 1980.
17. Aranda JV, Saheb N, Stern L, Avery ME: Arterial oxygen tension and retinal vasoconstriction in newborn infants. Am J Dis Child 122:189, 1971.
18. Rigatto H, Brady JP: Periodic breathing and apnea in the preterm infant. I. Evidence for hypoventilation possibly due to central depression. Pediatrics 50:202, 1972.
19. Steinschneider A: Prolonged sleep apnea and the sudden infant death syndrome: Clinical and laboratory observations. Pediatrics 50:646, 1972.
20. Aranda JV, Turmen T: Methylxanthines in apnea of prematurity. Clin Perinatol 6:87–108, 1979.
21. Miller MJ, Martin RJ, Carlo WA, et al: Oral breathing in newborn infants. Pediatrics 107:465–469, 1985.
22. Oliver TK Jr: Temperature regulation and heat production in the newborn. Pediatrics 50:646, 1972.
23. Roe CF, Santulli TV, Blair CS: Heat loss in infants during general anesthesia and operations. J Pediatr Surg 3:266, 1966.
24. Schedewie HE, Odell WD, Fisher DA, et al: Parathormone and perinatal calcium homeostasis. Pediatr Res 13:1, 1979.
25. Ward CF: Diseases of infants. In Katz J, Benumof JL (eds): Anesthesia and Uncommon Diseases. 2nd ed. Philadelphia, WB Saunders Co, 1981, chapter 4, pp 119–154.
26. Furman EB, Roman DG, Lemmer LAS, et al: Specific therapy in water, electrolyte, and blood volume replacement during pediatric surgery. Anesthesiology 42:187, 1975.
27. Snyder WH, Greaney EM: Congenital diaphragmatic hernia: 77 consecutive cases. Surgery 57:576, 1965.
28. Ban JL, Moore TC: Intrathoracic tension incarceration of stomach and liver through right-sided congenital posterolateral hernias. J Thorac Cardiovasc Surg 66:969–973, 1973.
29. Ravitch MM, Barton BA: The need for pediatric surgeons as determined by the volume of work and the mode of delivery of surgical care. Surgery 76:754, 1974.
30. Harrison MR, Bjordal RI, Langmark F, Knutrud O: Congenital diaphragmatic hernia: The hidden mortality. J Pediatr Surg 13:227, 1978.
31. Adelman S, Benson CD: Bochdalek hernias in infants: Factors determining mortality. J Pediatr Surg 11:569, 1976.
32. Greenwood RD, Rosenthal A, Nadas AS: Cardiovascular abnormalities associated with diaphragmatic hernia. Pediatrics 57:92, 1976.
33. Kent GM, Olley PM, Creighton RE, et al: Hemodynamic and pulmonary changes following surgical creation of a diaphragmatic hernia in fetal lamb. Surgery 72:427, 1972.
34. Murdock AI, Burrington JB, Swyer PR: Alveolar to arterial oxygen tension difference and venous admixture in newly born infants with congenital diaphragmatic herniation through the foramen of Bochdalek. Biol Neonate 17:161, 1971.
35. Rowe MI, Uribe FL: Diaphragmatic hernia in the newborn infant: Blood gas and pH considerations. Surgery 70:758, 1971.
36. Boles ET, Schiller M, Weinberger M: Improved management of neonates with congenital diaphragmatic hernias. Arch Surg 103:344, 1971.
37. Adams JG: Pediatric Anesthesia Case Studies. London, Henry Kimpton, 1976, p 155.
38. Lister J: Recent advances in the surgery of the diaphragm of the newborn. Prog Pediatr Surg 2:29, 1971.
39. Cullen ML, Klein MD, Philippart AI: Congenital diaphragmatic hernia. Surg Clin North Am 65:1115–1138, 1985.
40. Merin RG: Congenital diaphragmatic hernia: From the anesthesiologist's viewpoint. Anesth Analg 45:44, 1966.
41. Bray RJ: Congenital diaphragmatic hernia. Anaesthesia 34:567, 1979.
42. Wooley MM: Congenital posterolateral diaphragmatic hernia. Surg Clin North Am 56:317, 1976.
43. Creighton RE, Whalen JS, Conn AW: The management of congenital diaphragmatic hernia. Can Anaes Soc J 13:124, 1966.
44. Eger EI II, Saidman LJ: Hazards of nitrous oxide anesthesia in bowel obstruction and pneumothorax. Anesthesiology 26:61, 1975.
45. Boles ET Jr, Schiller M, Weinberger M: Improved management of neonates with congenital diaphragmatic hernia. Arch Surg 103:344, 1971.

46. deLorimier AA, Tierney DF, Parker HR: Hypoplastic lungs in fetal lambs with surgically produced congenital diaphragmatic hernia. Surgery 62:12, 1967.

47. Thein RMH, Epstein BS: General surgical procedures in the child with a congenital anomaly. In Stehling LC, Zauder HL (eds): Anesthetic Implication of Congenital Anomalies in Children. New York, Appleton-Century-Crofts, 1980, p 90.

48. Holder RM, Ashcraft KW: Congenital diaphragmatic hernia. In Ravitch MM, Welch KJ, Benson CD, et al (eds): Pediatric Surgery. 3rd ed. Chicago, Year Book Medical Publishers, Inc, 1979, p 439.

49. Ehrlich FE, Salzberg AM: Pathophysiology and management of congenital posterolateral diaphragmatic hernias. Am Surg 44:26, 1978.

50. Goetzman BW, Sunshine P, Johnson JD, et al: Neonatal hypoxic and pulmonary vasospasm: Response to tolazoline, J Pediatr 89:617, 1976.

51. Cohen D, Reid IS: Recurrent diaphragmatic hernia. J Pediatr Surg 16:42–44, 1981.

52. Reynolds M, Luck SR, Lapper R: The "critical" neonate with diaphragmatic hernia: A 21 year perspective. J Pediatr Surg 19:364–369, 1984.

53. Gibson C, Fonkalsrud EW: Iatrogenic pneumothorax and mortality in congenital diaphragmatic hernia. J Pediatr Surg 18:555–559, 1983.

54. Hansen J, Jones S, Burrington J, et al: The decreasing incidence of pneumothorax and improving survival in infants with congenital diaphragmatic hernia. J Pediatr Surg 19:385–388, 1984.

55. Cumming WA: Esophageal atresia and tracheoesophageal fistula. Radiol Clin North Am 13:277, 1975.

56. Calverly RK, Johnston AE: The anesthetic management of tracheoesophageal fistula: A review of ten years' experience. Can Anaesth Soc J 19:270, 1972.

57. Waterston DJ, Bonham Carter RE, Aberdeen E: Oesophageal atresia: Tracheoesophageal fistula: A study of survival in 218 infants. Lancet 1:819, 1962.

58. Chen H, Goei GS, Hertzler JH: Family studies on congenital esophageal atresia with or without tracheoesophageal fistula. Birth Defects 15:117, 1979.

59. Wyant GM, Cram RW: The management of infants with tracheoesophageal fistula. Can Anaesth Soc J 10:93, 1963.

60. Andrassy RJ, Mahour GH: Gastrointestinal anomalies associated with esophageal atresia or tracheoesophageal fistula. Arch Surg 114:1125, 1979.

61. Kluth D: Atlas of esophageal atresia. J Pediatr Surg 11:901, 1976.

62. Humphreys GH, Hogg BM, Ferrer J: Congenital atresia of the esophagus. J Thorac Surg 32:332, 1956.

63. Barry JE, Auldist AW: The VATER association: One end of a spectrum of anomalies. Am J Dis Child 128:769, 1974.

64. Koop CE, Schnaufer L, Broennel AM: Esophageal atresia and tracheoesophageal fistula: Supportive measures that affect survival. Pediatrics 54:558, 1974.

65. Randolph JG, Altman P, Anderson KD: Selective surgical management based upon clinical status in infants with esophageal atresia. J Thorac Cardiovasc Surg 74:335–342, 1977.

66. Grosfeld JL, Ballantine TVN: Esophageal atresia and tracheoesophageal fistula: Effect of delayed thoracotomy on survival. Surgery 84:394–402, 1978.

67. Louhimo I, Lindahl H: Esophageal atresia: Primary results in 500 consecutively treated patients. J Pediatr Surg 18:217–229, 1983.

68. Filston HC, Rankin JS, Grimm JK: Esophageal atresia: Prognostic factors and contribution of preoperative telescopic endoscopy. Ann Surg 199:532–537, 1984.

69. Cozzi F, Wilkinson AW: Low birth weight babies with oesophageal atresia or tracheo-oesophageal fistula. Arch Dis Child 50:791–795, 1975.

70. Baraka A, Slim M: Cardiac arrest during IPPV in a newborn with tracheoesophageal fistula. Anesthesiology 32:564–565, 1970.

71. Breveton RJ, Richwood MK: Esophageal atresia with pulmonary agenesis. J Pediatr Surg 18:618–620, 1983.

72. Haight C: Congenital esophageal atresia and tracheoesophageal fistula. In Mustard WT (ed): Pediatric Surgery. 2nd ed. Chicago, Year Book Medical Publishers, Inc, 1969.

73. Chatrath RR, El Shafie M, Jones RS: Fate of hypoplastic lungs after repair of congenital diaphragmatic hernia: Prediction of survival. J Pediatr Surg 8:815, 1973.

74. Raphaely RC, Downes JJ: Congenital diaphragmatic hernia: Prediction of survival. J Pediatr Surg 8:815, 1973.

75. Stogsdill WW, Miller JR, Stoelting VR: Review of anesthesia for congenital tracheoesophageal anomalies. Anesth Analg 46:1, 1967.

76. Grant DM, Thompson GE: Diagnosis of congenital tracheoesophageal fistula in the adolescent and adult. Anesthesiology 49:139, 1978.

77. Schneider KM, Becker JM: The "H-type" tracheoesophageal fistula in infants and children. Surgery 51:677, 1962.

78. Korones SB, Evans LJ: Measurement of intragastric oxygen concentration for the diagnosis of H-type tracheoesophageal fistula. Pediatrics 60:450, 1977.

79. Holder TM, McDonald VG, Woolley MW: The premature or critically ill infant with esophageal atresia: Increased success with a staged approach. J Thorac Cardiovasc Surg 44:344, 1962.

80. Hicks LM, Mansfield PB: Esophageal atresia and tracheoesophageal fistula. J Thorac Cardiovasc Surg 81:358–363, 1981.

81. Sosis M, Amoroso M: Respiratory insufficiency after gastrostomy prior to tracheoesophageal fistula repair. Anesth Analg 64:748–750, 1985.

82. Karl HW: Control of life-threatening air leak after gastrostomy in an infant with respiratory distress syndrome and tracheoesophageal fistula. Anesthesiology 62:670–672, 1985.

83. Salem MR, Wong AY, Lin TH, et al: Prevention of gastric distension during anesthesia for newborns with tracheoesophageal fistulas. Anesthesiology 38:82, 1973.

84. Jones TB, Kirchner SG, Lee FA, et al: Stomach rupture associated with esophageal atresia, tracheoesophageal fistula, and ventilatory assistance. Am J Radiol 134:675, 1980.

85. Hallman GL, Cooley DA: Surgical treatment of congenital heart disease. Philadelphia, Lea and Febiger, 1975.

86. Gersony WM, Peckham GJ, Ellison RC, et al: Effects of indomethacin in premature infants with patent ductus arteriosus: Results of a national collaborative study. Pediatrics 102:895–906, 1983.

87. Mavroudis C, Cook, LN, Fleischaker JW, et al: Management of patent ductus arteriosus in premature infants; indomethacin vs. ligation. Ann Thorac Surg 36:561–566, 1983.

88. Oxnard SC, McGough EC, Jung AL, et al: Ligation of the patent ductus arteriosus in the newborn intensive care unit. Ann Thorac Surg 23:564–567, 1977.
89. Hendren WH, McKee DM: Lobar emphysema of infancy. J Pediatr Surg 1:24–39, 1966.
90. Leape LL, Longino LA: Infantile lobar emphysema. Pediatrics 34:246–255, 1964.
91. Raynor AC, Capp MP, Sealy WC: Lobar emphysema of infancy: Diagnosis, treatment, and etiological aspects. Ann Thorac Surg 4:374–385, 1967.
92. Lincoln JCR, Stark J, Subramanian S, et al: Congenital lobar emphysema. Ann Surg 173:55–62, 1971.
93. Murray GF: Congenital lobar emphysema. Surg Gynecol Obstet 124:611–625, 1967.
94. Ryckman FC, Rosenkrantz JG: Thoracic surgical problems in infancy and childhood. Surg Clin North Am 65:1423–1454, 1985.
95. Pierce WS, DeParedes CG, Friedman S, et al: Concomitant congenital heart disease and lobar emphysema in infants: Incidence, diagnosis and operative management. Ann Surg 172:951–956, 1970.
96. Jones JC, Almond CH, Snyder HM, et al: Lobar emphysema and congenital heart disease in infancy. J Thorac Cardiovasc Surg 49:1–10, 1965.
97. Buntain WL, Woolley MM, Mahour GH, et al: Pulmonary sequestration in children: A twenty-five year experience. Surgery 81:413–420, 1977.
98. Heithoff KB, Shashikant M, Williams H, et al: Bronchopulmonary foregut malformations—a unifying etiological concept. Am J Roentgenol 126:46–55, 1976.
99. Martin JT: Case history number 93: Congenital lobar emphysema. Anesth Analg 55:869–873, 1976.
100. Cote CJ: The anesthetic management of congenital lobar emphysema. Anesthesiology 49:296–298, 1978.
101. Raynor AC, Capp MP, Sealy WC: Lobar emphysema of infancy. Ann Thorac Surg 4:374, 1967.
102. De Muth GR, Sloan H: Congenital lobar emphysema:
Long term effects and sequelae in treated cases. Surgery 59:601, 1966.
103. Ramenofsky ML, Leape LL, McCauley GK: Bronchogenic cyst. J Pediatr Surg 14:219–224, 1979.
104. DeParedes CG, Pierce WS, Johnson DG, et al: Pulmonary sequestration in infants and children: A 20-year experience and review of the literature. J Pediatr Surg 5:136–147, 1970.
105. Monclair T, Schistad G: Congenital pulmonary cysts versus a differential diagnosis in the newborn: Diaphragmatic hernia. J Pediatr Surg 9:417–418, 1974.
106. Nishibayashi SW, Andrassy RJ, Woolley MM: Congenital cystic adenomatoid malformation: A 30-year experience. J Pediatr Surg 16:704–706, 1981.
107. Rao CC, Krishna G, Grosfeld JL, et al: One lung pediatric anesthesia. Anesth Analg 60:450, 1981.
108. Vale R: Selective bronchial blocking in a small child. Br J Anaesth 41:453, 1969.
109. Cay DL, Csenderits LE, Lines V, et al: Selective bronchial blocking in children. Anaesth Intensive Care 3:117, 1975.
110. Johnson DG: Endoscopy. In Ravitch MM, Welch KJ, Bensdon CD, et al (eds): Pediatric Surgery. 3rd ed. Chicago, Year Book Medical Publishers, Inc, 1974, p 513.
111. Baraka A: Bronchoscopic removal of inhaled foreign bodies in children. Br J Anaesth 46:124, 1974.
112. Jordan WS, Graves CL, Elwyn RA: New therapy for postintubation laryngeal edema and tracheitis in children. JAMA 212:585, 1970.
113. Wood RE, Fink RJ: Applications of flexible fiberoptic bronchoscopes in infants and children. Chest 73:737, 1978.
114. Carden E, Raj PP: Special new low resistance to flow tube and endotracheal tube adapter for use during fiberoptic bronchoscopy. Ann Otol Rhinol Laryngol 84:631, 1975.

V

POSTOPERATIVE
CONSIDERATIONS

Early Serious Complications Specifically Related to Thoracic Surgery

18

I. INTRODUCTION

There are several life-threatening complications of major thoracic surgery that may occur in the immediate postoperative period and require prompt diagnosis and treatment. These include herniation of the heart through the pericardium following radical pneumonectomy, massive hemorrhage, blowout of a bronchial stump following pneumonectomy or lobectomy, respiratory insufficiency, right-sided heart failure, right-to-left shunting across a patent foramen ovale, arrhythmias, neural injuries, and total spinal anesthesia following intrathoracic intercostal nerve blocks. The order in which these complications are discussed is approximately related to the usual severity of symptoms and threat to life, with the most life-threatening complications considered first. The problem of appropriate fluid infusion and the relationship of fluid infusion to postpneumonectomy pulmonary edema is considered in chapter 13, and the complications of double-lumen tube insertion are discussed in chapter 8.

II. HERNIATION OF THE HEART

An intrapericardial approach may be employed for radical pneumonectomy in order to facilitate access to major vessels and allow a wider hilar dissection.[1] This technique may result in a large pericardial defect, which the surgeon is not able to close after the pneumonectomy is completed. There have been several reports of herniation of the heart through the pericardial opening into the empty hemithorax. The herniation can be into either the right or the left hemithorax,[2, 3] and herniations into

either side can cause profound function impairment; the mortality is 50 per cent.[4-6]

With a right-sided herniation, the entire heart protrudes through the defect and is displaced completely into the right hemithorax. The chest roentgenogram usually shows displacement of the cardiac silhouette into the right pleural cavity, with the apex of the heart pointing to the right side and at a right angle to the mediastinum, and the apex may touch the right chest wall.[7] In addition, the heart rotates on its mediastinal attachment, causing twisting and distortion of the structures in the mediastinal attachment. Twisting of the superior vena cava causes an acute superior vena cava syndrome, and twisting of the inferior vena cava causes acute cardiovascular collapse[8-11] (Fig. 18-1). Distortion of the distal trachea or left mainstem bronchus may cause wheezing, and obstruction of the pulmonary veins may cause pulmonary congestion and edema (Fig. 18-1). The electrocardiogram may reflect ischemia with changes in the S-T segments and T waves and shifts in the QRS axis[5, 12] (Fig. 18-1).

With left-sided herniation, the ventricular apex protrudes out of the pericardium, and the atrioventricular groove is constricted by the pericardium[2] (Fig. 18-1). The extrapericardial myocardium becomes ischemic and edematous and, if not reduced quickly, causes obstruction of ventricular outflow, ventricular arrhythmia, and myocardial infarction. Thus, left-sided herniations are much more likely to demonstrate ischemic electrocardiographic patterns with atrial and ventricular arrhythmias. Constriction of the atrioventricular groove may cause acute cardiovascular collapse. The chest roentgenogram usually shows that the heart has assumed

Herniation of the Heart Post Pneumonectomy
Causes (➡) and Effects (⇨)

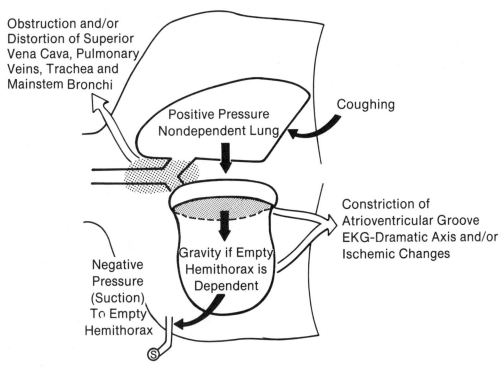

Figure 18–1. *Following a transpericardial radical pneumonectomy, the heart may herniate through a pericardial defect into the empty hemithorax. Factors that can cause this complication (solid arrows) are placing the empty hemithorax in a dependent position, which allows gravity to pull the heart through the defect; applying a high level of negative pressure suction to the empty hemithorax, which also pulls the heart through the defect; applying a high level of positive pressure ventilation to the remaining nondependent lung, which pushes the heart through the defect; and coughing, which also increases nondependent hemithorax pressure. The effects of herniation of the heart (open arrows) consist of obstruction and/or distortion of the mediastinal attachments (superior and inferior vena cava, pulmonary veins, and trachea and mainstem bronchi) and constriction of the atrioventricular groove by a tightly fitting pericardial defect. The EKG will show dramatic axis and/or ischemic changes.*

a spheric shape and has been displaced laterally and at a right angle to the mediastinum and that the apex is against the left chest wall.[7]

In most reports, herniation of the heart has occurred either immediately after the patient is turned from the lateral decubitus to the supine position (75 per cent) or during the first few hours of postoperative mechanical ventilation[6, 13] However, this complication can also occur as late as several days following surgery.[14] Events that increase intrapleural pressure in the non-surgical (ventilated) hemithorax or that decrease intrapleural pressure in the surgical (empty) hemithorax may predispose the patient to cardiac herniation. Placing the patient with the empty hemithorax in a dependent position allows the heart to be pulled by gravity into the empty hemithorax (Fig. 18–1). Use of high

levels of pressure and volume in the remaining lung can push the heart into the empty hemithorax (Fig. 18–1). Similarly, coughing can increase pleural pressure in the remaining lung and thereby promote displacement of the heart into the empty hemithorax (Fig. 18–1). Conversely, inadvertently applying suction to the chest drain in the empty hemithorax can pull the heart through a pericardial defect (tension vacuthorax)[6, 8] (Fig. 18–1).

The differential diagnosis consists of myocardial infarction, cardiac tamponade, massive pulmonary embolus, airway obstruction, and collapse of the remaining lung. When circulatory signs permit, the diagnosis can be confirmed by portable chest roentgenography. A diagnosis of cardiac herniation almost always requires immediate reexploration[4-6]; however, there is one report of herniation of the heart that caused only roentgenologic changes and no immediate clinical signs.[11]

There are three conservative measures that may improve cardiopulmonary function before and during transfer to the operating room (they are the reverse of the causes of herniation of the heart shown in Figure 18–1), and they should be instituted as soon as the diagnosis is entertained. First, the patient should be positioned so that the ventilated nonsurgical side is in a dependent position and the empty surgical side is in a nondependent position.[3, 14, 15] Gravity may return the heart and mediastinum to their normal anatomic positions. Even if the heart does not reenter the pericardium, the repositioning may decrease atriocaval kinking and increase cardiac output. Second, avoidance of high levels of pressure and volume in the ventilated lung may allow the return of the heart to the pericardium. Consequently, the tidal volume should be reduced, positive end-expiratory pressure (PEEP) should be removed, and the respiratory rate should be increased slightly. Third, suction to the empty hemithorax should be discontinued. Fourth, the pharmacologic support of the circulation should be provided as needed. Fifth, injecting 1 to 2 L of air into the surgical hemithorax may push the heart and mediastinum back to normal anatomic positions and may perhaps return the heart to the pericardium. Success with this latter technique has been variable.[13, 14, 16–18]

III. MAJOR HEMORRHAGE

Postoperative bleeding that necessitates emergency thoracotomy may occur in as many as 3 per cent of all thoracotomy patients.[19] The mortality of major postoperative bleeding is approximately 23 per cent.[19] There are several potential sources of major postoperative hemorrhage (Table 18–1), and these consist of bleeding from divided pulmonary arteries and veins due to slippage of surgical ligatures, diffuse bleeding from raw surfaces, and systemic arterial bleeding (bronchial and intercostal arteries).

Table 18–1. Potential Sites of Major Hemorrhage After Thoracotomy

1. Slippage of pulmonary artery and/or vein sutures or ligatures
2. Large raw surfaces
3. Bronchial arteries
4. Intercostal arteries

Table 18–2. Signs of Postoperative Intrathoracic Hemorrhage

1. Volume of blood in chest tube drainage
2. Hematocrit of blood in chest tube drainage
3. Signs of hypovolemia (tachycardia and decreased systemic blood pressure, systemic pulse pressure, central filling pressures, and urine output)
4. Signs of tension hemithorax (with nonfunctional chest tube)

Bleeding may be catastrophic if ligatures slip off a pulmonary artery or vein. Although these vessels are not highly pressurized, hemorrhage from these vessels is into a low pressure–high volume space and, therefore, may be massive. The risk of postoperative hemorrhage can be greatly diminished by adequate intraoperative exposure, and adequate intraoperative exposure may be greatly aided in most cases by one-lung ventilation and in a few cases by an intrapericardial approach to the hilum. In addition, branches of the pulmonary artery or vein should be directly oversewn with vascular suture material and/or should be doubly ligated, and then a transfixion suture or pursestring suture with a nonabsorbable material should be placed between the double ligation.[19]

Hemorrhage from raw surfaces is more common after pneumonectomy than after lobectomy because following lobectomy the apposition of the remaining lobes of lung against the chest wall and mediastinum may greatly diminish bleeding from these surfaces. Bleeding from raw pleural surfaces is especially likely when vascular adhesions between the visceral and parietal pleura have been divided. Hypertension is contributory to diffuse bleeding from raw surfaces.

Postoperative bleeding may be from systemic arteries, especially the bronchial arteries. Bleeding from bronchial arteries is encouraged by extensive mediastinal dissection that damages bronchial and mediastinal arteries. Bronchial artery bleeding will also occur when the bronchial artery is not included in the closure of a bronchial stump. If the free bronchial artery goes into spasm, then it may retract proximally. Subsequently, when the spasm is released postoperatively, the vessel will hemorrhage. In addition, the intercostal arteries may bleed if there has been inadvertent placement of periosteal sutures through an intercostal vessel.[20]

The drainage from a patent chest tube is an excellent monitor of the amount of intrathoracic bleeding (Table 18–2). In addition, the hematocrit of the usual fluid in the chest drainage is always less than 20 per cent, and intrathoracic bleeding will increase the hematocrit to some higher value (Table 18–2). Significant hemorrhage, of course, will be accompanied by the hemodynamic signs of hypovolemia, such as tachycardia, hypotension, and decrease in vascular filling pressures and urine output (Table 18–2).

Significant hemorrhage cannot always be ruled out by the absence of chest tube drainage, since the chest tube may be blocked by clotted blood or otherwise obstructed. Nevertheless, the patient will still show signs and symptoms of hypovolemia. In addition, if the chest tube is not draining well, there may be signs of significant shift in the mediastinum to the opposite side.

In extreme cases exsanguination may occur rapidly unless the bleeding is promptly controlled; indeed, immediate thoracotomy in the recovery room in order to obtain manual control of the bleeding site may be lifesaving. Once this has been accomplished, the patient can be returned to the operating room for closure under aseptic conditions. In all cases, blood, preferably fresh whole blood, should be administered. If time permits, the coagulation profile should be obtained, and specific coagulation factors and/or platelet concentrates should be administered as indicated by the laboratory findings.

IV. BRONCHIAL DISRUPTION

Development of a bronchopleural fistula is a serious complication of pulmonary resection and as recently as 1978 carried a mortality of 23 per cent.[21, 22] The term refers to any communication between the tracheobronchial tree and the pleural cavity and can result from dehiscence of the bronchial stump after lobectomy or pneumonectomy, from rupture of an inflammatory lesion or cavity within the lung into the pleura, or from trauma or neoplasm erosion. The symptoms and signs are variable and depend upon the size of the communication, the presence or absence of a chest drain, and whether or not there is fluid of any sort within the pleural space.

Gross disruption of a bronchial stump in the early postoperative period may result from technical error in bronchial closure, along with the use of high airway pressure for mechanical ventilation. The escape of gas is usually signaled by massive bubbling of gas through the chest tube drainage system. The patients quickly become hypoxemic and hypercarbic and develop a sympathomimetic cardiovascular response to these gas exchange changes. Immediate reexploration and revision of the bronchial closure is required. As soon as gross bronchial disruption is recognized, the chest tube should be removed from suction and left to under water seal only. If the leak continues to be large, strong consideration should be given to reinsertion of a double-lumen tube to prevent the escape of gas through the disrupted bronchial stump. The incidence of this postoperative catastrophe can be diminished intraoperatively (prior to chest closure) by the simple technique of filling the pleural space with irrigating solution and having the anesthesiologist exert 35 to 40 cm H_2O of pressure to demonstrate an airtight bronchial closure.

If the chest tube is obstructed, a tension pneumothorax with mediastinal shift will occur; the presence of a chest tube does not always prevent tension pneumothorax. High inflation pressures will be required for ventilation, and subcutaneous emphysema may become manifest (Fig. 18–2). A tension pneumothorax will shift the mediastinum, interfere with venous return, and decrease the cardiac output and blood pressure (Fig. 18–2). The chest roentgenogram is diagnostic, but if the clinical situation is critical, therapy should be instituted without taking one. Treatment consists of reestablishing the patency of the chest tube or inserting a needle or a trocar and cannula into the pleural cavity through the second intercostal space in the midclavicular line on the affected side.

Development of a chronic bronchopleural fistula may be expected to occur in 1 to 3 per cent of pulmonary resection patients.[21] A chronic bronchopleural fistula most frequently becomes evident within the first 2 weeks after operation, may be large, and may run a fulminating course characterized by sepsis, empyema, purulent sputum, and respiratory insufficiency. In a much smaller number of patients, bronchopleural fistulas may develop even later, usually are smaller, and usually occur in an insidious fashion, with malaise, fever, and the presence of multiple air fluid levels on chest roentgenograms. Factors that predispose to the formation of a bronchopleural fistula after pulmonary resection are preoperative irradiation, infection, residual neoplasm at the site of the closure, and presence of a long or avascular stump.

A large bronchopleural fistula that develops several days after pneumonectomy occurs dramatically. The onset is often abrupt, with a bout

Signs of Tension Pneumothorax

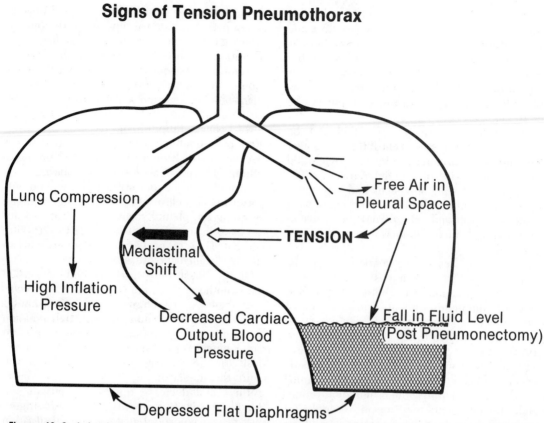

Figure 18–2. A tension pneumothorax will cause a mediastinal shift. The mediastinal shift compresses the contralateral lung (which causes poor compliance and high inflation pressures) and decreases venous return, cardiac output, and systemic blood pressure. Since both lungs are under pressure, the diaphragms are depressed and flat, and if the tension pneumothorax occurs postpneumonectomy, the free air in the pleural space will cause a fall in the postpneumonectomy fluid level.

of coughing and dyspnea precipitated by a change of posture that allows the operated side to be uppermost. Thin red-brown fluid that is characteristic of the contents of the empty hemithorax is both expectorated and inhaled into the remaining lung. This fluid is often infected and always irritant, so that it provokes bronchoconstriction and local inflammation, causing severe respiratory distress and hypoxemia. Signs of circulatory failure are usual too, probably caused by both hypoxemia and septicemia. The diagnosis is usually clear on clinical grounds alone. If confirmation is required, a chest roentgenogram will show a considerable fall in the fluid in the pneumonectomy hemithorax (fluid is replaced by air) and consolidation and collapse in the remaining lung.

Prompt resuscitation is essential and may need to include mechanical and differential lung ventilation with a double-lumen tube and support of the circulation. A functioning chest tube must be inserted immediately to evacuate the air (to prevent a tension pneumothorax) and fluid (to prevent further contamination of the

opposite lung) from the pneumonectomy cavity. Postural drainage and chest physiotherapy have no place in the management of a large bronchopleural fistula. The patient should be recumbent, with the normal side in a nondependent position. The stump must be closed surgically.[21]

At surgery, a double-lumen tube should be inserted to separate the two mainstem bronchi. The separation of the two mainstem bronchi prevents further contamination of the remaining or unoperated lung and allows positive-pressure ventilation of the remaining lung without loss of tidal volume through the fistula. The loss of tidal volume through the fistula can prevent effective ventilation in the remaining lung in three ways. First, tidal volume will be lost through the chest tube if the chest tube is functioning. Second, tension pneumothorax will develop if the chest tube is not functioning, which will cause mediastinal shift and compression of the remaining lung. Third, the escaping gas will pressurize the fluid in the empty hemithorax and force it to enter the fistula, which can cause contamination of the remaining lung.

From the foregoing considerations it is obvious that the lumen to the resected side must be occluded before positive-pressure ventilation is begun. The endobronchial lumen of the double-lumen tube should be in the contralateral main-stem bronchus. Surgical procedures for chronic bronchopleural fistula may include open drainage by rib resection, multiple rib thoracoplasty, coverage of the bronchial leak with muscle flaps, and additional pulonary resection; many patients require multiple procedures.[21]

If the chronic fistula is small, the symptoms are unobtrusive at first and consist of fever, tachycardia, and persistent cough with expectoration of small amounts of sputum, which is almost always blood tinged. Episodes of coughing at night and bouts of wheezy dyspnea are particularly suggestive of bronchopleural fistula. The chest roentgenogram at this stage (post-pneumonectomy) may show a decrease in the volume of fluid in the pleural space and an increase in the amount of air at the apex, or the fluid level may fail to continue rising as it normally does.

A small fistula after pneumonectomy may heal without surgery, provided infection is controlled and the patient can be positioned so that the fluid in the pleural space is below the level of the stump. Repeated aspiration of the pneumonectomy space will eliminate the chance of spilling of significant quantities of fluid into the tracheobronchial tree and is less likely to cause infection than a drain left in place continuously. However, surgery is usually necessary,[21] and a double-lumen tube (with the endobronchial lumen in the contralateral mainstem bronchus) should be used to separate the two lungs during surgery. Surgical procedures are as above.

V. RESPIRATORY INSUFFICIENCY

Acute respiratory insufficiency (within 30 days of resection) is probably the most common serious complication following pulmonary resection. Recent bronchial carcinoma resection data from a large thoracic surgery service indicate an incidence of 4.4 per cent, and in this study, the patients who developed acute respiratory failure had a mortality of 50 per cent.[23] Mortality from respiratory failure after right-sided pneumonectomy is greater than after pneumonectomy on the left side because the remaining functioning lung is smaller.[23] Chapter 3 discussed the mechanisms of hypoxemia and hypercarbia during anesthesia and surgery, and many of these mechanisms may continue to

function in the postoperative period. In addition, pulmonary resection per se involves additional new mechanisms of hypoxemia and hypercarbia.

Most of the mechanisms of hypoxemia during anesthesia and surgery involve a decrease in the functional residual capacity below the closing volume of the lung, causing either low ventilation-perfusion regions or atelectasis. First, postoperative pain will cause splinting of the chest wall, compression of the lungs, and a decrease in functional residual capacity. Second, splinting will also prevent coughing and deep breathing, which will promote retention of secretions, which, in turn, will decrease the functional residual capacity. These first two mechanisms of postoperative hypoxemia can be minimized by appropriate control of pain (see chapter 20). Third, the remaining lung in either hemithorax may be edematous and/or soiled with blood. The lung that was dependent during surgery may be edematous and/or may have aspirated blood (if a double-lumen tube was not used) owing to gravitational effects (in zones 3 and 4); the lung that was nondependent during surgery may be edematous and hemorrhagic owing to surgical compression and trauma. One-lung ventilation can minimize surgical trauma to the nondependent lung, and lung separation with a double-lumen tube will prevent aspiration of blood into the dependent lung. All of the remaining lung may be edematous because of infusion of excessive amounts of fluid to a now-diminished pulmonary vascular bed. The impact of diminishing the size of the pulmonary vascular bed should be predictable on the basis of preoperative pulmonary circulation and right ventricular testing results (see chapter 5). The major mechanism of carbon dioxide retention is fatigue of the respiratory muscles in attempting to move lungs that are now stiff, have a high airway resistance, and have a diminished gas exchange surface. The treatment of respiratory insufficiency is to institute mechanical ventilation, and while the patient is being mechanically ventilated (see chapter 19), the underlying causes of the failure should be diagnosed and reversed.

VI. RIGHT HEART FAILURE

Major pulmonary resection results in a decrease in the cross sectional area of the pulmonary vasculature and an increase in right ventricular afterload, which in some patients can result in acute right heart failure. Although patients at risk for developing right heart failure following pulmonary resection can usually be identified preoperatively,[24] right heart failure may also occur if additional stresses, such as infection and increased pulmonary blood flow and new active pulmonary vasoconstriction (such as caused by hypoxia, acidosis, and vasoactive amines and peptides), are placed on the right side of the heart. In addition, pulmonary hypertension and right ventricular afterload will be increased by increased pulmonary capillary and venous pressures, which may result from fluid overload and/or decreased left ventricular compliance (due to left ventricular ischemia and/or failure).

A pulmonary artery catheter should be used in any patient undergoing major pulmonary resection who is believed to be at risk for postoperative right- (or left-) sided cardiac failure; patients at risk for developing right-sided heart failure include those with an inferior wall myocardial infarction, which often involves the right ventricle, and those with preexisting pulmonary hypertension. The diagnosis of selective right heart failure is established when the right atrial pressure exceeds the left atrial pressure (i.e., the pulmonary artery wedge pressure) in the presence of an abnormally low cardiac output. In addition, pulmonary hypertension with a pulmonary artery diastolic-wedge pressure gradient will usually be present, along with the systemic signs of heart failure (oliguria, decreased mentation, and peripheral edema).

The treatment of acute right heart failure follows the same principles used in treating left-sided failure: control heart rate, optimize preload and the inotropic state of the ventricle, and reduce afterload (see chapter 13). Preload, as measured by central venous pressure, can be reduced by fluid restriction, by diuretics, or by a venous vasodilator such as nitroglycerin. Inotropic drug support should take into account the response of the pulmonary vasculature to the drug chosen. Thus dobutamine, a drug that tends to reduce pulmonary vascular resistance, is a reasonable choice in this setting.[25] Vasodilators that may be effective in reducing pulmonary vascular resistance include nitroglycerin, nitroprusside, and phentolamine. In addition to the above, treatment should include other measures aimed at reducing pulmonary arteriolar constriction. These include oxygen administration to reduce hypoxic pulmonary vasoconstriction, administration of aminophylline to relieve bronchospasm, antibiotic and chest physical therapy to clear infection (to diminish the size of the hypoxic compartment), and normalization of acid-base balance.

VII. RIGHT-TO-LEFT SHUNTING ACROSS A PATENT FORAMEN OVALE

Many adults have a patent foramen ovale; at autopsy, the incidence of a probe-patent foramen ovale is highest at 34 per cent during the first three decades of life and decreases to 20 per cent by the ninth and tenth decades.[26] There is normally no right-to-left shunting across the foramen ovale because left atrial pressure exceeds right atrial pressure, which keeps the one-way flap-valve of the foramen ovale pressed against the foramen ovale, resulting in a functionally competent seal. If the right atrial pressure exceeds left atrial pressure (as might occur during the use of PEEP[27]; in the course of pulmonary embolization,[28, 29] pulmonary hypertension,[28] chronic obstructive pulmonary disease,[30] pulmonary valvular stenosis,[27, 31] congestive heart failure,[27, 32] or cardiopulmonary bypass[28, 33, 34]; and during neurosurgical procedures complicated by air embolization[35]) the one-way flap-valve can open, and right-to-left shunting can occur through the foramen ovale (Fig. 18–3).

Several reports have documented new-onset right-to-left shunting across a patent foramen ovale or atrial septal defect following pneumonectomy[36–41] and lobectomy[42, 43] as a cause of otherwise unexplained postoperative dyspnea and systemic oxygen desaturation (Fig. 18–3). Mechanisms for the shunting across the patent foramen ovale include an increase in right atrial pressure to greater than left atrial pressure, which is caused by an increased pulmonary vascular resistance (due to the resection of vascular bed and/or anesthesia- and surgery-induced lung disease). In addition, a shift in the anatomic relationship of the inferior vena cava, right atrium, and intra-atrial septum due to the pulmonary resection can occur, so that the one-way flap-valve is functionally less competent and permits shunting across the foramen ovale (Fig. 18–3).

The diagnosis of right-to-left shunting across a patent foramen ovale should be suspected in any patient who is hypoxemic (with relatively normal chest roentgenogram findings) or who has a progressive PEEP-induced decrease in the arterial oxygenation tension (these latter patients likely have abnormal chest roentgenogram findings). In the latter circumstance PEEP

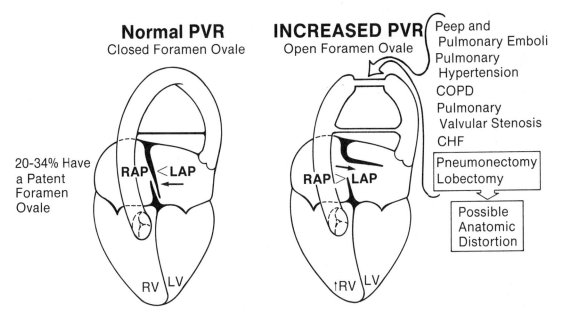

Figure 18–3. *Among the general population, 20 to 34 per cent have a patent foramen ovale. Normally, the patent foramen ovale remains functionally closed because left atrial pressure (LAP) exceeds right atrial pressure (RAP). When pulmonary vascular resistance is increased, such as following a pneumonectomy or lobectomy, right ventricular (RV) and right atrial pressures may be increased. If right atrial pressure exceeds left atrial pressure, then the foramen ovale opens and permits right-to-left shunting. (LV = left ventricle.)*

is presumably further increasing pulmonary vascular resistance and right ventricular and right atrial pressures, thereby increasing the right-to-left shunt across the foramen. In extubated patients the diagnosis should be suspected by otherwise unexplained clinically significant dyspnea and hypoxemia. Contrast two-dimensional echocardiography is an excellent, noninvasive method to diagnose this process, if suspected.[43] Contrast angiography and dye dilution curve analysis are the best definitive invasive diagnostic methods.[33]

Since surgical closure is stressful to the patient (it requires cardiopulmonary bypass) and, in the presence of pulmonary hypertension, may result in acute right ventricular failure, therapy should always first be nonsurgical and aimed at decreasing pulmonary vascular resistance and right ventricular and right atrial pressures. Thus, nonsurgical treatment consists of decreasing pulmonary vasoconstriction by clearing pulmonary infections, administering oxygen, reversing acidosis, eliminating conditions that release pulmonary vasoactive amines and peptides (such as hypotension and infection), using pulmonary vasodilators, and decreasing right-sided heart pressures by preload manipulation. These nonsurgical treatment modalities usually permit functional closure of the foramen ovale in the majority of patients.

The care of a patient with right-to-left intracardiac shunts must be meticulous. Avoidance of air bubbles in the intravenous lines is mandatory. Forceful flushing of poorly infusing venous catheters may result in systemic embolization.[32] Blood to be transfused should be filtered through a micropore filter to exclude particulate material. Since postoperative patients have an increased propensity to venous stasis, prophylactic anticoagulation should be considered to reduce the possibility of systemic thromboembolization.[32]

VIII. ARRHYTHMIAS

Supraventricular arrhythmias, primarily sinus tachycardia and atrial fibrillation and flutter, are frequent complications following major pulmonary resections, especially pneumonectomy.[44, 45] The potential causes of these arrhythmias following pulmonary resection include retraction and trauma to the heart and right ventricular and right atrial distension (due to increased pulmonary vascular resistance), perhaps compounded by preexisting cardiovascular disease, poor gas exchange, and sympathetic nervous system stimulation caused by pain. On occasion, especially in the aged,[46] these arrhythmias may cause circulatory embarrassment.[7]

General treatment consists of adequate sedation/analgesia and correction of hypoxia, hypercarbia or hypocarbia, and right heart failure (see Right Heart Failure above). Specific pharmacologic antiarrhythmia treatment is dependent on the particular arrhythmia[47] (see Table 13–8). Sinus tachycardia is treated with propranolol (0.5 mg every 2 minutes up to 5 mg). Paroxysmal atrial tachycardia can be treated with carotid sinus massage, along with edrophonium (2 to 10 mg) to improve the carotid massage response by increasing parasympathetic tone (first choice); neosynephrine (50 to 100 μg/dose), which will also make the carotid sinus massage more successful (second choice); verapamil (5 to 10 mg intravenously) (very close third); and propranolol (fourth choice). Treatment of atrial fibrillation is with digitalis (0.25 to 0.5 mg intravenously) if the patient is reasonably stable, verapamil (5 mg/dose) if the patient is moderately unstable, and externally synchronized cardioversion if the patient is extremely unstable. Treatment of atrial flutter consists of ouabain (0.1 to 0.2 mg intravenously) or verapamil (5 to 10 mg intravenously) (equal first choices), propranolol (second choice), and external cardioversion (third choice).

Ventricular arrhythmias, usually premature ventricular contractions, can be controlled with intravenously administered lidocaine and/or beta-blocking drugs. Ventricular fibrillation and tachycardia must be controlled by electric defibrillation, followed by xylocaine and, perhaps, propranolol and, rarely, bretylium administration. Temporary pacemaker insertion should be strongly considered for patients who have developed complete heart block.

IX. NEURAL INJURIES

During radical hilar dissection or excision of mediastinal tumors, phrenic, vagus, and recurrent laryngeal nerves may be injured accidentally or may be excised deliberately. Phrenic nerve injury causes respiratory embarrassment by a flail chest effect and also causes elevation of the ipsilateral hemidiaphragm. The diagnosis should be suspected in patients who have relatively clear chest roentgenograms, have adequate gas exchange, and cannot be weaned from the ventilator. The diagnosis can be confirmed by paradoxic movements of the diaphragm on fluoroscopy. Injury to the vagus nerve causes gastric and intestinal atony, which usually are

not problematic in the first few postoperative days. Bilateral partial injury of the recurrent laryngeal nerve causes adductor spasm of the vocal cords, which, following extubation, may result in upper airway obstruction. This must be diagnosed promptly and treated with immediate reintubation and possible tracheostomy until the dysfunction is resolved.

The recurrent laryngeal nerve or phrenic nerve usually shows return of function within 2 to 9 months after injury. If vocal cord function does not return after recurrent laryngeal nerve injury, the involved vocal cord may be injected with steroids, which often causes a return of function. In rare cases, surgical procedures, including the injection of Teflon, may have to be performed on the involved cord to improve its function. If phrenic nerve paralysis persists and continues to cause marked respiratory embarrassment due to paralysis of the diaphragm, it is possible to implant a phrenic nerve stimulator[48] or plicate the paralyzed diaphragm[20] to correct the respiratory insufficiency.

Aside from clamping of the thoracic aorta, there are two other causes of paraplegia following thoracotomy. First, damage to the spinal branches of intercostal arteries by dissection or diathermy at the posterior end of a rib will cause spinal cord ischemia.[49] This is most likely to occur with damage to the intercostal arteries of the left lower lobe.[50] Second, surgical dissection may create a communication between the epidural space and the pleural cavity. Clotted blood, or blood that can later clot, can then enter the epidural space and cause postoperative spinal cord compression and ischemia.[51]

There are other less serious neural injuries that are also specifically related to thoracic surgery. The brachial plexus is especially vulnerable to trauma during thoracic surgery and anesthesia.[52, 53] The brachial plexus has a potentially long superficial course in the axilla between two points of fixation, the vertebrae above and the axillary fascia below. If the two points of fixation are separated widely, stretching of the plexus will occur. Suspension of the arm from an ether screen in an excessive cephalad direction (see Fig. 10–1) in a paralyzed patient without muscle tone, which increases the distance between the two points of fixation, is the most common cause of stretching and damage to the brachial plexus. Stretching of the plexus is also promoted by extreme abduction, external rotation, and dorsal extension of the arm on an arm board.

The intercostal nerves are most exposed to injury during intrathoracic surgical procedures. A rib fracture occurring at the time of thoracotomy can compress the intercostal nerve, resulting in an intercostal neuritis, which is manifested by radicular pain in the postoperative period. When excessive stretching and tension are placed on the intercostal nerve roots while the chest is being opened, postoperative intercostal neuralgia may be quite severe. In addition, the chest tubes can produce a neuroma or neuritis by compression of the intercostal nerve.

X. COMPLICATIONS OF INTRATHORACIC INTERCOSTAL NERVE BLOCKS

The performance of intrathoracic intercostal nerve blocks under direct vision just prior to closure of the chest is a common method of securing immediate postoperative analgesia; in one large institution it has been estimated that these blocks are performed in 10 to 15 per cent of thoracotomy patients.[54] However, there have been case reports of total spinal anesthesia following this procedure.[54, 55] In these patients, following placement of intrathoracic intercostal nerve blocks at several different levels, there was an immediate profound decrease in blood pressure and pulse, persistent apnea, failure to regain consciousness, absence of reflexes, and dilated pupils, all of which are consistent with total spinal anesthesia. In addition, the temporal sequence of clinical recovery[56] and a clear-cut sensory level when the patient awakened also strongly indicate the occurrence of total spinal anesthesia.

There are several possible mechanisms for this complication. First, there can be outward prolongation of the subarachnoid space along the nerve roots. These dural cuffs can extend as far as 8 cm past the intervertebral foramen.[56] It is possible, then, that the local anesthetic was introduced into one or more dural cuffs surrounding the intercostal nerves. A second possibility is that the local anesthetic can spread centrally to the spinal fluid via the perineural spaces. A third possibility is that the local anesthetic could have been introduced directly into the subarachnoid space through an intervertebral foramen because of an unnoticed ill-placed angulation of the needle.

These reports constitute a relative contraindication to the performance of intercostal nerve blocks near the spinal cord with local anesthetics when the patient is under general anesthesia and when it is not possible to assess accurately the effect of the nerve blocks. These reports also emphasize the necessity of including spinal anesthesia in the differential diagnosis of postoperative cardiopulmonary and central nervous system depression when local anesthesia has been used in the vicinity of the spinal cord during general anesthesia.

REFERENCES

1. Allison PR: Intrapericardial approach to the lung root in the treatment of bronchial carcinoma by dissection pneumonectomy. J Thorac Cardiovasc Surg 15:99, 1946.
2. Yacoub, MH, Williams WG, Ahmad A: Strangulation of the heart following intrapericardial pneumonectomy. Thorax 23:261–265, 1968.
3. Gates GF, Sette RS, Cope JA: Acute cardiac herniation with incarceration following pneumonectomy. Radiology 94:561–562, 1970.
4. Takita H, Mijares WS: Herniation of the heart following intrapericardial pneumonectomy. Report of a case and review. J Thorac Cardiovasc Surg 59:443–446, 1970.
5. Beltrami V, Catenacci N: Cardiac herniation following intrapericardial pneumonectomy. Acta Chir Belg 76:293–295, 1977.
6. Deiraniya AK: Cardiac herniation following intrapericardial pneumonectomy. Thorax 29:545–552, 1974.
7. Kirsh MM, Rotman H, Behrendt DM, et al: Complications of pulmonary resection. Ann Thorac Surg 20:215, 1975.
8. McKlveen JR, Urgena RB, Rossi NP: Herniation of the heart following radical pneumonectomy: A case report. Anesth Analg 51:680, 1972.
9. Kirchoff AC: Herniation of the heart: Report of a case. Anesthesiology 12:774, 1951.
10. Grevel JA: Herniation of the heart—A hazard of thoracic surgery: Report of two fatal cases. Can J Surg 9:72, 1966.
11. Higginson JF: Block dissection in pneumonectomy for carcinoma. J Thorac Cardiovasc Surg 25:582, 1953.
12. Arndt RD, Frank CG, Schmitz AL, et al: Cardiac herniation with volvulus after pneumonectomy. Am J Roentgenol 130:155–156, 1978.
13. Gergely M, Urban AE, Deverall PB, et al: Herniation of the heart after intrapericardial pneumonectomy. Acta Chir Acad Sci Hung 18:129–132, 1977.
14. Cassorla L, Katz JA: Management of cardiac herniation after intrapericardial pneumonectomy. Anesthesiology 60:362, 1984.
15. Levin PD, Faber LP, Carleton RA: Cardiac herniation after pneumonectomy. J Thorac Cardiovasc Surg 61:104–106, 1971.
16. Wright MP, Nelson C, Johnson AM, et al: Herniation of the heart. Thorax 25:656–664, 1970.
17. Hidvegi RS, Abdulnour EM, Wilson JA: Herniation of the heart. J Can Assoc Radiol 32:185–187, 1981.
18. Rodgers BM, Moulder PV, DeLaney A: Thoracoscopy: New methods of early diagnosis of cardiac herniation. J Thorac Cardiovasc Surg 78:623–625, 1979.
19. Peterffy A, Henze A: Hemorrhagic complications during pulmonary resections: A retrospective review of

1428 resections with 113 hemorrhagic episodes. Scand J Thorac Cardiovasc Surg 17:283–287, 1983.

20. Cordel AR, Ellison RE: Complications of Intrathoracic Surgery. Boston, Little, Brown & Co, 1979, pp 240, 264, 284, 364.

21. Hankins JR, Miller JE, Attar S, et al: Bronchopleural fistula: Thirteen-year experience with 77 cases. J Thorac Cardiovasc Surg 76:755, 1978.

22. Malave G, Foster ED, Wilson JA, et al: Bronchopleural fistula. Present-day study of an old problem. Ann Thorac Surg 11:1–10, 1971.

23. Hirschler-Schulte CJW, Hylkema BS, Meyer RW: Mechanical ventilation for acute postoperative respiratory failure after surgery for bronchial carcinoma. Thorax 40:387–390, 1985.

24. Tisi GM: Preoperative evaluation of pulmonary function. Am Rev Respir Dis 119:293–310, 1979.

25. Harris P, Heath D: Pharmacology of the pulmonary circulation. In Harris P, Heath D (eds): The Human Pulmonary Circulation. New York, Churchill Livingstone, 1977, pp 182–210.

26. Hagen PT, Scholz DG, Edwards WD: Incidence and size of patent foramen ovale during the first 10 decades of life: An autopsy study of 965 normal hearts. Mayo Clin Proc 59:17–20, 1984.

27. Moorthy SS, Losasso AM: Patency of the foramen ovale in the critically ill patient. Anesthesiology 41:405–407, 1974.

28. Schroeckenstein RF, Wasenda GJ, Edwards JE: Valvular competent patent foramen ovale in adults. Minn Med 55:11–13, 1972.

29. Kovacs GS, Hill JD, Aberg T, et al: Pathogenesis of arterial hypoxemia in pulmonary embolism. Arch Surg 93:813–823, 1966.

30. Daly JJ: Venoarterial shunting in obstructive pulmonary disease. N Engl J Med 278:952–953, 1968.

31. Selzer A, Carnes WH: The role of pulmonary stenosis in the production of chronic cyanosis. Am Heart J 45:382–395, 1953.

32. Pieroni DR, Valdes-Cruz LM: Atrial right-to-left shunt in infants with respiratory and cardiac distress but without congenital heart disease: Demonstration by contrast echocardiography. Pediatr Cardiol 2:1–5, 1982.

33. Morthy SS, Losasso AM, Gibbs PS: Acquired right-to-left intracardiac shunts and severe hypoxemia. Crit Care Med 6:28–31, 1978.

34. Byrick RJ, Kolton M, Hart JT, et al: Hypoxemia following cardiopulmonary bypass. Anesthesiology 53:172–174, 1980.

35. Gronert GA, Messick JM Jr, Cucchiara RF, et al: Paradoxical air embolism from a patent foramen ovale. Anesthesiology 50:548–549, 1979.

36. Dlabel PW, Stutts BS, Jenkins DW, et al: Cyanosis following right pneumonectomy. Chest 81:370, 1982.

37. Holtzman H, Lippman M, Nakhjaran F, et al: Postpneumonectomy intraatrial right-to-left shunt. Thorax 35:307, 1980.

38. Schnabel GT, Ratto O, Kirby CK, et al: Postural cyanosis and angina pectoris following pneumonectomy: Relief by closure of an interatrial defect. J Thorac Surg 32:246, 1956.

39. Begin R: Platypnea after pneumonectomy. N Engl J Med 293:342, 1975.

40. LaBresh KA, Pietro DA, Coates EO, et al.: Platypnea syndrome after left pneumonectomy. Chest 79:605, 1981.

41. Seward JB, Hayes DL, Smith EC: Platypnea-orthodeoxia: Clinical profile, diagnostic workup, management, and report of seven cases. Mayo Clin Proc 59:221, 1984.

42. Springer RM, Gheorghiade M, Chakko CS, et al: Platypnea and intraatrial right-to-left shunting after lobectomy. Am J Cardiol 51:1802, 1983.

43. Vacek J, Foster J, Quinton RR, et al: Right-to-left shunting after lobectomy through a patent foramen ovale. Ann Thorac Surg 39:576–578, 1985.

44. Mowry F, Reynolds E: Cardiac rhythm disturbances complicating resectional surgery of the lung. Ann Intern Med 61:688, 1964.

45. Shields TW, Ujiki G: Digitalization for prevention of arrhythmias following pulmonary surgery. Surg Gynecol Obstet 126:743, 1968.

46. Breyer RH, Zippe C, Pharr WF, et al: Thoracotomy in patients over age seventy years: Ten-year experience. J Thorac Cardiovasc Surg 81:187, 1981.

47. Kaplan JA: Complications of thoracic surgery. In Kaplan JA (ed): Thoracic Anesthesia. New York, Churchill Livingstone, 1983, chapter 18, pp. 599–634.

48. Hatcher CR, Miller JI: Operative injuries to nerves during intrathoracic procedures. In Cordell RA, Ellison RG (eds): Complications of Intrathoracic Surgery. Boston, Little, Brown & Co, 1979, pp 363–365.

49. Henson RA, Parsons M: Ischemic lesions of the spinal cord: An illustrated review. Q J Med 142:205, 1967.

50. Mathew NT, John S: Iatrogenic ischemic paraplegia. Med J Aust 2:29, 1970.

51. Perez-Guerra F, Holland JM: Epidural hematoma as a cause of postpneumonectomy paraplegia. Ann Thorac Surg 39:282, 1985.

52. Clausen EG: Postoperative paralysis of the brachial plexus. Surgery 12:933–942, 1942.

53. Ewing MR: Postoperative paralysis in the upper extremity. Lancet 1:99–103, 1950.

54. Gallo JA, Lebowitz PW, Battit GE, et al: Complications of intercostal nerve blocks performed under direct vision during thoracotomy: A report of two cases. J Thorac Cardiovasc Surg 86:628–630, 1983.

55. Benumof JL, Semenza J: Total spinal anesthesia following intrathoracic intercostal nerve blocks. Anesthesiology 43:124–125, 1975.

56. Gillies IDS, Morgan M: Accidental total spinal analgesia with bupivacaine. Anesthesia 28:441–445, 1973.

57. Moore DC: Efocaine, complications following its use. West J Surg 61:635–638, 1953.

Mechanical Ventilation and Weaning

19

I. INTRODUCTION

The clearcut indications for postoperative mechanical ventilation (at least for a few hours) are numerous and include severe preexisting lung disease (see chapter 5), ventilatory depression due to residual anesthesia or paralysis (for example, the peak inspiratory force is less than 20 cm H_2O), presence of a significant amount of blood in the airway, massive intraoperative transfusion, following many pneumonectomies, large air leak following any resection (possible bronchopleural fistula), presence of flail chest, extensive surgical trauma to the lung remaining in the operative hemithorax, multiple and severe organ trauma, sepsis, and unacceptable arterial blood gas concentrations (perhaps due to the factors above). In addition to these obvious indications, continuing intubation and mechanical ventilation facilitates a smooth transition from the operating room to the intensive care unit (provided the patient is adequately anesthetized/sedated); allows the intraoperative use of high-dose narcotic anesthesia; enables adequate postoperative analgesia without concern for depression of respiration; allows a more aggressive approach to hemodynamic support (including intravascular volume loading) with-

out excessive concern for its effects on pulmonary function; avoids the need for application of intensive respiratory therapy in exhausted, stressed patients in the early postoperative period; allows restoration of functional residual capacity (FRC) prior to extubation, and facilitates return to the operating room if there are concerns about surgical complications. If postoperative mechanical ventilation is planned, even for only a few hours, the patient should continue to receive narcotics and be paralyzed, and the double-lumen tube should be changed to a single-lumen tube (except perhaps when there is a large bronchopleural fistula; see Differential Lung Ventilation below) prior to leaving the operating room.

The use of positive end-expiratory pressure (PEEP), constant positive airway pressure (CPAP), and intermittent mandatory ventilation (IMV), of either a spontaneously breathing or an apneic patient, and an increased understanding of the toxicity of unnecessarily high inspired concentrations of oxygen (F_IO_2) constitute the cornerstones of modern clinical mechanical ventilation management. This chapter describes, in a step-by-step manner, the current practice of mechanical ventilation, weaning, and extubation.[1-4] The recommendations for initial ventilator settings (see below) are based on the assumption that the patient's lungs are disordered and, therefore, require a considerable amount of support. In addition, it is assumed that a volume-limited ventilator is being used, the patient is adequately sedated, and the endotracheal tube and chest tubes are functioning properly.

II. INITIAL VENTILATOR SETTINGS: INTERMITTENT MANDATORY VENTILATION

Intermittent mandatory ventilation (IMV) means that the ventilator delivers a positive-pressure breath a mandatory number of times per minute while the patient does as much spontaneous breathing as desired between these mechanical breaths. The IMV mode of ventilation is at present the most commonly used and preferable ventilation mode for several reasons. First, because the patients are allowed to do, and usually are doing, some spontaneous ventilation, they are able to generate a more negative pleural pressure, which better maintains venous return and cardiac output (compared with simple intermittent positive-pressure ventilation [IPPV]). Second, and consequently, less intravenous fluid is usually required to maintain systemic pressure and perfusion. Third, since it is not necessary to eliminate these spontaneous breaths, sedation requirements are minimized, and paralysis requirements are eliminated. Fourth, the patients benefit psychologically because they know they are breathing on their own. Fifth, the respiratory muscles remain coordinated because they are exercised. Finally, when the weaning stage is reached, IMV allows a gradual transition from ventilator dependence to independence. There are a number of other mechanical ventilation modes that also facilitate mechanical ventilation and/or the transition from mechanical ventilation to weaning, such as pressure support (PS), mandatory minute ventilation (MMV), inverse ratio ventilation (IRV), and airway pressure release ventilation (APRV), which have recently been introduced; these will be discussed under Other New Mechanical Ventilation and Weaning Modes.

With conventional IMV, it is possible for the ventilator to begin to deliver a mechanical breath just as the patient is completing a spontaneous inhalation. This results in the stacking of a machine breath on top of a spontaneous breath and can lead to overdistension of the

lungs and high peak inspiratory pressures. This problem can be overcome by use of synchronized IMV (SIMV). With SIMV, the ventilator intermittently senses the onset of a spontaneous breath a mandatory number of times per minute and immediately causes a machine (positive-pressure) breath to occur. Consequently, the machine breath overrides the spontaneous breath, and stacking of breaths cannot take place.

Mechanical ventilation is initiated with a tidal volume of 12 ml/kg of lean body weight, an IMV respiratory rate so that the arterial carbon dioxide tension (P_aCO_2) is 40 mm Hg (which usually requires an initial rate of 8 to 12 breaths/min), and an inspired oxygen fraction (F_IO_2) of 1.0 (Table 19–1). Although patients may breathe spontaneously during IMV (which is especially helpful with regard to lowering pleural pressure and maintaining cardiac output), IMV should be regarded as providing total and full ventilatory support (i.e., the IMV breaths, not the spontaneous breaths, determine the minute ventilation).[5, 6] One hundred per cent oxygen should initially be used in order to update and document the level of right-to-left shunting and alveolar-arterial oxygen tension difference while minimizing the risk of unexpected hypoxemia. Administration of 100 per cent oxygen for a short period of time is not toxic (see below).

A tidal volume of 12 ml/kg is considered large tidal volume ventilation. Large tidal volume ventilation is desirable because it prevents the development of miliary atelectasis or microatelectasis that is associated with constant small tidal volume ventilation (for example, 6 ml/kg).[7] The miliary atelectasis or microatelectasis that is associated with small tidal volume ventilation results in a progressive increase in the alveolar-arterial oxygen tension difference and a progressive decrease in compliance. These deleterious changes associated with small tidal volume ventilation can be reversed by intermittent sighs. Large tidal volume ventilation, therefore, functions as frequent intermittent sighs and, thereby, minimizes the development of atelectasis. A smaller tidal volume of 8 to 10 ml/kg

Table 19–1. Initial Ventilator Settings

1. IMV or SIMV mode
2. Tidal volume 12 ml/kg
3. Respiratory rate so that P_aCO_2 = 40 mm Hg (usually 8 to 12 breaths/min)
4. F_IO_2 = 1.0
5. I/E = 1:2 to 3
6. Inspiratory flow rate 30 L/min

should be used in patients with bullous or cystic disease of the lung in an effort to minimize peak inspiratory pressures and risk of tension pneumothorax.

The respiratory rate should be set so that the patient has a normal arterial carbon dioxide tension (this rate is usually 8 to 12 breaths/min). Certainly, hypercarbia should be avoided in the vast majority of patients, since the accompanying acidosis is dangerous, and the hypoventilation necessary to produce hypercarbia may also cause hypoxemia. Mild degrees of hypercarbia (P_aCO_2 40 to 50 mm Hg) are indicated for patients who are chronic carbon dioxide retainers; mild hypercarbia helps to avoid changing the arterial and cerebrospinal fluid pH and bicarbonate levels from the values that the patient normally lives with. Hypocarbia should be avoided for multiple reasons. First, hypocarbia may cause a decrease in cardiac output via several mechanisms. In order to produce hypocarbia, an increased amount of positive-pressure ventilation will have to be used, which will decrease venous return. Hypocarbia also causes a withdrawal of sympathetic tone, which will decrease the inotropic state of the heart. Hypocarbia and alkalosis may decrease the level of ionized calcium, which will also decrease the inotropic state of the heart. Second, hypocarbia will also shift the oxygen-hemoglobin dissociation curve to the left, which increases the hemoglobin affinity for oxygen; at the tissue level, the increased hemoglobin-oxygen binding impedes the delivery of oxygen to the tissues. Third, hypocarbia and alkalosis will increase oxygen consumption. The increase in oxygen consumption is due to a pH-mediated uncoupling of oxidation from phosphorylation; the uncoupling requires more oxygen to be passed along the respiratory chain to generate the same amount of adenosine triphosphate.[8, 9] Quantitatively, at a P_aCO_2 of 40 mm Hg oxygen consumption is 250 ml/min, whereas at a P_aCO_2 of 20 mm Hg oxygen consumption is 500 ml/min. Thus, hypocarbia may increase tissue oxygen demand (as a result of increased oxygen consumption) at a time when it is not possible to increase tissue oxygen supply (oxygen-hemoglobin dissociation curve is shifted to the left and cardiac output is decreased). Fourth, hypocarbia may cause ventilation-perfusion abnormalities by inhibiting hypoxic pulmonary vasoconstriction and/or by causing bronchoconstriction and decreased lung compliance. Fifth, hyperventilation with alkalosis may cause ventricular irritability (perhaps due, in part, to a concomitant hypokalemia). However, the benefit of hyperventilation with hypocarbia to decrease an elevated intracranial pressure in head-injured patients may supersede the above cited physiologic disadvantages.

If the measured P_aCO_2 differs from the desired level, one can easily calculate the amount of change in minute ventilation needed to produce the desired change in P_aCO_2 by using the relationship:

$$V_E{}^2 = (P_aCO_2{}^1/P_aCO_2{}^2) \times V_E{}^1$$

where $V_E{}^2$ = the desired minute volume, $V_E{}^1$ = the actual minute volume, $P_aCO_2{}^2$ = the desired P_aCO_2, and $P_aCO_2{}^1$ = the actual P_aCO_2. Use of total minute ventilation, which includes both alveolar ventilation and dead space ventilation, instead of using only alveolar minute ventilation, is clinically acceptable since the dead space remains relatively constant with moderate changes in tidal volume.[10] A change in either respiratory rate or tidal volume, or both, can be used to change minute ventilation.

The use of large tidal volume ventilation usually makes it possible to achieve normocarbia with relatively slow respiratory rates (8 to 12 breaths/min). This is highly desirable in two ways. First, slow rates allow a decrease in the inspiration-expiration (I/E) ratio. A long expiratory time increases venous return and augments cardiac output; it facilitates full expiration and avoids air trapping and obstructive lung disease. The I/E ratio should be approximately 1:2 or 3 (except when airway resistance is high and an even longer exhalation period and lower I/E ratio are required). Second, slow respiratory rates also allow slower inspiratory flow while maintaining an appropriately low I/E ratio. The slower the inspiratory flow, the more laminar and less turbulent is the air stream. This decreases airway resistance, reduces airway trauma, and allows for a more even distribution of inspired gas to lung regions with different time constants. The inspiratory flow should be approximately 30 L/min.

III. GOAL #1: $\boxed{F_iO_2 < 0.5}$ AND P_aO_2 ACCEPTABLE

A. Why This Goal Is #1: Oxygen Toxicity

An inspired oxygen fraction (F_iO_2) greater than 0.5 is toxic to the lungs,[11, 12] and the first and compelling goal is to get the inspired oxygen fraction to less than 0.5 while maintaining an acceptable P_aO_2 (Table 19–2). The mechanism of oxygen-induced lung damage is the local accumulation of toxic, tissue-reactive free radicals, such as superoxide and hydrogen peroxide, which damage the pulmonary tissues. For this discussion, an acceptable P_aO_2 is defined as one that will be above the steep part of the oxygen-hemoglobin dissociation curve (see Fig. 3–29), and for all patients this will be a value greater than 60 mm Hg. A P_aO_2 value that is above the steep part of the oxygen-hemoglobin dissociation curve provides some margin of arterial oxygenation reserve and is protective against decreases in $P_{\bar{v}}O_2$. In addition, a P_aO_2 greater than 60 mm Hg will not cause or promote ventricular arrhythmias.

The rate of onset of oxygen-induced pulmonary damage is proportional both to the inspired tension of oxygen and to the duration of the exposure. In normal human volunteers, the first symptom after 6 hours of exposure to 100 per cent oxygen is substernal distress, which begins as a mild irritation in the area of the carina and may be accompanied by occasional coughing. As exposure continues, pain becomes more intense, and the urges to cough and deep breathe also become more intense. When the inspired oxygen tension has been 1.0 for greater than 12 hours, the pain, dyspnea, and paroxysmal coughing are severe. As toxicity progresses, these symptoms are accompanied by objective signs of lung compromise, such as a decreased vital capacity and lung compliance, and deterioration in blood gas concentrations. Finally, in animals, after days to weeks, acute respiratory failure occurs, and unless gas exchange is supported by mechanical ventilation, death ensues.

Pathologically, in animals, the lesion progresses from a tracheobronchitis (exposure for 12 hours to a day), to pulmonary interstitial edema (exposure for a few days to a week), to pulmonary fibrosis (exposure for greater than a week).[13] Often these pathologic changes are indistinguishable from those of the adult respiratory distress syndrome. Dose-time toxicity curves for humans indicate that oxygen toxicity does not occur when the inspired oxygen fraction is less than 0.5 (even for long periods of time).

B. How to Achieve Goal #1

PEEP is the treatment of choice of arterial hypoxemia due to right-to-left shunting through low ventilation-perfusion and atelectatic lung regions. PEEP increases end-expiratory lung volume (FRC), thereby preventing closure of airways at end-exhalation, and recruits alveoli and airways during inspiration (see Figs. 3–24 and 3–25). The prevention of airway closure and recruitment of alveoli increases ventilation-perfusion relationships and reverses atelectasis.[1] The beneficial effect of the application of PEEP and the deleterious effect of removal of PEEP on arterial oxygenation can be observed within minutes.[14, 15] The end-point for PEEP application is the lowest level of PEEP that provides an adequate P_aO_2 on an F_IO_2 of less than 0.5.[16] Increasing PEEP beyond this level to obtain optimal values for various other end-points, such as the production of maximum oxygen transport,[17] maximum static pulmonary compliance,[17] shunt less than 15 per cent,[18, 19] minimal arterial–end-tidal carbon dioxide gradient,[20] decreased mixed venous oxygen tension,[21] and minimal F_IO_2,[22] will not be clinically helpful and may cause harm[16] (see below). In addition, most of these other end-points require invasive monitoring, and/or vary independently of the PEEP level (i.e., they have multiple determinants and, therefore, have a fair amount

Table 19–2. Mechanical Ventilation and Weaning Plan

Goal (Temporal Sequence to Be Followed)	Goal				Achieved Primarily By
1. ↓ F_IO_2	↓ F_IO_2 <0.5			P_aO_2 >60 mm Hg	PEEP titration
2. ↓ PEEP	↓ F_IO_2 <0.5,	↓ PEEP <10 cm H_2O,		P_aO_2 >60 mm Hg	Respiratory care regimen
3. ↓ IMV rate	↓ F_IO_2 <0.5,	↓ PEEP <10 cm H_2O,	↓ IMV <1 breath/min,	P_aO_2 >60 mm Hg	Patient having adequate breathing power

of background variation), and/or respond sluggishly to changes in lung pathology.

The decrease in inspired oxygen concentration below 50 per cent is achieved by performing a dose (PEEP)–response (P_aO_2) titration. PEEP is progressively added (range 0 to 20 mm Hg) until the P_aO_2 is relatively normal for that patient (or at least above 60 mm Hg) with an F_IO_2 less than 0.5. PEEP should be raised in increments of 2.5 to 5.0 cm H_2O; the patient should be allowed to stabilize with regard to respiratory mechanics (peak inspiratory pressure, compliance), hemodynamics (pulse rate and rhythm, systemic and central filling pressures, and cardiac and urine output), and gas exchange (arterial blood gases). Usually each PEEP increment requires 0.5 to 1 hour to complete. Consequently, the performance of a PEEP–F_IO_2/P_aO_2 titration usually takes only several hours.

In many patients there appears to be a certain critical level of PEEP above which there is sudden and dramatic improvement in P_aO_2. In the vast majority of patients, levels of 5 to 12 cm H_2O are sufficient for substantial reversal of intrapulmonary shunting; it is seldom necessary to go as high as 15 cm H_2O. Of course, as the PEEP titration is being performed, other respiratory care modalities (see below), such as suctioning, turning, and administration of antibiotics, are instituted. The advent of fiberoptic bronchoscopy has eliminated the need for use of super-PEEP (PEEP greater than 20 to 25 cm H_2O) because regions of collapsed lung that are resistant to opening by PEEP are usually obvious on chest roentgenogram and can be suctioned and lavaged open under direct vision.

As the PEEP requirement increases, necessity for cardiovascular support and, therefore, monitoring requirements (central venous and pulmonary capillary wedge pressures and cardiac and urine output) generally increase.[23] It may be expected that hypovolemic patients will have a decrease in cardiac output as soon as PEEP is applied. Normovolemic patients will maintain cardiac output within normal limits up to a PEEP of 10 cm H_2O because compensatory peripheral venoconstriction maintains venous return. However, normovolemic patients will have a progressive decrease in cardiac output with a progressive increase in PEEP greater than 10 cm H_2O. Postpneumonectomy patients with an increased pulmonary vascular resistance may be expected to have a greater decrease in cardiac output at any given level of PEEP compared with patients with normal lungs.[24]

Again, in all patients, use of the IMV mode with some spontaneous ventilation is protective of the cardiac output.

The first cardiovascular support response to PEEP-induced impairment of hemodynamics should be a moderate augmentation of intravascular volume.[25] If fluid infusion does not restore satisfactory hemodynamic balance, then inotropic agents should be used to provide cardiovascular support. In patients with acute hypoxemic respiratory failure, dobutamine causes an increase in cardiac output with a decrease in pulmonary capillary wedge pressure and end-diastolic and end-systolic ventricular volumes (due to decreased afterload), whereas dopamine increases cardiac output, pulmonary capillary wedge pressure, and end-diastolic and end-systolic volumes (due to increased afterload).[26] Since even small increases in pulmonary capillary wedge pressure may increase the accumulation of pulmonary water in permeability pulmonary edema,[27–29] dobutamine appears to be the inotropic drug of choice.[26]

C. Mechanisms of PEEP-Induced Decreased Cardiac Output

One of the major limiting factors to the application of PEEP is a decrease in cardiac output. In the past several years, multiple mechanisms have been proposed for the PEEP-induced decrease in cardiac output; the following mechanisms have been reasonably well supported by experimental and clinical observations.

1. Decreased Venous Return [30, 31]

PEEP causes an increase in intrathoracic pressure, which decreases the gradient for blood to flow into the central intrathoracic veins from the peripheral veins (Fig. 19–1A). Up to a PEEP level of 10 cm H_2O in normovolemic patients and animals, sympathetically mediated venoconstriction increases peripheral venous pressure, thereby maintaining a normal pressure gradient for venous return. However, a progressive increase in PEEP greater than 10 cm H_2O causes a progressive decrease in cardiac output in normovolemic animals and patients. The decrease in cardiac output can usually be offset by fluid infusion only, which also results in increased peripheral venous pressure but at the expense of a hypervolemia relative to the blood volume that existed at 0 cm H_2O end-

Mechanisms of PEEP-Induced Decreased Cardiac Output

A. Decreased Venous Return

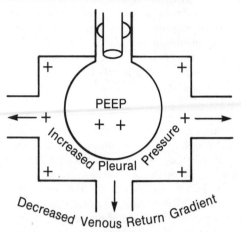

B. Increased Pulmonary Vascular Resistance and Right Ventricular Dysfunction

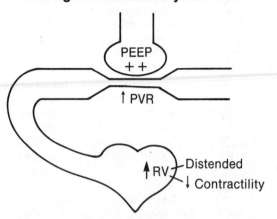

C. Leftward Displacement of Interventricular Septum

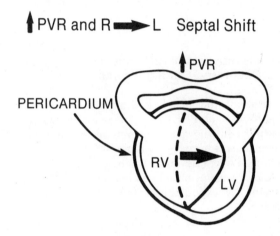

D. Decreased Transmural Ventricular Filling Pressure

E. Neural Reflexes

F. Humoral Reflexes

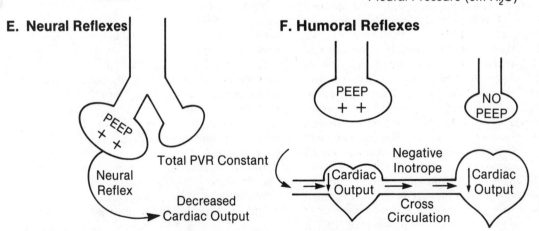

Figure 19-1. See legend on opposite page

expiratory pressure.[32] Because a sympathetically mediated venoconstriction at least partially offsets the hemodynamic effect of PEEP, it is not surprising that a significantly greater decrease in cardiac output at any given PEEP level can be caused by alpha-adrenergic blockade with phenyoxybenzamine.[30] Occasionally, infusion of a venoconstrictor (alpha-adrenergic stimulation) is necessary to restore satisfactory hemodynamics.[30]

2. Increased Pulmonary Vascular Resistance and Right Ventricular Dysfunction [33]

Pulmonary vascular resistance is a U-shaped function of increasing lung volume (see Fig. 3–13). The trough of the U-shaped total pulmonary vascular resistance curve occurs at normal functional residual capacity (FRC). As lung volume increases above FRC, the small intraalveolar vessels are compressed, and small vessel pulmonary vascular resistance increases, causing an increase in total pulmonary vascular resistance. As lung volume decreases below FRC, large vessel resistance increases, causing an increase in total pulmonary vascular resistance. The increase in large vessel resistance below FRC is due to hypoxic pulmonary vasoconstriction (small lungs are hypoxic); mechanical tortuosity of vessels is not thought to significantly contribute to the increased resistance.

It can be seen from Figure 3–13 that the effect of PEEP on pulmonary vascular resistance is dependent upon the initial lung volume at which the PEEP is applied (i.e., where the patient is on the U-shaped curve). If PEEP increases lung volume from a small volume to a normal FRC, pulmonary vascular resistance may decrease (due to a decrease in large vessel resistance), and cardiac output may increase. If PEEP increases lung volume from a normal FRC to a large value, pulmonary vascular resistance may increase greatly (due to an increase in small vessel resistance).

The increase in total pulmonary vascular resistance with large lung volumes increases the afterload on the right ventricle. The right ventricle is a thinly muscled cavity and can easily dysfunction (distend and have poor contractility)[34] when pulmonary vascular resistance (af-

terload) is greatly increased (Figs. 19–1 through 19–3). Consequently, a progressive PEEP-induced increase in pulmonary vascular resistance causes a progressive decrease in right ventricular output (Fig. 19–1B).

3. Leftward Displacement of Interventricular Septum [25]

Recent evidence has shown that progressively increasing PEEP causes the following sequence of events: increased pulmonary vascular resistance and right ventricular afterload; right ventricular free wall expansion and distension, which causes complete filling of the pericardial sac; and finally, movement of the interventricular septum into the left ventricle (Fig. 19–1 C). When the right ventricle has filled the pericardial sac, both ventricles must function within the common and unyielding stiffness of the pericardium, and the only structure that can give (allow further right ventricular expansion) in response to continued or increased pressure loading of the right ventricle is the interventricular septum. Compression by the overlying lungs may also prevent further right ventricular free wall expansion.

The right-to-left shift in the position of the interventricular septum causes the septum, which is normally convex toward the right ventricle, to become increasingly flat and perhaps concave toward the right ventricle. The displacement of the septum into the left ventricle interferes with left ventricular filling, compliance, and contractility.[35–39] Therefore, by its restraining influence on both ventricles, the pericardium enforces dynamic ventricular interaction[39, 40] through septal shifting, and left ventricular volume and diastolic pressure depend on the amount of right ventricular filling.[41] It is also apparent that at high PEEP levels the decrease in cardiac output may be due to acute biventricular failure.

4. PEEP-Induced Decreases in Transmural Ventricular Filling Pressures [42, 43]

The application of PEEP can cause a decrease in the transmural ventricular filling pressure (intracavitary pressure relative to pleural pres-

---

Figure 19–1. Mechanisms of PEEP-induced decreased cardiac output consist of decreased venous return (A), increased pulmonary vascular resistance and right ventricular dysfunction (B), leftward displacement of the interventricular septum (C), decreased transmural filling pressure (D), neural reflexes (E), and humoral reflexes (F). (+ = positive pressure (above atmospheric); PEEP = positive end-expiratory pressure; PVR = pulmonary vascular resistance; RV = right ventricle; R = right; L = left; LV = left ventricle; ZEEP = zero end-expiratory pressure.) See text for full explanation of each of these mechanisms.

↑ PVR ⟶ RV Distention

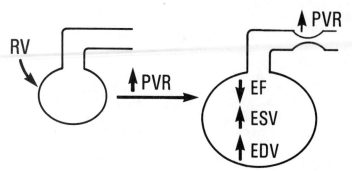

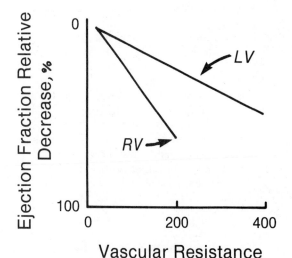

Figure 19–2. Increased pulmonary vascular resistance (PVR) causes a decrease in right ventricular (RV) ejection fraction (EF) and an increase in RV end-systolic volume (ESV) and end-diastolic volume (EDV). The increase in ESV and EDV results in right ventricular distension.

sure). Transmural ventricular filling pressures can decrease owing to differential (partial) transmission of the PEEP applied at the mouth to the pleural space and then from the pleural space to the cavities within the ventricles. Consider the example shown in Figure 19–1D. Initial conditions (pre-PEEP) consist of pressure of 0 cm H_2O at the mouth, pleural pressure of

Figure 19–3. The x-axis (vascular resistance per cent increase) and y-axis (ejection fraction relative decrease) in this diagram are constructed from data in reference 34 and refer to the combinations of pulmonary vascular resistance/right ventricle (RV) and systemic vascular resistance/left ventricle (LV). The right ventricle experiences a much more precipitous decrease in ejection fraction when pulmonary vascular resistance is increased compared with the decrease in left ventricular ejection fraction when the systemic vascular resistance is increased.

−5 cm H_2O, and a left ventricular end-diastolic filling pressure (relative to atmospheric pressure outside the body) of 5 cm H_2O, resulting in a transmural ventricular filling pressure (relative to pleural pressure) of 10 cm H_2O. Following the application of 10 cm H_2O of PEEP at the mouth, pleural pressure increases, but only by 7 cm H_2O, to a resultant 2 cm H_2O. Similarly, intracavitary ventricular filling pressure increases (relative to atmospheric pressure outside the body), but only by 4 cm H_2O, to a resultant 9 cm H_2O. However, the transmural ventricular filling pressure has now decreased to 7 cm H_2O. Thus, the 10 cm H_2O of PEEP applied at the mouth was only partially transmitted to the pleural space, and, in turn, was only partially transmitted to the cavities within the ventricles; the differential transmission of PEEP resulted in a decrease in the transmural ventricular filling pressure from 10 to 7 cm H_2O. Decrease in true transmural filling pressures of the ventricles decreases preload and cardiac output (leftward and downward move along a ventricular function curve).

5. Neural Reflex Cardiovascular Depression During Unilateral Lung Hyperinflation [44-46]

In experiments in open-chested dogs, acute unilateral pulmonary hyperinflation caused a decrease in cardiac output and heart rate. [44-46] Since the experimental design precluded changes in ventricular preload or afterload, these negative cardiovascular effects were attributed to a neural reflex (Fig. 19–1E). There are three known afferent receptors in the lung, and all can be stimulated by mechanically distending the lung. When stimulated, the stretch receptors evoke a modest increase in blood pressure and heart rate, the irritant receptors evoke no known cardiovascular response, and C-fiber receptors evoke a marked bradycardia and hypotension. Thus, the observed cardiovascular effects of unilateral lung hyperinflation in the dog experiments, namely a marked fall in heart rate and blood pressure and stroke volume, were likely the result of stimulation of C-fiber receptors within the lung itself.

6. Humoral Mediation of PEEP-Induced Decreases in Cardiac Output[45-51]

The PEEP-induced decrease in cardiac output may be caused by release of a cardiodepressant humoral substance or metabolite (Fig. 19–1F). For example, hyperinflation of in vitro and in vivo lung can release a variety of biologically active materials, such as the biogenic amines, polypeptides, proteolytic enzymes, and prostaglandins. Most of these substances can cause depression of cardiac function. A humoral mechanism of PEEP-induced decrease in cardiac output is further suggested by cross circulation experiments in animals, wherein 15 cm H_2O PEEP to one member of a cross circulated pair caused a decrease in the cardiac output of the other member, and by in vitro experiments that show that plasma from animals subjected to PEEP contains a negative inotropic agent, which is not present during zero end-expiratory pressure (Fig. 19–1F).

D. Differential Lung Ventilation

In the vast majority of patients with bilateral lung disease, the application of PEEP to both of the lungs increases the functional residual capacity of both lungs, thereby reversing atelectasis and increasing the ventilation-perfusion ratio of both lungs (see Figs. 3–24, 3–25, and 19–4). Similarly, in the vast majority of patients with unilateral lung disease, the application of PEEP to both of the lungs increases the functional residual capacity of the diseased lung toward normal while not excessively increasing the functional residual capacity of the normal lung (Fig. 19–5). However, in some patients with unilateral lung disease, PEEP to both of the lungs may fail to expand the diseased lung and excessively distend the normal lung. The distension of the normal lung may selectively increase pulmonary vascular resistance in the nondiseased lung and shunt blood flow to the diseased lung, thereby increasing the right-to-left shunt and causing a paradoxic decrease in the arterial oxygen tension[52, 53] (Fig. 19–6). Similarly, in some patients with bilateral lung disease, in which the disease is in the basilar regions (with normal apical regions), PEEP to both lungs may fail to expand the bases and may excessively distend apical regions (Fig. 19–7). The excessive distension of apical regions may selectively increase pulmonary vascular resistance in the apical regions and shunt blood flow to the atelectatic and low ventilation-perfusion ratio basilar regions, thereby increasing the right-to-left shunt and causing a paradoxic decrease in the arterial oxygen tension.[54, 55]

In situations in which PEEP increases the right-to-left shunt and decreases the arterial oxygen tension (unilateral or asymmetric lung disease and bilateral basilar disease), differential lung ventilation and PEEP can result in much more selective application of PEEP to the diseased area. In the first instance (unilateral lung

CONVENTIONAL TWO LUNG PEEP

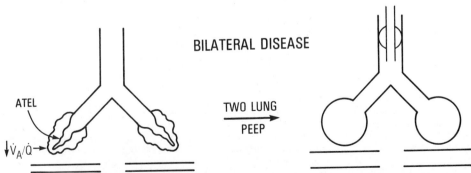

Figure 19–4. Application of PEEP to both lungs through a single-lumen tube in patients with bilateral lung disease usually results in a reversal of low ventilation to perfusion relationships and atelectasis in both lungs. (ATEL = atelectasis; ↓ V/Q = low ventilation-perfusion ratio.)

CONVENTIONAL TWO LUNG PEEP

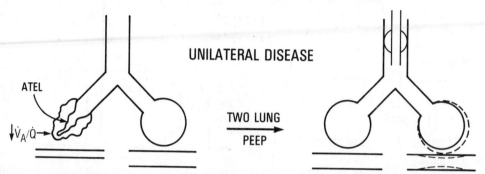

UNILATERAL DISEASE

ATEL

$\downarrow \dot{V}_A/\dot{Q}\rightarrow$

TWO LUNG
PEEP

Figure 19–5. Application of PEEP to both lungs through a single-lumen tube to patients with unilateral lung disease usually results in a reversal of low ventilation to perfusion relationships and atelectasis in the one diseased lung. (ATEL = atelectasis; $\downarrow \dot{V}_A/\dot{Q}$ = low ventilation-perfusion ratio.)

SELECTIVE APPLICATION OF PEEP TO NORMOXIC LUNG

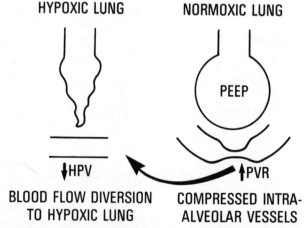

HYPOXIC LUNG   NORMOXIC LUNG

PEEP

$\downarrow$HPV $\uparrow$PVR

BLOOD FLOW DIVERSION   COMPRESSED INTRA-
TO HYPOXIC LUNG   ALVEOLAR VESSELS

Figure 19–6. Application of PEEP to both normoxic and hypoxic regions may fail to expand the hypoxic lung regions. This results in the selective application of PEEP to just the normoxic lung. The selective application of PEEP to only the normoxic lung can compress the small intra-alveolar vessels in the normoxic lung and increase normoxic lung pulmonary vascular resistance (PVR). The increase in normoxic lung PVR can cause diversion of blood flow to the hypoxic lung and effectively decrease hypoxic pulmonary vasoconstriction (HPV) in the hypoxic lung.

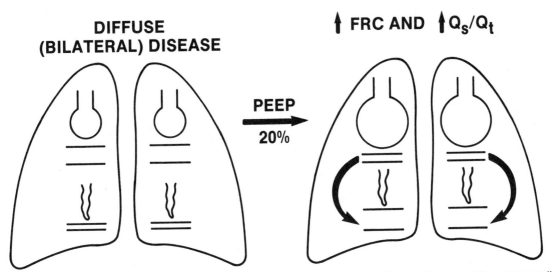

Figure 19–7. *The application of PEEP to both lungs, when both lungs contain diseased basilar regions, may result in distension of the apical regions, causing a selective increase in pulmonary vascular resistance in the apical regions, which results in a diversion of blood flow from the apical regions to the basilar regions. This may occur 20 per cent of the time that PEEP is applied to this kind of situation.[54, 55] The distension of the apices results in an increase in functional residual capacity (FRC), and the diversion of blood flow to the basilar regions results in an increase in shunt ($\dot{Q}_s/\dot{Q}_t$).*

disease), the application of PEEP to the two lungs (via a double-lumen tube) in an inverse proportion to their compliances should result in equal and normal functional residual capacities in both lungs[56] (Fig. 19–8). In this way a high level of PEEP is applied to only the diseased area in a much more economic and efficient manner. Since the PEEP is just being applied to part of the lung, the effects on cardiac output are much decreased.

In the second instance (bilateral basilar disease), reversal of atelectasis and improvement in ventilation-perfusion ratio in both lungs can be accomplished by placing the patient in the lateral decubitus position, ventilating each lung separately (via a double-lumen tube), and applying PEEP to only the dependent lung[57] (Fig. 19–9). The nondependent lung will improve its function by experiencing a low pulmonary vascular pressure, which results in a low blood

Differential Lung PEEP

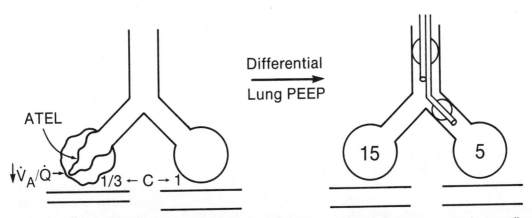

Figure 19–8. *Differential lung PEEP applies PEEP to each of the two lungs in an amount that is inversely proportional to the compliance of each of the lungs. Differential lung PEEP must be applied via a double-lumen tube. In this example the diseased lung has one third the compliance of the more normal lung and, therefore, receives three times as much PEEP. (ATEL = atelectasis; $\downarrow \dot{V}_A/\dot{Q}$ = low ventilation-perfusion ratio.)*

BILATERAL DEPENDENT BASILAR LUNG DISEASE

LATERAL DECUBITUS POSITION, DIFFERENTIAL LUNG VENTILATION, SELECTIVE DEPENDENT LUNG PEEP

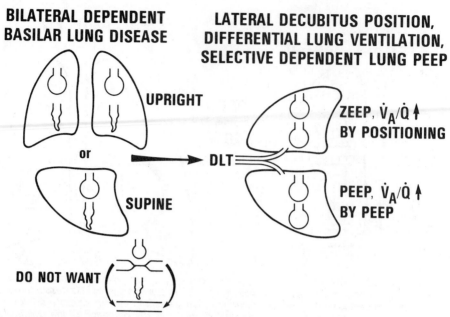

Figure 19–9. Schematic summarization of the results of the study in reference 57. Ventilation-perfusion ratios ($\dot{V}_A/\dot{Q}$) may be improved in patients with bilateral dependent basilar lung disease (viewed from either the upright or supine position) by turning the patient into the lateral decubitus position and ventilating the patient with differential lung ventilation via a double-lumen tube (DLT). The differential lung ventilation consists of zero end-expiratory pressure (ZEEP) to the nondependent lung and positive end-expiratory pressure (PEEP) to the dependent lung. The nondependent lung will improve its ventilation to perfusion relationship by virtue of being in a favorable nondependent position (see Figure 19–11), whereas the dependent lung will improve its ventilation to perfusion relationship by virtue of selectively receiving PEEP. This method avoids the problem of distension of the apical regions causing increased apical pulmonary vascular resistance resulting in blood flow diversion to basilar regions of the lung (see lower left-hand corner inset).

flow and shunt in the nondependent lung and a propensity to resorb fluid rather than transudate fluid in the nondependent lung. The dependent lung will improve its function by virtue of the application of selective PEEP to that lung. Again, the selective application of PEEP to only one lung minimizes effects on venous return and preserves the cardiac output.

The main criterion for initiation of differential lung ventilation is when PEEP to all of the lung causes an increase in shunt and a decrease in the arterial oxygen tension.[56, 57] Measurement of functional residual capacity cannot be used as a criterion, since functional residual capacity may be normal or increasing with the application of PEEP owing to distention of only the normal areas of lung (either the one lung or the apical regions), even though there is continued failure to expand the diseased areas of lung (either the other lung or the basilar regions) (Figs. 19–6 and 19–7). Of course, the chest roentgenogram must show either severe unilateral asymmetric lung disease or severe bilateral basilar disease. An additional specific indication for initiation of differential lung ventilation, which is independent of the PEEP-induced shunting issue, is the presence of a bronchopleural fistula that prevents positive-pressure ventilation because of loss of tidal volume through the fistula.

There are several methods for demonstrating a PEEP-induced increase in shunt with unilateral lung disease. First, shunt can be measured before and after the application of PEEP. Second, pulmonary angiograms, which provide a qualitative measure of regional lung blood flow, can be obtained via a pulmonary artery catheter injection.[53] Third, lung perfusion scans, which provide a quantitative measure of regional blood flow, can be performed with radioisotopes.[58]

The specific management of differential lung ventilation and PEEP for the patient with unilateral lung disease is as follows. Since it may be necessary to determine the position of the double-lumen tube with precision at any time (e.g., following any significant patient movement), a fiberoptic bronchoscope should be at the bedside. The most diseased lung should be placed in a nondependent position. The compliance of each lung should then be measured separately. The amount of PEEP applied to each lung should initially be inversely proportional to the compliance of each lung. For example, if one lung has one third the compliance of the other lung, then it would be reasonable to initially apply 15 cm H_2O to the diseased lung and 5 cm H_2O to the nondiseased lung. The tidal volume to each lung should be equal; equal tidal volumes will, of course, result in different peak inspiratory pressures. The application of PEEP inversely proportional to lung compliance and use of equal tidal volumes has most often resulted in equal functional residual capacities and blood flows to each lung. Poorer results have been obtained with ventilator settings resulting in equal end-tidal carbon dioxide concentrations or equal airway pressures.[59]

It was originally thought that the two lungs would have to be ventilated synchronously because asynchronous differential lung ventilation would cause mediastinal movements that would impair cardiovascular performance. However, experimental and clinical experience has not supported this hypothesis, and the two lungs do not have to be ventilated synchronously.[60, 61] In fact, some studies suggest that asynchronous or alternating differential lung ventilation actually improves compliance of each lung because one lung does not have to compete with the other during inspiration for space within the thorax.[60, 61] When the two lungs have achieved an equal compliance and the chest roentgenogram has improved, the double-lumen tube should be switched to a single-lumen tube, and treatment should proceed to goals 2 and 3 below.

The specific management of differential lung ventilation and PEEP for the patient with bilateral lung disease is similar to that for the patient with unilateral lung disease, except for a few important differences. First, the nondependent lung should receive none or a relatively low level of PEEP, and the dependent lung should receive a relatively high level of PEEP (which is the opposite from differential lung ventilation of the patient with unilateral lung disease in the lateral decubitus position). Second, the tidal volume to each lung should be proportional to the assumed perfusion to each lung.[57] Third, the patient should be turned from side to side every 2 to 3 hours so that each lung may be in a nondependent position for a time. Fourth, the need for fiberoptic bronchoscopy to check the position of the double-lumen tube is increased because of the much more frequent patient movement.

IV. GOAL #2: F_IO_2 <0.5, PEEP <10 cm H_2O, AND P_aO_2 ACCEPTABLE

A. Why This Goal is #2: Match Ventilation to Perfusion

If a patient requires more than 10 cm H_2O of PEEP to have a P_aO_2 greater than 60 mm Hg with an F_IO_2 of less than 0.5, then the ventilation-perfusion mismatch is so great that it is illogical to make the patient spontaneously ventilate with such disordered lungs. In other words, lungs that have F_IO_2 and PEEP requirements greater than 10 cm H_2O and 0.5, respectively, are inefficient to the point that the work of breathing is likely to be excessive, and the patient will fatigue and fail. When the PEEP requirement is less than 10 cm H_2O, the F_IO_2 is less than 0.5, and the P_aO_2 is adequate, the lungs are fulfilling their basic gas exchange function in a reasonably efficient manner, and it now makes sense to ask the patients to do some of the work of breathing on their own.

B. How to Achieve Goal #2

The second goal is to get the PEEP requirement to be less than 10 cm H_2O; of course, it is assumed that what was achieved before (F_IO_2 < 0.5, acceptable P_aO_2) is retained. This second goal is achieved primarily by instituting an intensive and aggressive respiratory care regimen utilizing coughing routines, frequent tracheal suctioning, fiberoptic bronchoscopy, chest physical therapy (chest percussion and vibration in various postures), humidification of the inspired gases, half-hourly to hourly turnings of the patient, care of diseased lung in a nondependent position as much of the time as possible, incentive spirometry, administration of antibiotics chosen according to culture and sensitivity studies, and, in selected patients, administration of bronchodilators (beta$_2$-agonists, aminophylline, steroids; see chapter 6), diuretics, and inotropic drugs (Fig. 19–10). Although there are no hard data to prove that any one of these respiratory care treatments is beneficial when used alone, there is a widespread consensus that when used together, and in the context of the other care necessary in the postoperative management of respiratory failure, they produce a clearing of atelectasis, eradication of infection, and a decrease in the PEEP requirements.[62, 63]

Goal #2 = $F_IO_2 \leq 0.5$, PEEP < 10 cm H_2O, PaO_2 adequate

Aggressive Respiratory Care Regimen

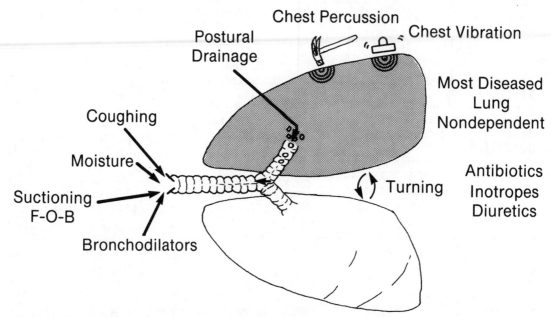

Figure 19-10. Goal #2 is to decrease the PEEP level to less than 10 cm of water while maintaining an F_IO_2 of less than 0.5 so that the PaO_2 is adequate. This is primarily achieved by the application of an intensive and aggressive respiratory care regimen. (FOB = fiberoptic bronchoscope.)

The only way patients can remove secretions from the tracheobronchial tree by themselves is by coughing, and effective voluntary coughing is the most efficient method of mobilizing and removing secretions.[64] However, many patients cannot or will not cough (due to depression by drugs, pain, or disease), and the secretions must be mechanically removed. Consequently, tracheal suctioning is often necessary and certainly mandatory whenever secretions are heard in the tracheobronchial tree by auscultation. The patients should be preoxygenated, and the maximum duration of suctioning should be 10 sec. Various angle-tipped catheters can improve the accuracy of cannulation of the mainstem bronchi,[65] and flexible fiberoptic bronchoscopy can be used for visually directed endobronchial suctioning.[66] Certainly, flexible fiberoptic bronchoscopy should be used whenever roentgenologically observable lobar obstruction is resistant to other standard medical therapy.[67] A balloon-tipped fiberoptic bronchoscope permits application of positive pressure to specific regions of the lung, in addition to enabling suction and lavage.[68]

Physically trying to shake the secretions loose from their alveolar and bronchial attachments by vibration and percussion, in conjunction with postural gravity drainage of the lungs, may increase the removal of secretions. External pressure may be applied to specific chest regions during exhalation in order to increase the expiratory flow of gas and may also increase the removal of secretions. Chest physical therapy appears to be especially beneficial for patients who are acutely ill, have large volumes of secretions, and cough ineffectively.[69] Chest physical therapy is also advantageous in patients with lobar atelectasis.[70] Chest physical therapy will not be beneficial in patients who do not have airway secretions. It should be realized that chest physical therapy in acutely ill patients may infrequently be associated with bronchoconstriction and hypoxemia.[69]

Dependent lung experiences higher pulmonary vascular pressures, and nondependent lung experiences lower pulmonary vascular pressures. The level of pulmonary vascular pressure has two important consequences for diseased lungs (Fig. 19–11). First, dependent

POSITION TREATMENT OF DISEASED LUNG

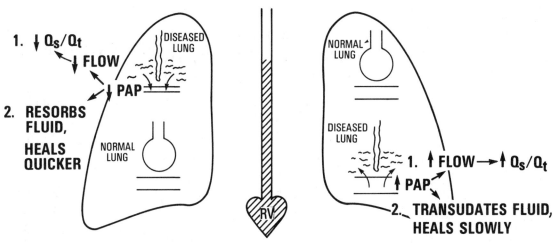

Figure 19–11. *The position of the patient can be used to treat lung disease. When diseased lung is placed in a nondependent position, it experiences a low pulmonary artery pressure (see chapter 3). The low pulmonary artery pressure means that blood flow to the region will be passively decreased, which will cause a decrease in shunt ($\dot{Q}_s/\dot{Q}_t$) through the diseased lung. In addition, the low pulmonary artery pressure causes the nondependent lung to have a propensity to resorb fluid and, therefore, heal more quickly. Conversely, when diseased lung is placed in a dependent position, it experiences a high pulmonary artery pressure. The high pulmonary artery pressure means that blood flow to the region will be passively increased, which will cause an increase in Q_s/Q_t through the diseased lung. In addition, the high pulmonary artery pressure causes a propensity to transudate fluid, resulting in more slowly healing lung or even a progressive deterioration in the lung.*

lung has a propensity to transudate fluid, whereas nondependent lung has a propensity to absorb fluid. Consequently, if diseased lung is placed in a dependent position, it may heal more slowly or actually become more diseased. Conversely, if diseased lung is placed in a nondependent position, it may heal more quickly. Second, dependent lung has a higher blood flow, and nondependent lung has a lower flow. Consequently, if diseased lung is placed in a dependent position, it will have a higher shunt because it is mechanically forced to have a higher blood flow. Conversely, if diseased lung is placed in a nondependent position, it will have a lower shunt because it is mechanically forced to have a lower blood flow. Thus, diseased lung should be in a nondependent position for as much time as possible.[71–74] Frequent turning of the patient will allow all parts of the lung to be placed in a nondependent position for their proportional share of the time.

Use of the respiratory care regimen outlined above usually allows the physician, within a few days, to decrease PEEP to less than 10 cm H_2O with continued maintenance of an adequate P_aO_2 with a low F_IO_2. Once the PEEP requirement is less than 10 cm H_2O, no special attempt

is made to reduce it further. Maintenance of some PEEP is desirable in terms of maintaining normal functional residual capacity and lung compliance, and providing a subjective sensation of good lung expansion. The achievement of an F_IO_2 less than 0.5 and a PEEP less than 10 cm H_2O with an acceptable P_aO_2 means that the blood and gas within the lungs is matched well enough so that the lungs perform their basic gas exchange function in a reasonably efficient manner. The patient is now a candidate for weaning from mechanical ventilation.

V. GOAL #3: $F_IO_2 < 0.5$, PEEP < 10 cm H_2O, IMV < 1 BREATH/MIN, P_aO_2 ACCEPTABLE

A. Why This Goal Is #3: Conversion from Intermittent Mandatory to Spontaneous Ventilation

Goals 1 and 2 were concerned with avoiding oxygen toxicity and matching ventilation to perfusion. Once ventilation-perfusion matching is achieved, it is reasonable to begin converting a patient who, in theory, required full ventilatory support (100 per cent dependent on the ventilator) to one who requires no ventilatory support (no dependence on the ventilator). The use of IMV weaning allows a gradual transition from 100 to 0 per cent ventilator dependence. During the transition, IMV is providing a progressively decreasing amount of partial ventilatory support.[6]

B. How To Achieve Goal #3

The third goal is to retain what was achieved before (F_iO_2 less than 0.5, PEEP less than 10 cm H_2O, and acceptable P_aO_2) and to get the IMV rate to be less than 1 breath/min. This weaning process is accomplished by a progressive decrease in the IMV rate. The rapidity by which the IMV rate can be reduced is dictated by and is directly proportional to the vital capacity (VC) and peak inspiratory force (PIF). Both of these breathing power indices can be rapidly and easily measured at the bedside with a spirometer (VC) and a dry gas manometer (PIF). The vital capacity is the volume exhaled forcefully after a maximal inspiration. The vital capacity maneuver requires cooperation, adequate lung compliance, and muscle strength. Since the vital capacity requires patient cooperation, it can give some indication of how much cooperation with breathing treatments will occur after extubation. The peak inspiratory force is the negative pressure generated at the airway when inspiration is artificially obstructed. This is a good indication of thoracic muscle strength. It may be more reliable than the vital capacity because it does not depend on patient motivation and may even be performed in the presence of coma. However, it provides little indication of subsequent voluntary activity. A poor vital capacity (dependent on cooperation, lung compliance, and muscle strength) coupled with a good peak inspiratory force (dependent on muscle strength) means that the patient is either poorly cooperating and/or has poor lung compliance.

The minimally adequate VC is 15 ml/kg (normal range 50 to 70 ml/kg), and the minimally adequate PIF is -20 to -25 cm H_2O (normal range -80 to -100 cm H_2O). The IMV rate may be decreased in 1 breath/min increments in patients who just achieve these minimal values (see below). Values much greater than these (more positive VC and more negative

PIF) mean that the IMV rate can be decreased more rapidly, and values much below these minimal ones (less positive VC and less negative PIF) mean that the IMV rate must be decreased much more slowly. When the decrease in IMV rate is begun, the head of the bed should be elevated as much as possible to reduce the pressure of the abdominal contents on the diaphragm and also to allow the patient to reestablish contact with the environment.

As the IMV rate is decreased, the patient is monitored by the spontaneous respiratory rate, VC, PIF, and P_aCO_2. When the rate of IMV withdrawal is appropriate and is being tolerated, the patient's spontaneous respiratory rate remains constant or only slightly increases, the VC and the PIF remain constant or improve, and the arterial blood gas concentrations do not deteriorate. Conversely, when the IMV withdrawal rate is too rapid and is not being tolerated, the spontaneous respiratory rate increases greatly (and is usually the first indication of intolerance), the VC and PIF decrease, and the arterial blood gas values deteriorate; the patient becomes hypertensive and tachycardiac, and may have arrhythmias. In patients who have a fresh incision and multiple indwelling catheters (nasogastric, urinary, and endotracheal tubes, intravenous and arterial lines), the pain input is high, and spontaneous respiratory rates are often between 20 and 30 breaths/min at the beginning of, and during, weaning.

The inability of a patient who has met the first two goals to tolerate the IMV withdrawal is usually because either the total clinical status requires full ventilatory support (for example, the patient is malnourished or has a neuromuscular problem) or the weaning system that is being used results in an intolerable increase in the work of breathing. Increased work of breathing is best indicated by negative fluctuations in inspiratory pressure greater than 2 cm H_2O during spontaneous breathing, which are usually indicative of inadequate inspiratory flow. Patients who fail to wean or take a long time to wean should be started on an intensive nutritional regimen.[75]

When P_aO_2 is adequate, with the F_iO_2 less than 0.5 (goal 1), the PEEP less than 10 cm H_2O (goal 2), VC greater than 15 ml/kg, PIF greater than -20 cm H_2O, IMV less than or equal to 1 breath/min, spontaneous respiratory rate less than 20 to 30/min, and P_aCO_2 approximately 40 mm Hg (goal 3); when no other major organ systems are in acute major failure or are unstable; and when the chest roentgenogram findings are reasonably equivalent to the premorbid findings or are rapidly improving and no new changes have appeared (such as infiltrates or pneumothorax), the patient is ready for extubation. It should be emphasized that throughout this entire mechanical ventilation and weaning process analgesics and sedatives must be administered and titrated so that the patient is comfortable, is not bucking on the endotracheal tube, and is without active expiratory efforts (see Fig. 3–37).

VI. SUMMARY OF MECHANICAL VENTILATION AND WEANING PROCEDURE

The logic of the above approach is that the patient's lungs are first required to have the ventilation and perfusion matched well enough, as indicated by an adequate or reasonable P_aO_2, with an F_IO_2 less than 0.5 and a PEEP level of less than 10 cm H_2O, so that the lungs function as an efficient gas exchange organ. Next the patient's lungs are required to sustain this efficient gas exchange without respirator aid as indicated by an adequate or reasonable VC, PIF, spontaneous respiratory rate, and P_aCO_2 on a low IMV. Finally, the process requires that no new complicating factor has occurred as indicated by lack of new chest radiographic findings, by resolution of previous pathologic chest radiographic findings, and by the absence of any significant disorder or complication in any of the other major organ systems.

VII. OTHER NEW MECHANICAL VENTILATION AND WEANING MODES

In the past few years a number of new mechanical ventilation modes have been introduced. The new modes are an outcome of microprocessor technology that enables the ventilator to monitor breath-by-breath flow, pressure, volume, and respiratory mechanics. The ability to sense and transduce these variables accurately, and on-line, allows the interaction between patient and ventilator to be much more sophisticated than ever before.

Pressure support (PS) ventilation is a ventilatory mode that provides additional inspiratory gas flow through a demand valve in response to a spontaneous breath. This additional gas flow keeps a positive inspiratory airway pressure (usually up to 30 cm H_2O above PEEP level) during inspiration and is discontinued when the patient's own inspiratory flow rate diminishes considerably, the exact point being determined differently in different ventilators. Thus, "supported" tidal volumes may vary according to the patient's inspiratory flow pattern. PS usually reduces the work of breathing,[76, 77] since the patient has only to trigger the demand valve, while part or all of the "spontaneous" breath itself is being supplied by the ventilator. When high levels of PS are used, it resembles the assist-control pressure-limited mode,[78] although the inspiration is not terminated once the preset pressure is achieved as in true pressure-limited devices. Some patients find PS to be a more comfortable ventilatory mode since it reduces the work of breathing and allows the patient to have more control over peak inspiratory flow rate, flow waveform, inspiratory time, and tidal volume.[79] PS may also be used as a weaning mode by gradually decreasing its level as the patient's own tidal volume improves. However, although perfectly practical in most cases, it does not seem to offer any improvement over existing weaning techniques and does require a reliable endogenous respiratory drive for ventilation. In addition, PS may also lead to a potentially harmful increase in airway pressure[78] as each and every breath is augmented by positive pressure.

Mandatory minute volume (MMV) and minimal minute ventilation (MiMv) are both methods that ensure the delivery of a preset minute volume, either by spontaneous breathing or by assistance from the ventilator itself. The difference between the two is that inadequate spontaneous ventilation of an MMV ventilator is supported by independent positive-pressure breaths, while during MiMv the mechanical assistance is only in the form of pressure support (i.e., the patient has to generate a spontaneous breath in order to be assisted). Current microprocessor ventilators supply MMV by continuously comparing the accumulating minute volume with the preset value and supplementing any deficit by mandatory mechanical breaths. The potential benefit of the MMV is clear; the patient is guaranteed a minimal minute ventilation regardless of her or his own spontaneous effort or drive and the weaning process becomes "automatic" (i.e., the patient passes "from artificial to spontaneous breathing without any attention to the controls being required"[80]). There are, however, no data describing such "automatic weaning" in groups of patients, probably because MMV has two main disadvantages that stem from the characteristics of its main parameter, namely, the minute volume. The first one is that it is difficult to estimate the right value of minute volume, as it would vary greatly according to the patient's dead space ventilation and carbon dioxide level. If the preselected minute volume value is too high, the patient will remain assisted by the ventilator, although he or she may be ready for extubation. A high preset minute volume value may also render the patient apneic because of a too low P_aCO_2 level. If the preselected minute volume value is too low, then the patient might be hypoventilated, distressed, and hypercarbic. The second problem associated with having minute volume as the preselected parameter is that minute volume is composed of both rate and tidal volume. Indeed, the patient may achieve the preselected minute volume value by shallow hyperventilation, which is not clinically acceptable and might signify impending respiratory catastrophe. Thus, it is difficult to see the practicality of MMV at this stage.

Two other new ventilatory modes that are specifically aimed at patients with the adult respiratory distress syndrome are inverse ratio ventilation (IRV)[81] and airway pressure release ventilation (APRV).[82] Inverse I/E ratio of up to 4:1 is claimed to achieve better oxygenation either by a straightforward increase in mean airway pressure or by a progressive alveolar recruitment and stabilization. APRV is the intermittent release of CPAP to ambient pressure for 1 sec. Consequently, the pressure waveform of IRV closely resembles that of APRV. The major difference between the two methods, besides the dominant airway pressure being "inspiratory" with IRV and "expiratory" with APRV, is that with IRV the patients do not breathe spontaneously, whereas with APRV the patient is allowed to breathe spontaneously. Thus, mean airway pressure is lower with APRV than with IRV. The technical details, indications, and clinical efficacy of these modes need to be further evaluated.

VIII. EXTUBATION OF THE TRACHEA

Additional criteria for extubation are that the patient should be alert, cooperative, and eager to be extubated. Prior to extubation of the trachea, the pharynx, nose, nasogastric tube (if present), and endotracheal tube should be suc-

tioned. Suctioning is followed by several positive-pressure sighs with 100 per cent oxygen. Extubation of the trachea should be accomplished by inflating the patient's lungs with 30 cm H_2O pressure, holding the pressure constant while the endotracheal tube cuff is rapidly deflated, and then immediately pulling the endotracheal tube out of the trachea (Fig. 19–12). This maneuver ensures that the first event following extubation is a forceful exhalation from total lung capacity (due to the elastic recoil of the chest wall); the forceful exhalation will blow out any material that has lodged on top of the endotracheal tube cuff and/or vocal cords that could not be reached by any of the other suction avenues (Fig. 19–12).

The patient is then asked to deep breathe and is observed for any laryngospasm or stridor. Humidified oxygen with an F_IO_2 0.1 greater than that used while the patient was intubated is administered by green face mask. Nasal prongs are most comfortable and do not interfere with eating, but they also do not provide an F_IO_2 greater than 0.3. When a higher F_IO_2 is required (which is usually the case), a face mask should be used, which with flow rates 5 to 10 L/min can yield an F_IO_2 between 0.3 and 0.5. Face masks with a reservoir bag can approach an F_IO_2 of 0.9. CPAP may also be administered by a tight fitting face mask. Of course, the expected F_IO_2 of all devices is dependent on appropriate positioning of the device on the patient's face. Arterial blood gas concentrations should be measured at 0.5 to 1 and at 4 to 6 hours postextubation, and a chest radiograph should be obtained 4 to 6 hours postextubation. Respiratory care measures instituted during the mechanical ventilation and weaning process are continued. In addition, incentive spirometry, which emphasizes a long increase in inspiratory transpulmonary pressure and lung volume (the ideal maneuver, Table 19–3), is the most cost-effective respiratory care measure and should be begun every hour. However, if a patient is experiencing significant postoperative pain, then it is unreasonable to expect good cooperation in performing this deep breathing maneuver; consequently, pain management must be effective (see chapter 20). The patient should be positioned upright, should be encouraged to cough, and should be encouraged to ambulate as soon and as much as possible. The nasogastric, urinary, and extraperipheral intravenous and arterial catheters and pleural tubes should be removed after 6 to 8 hours of trouble-free extubation.

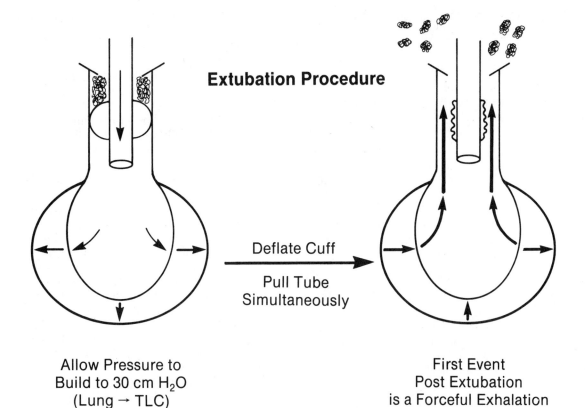

Extubation Procedure

Deflate Cuff

Pull Tube
Simultaneously

Allow Pressure to
Build to 30 cm H$_2$O
(Lung → TLC)

First Event
Post Extubation
is a Forceful Exhalation

Figure 19–12. The proper extubation procedure consists of allowing airway pressure to build to 30 cm of water so that the lung approaches total lung capacity (TLC). Then simultaneously, the endotracheal tube cuff is deflated and the endotracheal tube is pulled out. This procedure forces the first postextubation event to be a forceful exhalation (cough) due to the forceful elastic recoil of the lung from total lung capacity. The forceful exhalation can blow out of the airway any secretions and/or material that was lodged between the endotracheal tube cuff and the vocal cords, or on the vocal cords per se. In the author's experience this greatly diminishes the incidence of postextubation laryngospasm, breath holding, and choking-type respiration.

Table 19–3. Effects of Postoperative Respiratory Maneuvers

Maneuver	Alveolar Inflating Pressure	Time for Alveolar Inflation	Inflating Volume
Ideal maneuver	High (40–60 cm H$_2$O— preferably negative intrathoracic pressure)	Long (5–15 sec)	Largest possible (6–10 times tidal volume)
Expiratory maneuvers	Minimal (mostly deflating)	Minimal	Variable (not emphasized)
CO$_2$ hyperventilation	Moderate	Short (breathing deeper, but faster)	2–3 times tidal volume
IPPB	Preset (usually 15–20 cm H$_2$O positive airway pressure)	Long (5–10 sec)	Unknown (2–3 times tidal volume)
Sustained maximal inspiration	Maximal (30–50 cm H$_2$O negative intrathoracic pressure)	Long (5–10 sec)	Largest possible (2–6 times tidal volume)

IX. COMPLICATIONS OF MECHANICAL RESPIRATORY SUPPORT

The complications of mechanical respiratory support can be divided into those due to tracheal intubation and those due to mechanical ventilation.

I. Complications of tracheal intubation[83]
   A. During intubation
      1. Trauma to the eyes, cervical spinal column, nose, teeth, lips, tongue, larynx, and trachea
      2. Aspiration (of blood, tooth, laryngoscope bulb, gastric contents, and partial dentures)
      3. Esophageal intubation
      4. Endobronchial intubation
      5. Reflexes
         a. Sympathetic (hypertension, tachycardia, myocardial ischemia)
         b. Vagal (hypotension, bradycardia, cardiac arrest)
   B. With endotracheal tube in place
      1. Bronchospasm
      2. Tracheomalacia
      3. Tracheal perforation (by cuff, by tip of the tube)
      4. Inadequate secretion removal (possible obstruction of the tube)
      5. Trauma to all areas of contact (exacerbated by patient movement)
      6. Excessive inflation of cuff causing tube lumen narrowing
      7. Ruptured cuff
   C. During extubation
      1. Trauma to glottis by persistent inflated cuff
      2. Aspiration of supra–endotracheal tube cuff secretions
      3. Laryngospasm
      4. Respiratory obstruction by immediate edema of any part of the airway previously in contact with the endotracheal tube
   D. After extubation
      1. Sore throat, dysphagia
      2. Aphonia
      3. Paralysis of the hypoglossal and/or lingual nerve
      4. Vocal cord paralysis
      5. Ulceration, inflammation, infection, edema of any part of the airway previously in contact with the endotracheal tube
      6. Laryngeal granulomas and polyps
      7. Laryngotracheal membranes and webs
      8. Tracheal stenosis
      9. Sinusitis
II. Complications of mechanical ventilation[84]
   A. Complications attributable to operation of the ventilator
      1. Machine failure or disconnection
      2. Alarm failure
      3. Alarms not turned on
      4. Inadequate humidification
      5. Excessive inspired oxygen concentration
   B. Medical complications of positive-pressure breathing
      1. Inadequate positive-pressure breathing and alveolar hypoventilation
      2. Excessive positive-pressure breathing and alveolar hyperventilation
      3. Massive gastric distension
      4. Pneumothorax, pneumomediastinum
      5. Atelectasis
      6. Pneumonia
      7. Hypotension and decreased cardiac output
      8. Increased ventilatory dead space
      9. Antidiuretic hormone (ADH) secretion and water retention

Although this list of possible complications of mechanical respiratory support appears formidable, all are typically infrequent events, and more importantly, most are avoidable. Proper technique and adequate anesthesia should make the actual insertion of the endotracheal tube uncomplicated. Providing adequate sedation, using the minimum volume of air in the endotracheal tube cuff to effect sealing, frequently suctioning, and turning of the patient will render the presence of endotracheal tube benign. However, it is not possible to know about or eliminate pressure on the tissues in all areas of endotracheal tube contact. The volume of air in the endotracheal tube cuff should be checked for a minimum ("just") seal volume 1 hour after each inspired oxygen concentration change and only after the mouth has been suctioned. The endotracheal tube should be suctioned whenever breath sounds indicate the presence of tracheal or bronchial secretions.

REFERENCES

1. Shapiro BA, Cane RD, Harrison RA: Positive end-expiratory pressure therapy in adults with special reference to acute lung injury; A review of the literature and suggested clinical correlations. Crit Care Med 12:127–141, 1984.

2. Benumof JL: Update on mechanical ventilation. An epitome. West J Med 128:147, 1978.
3. Weisman IM, Rinaldo JE, Rogers RM, et al: State of the art: Intermittent mandatory ventilation. Am Rev Respir Dis 127:641, 1983.
4. Downs JB, Klein EF Jr, Desautels D, et al: Intermittent mandatory ventilation: A new approach to weaning patients from mechanical ventilators. Chest 64:331–335, 1973.
5. Shapiro BA, Cane RD: The IMV-AMV controversy: A plea for clarification and redirection (Editorial). Crit Care Med 12:472–473, 1984.
6. Cane RD, Shapiro B: Mechanical ventilatory support. JAMA 254:87–92, 1985.
7. Pontoppidan H, Geffin B, Lowenstein E: Acute respiratory failure in the adult. N Engl J Med 287:143, 690, 799, 1972.
8. Patterson RW: Effect of P_aCO_2 on O_2 consumption during cardiopulmonary bypass in man. Anesth Analg 5:269–273, 1976.
9. Cohen PJ, Alexander SC, Smith TC, et al: Effects of hypoxia and normocarbia on cerebral blood flow and metabolism in conscious man. J Appl Physiol 23:183, 1967.
10. Hedley-Whyte J, Pontoppidan H, Morris MJ: The response of patients with respiratory failure and cardiopulmonary disease to different levels of constant volume ventilation. J Clin Invest 45:1543, 1966.
11. Winter PM, Smith G: The toxicity of oxygen. Anesthesiology 37:210, 1972.
12. Lambertsen CJ: Effects of oxygen at high partial pressure. In Fenn WO, Rahn E. (eds): Handbook of Physiology, section 3. Respiration. vol 2. Baltimore, Williams & Wilkins Co, 1965, pp 1027–1046.
13. Nash G, Blennerhasset JB, Pontoppidan H: Pulmonary lesions associated with oxygen therapy and artificial ventilation. N Engl J Med 276:368, 1967.
14. De Campo T, Civetta JM: The effect of short-term discontinuation of high-level PEEP in patients with acute respiratory failure. Crit Care Med 7:47–49, 1979.
15. Rose DM, Downs JB, Heenan TJ: Temporal responses of functional residual capacity and oxygen tension to changes in positive end-expiratory pressure. Crit Care Med 9:79–82, 1981.
16. Albert RK: Least PEEP: Primum non nocere. Chest 87:2–3, 1985.
17. Suter PM, Fairley HB, Isenberg MD: Optimum end-expiratory pressure in patients with acute pulmonary failure. N Engl J Med 292:284–289, 1975.
18. Gallagher TJ, Civetta JM, Kirby RR: Terminology update: Optimal PEEP. Crit Care Med 6:323–326, 1978.
19. Kirby RR, Downs JB, Civetta JM, et al: High-level positive end-expiratory pressure (PEEP) in acute respiratory insufficiency. Chest 67:156–163, 1975.
20. Murray IP, Modell JH, Gallagher TJ, et al: Titration of PEEP by the arterial minus end-tidal carbon dioxide gradient. Chest 85:100–104, 1984.
21. Hurewitz A, Bergofsky EH: Adult respiratory distress syndrome. Med Clin North Am 65:33–51, 1981.
22. Weisman IM, Rinaldo JE, Rogers RM: Positive end-expiratory pressure in adult respiratory failure. N Engl J Med 307:1381–1384, 1982.
23. Powers SR Jr, Mannal R, Neclerio M, et al: Physiologic consequences of positive end-expiratory pressure (PEEP) ventilation. Ann Surg 178:265–272, 1973.
24. Lores ME, Keagy BA, Vassiliades T, et al: Cardiovascular effects of positive end-expiratory pressure (PEEP)

after pneumonectomy in dogs. Ann Thorac Surg 40:464–468, 1985.
25. Jardin F, Farcot J, Boisaute L, et al: Influence of positive end-expiratory pressure on left ventricular performance. N Engl J Med 304:387, 1981.
26. Molloy DW, Ducas J, Dobson K, et al: Hemodynamic management in clinical acute hypoxemic respiratory failure. Dopamine vs. dobutamine. Chest 39:636–640, 1986.
27. Prewitt RM, McCarthy J, Wood LDH: Treatment of acute low pressure pulmonary edema in dogs. J Clin Invest 67:409–418, 1981.
28. Cooligan T, Light RB, Wood LDH: Plasma volume expansion in canine pneumococcal pneumonia. Am Rev Respir Dis 126:86–90, 1982.
29. Molloy W, Ghignone M, Girling L, et al: Dobutamine and lasix in the treatment of oleic acid pulmonary edema in dogs. Fed Proc 42:733, 1983.
30. Schars SM, Ingram RH Jr: Influence of abdominal pressure and sympathetic vasoconstriction on the cardiovascular response to positive end-expiratory pressure. Am Rev Respir Dis 116:661–670, 1977.
31. Marini JJ, Culver BH, Butler J: Mechanical effect of lung distension with positive pressure on cardiac function. Am Rev Respir Dis 124:382–386, 1981.
32. Qvist J, Pontoppidan H, Wilson RS, et al: Hemodynamic responses to mechanical ventilation with PEEP. Anesthesiology 42:45–55, 1975.
33. Hobelmann CF Jr, Smith DE, Virgilio RW, et al: Hemodynamic alteration with positive end-expiratory pressure: The contribution of the pulmonary vasculature. J Trauma 15:951–959, 1975.
34. Weber KT, Janicki JS, Shroff SG, et al: The right ventricle: Physiologic and pathophysiologic considerations. Crit Care Med 11:323–328, 1983.
35. Brinker JA, Weiss JL, Lappe DL, et al: Leftward septal displacement during right ventricular loading in man. Circulation 61:626–633, 1980.
36. Weyman AE, Wann S, Feigenbaum H, et al: Mechanism of abnormal septal motion in patients with right ventricular volume overload: Cross-sectional echocardiographic study. Circulation 54:179–186, 1976.
37. Nichol PM, Gilbert BW, Kisslo JA: Two-dimensional echocardiographic assessment of mitral stenosis. Circulation 55:120–128, 1977.
38. Laver MB, Strauss WH, Pohost GM: Right and left ventricular geometry: Adjustments during acute respiratory failure. Crit Care Med 7:509–519, 1979.
39. Alderman EL, Glantz SA: Acute hemodynamic interventions shift the diastolic pressure-volume curve in man. Circulation 54:662–671, 1976.
40. Glantz SA, Misbach GA, Moores WY, et al: The pericardium substantially affects the left ventricular diastolic pressure-volume relationship in the dog. Circ Res 42:433–441, 1978.
41. Bemis CE, Serur JR, Borkenhagen D, et al: Influence of right ventricular filling pressure on left ventricular pressure and dimension. Cir Res 34:498–504, 1974.
42. Qvist J, Pontoppidan H, Wilson RS, et al: Hemodynamic responses to mechanical ventilation with PEEP: The effect of hypovolemia. Anesthesiology 42:45–55, 1975.
43. Harken AH, Brennan MF, Smith B, et al: The hemodynamic response to positive end-expiratory ventilation in hypovolemic patients. Surgery 76:786–793, 1974.
44. Cassidy SS, Eschenbacher WL, Johnson RL Jr: Reflex cardiovascular depression during unilateral lung hyperinflation in the dog. J Clin Invest 64:620–626, 1979.

45. Liebman PR, Patten MT, Manny J, et al: The mechanism of depressed cardiac output on positive end-expiratory pressure (PEEP). Surgery 83:594–598, 1978.
46. Cassidy SS, Robertson CH Jr, Pierce AK, et al: Cardiovascular effects of positive end-expiratory pressure in dogs. J Appl Physiol 44:743–750, 1978.
47. Said SI: Release of spasmogens from lungs by physical stimuli. Agents Actions 6:558–560, 1976.
48. Patten MT, Liebman PR, Hechtman HB: Humorally mediated decreases in cardiac output associated with positive end expiratory pressure. Microvasc Res 13:131–139, 1977.
49. Manny J, Grindlinger GA, Mathe AA, et al: Positive end-expiratory pressure, lung stretch, and increased myocardial contractility. J Surg 84:87–93, 1978.
50. Patten MP, Liebman PR, Manny J, et al: Humorally mediated alterations in cardiac performance as a consequence of positive end-expiratory pressure. J Surg 84:201–205, 1978.
51. Grindlinger GA, Manny J, Justice R, et al: Presence of negative inotropic agents in canine plasma during positive end-expiratory pressure. Circ Res 45:460–467, 1979.
52. Benumof JL, Rogers SN, Moyce PR, et al: Hypoxic pulmonary vasoconstriction and regional and whole-lung PEEP in the dog. Anesthesiology 51:503–507, 1979.
53. Carlon GC, Kahn R, Howland WS, et al: Acute life-threatening ventilation-perfusion inequality: An indication for independent lung ventilation. Crit Care Med 6:380–383, 1978.
54. Powers S, Mannal R, Neclerio M, et al: Physiologic consequences of positive end-expiratory pressure (PEEP) ventilation. Ann Surg 178:265–272, 1973.
55. Powers S, Dutton RE: Correlation of positive end-expiratory pressure with cardiovascular performance. Crit Care Med 3:64–68, 1975.
56. Carlon GC, Ray C Jr, Klein R, et al: Criteria for selective positive end-expiratory pressure and independent synchronized ventilation of each lung. Chest 74:501–507, 1978.
57. Hedenstierna G, Baehrendtz S, Frostell C, et al: Differential ventilation in acute respiratory failure. Indications and outcome. Bull Eur Physiopathol Respir 21:281–285, 1985.
58. Kanarek DJ, Shannon DC: Adverse effect of positive end-expiratory pressure on pulmonary perfusion and oxygenation. Am Rev Respir Dis 112:457–459, 1975.
59. East TD, Pace NL, Westenskow DR, et al: Differential ventilation with unilateral PEEP following unilateral hydrochloric acid aspiration in the dog. Acta Anaesthesiol Scand 27:356–360, 1983.
60. Muneyuki M, Konishi K, Horiguchi R, et al: Effects of alternating lung ventilation on cardiopulmonary function in dogs. Anesthesiology 58:353–356, 1983.
61. Hameroff SR, Caukins JM, Waterson CK, et al: High-frequency alternating lung ventilation. Anesthesiology 54:237–239, 1981.
62. Petty TL: Critical care for chronic air-flow limitation. Emphysema, chronic bronchitis, and cystic fibrosis. Semin Respir Med 3:263–274, 1982.
63. O'Donohue WJ: National survey of the usage of lung expansion modalities for the prevention and treatment of postoperative atelectasis following abdominal and thoracic surgery. Chest 87:76–80, 1985.
64. Oldenberg FA, Dolovich MB, Montgomery JM, et al: Effects of postural drainage, exercise and cough on mucus clearance in chronic bronchitis. Am Rev Respir Dis 120:739–745, 1979.
65. Wang KP, Wise RA, Terry PB, et al: A new controllable suction catheter for blind cannulation of the main stem bronchi. Crit Care Med 6:347–348, 1978.
66. Fulkerson WJ: Current concepts: Fiberoptic bronchoscopy. N Engl J Med 311:511–515, 1984.
67. Wanner A, Landa JF, Neiman RE Jr, et al: Bedside bronchofiberoscopy for atelectasis and lung abscess. JAMA 244:1281–1283, 1973.
68. Millen JE, Vandree J, Glauser FL: Fiberoptic bronchoscopic balloon occlusion and reexpansion of refractory unilateral atelectasis. Crit Care Med 6:50–55, 1978.
69. Kirilloff LH, Owens GR, Rogers RM, et al: Does chest physical therapy work? Chest 88:436–444, 1985.
70. Marini J, Pierson D, Hudson L: Acute lobar atelectasis: A prospective comparison of fiberoptic bronchoscopy and respiratory therapy. Am Rev Respir Dis 119:971–978, 1979.
71. Remolina C, Khan AU, Santiago TV, et al: Positional hypoxemia in unilateral lung disease. N Engl J Med 304:523–525, 1981.
72. Fishman AP: Down with the good lung. N Engl J Med 304:537–538, 1981.
73. Seaton D, Lapp NL, Morgan WKC: Effect of body position on gas exchange after thoracotomy. Thorax 34:518–522, 1979.
74. Douglas WW, Rehder K, Beynen FM, et al: Improved oxygenation in patients with acute respiratory failure: The prone position. Am Rev Respir Dis 115:559–566, 1977
75. Larca L, Greenbaum DM: Effectiveness of intensive nutritional regimens in patients who fail to wean from mechanical ventilation. Crit Care Med 10:297–300, 1982.
76. Kanak R, Fahey PJ, Vanderwarf C: Oxygen cost of breathing. Changes dependent upon mode of mechanical ventilation. Chest 87:126, 1985.
77. MacIntyre NR: Respiratory function during pressure support ventilation. Chest 89:677, 1986.
78. Banner MJ, Kirby RR: Similarities between pressure support ventilation and intermittent positive-pressure ventilation (letter). Crit Care Med 13:997–998, 1985.
79. Banner MJ, Kirby RR: Pressure support ventilation (letter). Crit Care Med 14:665–666, 1986.
80. Hewlett AM, Platt AS, Terry VG: Mandatory minute volume. A new concept in weaning from mechanical ventilation. Anaesthesia 32:163, 1977.
81. Gurevitch MJ, Van Dyke J, Young ES, et al: Improved oxygenation and lower peak airway pressure in severe adult respiratory distress syndrome. Treatment with inverse ratio ventilation. Chest 89:211, 1986.
82. Stock MC, Downs JB, Frolicher DA: Airway pressure release ventilation (APRV): A new ventilatory mode during acute lung injury (ALI). Crit Care Med 14:366, 1986.
83. Blanc VF, Tremblay NAG: The complications of trachea intubation: A new classification with a review of the literature. Anesth Analg 53:202–213, 1974.
84. Zwillich CW, Pierson DJ, Creagh CE, Sutton FD, Schatz E, Petty TL: Complications of assisted ventilation: A prospective study of 354 consecutive episodes. Am J Med 57:161–170, 1974.

Management of Postoperative Pain

20

I. INTRODUCTION

The treatment of pain following thoracotomy is important not only to ensure patient comfort but also to minimize pulmonary complications by enabling patients to breathe normally (without active exhalation and/or splinting) and deeply (so that they can cough) and to ambulate. Normal and deep breathing require stretching of the skin incision, which is painful. Postoperative patients will normally try to prevent stretching on the skin incision by reflexly contracting their expiratory muscles (splinting), which limits the stretch on the incision during inspiration, and by actively exhaling, which rapidly diminishes whatever stretch there is on the incision. Failing to cough avoids the deep inspiration prior to the forceful exhalation. Splinting, active exhalation, and failing to cough promote retention of secretions, airway closure, and atelectasis.

The systemic administration of narcotics can achieve the goals of relieving pain, diminishing splinting, and promoting coughing, but the therapeutic-respiratory depression window is small. Intercostal nerve blocks and thoracic epidural analgesia with local anesthetics are short-term, time consuming (require repeated injections), higher risk but efficacious procedures; they can be alternative to, or used in conjunction with, conventional narcotic treatment. Cryoanalgesia is a relatively new, safe, effective and long-lasting (3 to 4 weeks) pain management technique. Transcutaneous electric nerve stimulation may have beneficial effects when used as an adjunct to one of the above techniques. However, epidural narcotic administration has become the method of choice for providing pain relief for post-thoracotomy patients and is, therefore, the technique discussed at greatest length in this chapter.

II. SYSTEMIC NARCOTIC ADMINISTRATION

Systemic narcotic administration has traditionally been the most frequently utilized treatment for post-thoracotomy pain. Appropriate narcotic use achieves a balance between adequate patient comfort (which is usually indicated by an absence of active exhalation and splinting) and avoidance of excessive sedation or respiratory depression. Since active exhalation and/or splinting and unwillingness to cough can be observed, small doses of narcotic (e.g., 2 to 4 mg of morphine intravenously) can be administered to postoperative thoracotomy patients until it is evident that these unfavorable respiratory characteristics are minimized. Avoidance of administration of narcotics beyond these physiologic end points is important because narcotics can cause inhibition of coughing, decrease the frequency of signs, and tend to make breathing regular, all of which promote alveolar collapse and the development of atelectasis.[1] In addition, the opiates cause a marked desensitization of the central respiratory apparatus to the stimulating effects of hypercarbia and hypoxia; indeed, an increase of 20 per cent in the arterial carbon dioxide tension may be expected in patients adequately dosed with narcotic analgesics.[2, 3] The therapeutic range of systemic analgesics, when used as the sole method of pain relief and as defined above, is small and requires considerable physical attention (i.e., titration of drug to the desired effect).

The amount of drug required for pain relief is variable from patient to patient.[3] In patients undergoing abdominal surgery, a significant inverse correlation was found between the concentration of endorphins in the cerebrospinal fluid preoperatively and cerebrospinal fluid pethidine concentration achieved by patient-controlled analgesia postoperatively.[4] In other words, patients who had high cerebrospinal fluid levels of endorphins (presumably giving the patient natural analgesia) had low pethidine requirements, and patients who had low cerebrospinal fluid levels of endorphins (presumably rendering the patient without natural analgesia) had high pethidine requirements.[4] This strongly suggests that drug dosage requirement differences between patients are largely determined by preexisting and, perhaps, genetic neurochemical factors. Subsequent differences may be due to the variable presence of noxious stimuli unrelated to the incision, such as nasogastric tubes and Foley catheters. If adjunctive therapy is added, such as rectal indomethacin,[5] narcotic requirements can be greatly reduced and are, therefore, much less variable from patient to patient. Other factors that might be responsible for different patient-to-patient drug dosage requirements are differences in pain assessment methodology, patient population (such as age, sex, prior drug exposure), and placebo effects.

The amount of drug required for pain relief throughout an individual's hospital course decreases in an exponential manner.[3] This is because pain from the wound decays in an exponential manner. Thus, with intermittent intramuscular administration, mean narcotic doses typically reduce by one half every 1 to 2 days.[6] However, the usual interdosing interval of 3 to 4 hours gives a fast decay rate for pain relief, which is a poor match to the much slower decay rate of wound pain intensity, and periods of pain are likely to result. Patient-controlled (demand) analgesia and constant infusion systems can eliminate pain due to this discrepancy in the two decay rates.

Patient-controlled analgesia allows the patient, within certain limits, to determine how frequently a small dose of analgesic drug should be administered. The limits consist of the actual dose and a minimum dosing interval, which are set by the physician in charge of the treatment. Thus, the patient can fine tune to any critical drug level that equates with adequate analgesia at that particular moment. Extensive experience with patient-controlled analgesia has

shown that previously nonaddicted patients will select a critical drug level that assures complete alertness, even if it is accompanied by a certain amount of residual pain.[7] This amount of pain is quite well tolerated by the patient because it is the patient's choice that it should not be completely relieved, and he or she is assured that additional narcotic is available at a moment's notice if desired. Patient-controlled analgesia also confers psychologic benefit. Being able to control at least one important factor in their treatment calms and considerably relieves many patients.

Continuous narcotic infusion will also provide a constant analgesic level. By titrating the hourly dose to the patient's needs, a steady plasma concentration of narcotic may be achieved that will provide adequate analgesia. However, in practice, several problems remain. First, initial adequate analgesia can be obtained in about 80 per cent of patients, but in approximately 20 per cent it may be insufficient or excessive.[8] Thus, the problem of picking the right dose the first time still remains. Second, the patients still need to be monitored for signs of overdosage, and the respiratory rate must be checked frequently. However, once the appropriate hourly dose of narcotic can be determined, the patients do quite well.

III. INTERCOSTAL NERVE BLOCK

Intercostal nerve blocks with long-acting anesthetic agents (e.g., bupivacaine) are often employed as a means of treating postoperative pain after thoracotomy.[9-19] These blocks may be placed either intraoperatively (at the time of closure) under direct vision or postoperatively. Direct vision intraoperative blocks may be done by needle or by placement of catheters in the appropriate intercostal grooves for injection postoperatively when pain occurs.[17-20] A number of studies have shown that intercostal nerve blocks result in decreased postoperative pain and narcotic requirements,[9-11, 15] improvements in arterial blood gas values[11, 12, 14] and lung function,[9-11, 15, 16] and earlier discharge from the hospital.[10-12] Obviously, indwelling intercostal groove catheters can provide longer term and usually more accurate blocks than one-time direct vision needle block or intermittent percutaneous needle blocks.[16] These blocks have been used successfully in young patients (6-month-old infants) as well as in older children and adults.[10] Long-acting local anesthetics, such as bupivacaine with epinephrine, should be used for postoperative intercostal nerve blocks; three to five intercostal spaces should be blocked, with the middle space being the level of the incision.

The administration of intercostal nerve blocks, however, is not without an incidence of complications. Several reports have documented profound hypotension shortly following the intraoperative placement of intercostal nerve blocks.[21–24] In two of these reports the fall in blood pressure was thought to be due to paravertebral spread of the local anesthetic agent with resultant sympathetic blockade.[21, 22] The other two reports document total spinal block that was probably due to unrecognized dural puncture or perineural spread of the local anesthetic.[22–24] Although this complication can be avoided by administering the intercostal block at least 8 cm lateral to the intervertebral foramen,[24, 25] some authors advocate discontinuing altogether the placement of intercostal nerve blocks intraoperatively.[26] Potential problems with this technique, when performed postoperatively, include the hazards of pneumothorax,[12] rapid intravascular absorption of the local anesthetic, discomfort on injection, and the considerable time and skilled personnel required to perform the blocks. Although use of indwelling intercostal groove catheters decreases physician time and increases the safety of the procedure, the catheters tend to migrate, and the incidence of failed blocks increases.

IV. EPIDURAL LOCAL ANESTHETIC ADMINISTRATION

Thoracic epidural anesthesia (analgesia) essentially results in multiple intercostal nerve blocks after a single injection of a local anesthetic. It is not surprising, therefore, that this technique has the same beneficial effects on arterial blood gas values, results of pulmonary function tests, and narcotic requirement as conventional intercostal nerve blocks do.[27–30] Potential major complications of this technique include significant hypotension due to sympathetic blockade, cardiovascular and/or central nervous system toxicity due to intravascular injection of local anesthetic agents, headache due to inadvertent dural puncture (along with total spinal block if unrecognized), infection related to need for chronic catheterization, and trauma to the spinal cord. In addition, epidural analgesia with local anesthetic requires consid-

erable physician time and skill. The continuous infusion of 0.25 per cent bupivacaine in an epidural catheter has been investigated in an effort to prolong the block, minimize hypotension, and simplify treatment, but this technique did not provide adequate analgesia and/or was associated with a high incidence of major complications.[31–33] Consequently, and in view of the efficacy of cryoanalgesia and lumbar epidural narcotics (see below), the risks of epidural local anesthetic administration outweigh the benefits, and the technique is little used today.

V. CRYOANALGESIA

Extremely long-lasting intercostal nerve block may be obtained by intercostal nerve freezing (cryoanalgesia).[34–41] Direct application of an ice-ball to the nerve causes degeneration of nerve axons without damage to the support structure of the nerve (the neurolemma), thereby reversibly disrupting nerve activity. Thus, intraneural and perineural connective tissue are preserved, providing a scaffolding for regenerating capillaries, axons, and Schwann cells.[42] The area of anesthesia is along the dermatomes treated. During the next 2 to 3 weeks after nerve freezing, nerve structure and function begin to recover in parallel. Usually, from 1 to 3 months after freezing, there is full restoration of nerve structure and function, without untoward sequelae (neuritis or neuroma formation). The numbness that persists during this time period is not especially bothersome. Young women, however, have admitted to some distress during the period of axonal regeneration due to loss of sensation in the nipple area if the fifth and higher intercostal nerves have been frozen.[41]

Currently used cryoprobes are about the size of a pen; the core of the instrument has an exit port that permits rapid expansion of a gas (nitrous oxide). The rapid expansion of nitrous oxide cools a surrounding metal sheath. Since the metal sheath is in contact with a fluid, an ice-ball (temperature $-60°C$) forms at the tip of the cryoprobe. The cryoprobe is applied to the intercostal nerves as far posteriorly as possible from within the chest at the level of the incision, plus two or three interspaces above and below this level, just prior to closure of the thoracotomy wound. The nerves are approached from within the chest since the probe has to pierce the parietal pleura to reach the intercostal nerves in the subcostal groove. This is easily accomplished by the surgeon's lifting the nerve out of the groove with a small nerve hook. The cryoprobe is placed directly on the nerve and activated so that the center of the resultant ice-ball encapsulates the nerve. During the freeze, nerve tissue temperature is approximately $-20°C$.[41] If 2 to 3 mm of tissue remains between the tip of the cryoprobe and the nerve to be blocked, the nerve will not become adequately frozen and nerve function might not be totally eliminated. If the pleura is thickened, local peeling of the pleura is advisable.[41] Usually two 30-sec freeze cycles, which are separated by a 5-sec thaw period, are applied to each of the nerves selected. However, recent experience with one 30-sec freeze exposure has resulted in no loss of postoperative pain control with a significantly reduced period of numbness (from 3.0 months to 1.2 months).[41]

The use of cryoanalgesia in this way has effectively reduced postoperative narcotic requirements and has improved pulmonary function.[34, 36-39] Cryoanalgesia patients have had slight to moderate pain at the end of the first postoperative day, and only slight pain after that (as compared with patients receiving intravenous narcotics who experience moderate to severe pain at 24 hours). Most of the pain experienced by the cryoanalgesia patients has not been incisional discomfort, but rather shoulder or arm pain secondary to chest tube irritation of the pleura. Further advantage of the cryoanalgesia can be gained if the chest tubes can be placed within an intercostal space whose nerve has been subjected to cryoanalgesia.[41] Once the chest tubes are removed, usually on the second or third postoperative day, the pain in the cryoanalgesia patients has become barely noticeable. Consequently, these patients are more able to cooperate with the postoperative pulmonary physiotherapy maneuvers described in chapter 19. Return of sensation occurs in most patients by the thirtieth postoperative day. Long-term follow-up for 6 months has shown no adverse sequelae from the procedure.

Since cryoanalgesia causes temporary nerve damage, and the duration of the nerve damage far exceeds the duration of significant postoperative pain (even with a single 30-sec freeze, numbness persisted for a mean of 38 days),[41] cryoanalgesia cannot be considered a routine post-thoracotomy pain treatment. Cryoanalgesia may be a treatment of choice in thoracic pain situations that are expected to last a long time (e.g., pain from chest trauma) and significantly limit respiratory function.

VI. TRANSCUTANEOUS ELECTRIC NERVE STIMULATION

Pain transmitted by small unmyelinated C-fibers is inhibited by activation of large myelinated A-fibers. Low-voltage, high-frequency (80-Hz) transcutaneous electric impulses, which are continuous but variable, stimulate the large myelinated A-fibers. By placing the strip electrodes 2 cm from both sides of the thoracotomy and activating the power source, some diminution of post-thoracotomy pain occurs.

Transcutaneous electric nerve stimulation has the advantages of low cost, ease of application, and lack of undesirable side effects. However, although most patients obtain some relief, it is not complete, and some patients do not experience any pain relief. In those patients who do obtain analgesia, the duration of pain relief has varied from 1 hour,[43] to 1 day,[16] to 5 days.[35] Transcutaneous electric nerve stimulation may, however, reduce narcotic requirements,[44] help to improve pulmonary function,[44, 45] and decrease pulmonary complications.[44, 46] At the present time transcutaneous electric nerve stimulation is generally reserved for adjunctive use with narcotics to relieve postoperative pain from thoracotomy.

VII. EPIDURAL OPIOIDS

Since the use of epidural morphine for the treatment of pain was first reported in 1979,[47] this therapy has rapidly achieved widespread popularity.[48] Treatment of pain after thoracic surgery with epidural narcotics has several important advantages: first, there is no sympthetic blockade and neither motor nor sensory loss; second, success in relieving pain is usually predictable; and third, the duration of pain relief is generally much longer than that which results from using parenteral narcotics.[47, 49-54]

It appears that epidural and intrathecal opiates block the presynaptic and postsynaptic neurons in the substantia gelatinosa of the dorsal horn of the spinal cord. Epidural opiates gain access to the spinal cord by passive diffusion across the dura into the cerebrospinal fluid (CSF)[50, 55] and by absorption into arachnoid villi and posterior radicular arteries (which supply the dorsal horn region).[56] In support of these contentions are the high density of opiate receptors in the substantia gelatinosa of the dorsal horn[57, 58]; the high CSF–low plasma concentration ratio (40 to 100) of all narcotics after epidural and intrathecal use[50, 59]; and the fact that onset of action, potency, and duration of action are related to CSF narcotic concentration rather than plasma narcotic concentration.[50, 59] Blockade of the substantia gelatinosa results in a "selective" spinal block of pain conduction; does not block other sensations, such as external pressure, pin prick, temperature, and proprioception; and does not cause a sympathetic or motor block. Consequently, epidural narcotics cannot provide complete anesthesia during surgery.[60, 61] In contrast, epidural local anesthetics block nerve impulse conduction in the axons of nerve roots and long tracks in the spinal cord, resulting in blockade of sympathetic, sensory, and motor function, and can be used to provide complete anesthesia.

There is a close relationship between the lipid solubility of epidural narcotics and onset, duration, and extent of analgesia. High lipid solubility means that the narcotic leaves the epidural space and enters the subarachnoid CSF space rapidly; readily fixes to spinal opioid receptors, resulting in a rapid onset of action; does not diffuse widely throughout the epidural and cerebrospinal fluid space; and therefore results in a more segmental block (Fig. 20–1). High lipid solubility also means that the drug is absorbed into the vascular space from the epidural and CSF spaces more rapidly, resulting in a shorter duration of action (Fig. 20–1). The lipophilic narcotics are fentanyl, methadone, and meperidine (in decreasing order of lipid solubility); when administered in the epidural space at the segmental level of pain in doses of 0.1 mg, 5 mg, and 30 to 100 mg, respectively, they have a relatively short onset of action of less than 12 min, provide nearly complete pain relief in 20 to 30 min, and have a duration of action of 6 to 7 hours.[56, 62]

By contrast, morphine has a more complex molecular structure and a low lipid solubility. Low lipid solubility means that the narcotic leaves the epidural space and enters the subarachnoid space slowly; does not readily fix to the spinal opioid receptors, which results in a slow onset of action; diffuses widely throughout cerebrospinal fluid space; and therefore results in a relatively nonsegmental block (Fig. 20–1). Low lipid solubility also means that the drug is absorbed into the vascular space from the epidural and CSF spaces more slowly, resulting in a longer duration of action (Fig. 20–1). With an epidural dose of 5 mg, morphine has a relatively slow onset of action of 15 to 30 min, provides maximal pain relief in 40 to 60 min, and has a

duration of action often in excess of 12 hours. Since the lipophobic morphine spreads widely in the epidural and CSF spaces and causes a nonsegmental block, the level of epidural injection is not nearly as important for adequate pain relief (see below) as it is with the lipophilic narcotics. The wider spread of morphine is also responsible for an increased incidence of late respiratory depression compared with the lipophilic narcotics. All the narcotics have a positive epidural dose-response (intensity and duration of pain relief) relationship.[54, 64, 65]

The major advantage of "selective" blockade of spinal pain with narcotics lies in the avoidance of the major complications of local anesthetic blockade or parenteral narcotic administration described above. Contraindications to the use of both epidural and intrathecal narcotics include elevated intracranial pressure, preexisting peripheral neurologic disease, allergy to narcotics, infection at the site of injection, and perhaps gross disturbances of coagulation.

The use of intrathecal (subarachnoid) narcotics for pain relief is greatly limited by the inability to give repeated injections owing to the risks involved in leaving an indwelling catheter in the subarachnoid space. In an attempt to partially bypass this problem, single intrathecal injections of morphine have been successfully used preoperatively or intraoperatively to provide 18 to 24 hours of postoperative pain relief.[66–68] Intrathecal morphine results in extremely high CSF concentrations; subsequent slow (6 hours) passive circulation of CSF allows the lipophobic morphine to reach the cisterns of the brain and the respiratory center.[69] Thus, the use of intrathecal morphine appears to be associated with an increased occurrence of severe late respiratory depression (4 to 7 per cent compared with less than 1 per cent for epidural administration).[69] Since the epidural route can provide much longer-lasting analgesia with less risk, it has generally replaced the intrathecal route for treating postoperative pain.

The most serious complications of epidural opioids are early and late respiratory depression. The late respiratory depression can be life-threatening and is associated with decreased mentation and confusion; fortunately, the late respiratory depression is an infrequent occurrence (0.25 to 0.4 per cent[69] or lower[70] incidence) and is usually gradual in onset, allowing time for diagnosis and treatment.[56, 69] The early respiratory depression seems to be directly related to the plasma concentration of narcotic

Epidural Narcotics

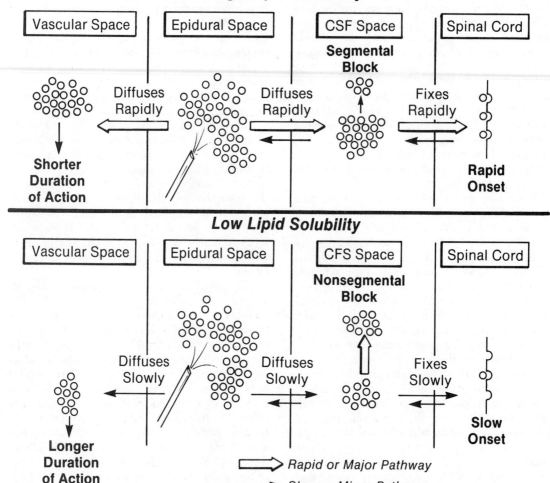

Figure 20–1. Epidural narcotics may be either of high or low lipid solubility. Narcotics with high lipid solubility diffuse rapidly into the cerebrospinal fluid (CSF) space and readily fix to spinal cord receptors, resulting in a rapid onset of a segmental block. In addition, high lipid solubility narcotics diffuse rapidly out of the epidural space into the vascular space, resulting in a shorter duration of action. Conversely, low lipid solubility narcotics diffuse slowly into the CSF space and do not readily fix to spinal cord receptors, resulting in a slow onset of a nonsegmental block. In addition, low solubility narcotics diffuse slowly out of the epidural space into the vascular space, resulting in a longer duration of action. The open arrows indicate rapid or major pathways, and the thin closed arrows indicate slow or minor pathways.

and has occurred in 30 min for some of the lipophilic narcotics and in 98 min for lipophobic morphine; the late respiratory depression has occurred in 6 to 10 hours for epidural morphine and is thought to be due to rostral spread of the hydrophilic morphine within the cerebrospinal fluid.[71] Results of quantitative studies of ventilatory responses to carbon dioxide, such as minute ventilation (V_E) and airway occlusion pressure, performed before and after epidural morphine administration are consistent with clinical experience and have shown 20 to 30 per cent decreases in V_E/CO_2 and P_{100}/CO_2 slopes.[72] The rapidity of onset, severity, and incidence of respiratory depression may be increased by other factors, such as inadvertent dural puncture,[54, 73] increased dosage and age,[69] position of the patient after injection,[74] raised intrathoracic and intra-abdominal pressures, and especially the administration of concomitant oral, intramuscular, or intravenous sedatives and/or narcotics.[69] Conversely, chronic administration of systemic opioids protects against the development of respiratory depression; indeed, there are no reports of respiratory depression in chronic pain patients previously made tolerant to opioids.[59, 75-77] Naloxone dramatically reverses both early and late respiratory depression.

The other side effects of epidural opioids are urinary retention, pruritus, and nausea and vomiting; these side effects are much more common but also far less serious than late respiratory depression. The incidence of these side effects increases with increasing dosage.[78] Thus, since the relationship between dose and intensity of analgesic response plateaus quickly, the risk-benefit ratio of increasing dosage rises rapidly once effective pain relief levels have been reached.[50, 67] The incidence of side effects may be minimized by continuous infusions of low doses of narcotics into the epidural space.

The incidence of postoperative patients' requiring bladder catheterization after epidural morphine has generally ranged around 15 per cent,[70] although considerable variability in this figure has been reported, and it can be as high as 53 per cent.[48, 79] The urinary retention occurs approximately 12 hours after beginning epidural morphine,[80] and is probably due to a sympathetically mediated increase in the tone of the bladder detrusor muscle and bladder neck sphincter; the incidence of the complication can be greatly decreased by administration of phenoxybenzamine.[79] The incidence of pruritus has also been variable and has been reported to be as low as 1 per cent,[56] although in most series it is considerably higher.[51, 70, 71] The pruritus is usually generalized,[81] but may be confined to just the areas affected by the epidural morphine.[82] The time of onset of pruritus is usually several hours after injection, and therefore histamine release is probably not causative. Nevertheless, the pruritus may occasionally be relieved by promethazine.[82] The mechanism of action of pruritus is most likely a generalized defect in the modulation of cutaneous sensation.[83] The incidence of nausea and vomiting has ranged from 17 to 50 per cent[70, 78, 84]; they occur when morphine reaches the chemoreceptor trigger zone in the fourth ventricle.[85] The incidence decreases with repeated dosing[75, 86]; presumably the brain becomes tolerant to these side effects, as it does to the respiratory depressant effect. Other factors that may contribute to the wide range in reported incidences of epidural morphine side effects are differences in clinical and experimental conditions, such as use of volunteers (increased frequency of complications) rather than patients, patient age, operative site, injection level, and dose of drug administered. Fortunately, the narcotic antagonist naloxone can reverse all of the above side effects. However, repeated injections of naloxone are sometimes necessary to eliminate recurring side effects and suggest that the binding of opiate to receptor is strong. Repeated use of naloxone can reverse the analgesic effects as well, so it must be used cautiously for this procedure.

Epidural opioids have had a moderately extensive trial in relief of post-thoracotomy pain. The epidural catheter may be placed prior to the induction of general anesthesia and checked for correct position by using a small dose of local anesthetic. Alternatively, it may be placed postoperatively prior to emergence from anesthesia, while the patient is still in the lateral decubitus position; the initial injection is made in the recovery room or intensive care unit. Several important clinical points have emerged from the post-thoracotomy epidural opioid analgesia experience.

First, although the thoracic epidural route has been used, the procedure has risks (primarily dural puncture and spinal cord damage), and the lumbar area for catheter insertion has been found to be just as satisfactory for pain relief if a slightly higher dose of morphine and adequate diluent volumes are used.[50, 53, 54, 75, 87-90] The reason morphine can be used with a lumbar epidural injection for the relief of thoracic pain is that morphine is lipophobic and will therefore remain in, and have time to spread throughout, the epidural and cerebrospinal fluid spaces. For relief of thoracic pain, instillation of 6 mg of morphine in 10 to 15 ml of diluent (preservative-free normal saline) in the lumbar epidural region has been used successfully.[53, 88] Although studied to a much smaller degree, fentanyl,[91, 92] methadone,[93] hydromorphone,[94] and nalbuphine[95] may also be used by either the thoracic or lumbar epidural route. Not surprisingly, the lumbar route requires a greater diluent volume to mechnically push the narcotic into a wider distribution, since these lipophilic narcotics will bind too quickly to a spinal cord at, and a few dermatomes above and below, the segmental level of introduction. Since the lumbar route is safer than the thoracic route and since fentanyl has not been associated with respiratory depression, the lumbar epidural route with fentanyl is the author's post-

Table 20–1. Epidural Narcotics for Postoperative Pain Management: Routes and Dosages

Site of Incision	Epidural Route	Drug	Dosage (Diluent Saline)	Reference
Thoracotomy	Thoracic	Fentanyl	1–2 µg/kg (10 ml) → 1–2 µg/kg/hour	88, 89
		Methadone	5 mg (10 ml)	90
		Pethidine	30–100 mg (10 ml)	53, 59
		Nalbuphine	10 mg (10 ml)	92
		Morphine	2–4 mg (8 ml) 0.1 mg/hour	31, 47, 50, 51, 72, 84–87
	Lumbar	Fentanyl	1–2 µg/kg (18 ml) → 1–2 µg/kg/hour	88, 89
		Morphine	6–8 mg (10–15 ml)	47, 50, 51, 72, 84–87
		Methadone	5 mg (10–15 ml)	84
Abdominal incison	Lumbar	Fentanyl	1–2 µg/kg (10 ml) → 1–2 µg/kg/hour	88, 89
		Morphine	2–6 mg (10 ml)	62
		Methadone	4–6 mg (18–20 ml)	90
		Hydromorphone	1.25–1.5 mg (10–15 ml)	91

thoracotomy pain management technique of choice. However, there remains a wide selection of drugs (and dosages) for use by the lumbar and thoracic epidural route (Table 20–1).

Second, epidural morphine[89] and fentanyl[75] have been reported to be effective following thoracic trauma. In patients with multiple fractured ribs, epidural morphine resulted in well over 6 hours of analgesia with each dose. Alternatively, continuous epidural infusion of fentanyl (1 to 2 µg/kg/hour following 2 µg/kg bolus) would appear to be a good choice in the thoracic trauma situation (as well as for post-thoracotomy pain) because it has a decreased likelihood of causing respiratory depression. Since there is no sympathetic blockade with epidural opioids, there is no need to lie the patient supine for top-up doses, and patients with some degree of hypovolemia may be managed more safely than with epidural local anesthetic administration.

Third, in the post-thoracotomy pain relief experience (summarized in Table 20–1), there have been relatively few significant side effects.

Fourth, catheters have been left in situ and used for as long as 5 days without the development of tolerance.[82]

Fifth, pain relief failures have usually been due to improper catheter localization since no pain relief could be demonstrated following injection of local anesthetics.[82]

Sixth, the expected increase in the mean post-thoracotomy expiratory flow rate, forced vital capacity, functional residual capacity, and ability to tolerate respiratory care maneuvers following epidural pain relief have been demonstrated to occur.[82] Even larger increases in ventilatory capacity have been demonstrated in the much larger experience with epidural pain relief after abdominal surgery.[63, 81] These increases are generally greater than, or equal to, those obtained by intravenous narcotics or epidural local anesthetic administration.

Finally, epidural narcotics have been used to treat intractable pain due to thoracic tumors.[59] Less dosage is required and longer duration of analgesia with each intermittent dose is obtained for intractable cancer pain compared with acute postoperative pain.[59] However, although results have been satisfactory after the first few series of injections for intractable pain, tolerance has developed, and dosages have had to be increased owing to continuous bathing of the spinal cord with a CSF concentration of opioid.[75] For treatment of chronic pain, permanent catheters have been implanted in the subarachnoid and epidural spaces and connected to reservoirs or perfusion pumps.[75, 96] These implants have been found to be effective, but again tachyphylaxis has been observed.[75]

REFERENCES

1. Egbert LD, Bendixen HH: Effect of morphine on breathing pattern: A possible factor in atelectasis. JAMA 188:485, 1964.
2. Weil JV, McCullough RE, Kline JS, et al: Diminished ventilatory response to hypoxia and hypercapnia after morphine. N Engl J Med 292:1103, 1975.
3. Bullingham RES: Optimum management of postoperative pain. Drugs 29:376–386, 1985.
4. Tamsen A, Hartvig P, Fagerlund C, et al: Patient-controlled analgesic therapy. II. Individual analgesic demand and analgesic plasma concentrations of pethidine in postoperative pain. Clin Pharmacokinet 7:164–175, 1982.

5. Keenan DJM, Cave K, Langdon L, et al: Comparative trial of rectal indomethacin and cryoanalgesia for control of early postthoracotomy pain. Br Med J 287:1335–1337, 1983.
6. Bullingham RES: Postoperative pain. Postgrad Med J 60:847–851, 1984.
7. Keeri-Szanto M: Drugs or drums: What relieves postoperative pain? Pain 6:217–230, 1979.
8. Church JJ: Continuous narcotic infusions for relief of postoperative pain. Br Med J 1:977–979, 1979.
9. Kaplan JA, Miller ED Jr, Gallagher EG Jr: Postoperative analgesia for thoracotomy patients. Anesth Analg 54:773–777, 1975.
10. Fleming WH, Sarafian LB: Kindness pays dividends: The medical benefits of intercostal nerve block following thoracotomy. J Thorac Cardiovasc Surg 74:273–274, 1977.
11. Delilkan AE, Lee LK, Yong NK, et al: Postoperative local analgesia for thoracotomy with direct bupivacaine intercostal blocks. Anaesthesia 28:561–567, 1973.
12. Bridenbargh PO, DuPen SL, Moore DC, et al: Postoperative intercostal nerve block analgesia versus narcotic analgesia. Anesth Analg 52:81–85, 1973.
13. Galway JE, Caves PK, Dundee JW: Effect of intercostal nerve blockade during operation on lung function and the relief of pain following thoracotomy. Br J Anaesth 47:730–735, 1975.
14. Faust RJ, Nauss LA: Post-thoracotomy intercostal block: Comparison of its effects on pulmonary function with those of intramuscular meperidine. Anesth Analg 55:542–546, 1976.
15. Toledo-Pereyra LH, De Meester TR: Prospective randomized evaluation of intrathoracic intercostal nerve block with bupivacaine on postoperative ventilatory function. Ann Thorac Surg 27:203–205, 1979.
16. de la Roche AG, Chambers K: Pain amelioration after thoracotomy: A prospective, randomized study. Ann Thorac Surg 37:239–242, 1984.
17. Restelle L, Movilia P, Bossi L, et al: Management of pain after thoracotomy: A technique of multiple intercostal nerve blocks. Anesthesiology 61:353–354, 1984.
18. Murphy DF: Continuous intercostal nerve blockade for pain relief following cholecystectomy. Br J Anaesth 55:521–524, 1983.
19. O'Kelly E, Garry B: Continuous pain relief for multiple fractured ribs. Br J Anaesth 53:989–991, 1981.
20. Olivet RT, Nauss LA, Payne WS: A technique for continuous intercostal nerve block analgesia following thoracotomy. J Thorac Surg 80:308–311, 1980.
21. Cottrell WM, Schick LM, Perkins HM, et al: Hemodynamic changes after intercostal nerve block with bupivacaine-epinephrine solution. Anesth Analg 57:492–495, 1978.
22. Skretting P: Hypotension after intercostal nerve block during thoracotomy under general anesthesia. Br J Anaesth 53:527–529, 1981.
23. Moore MC, Reitan JA: Sudden total spinal block after intraoperative intercostal injections. A case report. Anesth Rev 8:35–38, 1978.
24. Benumof JL, Semenza J: Total spinal anesthesia following intrathoracic intercostal nerve blocks. Anesthesiology 43:124–125, 1975.
25. Moore DC: Intercostal nerve block: Spread of India ink injected to the rib's costal groove. Br J Anaesth 53:325–329, 1981.
26. Gallo JA, Lebowitz PW, Battit GE, et al: Complications of intercostal nerve blocks performed under direct vision during thoracotomy: A report of two cases. J Thorac Cardiovasc Surg 86:628–630, 1983.
27. Spence AA, Smith G: Postoperative analgesia and lung function: A comparison of morphine with extradural block. Br J Anaesth 43:144–148, 1971.
28. Bromage PR: Extradural analgesia for pain relief. Br J Anaesth 39:721–729, 1967.
29. Shuman RL, Peters RM: Epidural anesthesia following thoracotomy in patients with chronic obstructive airway disease. J Thorac Cardiovasc Surg 71:82–88, 1976.
30. James EC, Kolberg HL, Iwen GW, et al: Epidural analgesia for post-thoracotomy patients. J Thorac Cardiovasc Surg 82:898–903, 1981.
31. Griffiths DPG, Diamond AW, Cameron JD: Postoperative extradural analgesia following thoracic surgery: A feasibility study. Br J Anaesth 47:48–55, 1975.
32. Conacher ID, Paes ML, Jacobson, L, et al.: Epidural analgesia following thoracic surgery. A review of two years' experience. Anaesthesia 38:546–551, 1983.
33. El-Baz NM, Faber LP, Jensik RJ: Continuous epidural infusion of morphine for treatment of pain after thoracic surgery: A new technique. Anesth Analg 63:757–764, 1984.
34. Katz J: The management of pain. In Benumof JL (ed): Clinical Frontiers in Anesthesiology. San Diego, Grune and Stratton, 1983.
35. Rooney S, Jain S, McCormack P, et al: A comparison of pulmonary function tests for postthoracotomy pain using cryoanalgesia and transcutaneous nerve stimulation. Ann Thorac Surg 41:204–207, 1986.
36. Glynn CJ, Lloyd JW, Barnard JDW: Cryoanalgesia in the management of pain after thoracotomy. Thorax 34:325–327, 1980.
37. Katz J, Nelson W, Forest R, et al: Cryoanalgesia for post-thoracotomy pain. Lancet 1:512–513, 1980.
38. Maiwand O, Makey AR: Cryoanalgesia for relief of pain after thoracotomy. Br Med J 282:1749–1750, 1981.
39. Nelson KM, Vincent RG, Bourke RS, et al: Intraoperative intercostal nerve freezing to prevent post-thoracotomy pain. Ann Thorac Surg 18:280–284, 1974.
40. Orr IA, Keenan DJM, Dundee JW: Improved pain relief after thoracotomy: Use of cryoprobe and morphine infusion. Br Med J 283:945, 1981.
41. Maiwand MO, Makey AR, Rees A: Cryoanalgesia after thoracotomy. Improvement of technique and review of 600 cases. J Thorac Cardiovasc Surg 92:291–295, 1986.
42. Myers RR, Powell HC, Heckman HM, et al: Biophysical and pathological effects of cryogenic nerve lesion. Ann Neurol 10:478–485, 1981.
43. VanderArk GD, McGrath KA: Transcutaneous electrical stimulation in treatment of postoperative pain. Am J Surg 130:338–340, 1975.
44. Ali J, Yaffe CS, Serrette C: The effect of transcutaneous electric nerve stimulation on postoperative pain and pulmonary function. Surgery 89:507–512, 1981.
45. Stratton SA, Smith MM: Postoperative thoracotomy: Effect of transcutaneous electrical nerve stimulation on forced vital capacity. Phys Ther 60:45–47, 1980.
46. Hymes AC, Raab DE, Yonehiro EG, et al: Acute pain control by electrostimulation: A preliminary report. Adv Neurol 4:761–767, 1974.
47. Behar M, Olshwang D, Magora F, et al: Epidural morphine in the treatment of pain. Lancet 1:527–529, 1979.
48. Torda TA: Management of acute and postoperative pain. Int Anesthesiol Clin 21:27–47, 1983.
49. Torda TA, Pybus DA: Comparison of four narcotic

analgesics for extradural analgesia. Br J Anaesth 54:291–294, 1982.

50. Nordberg G, Hedner T, Mellstrand T, et al: Pharmacokinetic aspect of epidural morphine analgesia. Anesthesiology 58:545–551, 1983.

51. Pybus DA, Torda TA: Dose-effect relationships of extradural morphine. Br J Anaesth 54:1259–1262, 1982.

52. Magora F, Olshwang D, Eimerl D, et al: Observations on extradural morphine analgesia in various pain conditions. Br J Anaesth 52:247–251, 1980.

53. Shulman MS, Brebner J, Sandler A: The effect of epidural morphine on post-operative pain relief and pulmonary function in thoracotomy patients. Anesthesiology 59:A192, 1983.

54. Rawal N, Sjostrand U, Dahlstrom B: Postoperative pain relief by epidural morphine. Anesth Analg 60:726–731, 1981.

55. Snyder SH: Opiate receptors and internal opiates. Sci Am 236:44–56, 1977

56. Cousins MJ, Mather LE: Intrathecal and epidural administration of opioids. Anesthesiology 61:276–310, 1984.

57. Pert CB, Snyder SH: Opiate receptors: Demonstration in nervous tissue. Science 179:1011–1014, 1973.

58. Atweh SF, Kuhar MJ: Autoradiographic localization of opiate receptors in rat brains. I. Spinal cord and lower medulla. Brain Res 124:53–67, 1977.

59. Glynn CJ, Mather LE, Cousins MJ, et al: Peridural meperidine in humans: Analgetic response, pharmacokinetics and transmission into CSF. Anesthesiology 55:520–526, 1981.

60. Holland AJC, Srikantha S, Tracey JA: Epidural morphine and postoperative pain relief. Can Anaesth Soc J 28:453–457, 1981.

61. Chayen MS, Rudick V, Borvine A: Pain control with epidural injection of morphine. Anesthesiology 53:338–339, 1980.

62. Martin J, Lamarche Y, Tetrault JP: Epidural and intrathecal narcotics. Can Anaesth Soc J 30:662–673, 1983.

63. Reference withdrawn.

64. Crawford RD, Batra MS, Fox F: Epidural morphine dose response for postoperative analgesia. Anesthesiology 55:A150, 1981.

65. Martin R, Salbaing J, Blaise G, et al: Epidural morphine for postoperative pain relief. A dose response curve. Anesthesiology 56:423–426, 1982.

66. Mathews ET, Abrams LD: Intrathecal morphine in open heart surgery. Lancet 1:543, 1980.

67. Katz J, Nelson W: Intrathecal morphine for postoperative pain relief. Reg Anaesth 6:1–3, 1981.

68. Fromme GA, Gray JR: A comparison of intrathecal and epidural morphine for treatment for post-thoracotomy pain. Anesth Analg 64:185–304, 1985.

69. Gustafsson LL, Schildt B, Jacobsen K: Adverse effects of epidural and intrathecal opiates: Report of a nationwide survey in Sweden. Br J Anaesth 54:479–486, 1982.

70. Reiz S, Westberg M: Side effects of epidural morphine. Lancet 2:203–204, 1980.

71. Weddel S, Ritter R: Serum levels following epidural administration of morphine and correlation with relief of post-surgical pain. Anesthesiology 54:210–214, 1981.

72. Knill RL, Clement JL, Thompson WR: Epidural morphine causes delayed and prolonged ventilatory depression. Can Anaesth Soc J 28:537–543, 1981.

73. Welch DB: Epidural narcotics and dural puncture. Lancet 1:55, 1981.

74. Colpaert FC: Can chronic pain be suppressed despite purported tolerance to narcotic analgesia? Life Sci 24:1201–1210, 1979.

75. Coombs DW, Saunders RL, Gaylor M, et al: Epidural narcotic infusion: Implantation technique and efficacy. Anesthesiology 55:469–473, 1981.

76. Zenz M, Piepenbrock S, Schappler-Scheele B, et al: Epidural morphine analgesia (PMA). III. Cancer pain. Anaesthetist 30:508–513, 1981.

77. Zenz M, Schappler-Scheele B, Neuhans R, et al: Long term peridural morphine analgesia in cancer pain. Lancet 1:91, 1981.

78. Bromage PR, Camporesi EM, Durant PAC, et al: Nonrespiratory side effects of epidural morphine. Anesth Analg 61:490–495, 1982.

79. Evron S, Magora F, Sadovsky E: Prevention of urinary retention with phenoxybenzamine during epidural morphine. Br Med J 288:190, 1984.

80. Petersen TK, Husted SE, Rybro L, et al: Urinary retention during I.M. and extradural morphine analgesia. Br J Anaesth 54:1175–1177, 1982.

81. Bromage PR, Camporesi E, Chestnut D: Epidural narcotics for postoperative analgesia. Anesth Analg 59:473, 1980.

82. Torda TA, Tybus DA: Clinical experience with epidural morphine. Anaesth Intensive Care 9:129–134, 1981.

83. Bromage PR: The price of intraspinal narcotic analgesia. Anesth Analg 60:461–463, 1981.

84. Lanz E, Theiss D, Riess W, et al: Epidural morphine for postoperative analgesia: A double-blind study. Anesth Analg 61:236–240, 1982.

85. Bromage PR, Camporesi EM, Durant PA, et al: Rostral spread of epidural morphine. Anesthesiology 56:431–436, 1982.

86. Bowen-Wright RM, Goroszeniuk T: Epidural fentanyl for pain of multiple fractures. Lancet 2:1033, 1980.

87. Welch DB, Hrynaszkiewicz AT: Postoperative analgesia using epidural methadone. Administration by the lumbar route for thoracic pain relief. Anaesthesia 36:1051–1054, 1981.

88. Steidl LJ, Fromme GA, Danielson DR: Lumbar versus thoracic epidural morphine for post-thoracotomy pain. Anesth Analg 63:277, 1984.

89. Johnston JR, McCaughey W: Epidural morphine: A method of management of multiple fractured ribs. Anaesthesia 35:155–157, 1980.

90. Fromme GA, Steidl LJ, Danielson DR: Comparison of lumbar and thoracic epidural morphine for relief of postthoracotomy pain. Anesth Analg 64:454–455, 1985.

91. Lomessy A, Magnin C, Viale J, et al: Clinical advantages of fentanyl given epidurally for postoperative analgesia. Anesthesiology 61:466–469, 1984.

92. Wolf MJ, Davies GK: Analgesic action of extradural fentanyl. Br J Anaesth 52:357–358, 1980.

93. Welch DB, Hrynaszkiewicz A: Postoperative analgesia using epidural methadone. Administration by the lumbar route for thoracic pain relief. Anaesthesia 36:1051–1054, 1981.

94. Wakerlin G, Shulman MS, Yamaguchi LY, et al: Experience with lumbar epidural hydromorphone for pain relief after thoracotomy. Anesth Analg 65:S163, 1986.

95. Mok MS, Louie BW, Hwong BF, et al: Epidural nalbuphine for the relief of pain after thoracic surgery. Anesth Analg 64:S258, 1985.

96. Coombs DW, Saunders RL, Pageau MG: Continuous intraspinal narcotic analgesia. Technical aspects of an implantable infusion system. Reg Anaesth 7:110–113, 1982.

INDEX

Note: Numbers in *italics* refer to figures; numbers followed by (t) refer to tables.

a waves, *193*
  giant, *194*
Abdomen, closure of, 415
Abdominal aorta, *19*
Abdominal bleeding, emergency room thoracotomy for, 398
Abdominal depression, in penetrating abdominal injuries, 398
Abdominal incision, in esophageal and aortic surgery, 270
Abdominal surgery, complications of, 157–158
Abdominal viscera, through diaphragmatic defects, 394
Abscess, bronchopleural fistula and, 390
  distal to airway obstructing tumor, 344
  lung. *See* Lung abscess.
  one-lung ventilation and, 424
Absorption atelectasis in dependent lung, inspired oxygen concentration and, 272, 273, *274*
  lateral decubitus position and, 121
  volume loss and, 110
ACD. *See* Acid-citrate-dextrose.
Acetylcholine, persistence of fetal circulation and, 408
Acetylcholine receptors, myasthenia gravis and, 367, 368
Acetylcysteine, 161
Acid-base balance, 72–73
Acid-citrate-dextrose, 72
Acidosis, cerebral, 99
  metabolic, diaphragmatic hernia and, 416
    hypercapnia and, 98
  pulmonary vascular resistance and, 187
ACT. *See* Activated clotting time.
ACTH, 81(t)
Activated clotting time, 311
  aortic dissection and, 387
Activated partial thromboplastin time, 311, 312
Active expiration, 87–88. *See also* Expiration.
Acute respiratory failure, 187. *See also* Respiratory distress.
Adenine nucleotides, 79(t)
Adenocarcinoma. *See also* Carcinoma(s).
  esophageal, 152
  lung, 132(t)
    cytology and, 135
Adenoma, 81(t)

Adenomatoid malformations, cystic, 422, 423, 424
Adenosine triphosphate, 117
ADH. *See* Arginine vasopressin.
Adhesion, between visceral and parietal pleura, 263
Adjunct(s), anesthetic, airway reactivity and, 203(t)
  cardiovascular function and, 207(t)
Adrenergic compounds. *See also* Beta-blocker(s).
  ciliary activity and, 161
  positive end-expiratory pressure and, 451
α-Adrenergic receptor stimulation, 78, 451
Adrenocorticosteroids, 81(t), 161
Adriamycin. *See* Doxorubicin.
Adult respiratory distress syndrome, differential lung ventilation in, 13
  hypoxemia and, 92–94, *93*
  new ventilatory modes and, 462
  pulmonary circulation and vasomotion in, 52
Advance information sheet for intensive care unit, 320(t)
Advanced intraoperative monitoring, 179–199. *See also* Intraoperative monitoring.
Aerosol(s), in cannisters, 304
  steroids as, 305
  ultrasonic, 204
Afterload, 96
  right heart failure and, 439–440
Aged, 83, 169
β-Agonists, 304–305, 304(t), *314*
  fiberoptic bronchoscope and, 328
  postoperative positive end-expiratory pressure goals and, 457
Air bubbles, hazards of, 441
Air cysts, 355–357
Air embolism, central venous access and, 197(t), 198
  high inspired oxygen concentrations and, 97
  mediastinoscopy and, 338
Air flow, pattern of, 59
Air flow resistance, 61, *62*. *See also* Airway resistance.
  measurement of, 181
Air fluid level, in mediastinal cyst, 423
Air injection, in herniation of heart, 436
Air leak, 293–295
Air spaces, anatomy of, 26–29
Air trapping, inhaled foreign body and, 399

Fibrosis, hemothorax and, 395
  myocardial, left ventricular compliance and, 182
  pulmonary, oxygen toxicity and, 448
Fick principle, 76–77
Filling pressure(s), 207
  abnormal heart, 189–190
  transmural ventricular, positive end-expiratory
    pressure-induced decreases in, 450, 451–452
Fires, airway, 344
Fissure, horizontal or oblique, 21, 22, 23, 25
Fistula, bronchopleural, 224, 225
    cutaneous, 224
    differential lung ventilation and, 456
    emergency surgery for, 387–390
    high-frequency ventilation in, 13, 293–295
    one-lung ventilation and, 424
    postoperative development of, 437
    tracheobronchial disruptions and, 393
  tracheoesophageal, 415(t), 417–420
Flail chest, 391–392, 394, 396
  diaphragmatic disruptions and, 394
Flaps of muscles or omentum, bronchopleural fistula and, 388
Fleming, A., 8
Flexible fiberoptic bronchoscopy, 327
  in massive hemoptysis, 378
  in pediatric population, 428
Flexible fiberoptic esophagoscopy, 340
Flow interrupter, 291
  high-frequency ventilation, 295
Flowmeter, fractured or sticking, 84
Flow-tube sensor in measuring gas volume passing from
    chest tube, 389
Flow-volume curves in tracheal obstruction, maximal in-
    spiratory and expiratory, 351
Flow-volume loop, mediastinal tumors and, 365
  tracheal resection and, 350
Fluid(s), for premature and newborn, 410–411
  postoperative infusion of, 449
  restriction of, 440
  transuding into dependent lung, 272
Fluoroscopy, bronchial blocker and, 425, 425
  inhaled foreign body and, 399
  mainstem bronchial intubation and, 426, 426
Fluroxene, 209, 210(t)
  cardiovascular responses to hypercapnia and, 98(t)
Flutter, atrial, 441, 442
Fogarty occlusion or embolectomy catheter, 253–256,
    293, 424–425
  foreign body removal and, 400
  massive hemoptysis and, 378
Foley catheter, 256
Foramen of Morgagni, diaphragmatic hernia through, 413,
    414, 415
Foramen ovale, closure of, 407
  patent, 57, 407
    general population and, 440, 441
    right-to-left shunting across, 440–441
Forced expiration, during anesthesia, 87–88
  pressure gradients and, 64–65
Forced expired volume, in minimal pulmonary function
    test criteria, 141(t)
  in one second, 157
    after bullectomy, 356
    lateral position test and, 144
    radiospirometry and, 144
  in one second/forced vital capacity, 141
Forced midexpiratory flow between 25 and 75 per cent,
    141, 142

Forced vital capacity, preoperative, 141, 141
Foreign body in tracheobronchial tree, anesthetic consid-
    erations for, 400(t)
  bronchoscopy and, 427
  esophagoscopy and, 340
  inhaled, main bronchi and, 25
    types of, 399
  physical characteristics of, 401
  removal of, 399–401
    rigid ventilating bronchoscope and, 332
Fraction of inspired oxygen, anesthesia and, 90
  atelectatic hypoxic pulmonary vasoconstriction and, 117
  dependent-lung volume loss and, 110
  mucociliary flow and, 91
  one-lung ventilation and, 112
  right-to-left transpulmonary shunt and, 73
Fracture, chest wall, 391–392, 394, 396
  of teeth, 333
  rib, 393
Frank-Starling principle, 181, 181
FRC. See Functional residual capacity.
Fresh frozen plasma, 313
  in massive transfusion hemostatic defects, 312
  massive hemoptysis and, 379
Frictional resistance, work of breathing and, 61, 62
FSP. See Fibrin split products.
Fuji Systems, 256
Full stomach, double-lumen tube and, 253
Functional residual capacity, 53, 275
  absorption atelectasis and, 90
  active expiration and, 87–88
  airway management for tracheal resection and, 354
  airway resistance and, 88, 89
  closing capacity and, 67–68
  differential lung continuous positive airway pressure/
    positive end-expiratory pressure and, 283
  excessive intravenous fluids and, 88–90
  hypoxemia during anesthesia and, 85–91
  immobility and, 88–90
  inspired oxygen concentration and, 90
  intraoperative monitoring of, 181
  lateral position test and, 144
  light or inadequate anesthesia and, 87–88
  lung volumes and, 62–63
  mucociliary flow and, 91
  of anesthetized patient in lateral decubitus position,
    107–109
  paralysis and, 87
  postoperative increased pulmonary vascular resistance
    and, 451
  preoperative assessment and, 142
  rapid shallow breathing and, 90–91
  respiratory effects of anesthetics and, 83, 84
  right ventricular dysfunction and, 451
  secretion removal and, 91
  supine position and, 85, 88–90
  surgical position and, 90
  thoracic cage muscle tone and, 85–87
  ventilatory history and, 90–91
FVC. See Forced vital capacity.

Gale, J.W., 8, 9
Gamma Med catheter, 349
Gangrene, artery dissection and, 383
Garcia, M., 7
Gargle, viscous lidocaine pharyngeal, 330
Garnet, in laser, 344–347

Malignant spread. *See* Metastasis.
Malignant tumors, of tracheobronchial tree, 343. *See also* Lung cancer.
Mallinkrodt double-lumen tube, 249
Malnutrition, 163, 317, 317(t)
Malposition, of double-lumen tube, 236–237, *236*
Mammary artery and vein, mediastinum and, *36*
Mandatory minute volume, 461–462
Manometer, continuous positive airway pressure systems and, *279, 280*
 dry gas, conversion from intermittent mandatory ventilation and, 460
Manubrium, 15, *18*
Mapleson circuits, 95
Marfan's syndrome, 382
Martin, channels of, 29
Mass spectrometer, 180
Massaging of chest tubes, 322
Massive hemoptysis, chest x-ray and, 377
 conservative treatment in, 376, 377
 cystic fibrosis and, 378
 surgery in, emergency, 376–381
  indications for, 376–377
 treatment algorithm for, *377*
Massive transfusion, hemostatic defects in, 312, 312(t)
 intraoperative monitoring and, 169
 management of, 312–313, *313*
Mass-movement oxygenation, apneic, 296
Matas, R., 7
Maximal inspiratory and expiratory flow-volume curves in tracheal obstruction, *351*
Maximum breathing capacity, 157
 in minimal pulmonary function test criteria, 141(t)
 preoperative assessment of, 142
Maximum midexpiratory flow rate, 141, 142
MBC. *See* Maximum breathing capacity.
McKesson, I., 7
Mean arterial pressure, 323
 in pulmonary artery, cardiac output and, *147*
 intraoperative monitoring of, 179
Mean transit time, lung water measurement and, 198–199
Mechanical failure of equipment, 83–85
Mechanical ventilation, 419, 445–466
 arterial oxygen tension and, 447–457
 cardiac output and, 449–453, *450*
  differential lung ventilation and, 453–457
  humoral mediation of, *450*, 453
  interventricular septum displacement and, *450, 451*
  pulmonary vascular resistance and, *450, 451, 452*
  right ventricular dysfunction and, *450, 451, 452*
  transmural ventricular filling pressures and, *450,* 451–452
  venous return in, 449–451
 complications of, 464
 conversion from, to spontaneous ventilation, 459–461
 development of, 11
 diaphragmatic hernia and, 416
 differential lung ventilation in, 453–457
 extubation of trachea and, 462–463, *463*
 first operating room use of, 11
 flail chest and, 391–392
 hemothorax and, 396
 initial ventilatory settings in, 446–447, 446(t)
 inspired oxygen concentration goal in, 448–461
  cardiac output and, 449–453, *450*
  conversion to spontaneous ventilation and, 459–460
  differential lung ventilation in, 453–457
  how to achieve, 448–449, 457–459, 460–461
  oxygen toxicity and, 447–448
  ventilation-perfusion mismatch and, 457

Mechanical ventilation (*Continued*)
 intermittent mandatory ventilation in, 446–447, 446(t)
  conversion from, 459–461
 myasthenia gravis and, 370
 new methods of, 461–462
 oxygen toxicity and, 447–449
 postoperative, 319
 postpneumonectomy bronchopleural fistula and, 438
 respiratory insufficiency and, 439
 superior vena cava syndrome and, 367
 ventilation to perfusion match in, 457–459
 weaning modes for, 461–462
 weaning plan for, 448(t)
 weaning procedure and summary of, 461
Median sternotomy, 350
 aortic dissection and, 383
 bronchopleural fistula and, 388
 incisions in, 266–267, *267*
 myasthenia gravis and, 369
 pulmonary resection via, 226
 superior vena cava syndrome and, 366
Mediastinotomy, 263
Mediastinal bounce, high-frequency ventilation and, 291, 295
Mediastinal cyst, bronchogenic, 423
Mediastinal emphysema, 293
 high-flow ventilation and, 299
Mediastinal fibrosis, idiopathic, 366
Mediastinal granuloma, 366
Mediastinal lymph node, 33, *34*
 inspection and biopsy of, 335
Mediastinal mass(es), 363–367
 location of, *150*
 management principles for, 364–365, 364(t)
 massive hemoptysis and, 376(t)
 preoperative cardiopulmonary evaluation in, 150–152
 symptoms of, 151
Mediastinal organ functions, intraoperative monitoring and, 169
Mediastinal shift, congenital lobar emphysema and, 422
 diaphragmatic disruptions and, 394
 diaphragmatic hernia and, 413, *414*, 415
 inhaled foreign body and, 399
 physiology of, 104–105
 pneumothorax and, 393
 postpneumonectomy, tension pneumothorax and, *438,* 438
 schematic representation of, *105*
Mediastinal tamponade, central venous access and, 197(t), 198
Mediastinal tumor. *See* Mediastinal mass(es).
Mediastinal vein, 34
Mediastinal widening, lung cancer and, 133
Mediastinitis, tracheobronchial disruptions and, 393, 394
Mediastinoscopy, 263, 335–338, *336*
 anesthetic technique for, 337
 complications of, 337–338, 337(t)
 contraindications to, 335–337
 esophageal tumors and, 152–153
 indications for, 335–337
 lung cancer and, 137, 138
Mediastinotomy, anterior, 335, 337
 lung cancer and, 138
Mediastinum, anatomy of, 35–37
 anterior, 35, 264
  borders of, 36
 division of, 35–36
 lobectomy and, 269
 middle, *35*
  borders of, 36

Wright spirometer, 141, 175
   lung lavage and, 360

^{133}Xe. *See* Xenon-133.
Xenon-133, closing capacity measurement by, 65, *66*
   preoperative assessment and, 143–144
Xiphoid process, 15, *18*, 267
   mediastinum and, *35*

X-ray(s), chest. *See* Chest radiograph.
   history of, 6
Xylocaine. *See* Lidocaine.

Yttrium, in laser, 344–347

Zero end-expiratory pressure, 110–111, 205
Zones of lung, 40, *41*, *42*, 45, 46